Essentials of Gynaecology
Second Edition

Essentials of
Gynaecology

Second Edition

Lakshmi Seshadri, MD
Senior Consultant in Obstetrics and
   Gynaecology
Thirumalai Mission Hospital, Vellore
Formerly
Professor and Head of the Department
Christian Medical College Hospital
Vellore, Tamil Nadu

. Wolters Kluwer

Publishing Manager: P Sangeetha
Development Editor: Dr Vallika Devi Katragadda
Production Editor: K Annie Devi
Assistant Manager-Manufacturing: Sumit Johry

10th Floor, Tower C, Building No. 10
Phase – II, DLF Cyber City, Gurgaon, Haryana – 122002

Second Edition, 2017

ISBN-13: 978-93-5129-698-0

Published by Wolters Kluwer (India) Pvt. Ltd., Gurgaon
Compositor: Chitra Computers, Delhi
Printed and bound at Nutech Print Services-India

For product enquiry, please contact – Marketing Department (marketing@wolterskluwerindia.co.in) or log on to our website www.wolterskluwerindia.co.in.

Preface to the Second Edition

The first edition of *Essentials of Gynaecology* was written with a view to provide the medical students with a simple textbook which gives them a good understanding of basic anatomy, physiology, clinical symptomatology, diagnosis and management of gynaecological conditions, in a user-friendly format. The book served this goal to a large extent and was well received and appreciated for the unique features such as flowcharts, simple diagrams, clinical photographs, summary boxes and key points. In the second edition, these important features have been retained. In addition, clinical guidelines, classifications of diseases, staging of malignancies and management have been updated. A new look has been given to match its companion, *Essentials of Obstetrics*.

I am very appreciative of the help from my colleague Dr Aruna Kekre who has given valuable suggestions. The team at Wolters Kluwer consisting of Dr Vallika Devi Katragadda, Ms Sangeetha Parthasarathy, Ms Pooja Chauhan, and Ms Annie Devi have done an exemplary job.

Dear students and friends – Welcome to the second edition of *Essentials of Gynaecology*.

Lakshmi Seshadri

Preface to the First Edition

The study of gynaecology at the undergraduate level can be confusing. The final year student in India is suddenly confronted with complex scenarios, having studied anatomy and physiology in the first year and refreshed these during short postings in the second and third years. He or she then struggles with heavy reference volumes intended for the postgraduate student or the practising clinician, full of contemporary research, mind-boggling detail and sometimes exotic cases. Then the exams confront the student, where one is forced to simplify, condense and remember—not to mention how to formulate clear answers for theory questions and how to answer to the point in the clinical examination and viva voce.

Over three decades as a practising clinician, teacher and examiner, I have noticed that a number of my undergraduate students are at a loss for a simple, yet adequate, textbook. The undergraduate medical student reading a subject for the first time must thoroughly understand the basic anatomy, pathophysiology and clinical symptomatology in the discipline. He or she should know how to evaluate patients clinically, how to choose appropriate investigations and how to manage patients on the basis of available evidence. All these inputs should be provided in a precise, clear and easily understandable format.

This book tries to meet these needs in a number of ways. Relevant and important points have been highlighted or given in boxes for easy reading. Flowcharts, diagrams, clinical photographs and radiological images are liberally provided to enable easy understanding. Illustrative cases are discussed at the end of each chapter to sustain interest. The questions provided at the end of each chapter are designed to stimulate the student to brush up those areas which he or she has not clearly understood in the first reading of the chapter. These questions should be helpful for students not only in preparing them for examinations but also for the day-to-day management of patients later on in their career.

With regard to clinical practice, guidelines for management keep evolving as new evidence is found. It is important that undergraduates are aware of current evidence-based guidelines. In this book I have attempted to include the most relevant and updated classifications, staging of tumours and management guidelines.

It is hoped that students will find this useful not only while preparing for their examinations, but also when managing patients and brushing up their basics during postgraduation.

I would like to thank all my colleagues for making this book a possibility and all my students for making it a necessity. They have contributed by providing feedback, editing some chapters, taking clinical photographs and, most importantly, by sustaining my interest in teaching.

Lakshmi Seshadri

Contents

Preface to the Second Edition   *v*
Preface to the First Edition   *vii*

Section 1   Basic Science in Gynaecology   1

  1. Anatomy of the Female Reproductive Tract   2
  2. Development of the Female Genital Tract: Normal and Abnormal   23
  3. Female Reproductive Physiology   37

Section 2   Gynaecological Evaluation   55

  4. Gynaecological History and Physical Examination   56
  5. Imaging in Gynaecology   76
  6. Gynaecological Symptoms and Differential Diagnosis   91

Section 3   Benign Gynaecology   109

  7. Abnormal Uterine Bleeding   110
  8. Disorders Associated with Menstrual Cycle   127
  9. Benign Diseases of the Vulva, Vagina and Cervix   135
 10. Benign Diseases of the Uterus   147
 11. Benign Diseases of the Ovary and Fallopian Tube   169
 12. Infections of the Lower Genital Tract   183
 13. Infections of the Upper Genital Tract   198
 14. Tuberculosis of the Female Genital Tract   210
 15. Endometriosis   217
 16. Chronic Pelvic Pain   233

Section 4   Gynaecological Endocrinology and Infertility   243

 17. Paediatric and Adolescent Gynaecology   244
 18. Primary Amenorrhoea   254
 19. Secondary Amenorrhoea and Polycystic Ovarian Syndrome   264
 20. Hirsutism and Virilization   278
 21. Menopause   291
 22. Infertility   305
 23. Hormone Therapies in Gynaecology   329

Section 5   Disorders of the Pelvic Floor and Urogynaecology   351

24. Pelvic Organ Prolapse   352
25. Urogynaecology   370
26. Urinary Tract Injuries, Urogenital Fistulas; Anal Sphincter Injuries and
     Rectovaginal Fistulas   386

Section 6   Gynaecological Oncology   401

27. Preinvasive and Invasive Diseases of the Vulva and Vagina   402
28. Premalignant Diseases of the Cervix   414
29. Malignant Diseases of the Cervix   435
30. Premalignant and Malignant Diseases of the Uterus   455
31. Malignant Diseases of the Ovary and Fallopian Tube   472
32. Gestational Trophoblastic Disease   500

Section 7   Operative Gynaecology   517

33. Preoperative Preparation and Postoperative Management   518
34. Gynaecological Surgery   530

Index   561

Section 1

Basic Science in Gynaecology

1

Anatomy of the Female Reproductive Tract

Case scenario

Mrs KL, 48 was brought to the emergency room in shock 6 hours after abdominal hysterectomy. Her pulse was not felt and blood pressure was 70/40 mmHg. She was accompanied by a local gynaecologist who had performed the surgery. Examination revealed signs of internal bleeding and the patient was taken for relaparotomy after resuscitation. Laparotomy revealed 1.5 L of blood in the peritoneal cavity, generalized oozing in the pelvis and active bleeding from the stump of the right uterine artery. The vessel had retracted and was difficult to clamp. A senior consultant had to be called in to perform ligation of internal iliac vessels.

Introduction

A thorough knowledge of anatomy of the reproductive tract (internal genital organs, their relation to important structures, course of ureter and anatomy of blood vessels and nerves that supply the pelvic structures) is essential for performing gynaecological surgery and managing surgical emergencies. The reproductive tract consists of external and internal genital organs. They are located between the urinary and gastrointestinal tracts. They are also closely related developmentally; therefore, developmental abnormality and pathology in one organ can affect the other as well.

External genitalia (vulva)

Vulva or the external genitalia includes all structures from mons pubis to perineal body as listed in Box 1.1 (Fig. 1.1).

Mons pubis

This is the triangular area anterior to the pubic bones and is continuous above with abdominal wall and below with the labia. It is filled with adipose tissue and covered by hairy skin.

Labia majora

These are folds of fatty tissue covered by skin that extend from mons pubis to perineum, to

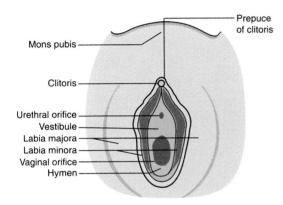

Figure 1.1 Structures in the vulva.

meet in front of the anus forming the posterior fourchette. The skin on the lateral aspect of labia majora is pigmented and covered by hair. Inner aspect is smooth and shiny, and contains apocrine, sweat and sebaceous glands.

Labia minora

Labia minora are folds of skin that lie medial to the labia majora, encircling the urethral and vaginal orifices. Posteriorly they fuse with the posterior fourchette but anteriorly divide to form a hood or prepuce and a frenulum for the clitoris.

Clitoris

Clitoris is the homologue of the penis and is formed by two corpora cavernosa and erectile tissue. It is about 1.5–2 cm in length and is located anterior to the urethral orifice between the anterior folds of labia minora.

Vestibule

The area between the labia minora is referred to as the vestibule. This is perforated by urethral and vaginal orifices.

Urethral orifice

The urethral orifice (meatus) is a vertical opening above the vaginal orifice. The ducts of Skene (paraurethral) glands open just inside or outside the meatus.

Vaginal orifice

This lies between the labia minora and is partially covered by a thin membrane called hymen. The ducts of Bartholin glands open into the vaginal orifice laterally between the hymen and the labia minora.

Hymen

Hymen is the thin membrane that covers the vaginal orifice. This ruptures during the first intercourse and remains as small, rounded tags.

Bartholin glands

These are small glands located on the posterolateral aspect of vaginal orifice, beneath the bulbospongiosus muscle, at 4 and 8 o'clock positions. The glands are about 1 cm in size and not palpable normally. The ducts are 2 cm long and open into the vaginal orifice superficial to the hymen. The glands are compound racemose, lined by cuboidal epithelium. Ducts are lined by cuboidal epithelium proximally and transitional epithelium distally. The secretions provide lubrication during sexual intercourse.

Skene glands

These are paraurethral glands that are homologous of the prostate and are located on either side of the distal urethra. The ducts open into the urethra close to the external meatus.

Vestibular bulbs

These are elongated masses of erectile tissue located beneath the bulbospongiosus muscle on either side of the vaginal orifice. They meet anteriorly as a narrow strip.

Perineum

The anatomical or true perineum is a diamond-shaped area that extends from the pubis anteriorly to the coccyx posteriorly and the ischial tuberosities laterally (Fig. 1.2). This is divided by an imaginary line between the two ischial tuberosities into anterior or urogenital triangle and posterior or anal triangle.

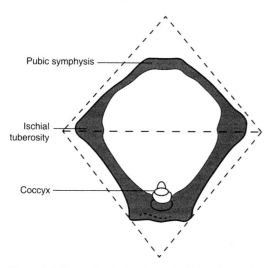

Figure 1.2 The anatomical perineum. This is a diamond-shaped area that extends from the pubis anteriorly to the coccyx posteriorly and the ischial tuberosities laterally.

The urogenital triangle

The urogenital triangle forms the anterior triangle of the perineum.

Boundaries
- **Anterior:** Subpubic angle
- **Posterior:** Superficial transverse perinei muscles

- **Lateral:** Ischiopubic rami and ischial tuberosities (Fig. 1.3)

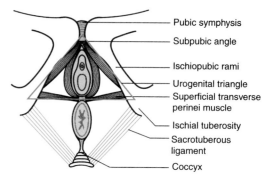

Figure 1.3 The urogenital triangle. The boundaries are subpubic angle anteriorly, superficial transverse perinei muscle posteriorly, and ischiopubic rami and the ischial tuberosities laterally.

Contents

The contents of the urogenital triangle are listed in Box 1.2.

Box 1.2 Contents of the urogenital triangle

- Vulva and its contents
- Urogenital diaphragm
- Superficial perineal muscles
- Deep perineal muscles
- Blood vessels, nerves and lymphatics

Muscles of the perineum

They fall into two groups: Superficial and deep (Box 1.3). The perineal membrane separates the superficial perineal muscles that lie below the membrane (Fig. 1.4) from the deep muscles that lie above it.

Box 1.3 Muscles of the perineum

- Superficial perineal muscles
  - Ischiocavernosus
  - Bulbospongiosus
  - Superficial transverse perinei
- Deep perineal muscles
  - Deep transverse perinei
  - Urethral sphincter

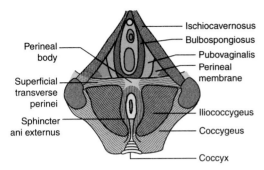

Figure 1.4 Superficial muscles of the perineum.

Superficial perineal muscles

The features of the superficial muscles are listed in Boxes 1.4–1.6.

Box 1.4 Ischiocavernosus

- Origin: Ischial tuberosity
- Insertion: Ischiopubis
- Functions
  - Compression of clitoris
  - Venous congestion
  - Erection of clitoris

Box 1.5 Bulbospongiosus

- Origin: Perineal body
- Insertion: Clitoris
- Location: Lies over vestibular bulb
- Functions
  - Compression of vestibular bulb
  - Compression of dorsal vein of clitoris

Box 1.6 Superficial transverse perinei

- Origin: Ischial tuberosity
- Insertion: Perineal body and central tendon
- Function
  - Fixes the perineal body

Deep perineal muscles

The features of deep perineal muscles are given in Boxes 1.7 and 1.8.

Perineal membrane

Perineal membrane is a dense triangular condensation of fascia that stretches between the two ischiopubic rami and is pierced by the

---

Box 1.7 Deep transverse perinei

- Origin: Ischial bone
- Insertion: Lateral vaginal wall
- Location: Above the perineal membrane
- Function: Support the lower vagina

Box 1.8 Urethral sphincter

- Origin: Ischiopubis
- Insertion: Urethra and vagina
- Function: Compression of urethra

---

urethra and the vagina. This membrane separates the superficial from the deep compartment of the perineum. The perineal membrane and the deep transverse perinei muscles attach the lower vagina and the urethra to pubic rami and provide support to these structures. Perineal membrane with the muscle above it was known as **urogenital diaphragm**, but this terminology is not used now.

The anal triangle

Boundaries

- **Anterior:** Superficial transverse perineal muscles
- **Posterior:** Coccyx
- **Lateral:** Ischial tuberosities and sacrotuberous ligaments (Fig. 1.5)

Contents

Contents of anal triangle are listed in Box 1.9.

Anal canal

Anal canal extends from the anorectal junction to the anal verge and is approximately 4 cm in

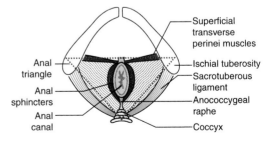

Figure 1.5 The anal triangle. The boundaries are superficial transverse perinei muscles anteriorly, coccyx posteriorly, and ischial tuberosities and sacrotuberous ligaments laterally.

length. The dentate line is located 2 cm from the anal verge. The canal is lined by columnar epithelium above the dentate line and squamous epithelium below the dentate line.

The anal sphincters

There are two anal sphincters—External and internal. The *external anal sphincter* is made of skeletal muscle and has three parts—Subcutaneous, superficial and deep. The fibres of external anal sphincters merge with each other and are attached to perineal body anteriorly and to puborectalis and anococcygeal body posteriorly.

Anococcygeal body (raphe)

Anococcygeal body is a fibromuscular structure located between the anus and the coccyx. The fibres of the levator ani and anal sphincters are attached to it.

Ischiorectal fossae

These lie on either side of the anal canal. They are wedge-shaped, fat-filled spaces. Boundaries and contents of the fossae are given in Box 1.10 and Fig. 1.6.

Perineal body

This is a fibromuscular structure between the anus and the lower vagina. Several muscles are inserted into it (Box 1.11; Fig. 1.7).

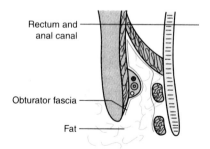
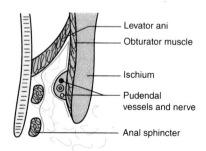

Rectum and anal canal

Obturator fascia

Fat

Levator ani

Obturator muscle

Ischium

Pudendal vessels and nerve

Anal sphincter

Figure 1.6 Coronal section of the ischiorectal fossae. These are wedge-shaped spaces on either side of the anal canal.

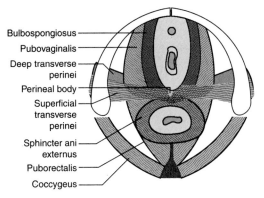

Figure 1.7 Various muscles that form the perineal body.

Internal genital organs

The internal genital organs consist of those given in Box 1.12.

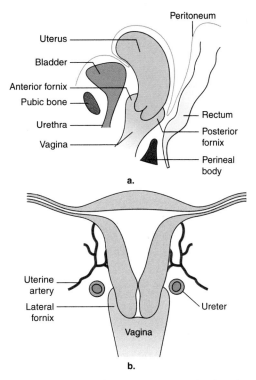

Figure 1.8 Vagina. a. Sagittal section showing the axis of the vagina, the anterior and posterior fornices, and the relationship to bladder and urethra. b. Coronal section showing the lateral fornices and their proximity to ureters.

Box 1.12 Internal genital organs

- Vagina
- Uterus
- Fallopian tubes
- Ovary

Vagina

Vagina is the fibromuscular tube that extends from vestibule to uterine cervix (Box 1.13).

The attachment of the vagina to the cervix is at its middle (Fig. 1.8a and b). Therefore, a gutter is formed all around the cervix between it and the vagina, called **fornices**. Ureter and uterine artery are in close proximity to lateral fornices. The posterior attachment is at a higher level, making the posterior fornix deep. The anterior wall of the

vagina is, therefore, shorter than the posterior wall. The opening at the vestibule is partially covered by hymen. The vaginal walls have rugae, which allow stretching during parturition. The axis of the vagina is horizontal. There are three sulci on the anterior vaginal wall: Submeatal sulcus, bladder sulcus and transverse vaginal sulcus. These are described in Chapter 24, *Pelvic organ prolapse*.

Structure

Vaginal wall is composed of three layers (Box 1.14).

Box 1.13 Vagina

- Fibromuscular tube from vestibule to cervix
- Axis horizontal
- Closely applied to
  - Anteriorly
    - Bladder
    - Urethra
  - Posteriorly
    - Posterior cul-de-sac
    - Rectum
    - Anal canal
    - Perineal body
- Anterior and posterior walls in apposition

Box 1.14 Structure of vagina from within to outwards

- Mucosa
  - Stratified squamous epithelium
  - Subepithelial connective tissue
- Muscle layer
  - Outer longitudinal
  - Inner circular
- Condensed endopelvic fascia

<table>
<tr><td>

Clinical implications

The clinical implications of the *anatomy of vagina* are given as follows:
- *Vaginal rugae:* Evidence of oestrogenization
- *Bladder sulcus:* For diagnosis of vaginal elongation of cervix
- *Transverse vaginal sulcus:* Location of bladder neck
- *Depth of fornices:* Diagnosis of prolapse/elongation of cervix

</td></tr>
</table>

Uterus

Uterus is a pear-shaped hollow viscus, located between the bladder and the rectum. It is divided into **cervix** and **uterine corpus**, the dividing line being the internal os.

Cervix

The cervix is the lower part of the uterus. It is continuous with the uterus above and is attached to the vagina below. The attachment of the vagina divides the cervix into upper supravaginal cervix and lower portiovaginalis (Fig. 1.9). It has an external os and an internal os, and a cervical canal in between. Total length is 2.5–3 cm (Box 1.15). The external os is circular in the nullipara, but becomes a transverse slit after childbirth. Anatomical features of the cervix are given in Box 1.15.

Box 1.15 Cervix

- Constitutes the lower part of uterus
- Total length: 2.5–3 cm
- Divided into
  - Supravaginal cervix
  - Portiovaginalis
- Has
  - External os
  - Internal os
  - Endocervical canal between the two
- Structure
  - Fibromuscular wall
  - Endocervical canal—Columnar epithelium
  - Ectocervix—Stratified squamous epithelium
  - Glands—Secrete mucus

Uterine corpus

The size and shape of the **uterus** changes with changes in hormone levels associated with puberty and pregnancy. The dimensions of nulliparous uterus are given in Box 1.16. The uterus is normally anteverted and anteflexed. Flexion is the angle between the uterus and the cervix, and version is the angle between the uterus and the vagina.

Structure

The uterine wall consists of three layers: Inner endometrium, outer serosa and a middle layer

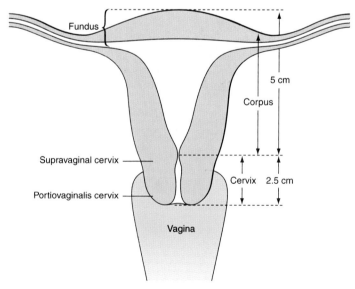

Figure 1.9 Uterus and cervix. Uterine fundus is the part above the line of attachment of the fallopian tubes. The part of the cervix above the attachment of the vagina is supravaginal cervix and below this is portiovaginalis cervix.

composed of smooth muscles called myometrium. The endometrial cavity is continuous with that of the tubes, cervix and vagina. The endometrium including glands and stroma is very sensitive to oestrogen and progesterone and undergoes changes during menstrual cycle and pregnancy. The myometrium consists of three layers. The outer longitudinal fibres of the myometrium are continuous with those of the tubes. The middle layer of interlacing fibres is important for uterine contraction and retraction. The blood vessels pass through this layer, and contraction of these fibres occludes the vessels and stops bleeding after parturition. The inner circular layer is thin and insignificant. The serosa or peritoneum covering the uterus stops at the uterovesical junction anteriorly but extends down to form the cul-de-sac or pouch of Douglas posteriorly (Box 1.17).

The cul-de-sac is the most dependent part of the pelvis, and, therefore, fluids, pus and blood collect here to form abscess or haematocele.

This can be easily accessed through the posterior fornix.

Fallopian tubes

The fallopian tubes are about 10 cm in length and extend laterally from the corneal ends of the uterus into the peritoneal cavity. Each tube is divided into four regions (Box 1.18; Fig. 1.10). The infundibulum has fimbriae with cilia to aid in ovum pick-up.

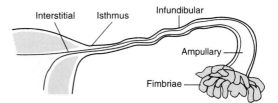

Figure 1.10 Parts of the fallopian tube. The tube is narrow at the isthmus and broader at the ampullary part.

Structure

The structure of the tube is given in Box 1.19. The tube has three layers: Inner mucosa, outer serosa and muscularis layer between the two.

Box 1.19 Structure of fallopian tube

- Mucosa
- Ciliated columnar epithelium
- Muscularis
  - Outer longitudinal
  - Inner circular
- Outer serosa

Clinical implications

The clinical implications of *fallopian tubes* are given as follows:
- Narrow intramural part
  - Early rupture of ectopic gestation
- Isthmus
  - Site for tubal sterilization

Ovaries

The tube and ovary together are referred to as **adnexa**. The ovaries are the female gonads. The size of the ovaries varies with age, sex steroid hormone levels and certain medications. The ovaries are located on either side of the uterus, close to the infundibulum of the tubes. They are connected to the uterine cornu by the ovarian ligaments and to the broad ligament by mesovarium (Fig. 1.11). The **hilum** of the ovary is located along the mesovarium, and the vessels and nerves enter the ovary through the hilum. The ovarian vessels are carried in a fold of peritoneum, called the infundibulopelvic ligaments, from the lateral pelvic wall to the ovary (Box 1.20).

Vestigial remnants of the cephalic and caudal ends of the Wolffian structures persist as **epoophoron** and **paroophoron** that can occasionally enlarge and form cysts.

Structure

The ovary is divided into an outer cortex and an inner medulla (Box 1.21; Fig. 1.12). The cortex contains the specialized stroma and the follicles and is responsible for the important functions of ovulation and steroid hormone production. The ovarian medulla is the stroma of the ovary and is highly vascular. It is developed from the embryonic mesenchyme and contains blood vessels, lymphatics and nerves.

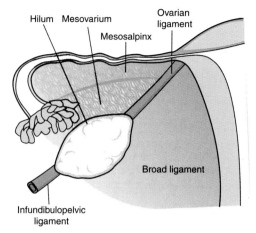

Figure 1.11 Attachments of the ovary. Infundibulopelvic ligament attaches the ovary to the lateral pelvic wall and the ovarian ligament to the uterine cornu. Mesovarium lies between the ovary and the broad ligament.

Box 1.20 Ovaries

- Size
  - 3 × 2 cm
- Mesovarium (mesentery)
  - Posterior surface of broad ligament
- Ovarian ligament
  - Uterine cornu
- Infundibulopelvic ligament
  - Lateral pelvic wall

Box 1.21 Structure of the ovary

- Cortex
  - Cuboidal surface epithelium
  - Specialized stroma
  - Follicles
- Medulla
  - Fibromuscular tissue
  - Blood vessels

Clinical implications

Clinical implications of *structure of the ovary* are given as follows:
- Ovarian cortex contains the primordial follicles; hence, as much of cortex as possible should be preserved during wedge resection of ovary.
- Clamping the infundibulopelvic ligament compromises blood supply to the ovary.
- Due to proximity of ovary to the tube, infection and malignancy spread from one structure to another very early.

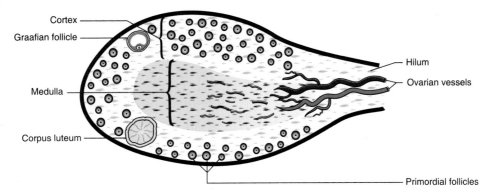

Figure 1.12 Cut section of the ovary, revealing the cortex and medulla. The Graafian follicles are located in the cortex.

Endopelvic fascia

The endopelvic fascia is a fascial covering or sheath around the pelvic viscera, blood vessels and other structures that enter and exit the peritoneal cavity. It is divided into **parietal layer** that forms the sheaths of the pelvic muscles and **visceral layer** that ensheathes the pelvic viscera. The space between the peritoneum and the pelvic is filled with loose pelvic cellular tissue. The pelvic cellular tissue is continuous with the tissue of the perinephric space, the tissue above the levator ani and obturator internus, and extends along the sheaths of vessels and other structures. Fluid or pus collected in the cellular tissue can thus spread along this plane in case of infection.

Ligaments

The endopelvic fascia condenses in some areas to form ligaments that support the uterus and other pelvic structures (Box 1.22; Fig. 1.13).

Box 1.22 Ligaments of the uterus and cervix

- Cardinal ligaments
- Pubocervical ligaments
- Uterosacral ligaments
- Round ligaments
- Broad ligaments
- Ovarian ligaments
- Infundibulopelvic ligaments

Cardinal or Mackenrodt ligaments

These extend from the lower part of the uterus and supravaginal cervix and lateral vaginal fornix to the lateral pelvic wall. The loose cellular

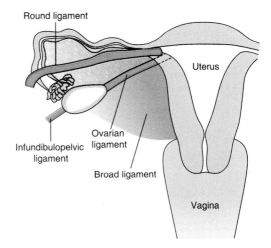

Figure 1.13 Round, infundibulopelvic, ovarian and broad ligaments.

tissue in this area is referred to as **parametrium**. The ureter, before entering the bladder, traverses this ligament and is encased in a fascial sheath, called **ureteric tunnel**, which lies 2 cm lateral to the cervix. The uterine artery crosses to the uterus above the ureter at this point. The descending cervical branch of the uterine artery courses through this ligament. The lymphatics from the upper vagina and cervix also course through the ligament and some drain into the parametrial node. Frankenhauser plexus, which consists of sympathetic ganglia and nerves, also extends into the parametrium (Box 1.23; Fig. 1.14).

Spread of infection and malignancy into the parametrium and cardinal ligaments occurs via the lymphatics. Parametrial extension of malignancy is important in staging of cervical cancer.

Box 1.23 Contents of cardinal ligaments and parametrium

- Ureteric canal
- Descending cervical artery
- Lymphatics and lymph node
- Frankenhauser plexus

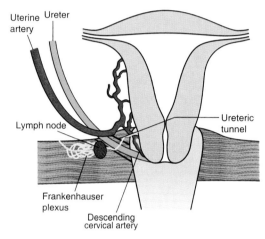

Figure 1.14 Structures in the cardinal ligament—Descending cervical branch of the uterine artery, ureter in the ureteric tunnel, lymph node and Frankenhauser plexus.

Pubocervical ligament

This condensation of the pubovesicocervical fascia passes from the anterolateral aspect of the cervix to the posterior surface of the public bone. Some fibres extend from the bladder and the pubis and form the bladder pillars. Pubocervical ligaments merge posterolaterally with the cardinal ligaments.

Uterosacral ligaments

These ligaments extend from the posterior part of the supravaginal cervix to the sacrum. They lie on either side of the rectosigmoid. Anterolaterally, they merge with cardinal ligaments. Frankenhauser plexus of nerves is located mainly along these ligaments.

The three ligaments together are referred to as **triradiate ligaments** (Fig. 1.15).

Round ligaments

These are vestiges of the gubernaculums and are made of fibromuscular tissue. They extend laterally from the uterine cornu extraperitoneally, to enter the inguinal canal and finally merge with

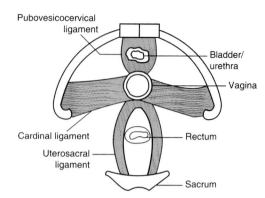

Figure 1.15 Ligaments attached to the lower uterus and cervix—Cardinal, pubocervical and uterosacral ligaments.

the skin and connective tissue of the mons pubis and labia majora. The ligament contains a blood vessel arising from uterine/ovarian artery and should be ligated during surgery.

Broad ligaments

The peritoneum on the anterior and posterior surfaces of the uterus spreads out laterally towards the pelvic wall to form the broad ligaments. Between the two layers of the peritoneum is the pelvic cellular tissue containing ureter and the plexus formed by the anastomosis of uterine and ovarian vessels. The round ligaments, tubes and ovarian ligaments are covered by the peritoneum of the broad ligament and are contained in its upper part.

Ovarian ligaments

They pass from the medial pole of the ovaries to the uterine cornu posterior to the attachment of the tubes.

Infundibulopelvic ligaments

These are lateral extensions of the broad ligaments between the ovary and the pelvic wall. They contain the ovarian vessels.

Clinical implications

Clinical implications of *cardinal and uterosacral ligaments* are given as follows:

- Congenital or acquired weakening of cardinal and uterosacral ligaments causes descent of the uterine cervix and uterus, leading to pelvic organ prolapse.
- While clamping the cardinal ligament during hysterectomy, care must be taken to avoid the ureter in the ureteric tunnel.

Pelvic floor

The pelvic organs are supported in the upright position by a fibromuscular floor that includes the levator ani, coccygeus muscle, external anal sphincter, urethral sphincter and deep perineal muscles.

Pelvic diaphragm

Pelvic diaphragm consists of levator ani muscle covered by pelvic fascia. The muscle covers the space from the pubic bone to the coccyx and from one pelvic side wall to another, forming a funnel-shaped support. The muscle has three components—The puborectalis, pubococcygeus and iliococcygeus (Box 1.24; Fig. 1.16). Fibres of the puborectalis that are inserted into the vagina are known as pubovaginalis. The coccygeus, formerly called ischiococcygeus, extends from the ischial spine to the coccyx but is not a part of levator ani.

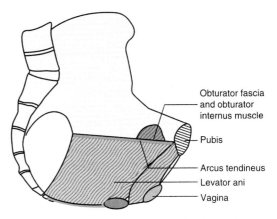

Figure 1.17 Arcus tendineus fascia pelvis. It extends from the pubic bone to the ischial spine.

Box 1.24 Components of levator ani

• Puborectalis
• Pubococcygeus
• Iliococcygeus

The muscle fibres of the levator ani muscles arise from the **arcus tendineus fascia pelvis** or **white line**, which is a thickening of the fascial covering of the obturator internus muscle and extends from the public bone to the ischial spine (Fig. 1.17). The fibres of the levator ani pass backwards and medially and fuse in the midline forming the **levator plate**. Urogenital hiatus is the space between the levator ani muscles; the urethra, vagina and anal canal are enclosed in this hiatus.

The fibres of the puborectalis arise from the pubic bone, form a sling around the vagina and rectum and are inserted into perineal body, rectal wall and anococcygeal raphe. The medial and anterior fibres that cross the lateral vaginal wall between the middle and lower third and are inserted into the vaginal wall and perineal body are referred to as pubovaginalis. Some fibres decussate behind the urethra (pubourethralis) as well. These muscle fibres form a sling around the urethra, vagina and rectum, pulling these structures anteriorly towards the pubis. When the muscle contracts, the urethra, vagina and rectum are kinked and narrowed. The contraction of the levator ani also maintains the vagina in its horizontal position at rest.

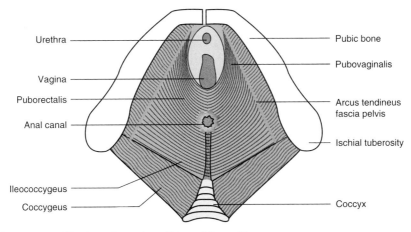

Figure 1.16 Components of levator ani muscles—Puborectalis and iliococcygeus.

The pubococcygeus muscle fibres also arise from the posterior surface of the pubis and are inserted into the rectum, anococcygeal raphe and coccyx.

The ischiococcygeus, though not part of the levator ani as already mentioned, also forms the posterior part of the pelvic floor and pelvic support. It originates from the ischial spine and sacrospinous ligament and is inserted into the lateral part of the lower sacrum and coccyx.

The uterus and vagina lie horizontally on the pelvic floor. The levator ani muscle has a resting tone that keeps the pelvic floor closed and prevents herniation of the uterus and cervix. When the muscle is damaged, as happens after multiple vaginal deliveries, the resting tone is lost and herniation or pelvic organ prolapse results.

> **Clinical implications**
>
> The clinical implications of the *structure and shape of pelvic floor* are as follows:
> - The resting tone of the fibres of levator ani provides support for pelvis viscera.
> - They help in maintaining urinary and rectal continence during increase in intra-abdominal pressure.

Supports of the uterus

Uterus is supported by **ligaments and pelvic floor**. The round and broad ligaments are weak ligaments, but the cardinal and uterosacral ligaments support the cervix and upper vagina. Stretching of these ligaments with childbirth or postmenopausal atrophy leads to prolapse of the cervix or vaginal apex. The **levator ani** muscle is the main structure that supports the uterus and holds it in its position. Weakening or loss of tone of this muscle plays a major role in the pathogenesis of prolapse.

Supports of the vagina

Vaginal supports also hold the bladder, rectum and urethra in their position. The vaginal supports are divided into level I, II and III (De Lancey). Weakening of these supports causes prolapse of the cervix or vaginal apex, cystocele, rectocele or urethrocele (*see* Chapter 24, *Pelvic organ prolapse*). Level I supports are the **uterosacral** and **cardinal ligaments** and support the upper vagina and cervix. The lateral vagina and endopelvic fascia around the middle third of the vagina are attached to the **arcus tendineus fascia pelvis** laterally. The lateral vaginal sulcus represents this line of attachment that runs from the pubic bone to the ischial spine on either side. This forms the lateral support at level II. Posteriorly, there is a condensation of the endopelvic fascia on the levator ani that extends from the arcus tendineus fascia pelvis to the perineal body and is known as **arcus tendineus fascia rectovaginalis**. The attachment of the posterior vaginal muscularis to this forms the posterior support at level II. The **perineal body**, **superficial** and **deep perineal muscles** and **perineal membrane** that support the lower third of the vagina constitute level III supports.

> **Clinical implications**
>
> The clinical implications of *supports of vagina* are listed as follows:
> - Cardinal and uterosacral ligaments
>   - Pathogenesis of prolapse
>   - Surgical correction of prolapse
> - Levator ani
>   - Pathogenesis of prolapse
> - Cardinal ligaments
>   - Dissection during radical hysterectomy

Pelvic ureters

The ureters are located retroperitoneally and run from the renal pelvis to the urinary bladder. The abdominal segments lie on the psoas muscle and run downwards and medially. They enter the pelvis by crossing the common iliac vessels from lateral to medial aspect at their bifurcation. Here the ureters lie just medial to the ovarian vessels that cross over the ureters soon after to supply the ovaries (Fig. 1.18). They can be found attached to the posterior peritoneum during dissection. At the level of the ischial spines, they turn forwards and medially towards the base of the broad ligament. They then enter the ureteric canal in the cardinal ligament, crossing under the uterine vessels (Fig. 1.19). Here, they are 2 cm lateral to the cervix. The ureters run medially and enter the bladder close to the anterior vaginal wall (Box 1.25).

The ureters receive rich blood supply from all the blood vessels in the pelvis. These vessels anastomose to form a plexus on the adventitia of the ureters before entering it. Therefore, it is protected from devascularization unless it is skeletonized.

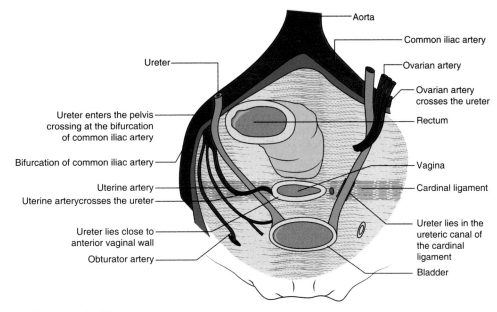

Figure 1.18 Course of pelvic ureters.

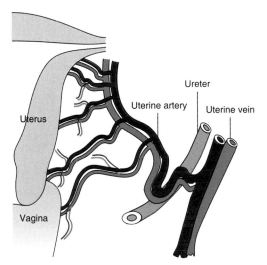

Figure 1.19 Uterine artery and ureter. The ureter crosses under the uterine artery (water under the bridge).

Clinical implications

The ureter lies in close association with several pelvic structures and is, therefore, susceptible to injury during a variety of pelvic surgical procedures. It is important to know the points at which there is close proximity so that care can be taken to avoid such injury and formation of fistula (Box 1.26). Its close proximity to ovarian and uterine vessels (Fig. 1.20) makes it prone to injury during common gynaecological procedures such as hysterectomy and oophorectomy.

Box 1.25 Course of the pelvic ureters

- Cross the common iliac at bifurcation
- Lie medial to ovarian vessels that cross over it soon after
- Lie attached to the posterior peritoneum
- Reach the level of uterosacral ligaments
- Turn forwards at ischial spine
- Enter the base of broad ligaments
- Cross under the uterine vessels
- Enter ureteric canal in cardinal ligaments
- Run forwards to enter the bladder
- Lie close to the anterior vaginal wall

Box 1.26 Points at which ureter is prone to injury

• Pelvic brim	Clamping infundibulopelvic ligaments
• Bifurcation of common iliac	Internal iliac artery ligation
• Broad ligament	Uterine artery ligation
• Cardinal ligament	Dissection of ureteric tunnel Clamping cardinal ligament
• Upper vagina	Clamping vaginal angle
• Devascularization	All through the course in pelvis

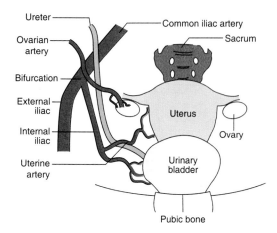

Figure 1.20 Relations of the pelvic ureter. It crosses the bifurcation of vessels and then crosses under the uterine artery to enter the ureteric tunnel.

Urinary bladder and urethra

The urinary bladder and urethra are in close proximity to the anterior surface of the uterus and vagina. The proximity and susceptibility to injury varies with the amount of urine in the bladder. The superior surface of the bladder is adjacent to the anterior uterine surface. Base of the bladder is located adjacent to the anterior vaginal wall. Bladder neck and urethra lie anterior to the anterior vaginal wall. The space between the bladder and the pubic symphysis is called **space of Retzius**.

Clinical implications

The clinical implications of *urinary bladder and urethra* are listed as follows:
- Bladder closely applied to the uterus
  - Injury while pushing the bladder down
  - Adhesion due to previous surgery
- Space of Retzius
  - Approach for surgical correction of stress incontinence

Blood supply

The internal and external genitalia have a rich blood supply in order to allow for the needs of pregnancy and labour. There are some unique characteristics to be remembered that are listed in Box 1.27.

Box 1.27 **Unique characteristics of pelvic vasculature**

- Arteries are paired
- Significant anatomical variation in vasculature is seen
- Arteries enter the organs from lateral aspect
- Rich collateral circulation is present
- Veins form a basket of plexuses around viscera

Ovarian vessels

The ovaries are supplied by ovarian vessels. The ovarian arteries arise from the aorta just below the renal vessels. They descend retroperitoneally, cross the ureter anteriorly and enter the infundibulopelvic ligaments. After supplying the ovary, they give off branches to supply the fallopian tube and finally anastomose with ascending branch of the uterine artery near the uterine cornu in the broad ligament. The right ovarian vein drains into the inferior vena cava, but the left ovarian vein joins the left renal vein.

Internal iliac (hypogastric) vessels

The aorta bifurcates into common iliac arteries at the level of L4 vertebra. Common iliac arteries divide into external and internal iliac arteries at the sacroiliac joints. The ureters cross the common iliac arteries at their bifurcation.

The internal iliac (hypogastric) artery lies posteromedial to the external iliac vessels. The ureter is anterior and the internal iliac vein is posterior to the artery. The artery on each side divides into anterior and posterior divisions. The posterior division exits the pelvis and does not give off any visceral branches. The anterior division gives rise to several branches that supply the internal and external genitalia (Box 1.28; Fig. 1.21).

The obturator and superior vesical arteries are the first two branches of the anterior division, followed by the uterine artery. The vaginal artery also arises from the internal iliac artery but occasionally arises from the uterine artery. After giving off these branches in the pelvis, the internal iliac artery continues as internal pudendal artery that hooks behind the ischial spines to enter the pudendal canal in the ischiorectal fossa. Here it gives off two more branches: The inferior rectal and perineal arteries. The vessel then ends as dorsal artery of the clitoris. The parietal branches supply the respective muscles and tissues.

Box 1.28 Branches of the anterior division of the internal iliac artery

- Parietal branches
  - Obturator
  - Inferior gluteal
  - Internal pudendal
    - Inferior rectal
    - Perineal
    - Dorsal artery of the clitoris
- Visceral branches
  - Superior vesical (umbilical)
  - Uterine
  - Vaginal
  - Middle vesical
  - Middle rectal
  - Inferior vesical

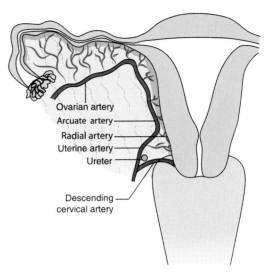

Figure 1.22 Branches of the uterine artery and its anastomosis with branches of ovarian artery.

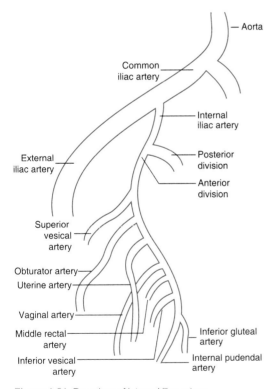

Figure 1.21 Branches of internal iliac artery.

descending cervical branches. The arcuate arteries give off several branches to the uterus that run transversely, called **radial arteries**. The terminal part of the uterine artery ultimately anastomoses with the ovarian vessels. The descending branch runs in the cardinal ligament to supply the cervix and vagina.

Blood supply to the vulva

The vessels that supply the structures of the vulva are as listed in Box 1.29. The internal pudendal artery hooks around the ischial spine to enter the Alcock canal and reaches the perineum (Fig. 1.23). There it gives rise to two main branches, the inferior rectal and perineal arteries, before terminating as dorsal artery of the clitoris (Fig. 1.24).

Box 1.29 Blood supply to the vulva

- External pudendal arteries from femoral vessels
- Perineal arteries from internal pudendal vessels
- Dorsal artery of the clitoris from internal pudendal vessels

Uterine arteries

The uterine arteries run medially, and cross over the ureter about 2 cm lateral to the internal os in the broad ligament. At the lateral border of the uterus, they turn sharply upwards and run along the side of the uterus as **arcuate artery** (Fig. 1.22). Before turning upwards, they give off the

Sacral vessels

The middle sacral artery that arises from the aorta and lateral sacral arteries from the internal iliac anastomose to form a rich sacral plexus along the sacral vertebrae retroperitoneally.

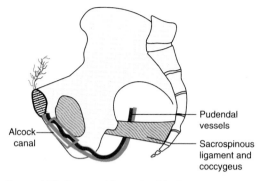

Figure 1.23 Course of the pudendal artery.

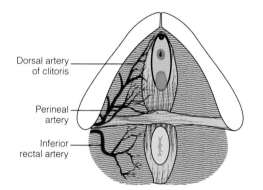

Figure 1.24 Course of the perineal artery.

Venous drainage is along the same arteries that supply the various structures of the pelvis and vulva.

Clinical implications

The clinical implications of *blood supply to the pelvis* are given as follows:

- Rich collaterals — Ligation of internal iliac/uterine arteries possible

- Rich anastomoses at sacrum — Bleeding during dissection

- Close proximity to ureter — Risk of ureteric injury

- Descending cervical/vagina — Prone to haemorrhage if not carefully ligated

- Rich blood supply to clitoris — Risk of bleeding during surgery

- Proximity of pudendal artery to ischial spine — Prone to injury during sacrospinous fixation

---

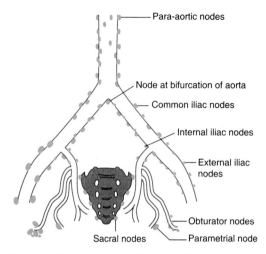

Figure 1.25 Lymph nodes of the pelvis that drain the genital organs.

Lymphatic drainage

Lymphatic drainage is usually along the veins that drain the organs. There are groups of lymph nodes along all the major vessels (Fig. 1.25). In addition, constant nodes are present in some locations (Box 1.30).

Box 1.30 Constant lymph nodes

- Obturator—In the obturator fossa
- Parametrial—At the crossing of ureter and uterine artery
- Node of Cloquet—Deep inguinal at the opening of femoral canal

---

The nodes that drain the various organs are listed in Table 1.1. Lymphatics from vulva and lower vagina that are supplied by branches of femoral and internal iliac vessels drain into inguinal, external and internal iliac nodes. The lymphatics from upper vagina and cervix drain into obturator, internal iliac, external iliac and along the uterosacral ligaments to the sacral nodes. Lymphatics from the uterine body drain into iliac nodes but, along the ovarian vein, reach the para-aortic nodes as well. Occasionally, some lymphatics that run along the round ligament from the uterine fundus may drain into the inguinal nodes. The primary nodes of drainage for ovary are the para-aortic nodes since ovarian vessels arise from aorta.

Table 1.1 Lymph nodes draining the pelvic viscera		
Organ	Primary nodes	Secondary nodes
Vulva	Superficial inguinal	Common iliac
Lower vagina	• Deep inguinal • External iliac	Para-aortic
Upper vagina	External iliac	Common iliac
Cervix	• Internal iliac • Obturator • Sacral	Para-aortic
Uterus	• Internal iliac • Para-aortic	Para-aortic
Ovary and tube	• Para-aortic • Inguinal (rare)	Supraclavicular

Clinical implications

Clinical implications of *lymphatic drainage of the pelvis* are given as follows:

• Malignancies of the genital tract	Dissection of primary nodes
• Close proximity of nodes to vessels	Risk of injury during dissection

Nerve supply

The pelvis is supplied by somatic nerves and autonomic nervous system (Fig. 1.26).

Somatic innervation

This is from T12 to S4 through the nerves listed in Box 1.31. They supply the levator ani, perineal muscles, obturator and muscles of the lower

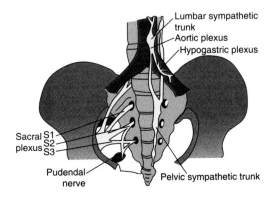

Figure 1.26 Splanchnic and somatic nerves of the pelvis.

anterior abdominal wall. The cutaneous nerves supply the perineum, thighs and abdominal wall.

Box 1.31 Somatic innervation

- Lumbosacral trunk: T12, S1–S5
- Obturator: L2, L3, L4
- Pudendal: S2, S3, S4
- Iliohypogastric: T12, L1
- Ilioinguinal: L1
- Genitofemoral: L1, L2
- Posterior femoral cutaneous: S1, S2, S3

The lumbosacral trunk, obturator and pudendal nerves supply the muscles of the pelvis, gluteal region and thigh, obturator muscle, pelvic and urogenital diaphragm and perineal muscles. The sensory nerve supply to the mons pubis and labia majora is from the ilioinguinal and genitofemoral nerves. Perianal area, perineum, vestibule of the vagina and clitoris are supplied by the pudendal nerve.

Autonomic innervation

The autonomic nervous system controls the contraction and relaxation of the smooth muscles of the uterus, bladder, rectum and the blood vessels. *Sympathetic system* stimulates contraction, and *parasympathetic system* causes relaxation. The fibres of sympathetic and parasympathetic nerves are intermingled (Fig 1.27).

Sympathetic system The sympathetic nerve supply arises from T10 to L2. The sympathetic ganglia are located in the lumbar and sacral regions. The lumbar sympathetic plexus lies along the aorta. This continues downwards to form the superior hypogastric plexus. Nerves from this plexus descend to form the inferior hypogastric plexus at the bifurcation of the common iliac. This divides into two lateral portions. They then continue downwards and are joined by the parasympathetic fibres S2, S3 and S4 to form the pelvic plexuses at the base of the broad ligament (Box 1.32). The Frankenhauser plexus along the uterosacral and cardinal ligaments is formed by nerves from the pelvic plexus. These two plexuses together supply the uterus, cervix, vagina, anus, rectum and urinary bladder. Ovary is supplied by ovarian plexus, which is derived from nerves from the renal plexus. Sympathetic nerves control the smooth muscles of the uterus and bladder and cause vasoconstriction.

Labels on figure: Lumbar sympathetic trunk; Aortic plexus; Hypogastric plexus; Sacral plexus S1 S2 S3; Pudendal nerve; Pelvic sympathetic trunk

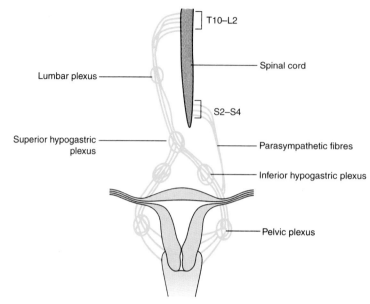

Figure 1.27 Autonomic innervations of the reproductive tract. The sympathetic nerves arise from T10–L2, and form the superior and interior hypogastric plexuses; they are joined by parasympathetic fibres from S2, S3 and S4 to form pelvic plexuses.

Box 1.32 Autonomic innervation

- Sympathetic
  - Lumbar plexus
  - Superior hypogastric plexus (T11–L2)
  - Inferior hypogastric plexus
  - Pelvic plexus
  - Frankenhauser plexus
  - Ovarian plexus
- Parasympathetic
  - From S2, S3, S4 (pelvic plexus)

Parasympathetic system The efferent parasympathetic nerve supply to the pelvis emerges with the ventral rami of S2–S4 as myelinated, preganglionic nerves and joins the sympathetic fibres from the hypogastric plexus to form the pelvic plexuses. They have an inhibitory effect on the rectum, urinary bladder and erectile tissue of the clitoris and cause vasodilatation of the ovarian and uterine vessels.

Afferent sensory nerve fibres from the uterus, bladder and rectum travel via the sympathetic and parasympathetic nerves to reach the spinal cord and cranial ganglia. They transmit visceral sensations such as bladder and rectal distension, and pain of cervical stretching and uterine contractions. Pain from the perineum, labia, clitoris and anus is transmitted through the pudendal nerve to spinal segments S2–S4.

Physiological actions of autonomic system

The sympathetic and parasympathetic systems have opposite actions (Box 1.33).

Box 1.33 Physiological actions of autonomic system

- Sympathetic
  - Muscular contraction
  - Vasoconstriction
- Parasympathetic
  - Muscular relaxation
  - Vasodilatation

Clinical implications

The clinical implications of *pelvic innervation* are listed as follows:

• Pudendal nerve at ischial spine	Nerve block for obstetric procedures
• S2, S3, S4 segments supplying uterus	Uterine pain felt at the back
• Frankenhauser plexus	Uterosacral nerve ablation

Key points

- The reproductive tract consists of external and internal reproductive organs.
- The external reproductive organs include the structures of the vulva and the gynaecological perineum.
- The clitoris is the homologue of the penis.
- The vaginal orifice is in the vestibule, lies between the two labia minora and is partially covered by hymen.
- The Bartholin glands are located in the posterolateral aspect of the vaginal orifice and are not palpable unless enlarged.
- Muscles of the perineum are separated by the perineal membrane into superficial and deep muscles. Superficial muscles cause venous congestion, compression of vestibular bulb and clitoris and erection of clitoris.
- Deep perineal muscles are the sphincter urethrae and deep transverse perinei muscles. They compress the urethra and support the lower vagina, respectively.
- Internal genital organs consist of the vagina, uterus, fallopian tubes and ovaries.
- The axis of the vagina is horizontal when the woman is standing. The anterior wall is shorter than the posterior wall.
- The cervix uteri has an upper, supravaginal part and lower portiovaginalis. Endocervical canal is lined by columnar epithelium and ectocervix by stratified squamous epithelium.
- Uterus is pear shaped with a length of 7 cm and anteroposterior width of 2.5 cm. The endometrium is very sensitive to oestrogen and progesterone and undergoes changes during menstrual cycle and pregnancy.
- The myometrium plays a major role in contraction during parturition and contraction and retraction after delivery.
- The fallopian tubes are 10 cm long and are divided into four regions. Fertilization of the ovum takes place in the tube, and the fertilized ovum is then transported to the uterine cavity.

- The ovaries are the female gonads and are located on either side of the uterus. Histologically, each ovary is divided into vortex and medulla. The cortex contains the specialized stroma and follicles and is responsible for ovulation and steroid hormone production.
- The ligaments that support the uterus and vagina are formed by condensation of the endopelvic fascia.
- The cardinal ligament is the most important ligament and supports the upper vagina and supravaginal cervix. Important structures including the ureter, descending artery, lymphatics and Frankenhauser plexus are contained in it.
- The pelvic floor supports the pelvic organs. Levator ani muscle is the most important component of the pelvic floor.
- The components of the levator ani are pubococcygeus and ileococcygeus. They support the mid-vagina and bladder neck.
- The ovaries are supplied by ovarian arteries, which arise from the aorta and are carried in the infundibulopelvic vessels. The rest of the genital organs are supplied mainly by branches of the internal iliac artery. There is rich anastomosis between the arteries.
- The pelvic ureter is closely related to the ovarian and uterine vessels during its course in the pelvis. There are several points where it is prone to injury. Care should be taken to avoid injury to the ureter during pelvic surgeries.
- The lymphatics that drain the various parts of the genital tract lie along the respective blood vessels.
- The pelvic structures are supplied by somatic nerves and autonomic nervous system. The sensory motor nerve supply is through the lumbosacral trunk, pudendal ilioinguinal and genitofemoral nerves from T12 to S5. Autonomic supply is both parasympathetic and sympathetic. They control smooth muscle functions of the rectum, bladder and uterus, and afferent fibres carry sensations to the brain.

Self-assessment

Case-based questions

Case 1

A 45-year-old lady with diagnosis of cervical cancer is taken up for radical hysterectomy with pelvic lymphadenectomy. Due to prior laparotomy, there are adhesions in the pelvis.

1. What are the points at which ureteric injury can occur?
2. Which are the primary and secondary nodes that you will remove?

3. What are the structures in the cardinal ligament that you will encounter during dissection?

Case 2

A 25-year-old lady presents with clinical features suggestive of acute pelvic inflammatory disease. On examination, there is a fullness in the pouch of Douglas with bogginess.

1. What is your diagnosis?
2. Why does this occur?
3. What approach will you use to drain the abscess?

Answers

Case 1

1. At the pelvic brim, close to infundibulopelvic ligament; during node dissection, as it crosses the common iliac vessels; in the broad ligament; in the cardinal ligament; at the vaginal vault. Devascularization can occur anywhere in the pelvis.
2. (a) Primary nodes—Internal iliac, external iliac, obturator and sacral nodes
   (b) Secondary nodes—Common iliac and nodes at aortic bifurcation
3. Ureter, descending cervical branch of the uterine artery, nerve plexus and lymph node.

Case 2

1. Pelvic abscess. Clinical features of acute pelvic inflammatory disease and bogginess in the pouch of Douglas, which is a characteristic sign of pelvic abscess.
2. The peritoneum on the posterior surface of the uterus extends down to the posterior vagina before it is reflected onto the anterior surface of the rectum. This forms a cul-de-sac or pouch of Douglas. This is the most dependent part of the pelvis, and pus tends to collect in this pouch.
3. Pouch of Douglas can be approached through the posterior fornix of the vagina. The abscess is separated from the vaginal fornix only by vaginal wall and peritoneum.

Long-answer questions

1. Describe the course of pelvic ureter. What are the anatomical sites where it is susceptible to injury?
2. Describe the blood supply to the internal and external genital organs with appropriate diagrams.

Short-answer questions

1. Anatomy of fallopian tube
2. Pelvic lymphatic drainage
3. Levator ani
4. Lymphatic drainage of cervix
5. Supports of uterus
6. Perineal body
7. Cardinal ligaments
8. Pouch of Douglas
9. Internal iliac artery

2

Development of the Female Genital Tract: Normal and Abnormal

Case scenario

A 1-year-old child was brought to the clinic by parents with ambiguous genitalia. The parents had noticed this at birth, but were assured by the local midwife who conducted the delivery that the child was a male and the genitalia would become normal in course of time. But there was no change with time. The parents wanted to know the gender of the child since they had to make a decision about sex of rearing.

Introduction

Embryological development of female external and internal genitalia and gonad is a complex and coordinated process of differentiation, regression, maturation, migration, fusion and canalization, controlled by genetic and hormonal factors. It is closely associated with the development of kidneys and urinary tract. Therefore, anatomical and developmental abnormalities in female genital tract are often associated with abnormalities in urinary tract as well and should be specifically looked for.

Development of the gonad

The sex chromosomes (XX or XY) determine the development of the gonads: 46 XX will develop into a female and 46 XY will develop into a male. The type of gonad present determines the phenotypic sex. However, it is the presence or absence of Y chromosome that determines the development of the gonad into testis or ovary. Genetic basis of gonadal development is described in Box 2.1.

Box 2.1 Genetics of gonadal development

- Y chromosome determines the development of testis
- In the absence of Y chromosome, gonad develops into ovary
- Two X chromosomes are essential for optimal ovarian development
- In the absence of second X chromosome, ovary is devoid of oocytes
- Other genes on other chromosomes are also involved in gonadal differentiation

Embryologically, the gonadal development proceeds described as follows:

- Around the fifth week after fertilization, two gonadal ridges appear on either side of the midline in the dorsal aspect of the embryo. These are formed by the proliferation of coelomic epithelium.
- The primordial germ cells are formed in the yolk sac and migrate along the mesentery of the hindgut into these gonadal ridges by the sixth week (Fig. 2.1).

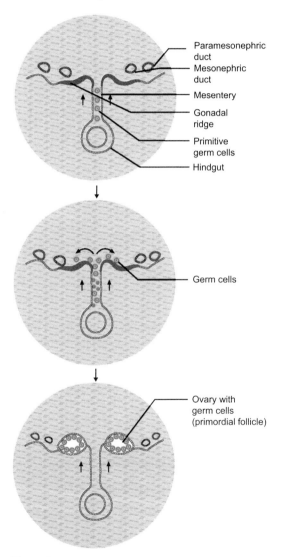

Figure 2.1 Development of ovary. Gonadal ridges appear on either side of the midline. Primordial germ cells, formed in the yolk sac, migrate along the mesentery of the hindgut into the gonadal ridges.

- The gonadal swellings (ridges) differentiate into testis or ovary depending on the sex chromosomes.
- The cells of the coelomic epithelium differentiate into pregranulosa cells in the female. The germ cells form the oocytes and are surrounded by ring of pregranulosa cells and later by granulosa cells to form primordial follicles by 20 weeks' gestation. They arrange themselves in the ovarian cortex, while the ovarian medulla consists mainly of connective tissue.
- The gonads later descend into the pelvis.
- Several follicles undergo atresia. At birth, there are about 1 million normal follicles and no new follicles develop after birth.

The gonads produce sex hormones. Ovary produces oestrogen, and testis produces testosterone and anti-Müllerian hormone (AMH). Development of internal genital organs is dependent on the production of these hormones.

Development of the internal genital organs

The internal genital organs develop from the mesoderm.

- Two pairs of genital ducts, the Wolffian (mesonephric) and Müllerian (paramesonephric) ducts, are formed in the dorsal mesoderm in both sexes by the sixth week.
- The Wolffian ducts precede the Müllerian ducts. They are medial, arise in the lower thoracic and upper lumbar region, and run caudally to enter the urogenital sinus.
- The Müllerian ducts arise laterally and run parallel to the Wolffian ducts. Their cephalic ends open into the coelomic cavity, but caudal ends meet and fuse with the fellow of the opposite side.
- The open cephalic parts of the Müllerian ducts form the fallopian tubes; fused lower part becomes the uterus and cervix and the intervening septum disappears later (Fig. 2.2). The fused lower part enters the urogenital sinus by 9 weeks' gestation.
- In the female, the Wolffian ducts regress due to lack of testosterone. In the male, Müllerian ducts degenerate due to production of AMH and Wolffian ducts develop into male internal genitalia.

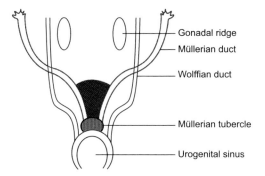

Figure 2.2 Development of the uterus and tubes. The caudal portions of the two Müllerian ducts fuse in the midline to form the uterus and cervix, while the unfused cephalic portion becomes the tubes.

Development of the vagina

The vagina has a dual origin described as follows:

- Where the Müllerian ducts enter the urogenital sinus, a swelling appears from the lower end of the fused Müllerian ducts and is referred to as Müllerian tubercle (Figs 2.2 and 2.3a and b).

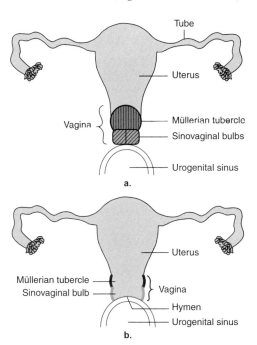

Figure 2.3 Development of the vagina. a. Müllerian tubercle forms at the caudal end of the fused Müllerian duct where it joins the urogenital sinus. b. Two sinovaginal bulbs arise from the urogenital sinus to meet the Müllerian tubercle. Vagina is formed by canalization of both these structures.

- Paired outgrowths called sinovaginal bulbs arise from the urogenital sinus to meet the Müllerian tubercle, and these fuse, elongate and canalize to form the vagina.
- Vagina, therefore, develops from Müllerian duct as well as urogenital sinus. The junction of sinovaginal bulbs with the urogenital sinus is marked by the hymen.

Defects in fusion and canalization of any of these structures can lead to anomalies in the uterus, cervix and vagina. Remnants of Wolffian structures can be seen as epoophoron and paroophoron (small tubular structures) in meso-varium or mesosalpinx and Gartner duct in lateral vaginal wall.

Structures from which gonads and internal genitalia develop are listed in Box 2.2.

Box 2.2 Development of ovaries and internal genitalia

- Gonadal ridge—Ovary
- Primitive germ cells—Oocytes
- Müllerian ducts
  - Cephalic unfused portion—Fallopian tubes
  - Caudal fused portion—Uterus and cervix
- Müllerian tubercle—Upper vagina
- Sinovaginal bulbs—Lower vagina

Development of the external genitalia

The caudal end of the urogenital sinus is covered by cloacal membrane. A longitudinal septum appears in the urogenital sinus called urorectal septum. This septum grows caudally and meets the cloacal membrane, dividing the cloaca into anal canal and urogenital canal. The cloacal membrane breaks down to form anal and vaginal openings (Fig. 2.4a–d). The point where the urorectal septum meets the cloacal membrane develops into the perineal body.

The genital tubercle forms as a prominence at the tip of the cloacal membrane. On either side of the anterior part of the cloacal membrane, a pair of genital folds appears and lateral to these develops a pair of genital swellings. Development is the same in both sexes up to this point (about 10 weeks' gestation). In the absence of androgens, the genital folds become the labia minora and

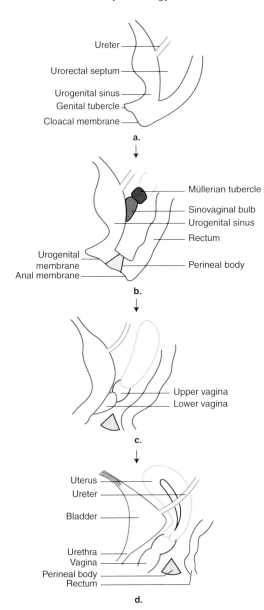

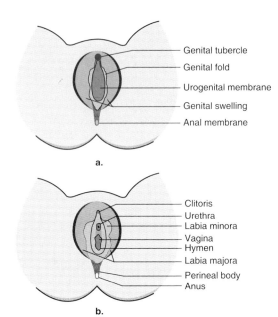

Figure 2.5 Development of external genitalia. a. Genital swellings and genital folds form on either side of the urogenital membrane. Genital tubercle forms at the tip of the membrane. b. The labia majora and minora develop from the genital swellings and genital folds. Genital tubercle develops into the clitoris.

forms the urethra. These changes take place in the second trimester. Structures from which external genitalia develop are given in Box 2.3.

Box 2.3 Development of female external genitalia

- Genital tubercle—Clitoris
- Genital folds—Labia minora
- Genital swellings—Labia majora

The external genitalia are very sensitive to androgens. The degree of masculinization depends on the gestational age at exposure to androgen and local tissue sensitivity. Early exposure leads to labioscrotal fusion, but exposure later causes only enlargement of clitoris.

Abnormal development

Various abnormalities due to the presence or absence of androgens and AMH are shown in Fig. 2.6. These occur due to abnormalities in one

Figure 2.4 Development of bladder, vagina and anal canal. a. Caudal end of the urogenital sinus is covered by cloacal membrane. Vertical urorectal septum grows towards this membrane. b. Urorectal septum divides the urogenital sinus into urogenital canal and anal canal. c. Sinovaginal bulbs arise from the posterior aspect of the urogenital sinus to form the vagina. d. Urethra and urinary bladder lie anteriorly, anal canal lies posteriorly and the vagina is in between the two.

genital swellings develop into the labia majora. Genital tubercle forms the clitoris (Fig. 2.5a and b). Urethral groove develops anteriorly and later

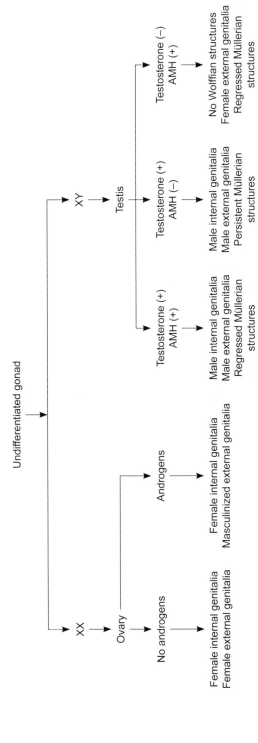

Figure 2.6 Abnormalities due to the presence (+) or absence (–) of androgens and AMH. *AMH*, anti-Müllerian hormone; *XX, XY*, sex chromosomes.

of the several genes involved in gonadal development, such as the *SRY, SOX9, WT-1, DHH* and *SF-1* genes. Turner syndrome (45X0) and other forms of gonadal dysgenesis are discussed in Chapter 18, *Primary amenorrhoea.*

Combinations of female, male or absent internal genitalia with male or female external genitalia are possible. In general, developmental abnormalities can be classified as in Box 2.4.

Box 2.4 Classification of developmental anomalies of genital tract

- Ambiguous genitalia
- Developmental disorders of the vagina
- Developmental disorders of the cervix and uterus

Ambiguous genitalia

This may be classified as in Box 2.5.

Box 2.5 Classification of ambiguous genitalia

- Female pseudohermaphroditism
- Male pseudohermaphroditism
- True hermaphroditism

Female pseudohermaphroditism This, by definition, is female genotype, normal ovaries but with virilization of external genitalia (Fig. 2.7). Exposure to endogenous androgens as in congenital adrenal hyperplasia is the most common cause. This may be a neonatal emergency due to electrolyte disturbances.

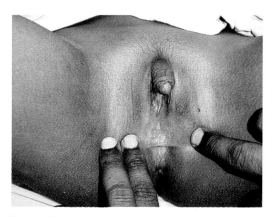

Figure 2.7 Female pseudohermaphroditism. Virilization of female external genitalia in a newborn infant with congenital adrenal hyperplasia.

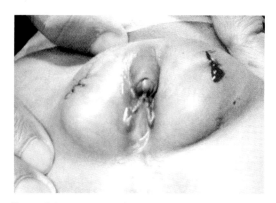

Figure 2.8 Male pseudohermaphroditism. Testes are seen in the labia and the penis is underdeveloped with hypospadias—Partial androgen-insensitivity syndrome.

Male pseudohermaphroditism In this condition, the genotype is male, but there is inadequate masculinization of external genitalia (Fig. 2.8).

This can be due to the following defects:

- Inadequate testosterone production due to enzyme defects
- Inadequate testosterone metabolism as in 5α-reductase deficiency (partial androgen-insensitivity syndrome)
- Inadequate testosterone receptors as seen in androgen-insensitivity syndrome

There is another situation where AMH is deficient. In addition to Wolffian structures and normal male external genitalia, uterus and tubes are also present in this condition.

True hermaphroditism These children are born with testis on one side, ovary on the other side or ovotestes on both sides. Karyotyping may reveal 46XX,XY or mosaics with any combination. Müllerian structures are generally present due to deficient AMH, and masculinization of external genitalia is not complete. Pure and mixed gonadal dysgeneses are the other conditions where sexual infantilism is seen along with absent or streak gonads.

Evaluation and management

Evaluation of ambiguous genitalia should be as shown in Box 2.6.

Management depends on the diagnosis. Infants with congenital adrenal hyperplasia require immediate correction of electrolyte disturbances. Sex of rearing, genital reconstruction and psychological issues have to be decided upon in consultation with the parents. Corrective surgery, hormone therapy and gonadectomy may be required at or after puberty. Following points must be remembered:

- All infants with XX karyotype and congenital adrenal hyperplasia should be reared as girls and corrective surgery performed for clitoromegaly and labial fusion at the appropriate time.
- Children with complete androgen insensitivity should also be raised as females.
- Y chromosome–bearing gonads, if not descended, are susceptible to malignancy and should be removed.
- Others (except those with complete androgen insensitivity) with XY chromosome will have partial development of male external genitalia and further development at puberty. These children should be raised as males.

- Surgical correction can wait till puberty in most cases.

Developmental abnormalities of the genital tract

When dealing with developmental abnormalities of the genital tract, it must be remembered that

- Development of the internal and external genital organs is independent of the development of the gonad, though controlled by the hormones from the gonad. Therefore, women with normal gonads may have congenital uterovaginal anomalies.
- Since the development of the reproductive system is closely linked to that of the urinary system, abnormalities of the two systems may coexist.

Developmental abnormalities of the vagina

Developmental abnormalities of the vagina arise from noncanalization of the upper vagina that is Müllerian in origin or the lower vagina that arises from sinovaginal bulbs. At the junction between the upper and lower parts of the vagina or between the two Müllerian ducts, septae may be present. The various abnormalities are given in Box 2.7 and Fig. 2.9.

Vaginal agenesis

Complete/total vaginal agenesis Failure of canalization of the vagina results in vaginal agenesis. This is usually associated with Müllerian agenesis, also known as Mayer–Rokitansky–Kuster–Hauser (MRKH) syndrome. Renal and vertebral anomalies are often seen in association

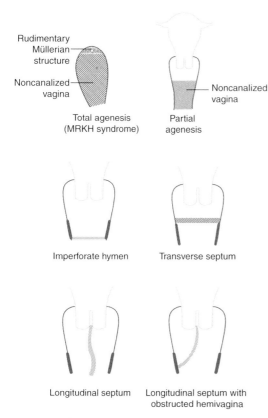

Rudimentary
Müllerian
structure

Noncanalized
vagina

Total agenesis
(MRKH syndrome)

Noncanalized
vagina

Partial
agenesis

Imperforate hymen

Transverse septum

Longitudinal septum

Longitudinal septum with
obstructed hemivagina

Figure 2.9 Developmental anomalies of vagina.

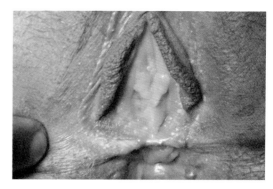

Figure 2.10 Vaginal atresia. There is no vaginal orifice but a dimple can be seen.

with this condition. They present at puberty with primary amenorrhoea. Fibromuscular Müllerian remnants are usually present and the vagina is totally noncanalized. A small dimple or a very short vagina may be identified. In 7–10% of women, the uterus may be normal with functional endometrium. They usually develop haematometra after menarche and present with cyclic abdominal pain.

Partial vaginal agenesis Failure of canalization of the lower part of the vagina, distal to the normal uterus, cervix and upper vagina, leads to this anomaly. This occurs due to abnormal development of the sinovaginal bulbs. Menstrual blood distends the uterus and upper vagina, and, therefore, these girls present with abdominal pain and pelvic mass at puberty (cryptomenorrhoea; Fig. 2.10). Vaginal dimple may be visualized.

Imperforate hymen

Hymen is situated at the junction between sinovaginal bulbs and urogenital sinus. Noncanalization

of this leads to mucocolpos in the neonatal period or haematocolpos at puberty. Girls with imperforate hymen, therefore, present with primary amenorrhoea, abdominal pain and pelvic mass (cryptomenorrhoea). A bluish bulging membrane is seen just above the introitus.

Microperforate and cribriform hymen are other anomalies of the hymen. They are usually asymptomatic, although some present with difficulty in coitus.

Anomalies of vertical fusion

Transverse vaginal septum Transverse septum is due to noncanalization at the junction between the two developmental parts of the vagina: Müllerian tubercle and sinovaginal bulbs. The septum may be present at the lower, middle or upper third of the vagina, but is seen most often at the upper or middle third. It is rarely associated with uterine anomalies. The septae are less than 1 cm thick. Clinical presentation is similar to partial vaginal agenesis. A short vagina is present below the septum.

Anomalies of lateral fusion

Longitudinal vaginal septum The septum may be complete or partial. Other anomalies of fusion of Müllerian ducts such as septate or bicornuate uterus or uterus didelphys are usually associated. They may present with dyspareunia or the septum may be diagnosed on routine pelvic examination.

Obstructed hemivagina The vertical septum may fuse with the lateral vaginal wall (right or left) in the lower third. This leads to obstructed hemivagina. This results in collection of blood in the obstructed part of the vagina (hemihaematocolpos) with dysmenorrhoea and pelvic mass. The condition is commonly associated with ipsilateral renal agenesis.

Clinical evaluation and investigations

Clinical evaluation is as given in Box 2.8. Rectal examination is very useful for diagnosing haematocolpos. A bulge is felt anteriorly and the uterus above it. When the patient is uncooperative, examination under anaesthesia may be required. Ultrasonography may be sufficient to diagnose the type of anomaly in some girls, but magnetic resonance imaging (MRI) is a very useful investigation. The exact nature of the anomaly, level of atresia and associated haematosalpinx can be visualized (Fig. 2.11) on MRI. Renal system should also be evaluated.

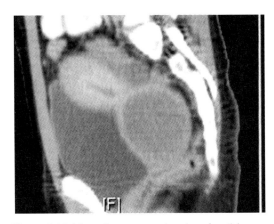

Figure 2.11 Magnetic resonance imaging of partial vaginal atresia. Sagittal view of the uterus and vagina with haematocolpos and haematometra. The upper vagina is grossly distended with blood.

Box 2.8 Evaluation of vaginal anomalies

- Clinical evaluation
  - Examination of external genitalia
  - Per rectal examination to look for haematocolpos and uterus
  - Examination under anaesthesia
- Investigations
  - Ultrasonography
  - Magnetic resonance imaging, if required

Box 2.9 Surgical management of vaginal anomalies

- Imperforate hymen
  - Cruciate incision
- Transverse vaginal septum
  - Excision of septum
- Longitudinal septum
  - Excision of septum
- Vaginal agenesis with haematocolpos
  - Drainage of haematocolpos
  - Vaginal reconstruction
- Total vaginal atresia (MRKH)
  - Nonsurgical
    - Gradual dilatation
  - Surgical
    - McIndoe vaginoplasty
    - Williams vulvovaginoplasty
    - Sigmoid vaginoplasty

MRKH, Mayer–Rokitansky–Kuster–Hauser.

Treatment

Surgical correction or creation of neovagina is required for most of these patients. The various methods are listed in Box 2.9. Imperforate hymen is managed by a cruciate incision on the hymen and drainage of the collected blood. Transverse and longitudinal vaginal septae should be excised.

In women with total vaginal atresia, vagina should be created when sexual activity is anticipated.

Nonsurgical treatment

Gradual dilatation using graduated hard dilators (Frank or Ingram procedure) should be offered to all women with vaginal atresia. The dilatation should continue for 3–4 months and has a success rate of 80%.

Surgical treatment

Neovagina can be created surgically by dissecting the space between the urethra and the rectum and using a mould, skin graft (McIndoe operation), amniotic membrane or part of the sigmoid colon (sigmoid vaginoplasty) to line the cavity. Williams vaginoplasty involves the creation of a perineal pouch using skin flaps from labia minora. Fibrosis and closure of the newly constructed vagina is common following vaginoplasty. Therefore, surgery is generally performed just before the girl plans regular sexual activity. Prognosis for conception depends on the degree of agenesis, degree of damage to the endometrium and tubes due to endometriosis and infection.

Developmental anomalies of the uterus and cervix

These are grouped under Müllerian duct anomalies. They result from defective fusion or canalization. The defect may involve the entire length of the Müllerian ducts, but more often they are segmental. A useful classification devised by Buttram and Gibbons in 1979 and modified by American Fertility Society (AFS) in 1988 is given in Box 2.10. This is currently adopted by the American Society of Reproductive Medicine (ASRM).

The anomalies according to ASRM classification are depicted in Fig. 2.12. Class I anomalies include vaginal anomalies, which have already been discussed. It is important to remember that many of these anomalies produce no symptoms

and, therefore, may go unnoticed. The most common anomaly is septate uterus.

Gynaecological and obstetric problems associated with Müllerian anomalies are presented in Box 2.11. Most women with Müllerian anomalies with outflow obstruction present with amenorrhoea and abdominal pain at puberty. Total nonfusion anomalies produce no symptoms; anomalies such as arcuate uterus are generally undiagnosed.

> ### Box 2.11 Clinical problems of Müllerian anomalies
>
> - Gynaecological
>   - Primary amenorrhoea
>   - Outflow obstruction
>   - Dyspareunia
>   - Infertility
>   - Ectopic pregnancy
> - Obstetric
>   - Recurrent pregnancy loss
>   - Preterm labour
>   - Malpresentations
>   - Foetal growth restriction
>   - Dystocia
>   - Ruptured uterus
>   - Retained placenta
>   - Postpartum haemorrhage

> ### Box 2.10 ASRM classification of Müllerian anomalies
>
> - Class I
>   - Segmental or complete Müllerian agenesis or aplasia
>   - Vaginal
>   - Cervical
>   - Fundal
>   - Tubal
>   - Combined
> - Class II
>   - Unicornuate uterus with or without a rudimentary horn
>   - With rudimentary horn
>   - With communicating endometrial cavity
>   - Noncommunicating cavity
>   - With no cavity
>   - Without rudimentary horn
> - Class III
>   - Uterus didelphys
> - Class IV
>   - Bicornuate
>   - Complete
>   - Partial
> - Class V
>   - Septate uterus
>   - Complete
>   - Partial
> - Class VI
>   - Arcuate uterus
> - Class VII
>   - DES-related abnormalities
>   - T-shaped uterus with or without dilated horns

ASRM, American Society of Reproductive Medicine; *DES*, diethylstilbestrol.

Evaluation and management

Evaluation of women with Müllerian anomalies is given in Box 2.12. Women with Müllerian anomalies have normal external genitalia and secondary sexual characteristics since ovaries are normal. Investigations will depend on the nature of anomaly suspected and the clinical presentation. Ultrasonography is useful to confirm the presence of ovaries or the absence

> ### Box 2.12 Evaluation of Müllerian anomalies
>
> - Clinical evaluation
>   - History
>   - Examination of secondary sexual characteristics
>   - External genitalia
>   - Per vaginal and per rectal examination
> - Investigations
>   - Ultrasonogram—Pelvic and renal
>   - Magnetic resonance imaging
>   - Laparoscopy, hysteroscopy
>   - Hysterosalpingogram

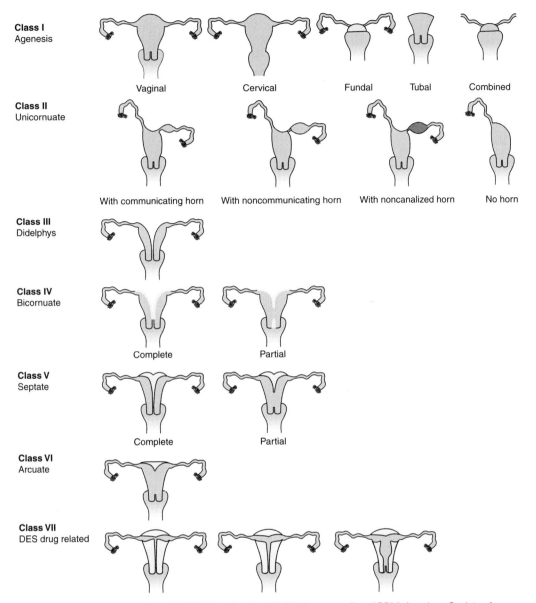

Figure 2.12 Pictorial representation of ASRM classification of Müllerian anomalies. *ASRM*, American Society of Reproductive Medicine; *DES*, diethylstilbestrol.

of uterus. Some anomalies such as bicornuate uterus can be clearly visualized (Fig. 2.13). MRI is very useful for visualizing the anomalies of uterus and vagina and is currently recommended as the investigative modality of choice (Fig. 2.14a and b). Hysteroscopy, laparoscopy or both can help in differentiating between septate and bicornuate uterus if MRI is not available (Fig. 2.15a and b). Hysterosalpingogram may be used as an initial step in evaluation when Müllerian anomaly is suspected (Fig. 2.16a–c), but MRI or endoscopy is required to confirm the diagnosis and identify the exact nature of anomaly in most cases. Urinary tract should be evaluated as well, since urinary tract anomalies are often associated with Müllerian anomalies.

Management depends on the type of anomaly. In women with vaginal agenesis, vaginal

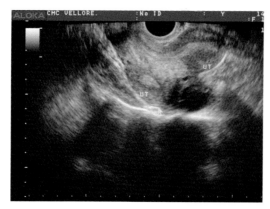

Figure 2.13 Transvaginal ultrasonography showing bicornuate uterus (class IVb). Uterine cavity is visible in both horns of the uterus. *UT*, uterine horn.

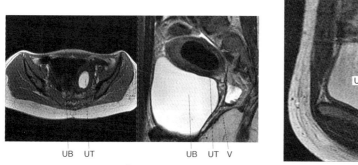

UB   UT   UB   UT   V

a.

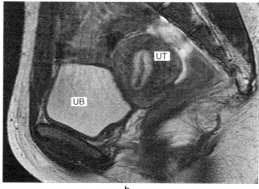

b.

Figure 2.14 Müllerian anomalies as seen on magnetic resonance imaging. a. Unicornuate uterus with haematometra (class IId). Coronal section is T1-weighted image showing uterine horn (*UT*) and bladder (*UB*). Sagittal section is a T2-weighted image and shows noncanalized vagina (*V*), unicornuate uterus with haematometra (*UT*) and bladder (*UB*). b. Sagittal section showing uterus with haematometra (*UT*) and agenesis of cervix and vagina (class Ia). Urinary bladder (*UB*) is seen anteriorly.

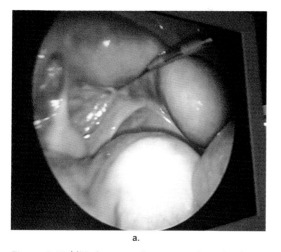

a.

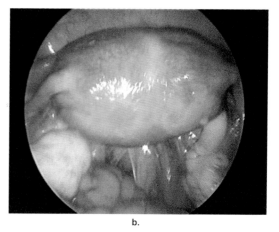

b.

Figure 2.15 Müllerian anomalies as seen through a laparoscope. a. Bicornuate uterus. Both the uterine horns are visible. b. Septate uterus. Uterus with broad fundus and a sagittal line indicating the septum is seen.

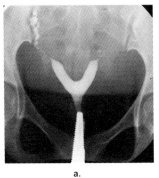 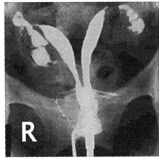 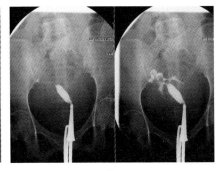

a.   b.   c.

Figure 2.16 Müllerian anomalies seen on hysterosalpingography. a. Bicornuate uterus—Partial (class IVb). b. Bicornuate uterus—Complete (class IVa). c. Unicornuate uterus (class IId).

reconstruction is performed. Rudimentary horn with signs of obstruction should be excised. Uterine septum can be excised hysteroscopically. Strassman metroplasty consists of wedge resection of the septum and reconstruction of the uterus and may be indicated in women with bicornuate uterus. Surgical procedures for various anomalies are listed in Box 2.13.

Counselling regarding sexual function, reproductive capability, obstetric and other complications is an important aspect of managing women with developmental anomalies of the genital tract. Appropriate treatment should be undertaken at the right time, not too early or too late. Many women with appropriate treatment can lead normal or near-normal lives.

Box 2.13 Surgical management of Müllerian anomalies

- Class I
  - Vaginal reconstruction
- Class II
  - Excision of rudimentary horn
- Class III
  - Occasionally metroplasty
- Class IV
  - Strassman metroplasty
- Class V
  - Hysteroscopic septal resection
- Class VI
  - No surgery required
- Class VII
  - Depends on anomaly
  - May not require surgery

Key points

- The sex chromosomes determine the development of gonads. Two X chromosomes are essential for optimal development of ovary.

- The primordial germ cells migrate from the hindgut into the gonadal ridge and form the oocytes.

- Ovary produces oestrogen and testes produce testosterone and anti-Müllerian hormone.

- The Wolffian ducts regress and the Müllerian ducts develop into uterus and tubes.

- The vagina is formed by canalization of Müllerian tubercle and sinovaginal bulbs.

- The cloaca is divided by urorectal septum into rectum and urogenital sinus. The urinary bladder develops from the urogenital sinus.

- External genitalia develop from genital folds, genital swellings and genital tubercle.

- The hymen is formed at the junction of the sinovaginal bulbs with the urogenital sinus.

- Various abnormalities of the genital tract develop due to the presence or absence of androgens and anti-Müllerian hormone.

- Developmental anomalies of the reproductive tract are broadly classified into ambiguous genitalia, developmental disorders of the vagina and developmental disorders of the uterus and cervix.

- Ambiguous genitalia may be due to female pseudohermaphroditism, male pseudohermaphroditism or true hermaphroditism.

(Continued)

Key points *(Continued)*

- Y chromosome–bearing gonads, if not descended, are susceptible to the development of malignancy and must be removed. Surgical correction can wait till puberty in most girls.
- Vaginal anomalies and Müllerian anomalies are best evaluated by magnetic resonance imaging.

- Surgical correction depends on the nature of the anomaly.
- Imperforate hymen leading to haematocolpos is the most common anomaly encountered and is managed by cruciate incision.

Self-assessment

Case-based questions

Case 1

A 15-year-old girl is brought with a history of not having attained menarche and of cyclic abdominal pain.

1. How will you evaluate clinically?
2. What investigations will you order?
3. If a haematocolpos with haematometra is diagnosed, how will you proceed?
4. If you find a bluish membrane above the introitus, what is your diagnosis and how will you manage?

Case 2

A 26-year-old lady presents with a history of four miscarriages at 16–18 weeks' gestation. Pelvic examination reveals a vertical septum in the vagina.

1. How will you evaluate the patient further?
2. Evaluation reveals a bicornuate uterus with septate vagina. According to ASRM classification, how will you classify this anomaly?
3. How will you manage?

Answers

Case 1

1. General examination—Breast development, axillary and pubic hair, external genitalia, per abdominal and per rectal examination.

2. Pelvic ultrasonography and renal ultrasonography.
3. Examination under anaesthesia.
4. Cruciate incision on the hymenal membrane and drainage of haematocolpos and haematometra.

Case 2

1. Ultrasonography of pelvis and renal system, hysterosalpingography.
2. ASRM class IV, complete or partial.
3. Strassman metroplasty with excision of vaginal septum.

Long-answer questions

1. Describe the embryological development of the uterus and vagina.
2. Discuss the classification of Müllerian anomalies. What are the obstetric complications associated with Müllerian anomalies?

Short-answer questions

1. Imperforate hymen
2. Bicornuate uterus
3. Developmental anomalies of the vagina
4. ASRM classification of Müllerian anomalies
5. Evaluation of uterovaginal anomalies

3

Female Reproductive Physiology

Case scenario

Miss GK, 28, presented with a history of scanty menstruation for 3 years. Further questioning revealed that her menarche was at 14 years of age, and menstrual cycles were regular for 5 years after menarche, but had become progressively infrequent. For the past 3 years she had no spontaneous menstruation, only withdrawal bleeding after administration of hormones. Evaluation at a local hospital revealed grossly elevated serum follicle-stimulating hormone level and low serum oestradiol level. She was referred to our clinic for further management.

Introduction

Normal reproductive function involves a complex interaction between the hypothalamus, pituitary, ovary and uterus. Menstrual cycle is an external manifestation of this interaction. The cyclic events leading to menstruation are controlled by various hormones. An understanding of the physiology of reproduction is important for the management of menstrual irregularities, disorders of puberty, infertility and menopause.

Physiology of hypothalamic–pituitary function

Hypothalamus

The hypothalamus is located at the base of the brain just above the pituitary gland. The neuroendocrine function of the hypothalamus is the key factor in the regulation of menstrual cycle. The hypothalamus is connected to other areas of the brain including thalamus, pons and limbic system and to the pituitary gland.

- The hypothalamus secretes various releasing hormones including gonadotropin-releasing hormone (GnRH). These releasing hormones are transported to the anterior pituitary through the hypothalamohypophyseal portal system of veins.
- In addition, the hypothalamus also secretes dopamine, which is an inhibitor of prolactin. Thus, secretion of gonadotropin, thyrotropin, adrenocorticotropin and growth hormone by the pituitary gland is stimulated by the hypothalamus, but secretion of prolactin is inhibited by the hypothalamus.
- Secretion of releasing hormones by the hypothalamus is under the feedback control by the target hormones from the ovary, thyroid or adrenal gland and by neurotransmitters and impulses from higher brain centres (Box 3.1).
- Neurotransmitters play an important role in the neuroendocrine regulation of reproduction. There are several neurotransmitters, including biogenic amines, neuropeptides and excitatory and inhibitory amino acids.
- Endorphin, an endogenous opioid, is a neuropeptide that can increase prolactin and inhibit GnRH secretion and is an important mediator in hypothalamic amenorrhoea.

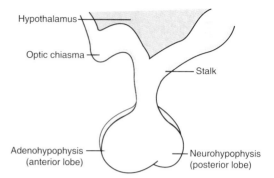

Figure 3.1 The pituitary gland. It consists of anterior and posterior lobes. The gland is connected by a stalk to the hypothalamus.

the hypothalamus. Cells that secrete gonadotropins, namely luteinizing hormone (LH) and follicle-stimulating hormone (FSH), are called **gonadotrophs**, whereas prolactin-secreting cells are called **mammotrophs**.

The posterior pituitary consists of the axons of the neurons from the supraoptic and paraventricular nuclei of the hypothalamus. Two hormones, oxytocin and arginine vasopressin, are secreted by the posterior pituitary. Precursors for these hormones are produced in the hypothalamic nuclei and transported along the axons to the posterior pituitary. The precursors are cleaved and activated during transport.

The anterior pituitary receives its blood supply entirely through a plexus of vessels from the hypothalamus through the stalk (Fig. 3.2). This is

---

Box 3.1 Hypothalamus

- Located at the base of the brain
- Connected to
  - Pituitary gland
  - Other parts of the brain
- Secretes
  - Releasing hormones
  - Dopamine
- Controlled by
  - Hormonal feedback
  - Neurotransmitters
  - Impulses from other parts of the brain

Pituitary gland

The pituitary gland has an anterior adenohypophysis developed from epidermal ectoderm and a posterior neurohypophysis developed from neuroectoderm (Fig. 3.1). The posterior pituitary is an extension of the hypothalamus. The anterior pituitary contains specialized cells that synthesize hormones when stimulated by

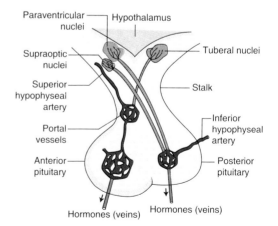

Figure 3.2 Blood supply of pituitary gland. The anterior pituitary receives its blood supply through a plexus of vessels (portal system) through the stalk. The posterior pituitary is supplied by the hypophyseal arteries. The hormones are transported into the circulation by the veins.

- Connected to the hypothalamus by a stalk
- Divided into
  - Anterior: Adenohypophysis
  - Posterior: Neurohypophysis
- Adenohypophysis
  - Secretes
    - Gonadotropins
    - Prolactin
    - Other trophic hormones
  - Supplied by portal system
- Neurohypophysis
  - Secretes
    - Oxytocin
    - Arginine vasopressin
  - Supplied by hypophyseal arteries

a portal system through which the releasing hormones from the hypothalamus to the pituitary and feedback hormones from the pituitary to the hypothalamus are transported. The posterior pituitary is supplied by hypophyseal arteries (Box 3.2).

Gonadotropin-releasing hormone

It is a peptide hormone secreted by the arcuate nucleus of the hypothalamus and controls the production of both FSH and LH. It is secreted in a pulsatile fashion (Fig. 3.3). The amplitude and frequency of the pulses vary with the time of menstrual cycle and determine the release of FSH or LH (Box 3.3). Low-amplitude, high frequency pulses stimulate FSH, while high-amplitude, low-frequency pulses stimulate LH. If GnRH is administered continuously, there

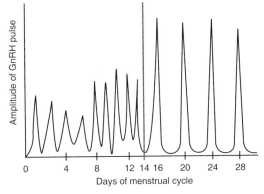

Figure 3.3 Gonadotropin-releasing hormone (GnRH) is released in a pulsatile fashion. In the follicular phase, the amplitude is low and frequency is high; in the luteal phase, the amplitude is high and frequency is low.

Box 3.3 Gonadotropin-releasing hormone

- Peptide hormone
- Secreted by the hypothalamus
- Half-life: 2–4 minutes
- Stimulates secretion of FSH and LH by pituitary
- Released in pulsatile fashion
  - Follicular phase
    - Once in 60 minutes
    - Low amplitude
  - Luteal phase
    - Once in 90–120 minutes
    - High amplitude

FSH, follicle-stimulating hormone; LH, luteinizing hormone.

is suppression of gonadotropin secretion and this phenomenon is called **downregulation**. Intermittent or pulsatile administration causes **upregulation** and release of gonadotropins.

Gonadotropins

FSH and LH are glycoprotein hormones that share a common α subunit but differ in their β subunits. The production of LH is dependent on GnRH pulse frequency and amplitude, but the production of FSH is influenced by levels of peptides—Inhibin, activin and follistatin in addition to the GnRH pulse.

Follicle-stimulating hormone

FSH is stimulated by GnRH and suppressed by oestrogen and inhibin, which are produced by the ovarian follicle and corpus luteum, respectively (Box 3.4).

Box 3.4 Follicle-stimulating hormone

- Glycoprotein
- Stimulated by GnRH production
- Suppressed by oestrogen and inhibin
- Two peak levels during menstrual cycle
  - Follicular phase (6th day)
  - Preovulatory phase (12th day)
- Functions
  - Recruitment of follicles
  - Follicular growth
  - Acts on granulosa cells
    - Increase in number
    - Increase in LH receptors
    - Increase in aromatase activity

GnRH, gonadotropin-releasing hormone; LH, luteinizing hormone.

- The level of FSH begins to rise in the latter half of the luteal phase, with the loss of function of corpus luteum. This rise in FSH is responsible for recruitment of follicles for the next menstrual cycle.
- Of the recruited follicles, one follicle has a higher number of FSH receptors and this is destined to be the dominant follicle. The developing follicles produce increasing amounts of oestrogen and inhibin B. These hormones inhibit FSH production by the gonadotrophs such that FSH levels start falling after reaching a peak on day 6 of the menstrual cycle (Fig. 3.4). In spite of the lower FSH concentration, the dominant follicle that has the maximum number of FSH receptors continues to grow, while the other follicles that have fewer FSH receptors become atretic.
- There is a second FSH peak just before ovulation, on day 12. This is in response to increased GnRH output by the hypothalamus. Concurrent with this, there is a preovulatory LH surge.
- The level of FSH decreases with ovulation and remains so till the late luteal phase due to suppression by progesterone, oestrogen and inhibin A produced by the corpus luteum. By day 22, with the failing function of corpus luteum, level of FSH begins to rise again.

Luteinizing hormone

LH production is suppressed by a moderate level of oestrogens but stimulated by high levels.

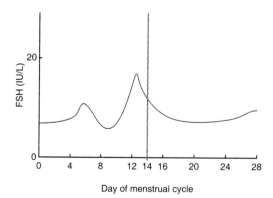

Figure 3.4 Graph showing FSH secretion during menstrual cycle. The level peaks on day 6, falls immediately thereafter and peaks again on day 12. The level decreases again and starts rising by day 22 to peak on day 6 of the next cycle. *FSH*, follicle-stimulating hormone.

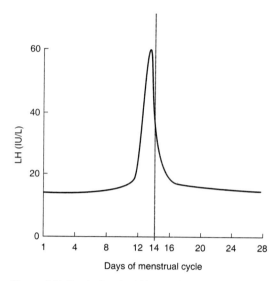

Figure 3.5 Graph showing LH secretion during menstrual cycle. LH is present at low basal levels throughout the cycle but peaks 24–36 hours before ovulation and returns to basal level immediately after ovulation. This is called the LH surge. *LH*, luteinizing hormone.

Thus, oestrogens have a dual effect on LH secretion depending on the circulating oestrogen concentration.

- It is present at low levels throughout the menstrual cycle.
- Peak secretion called LH surge occurs 24–36 hours before ovulation. This surge triggers ovulation (Fig. 3.5).
- LH also stimulates production of androgens by the theca cells. These androgens are aromatized to oestrogens by the granulosa cells (Box 3.5).

Box 3.5 Luteinizing hormone

- Glycoprotein
- Stimulated by GnRH and high level of oestrogen
- Suppressed by moderate level of oestrogen
- Present in low levels throughout menstrual cycle
- Peak level 24–36 hours before ovulation
- Functions
  - Triggers ovulation
  - Stimulates androgen production by theca cells
  - Stimulates synthesis of progesterone by corpus luteum

GnRH, gonadotropin-releasing hormone.

Prolactin

Prolactin is a polypeptide hormone primarily responsible for the synthesis of milk by the breast. The size of prolactin molecules varies, and, accordingly, they are classified into microprolactins and macroprolactins. Unlike the gonadotropins that are stimulated by the hypothalamus, prolactin is under inhibitory control of the hypothalamus (Box 3.6). Prolactin secretion is stimulated by thyrotropin-releasing hormone (TRH), vasopressin, vasoactive intestinal peptides and endogenous opioids. Hyperprolactinaemia is discussed in Chapter 19, *Secondary amenorrhoea and polycystic ovarian syndrome.*

Box 3.6 Prolactin

- Polypeptide hormone
- Controls milk secretion by breast
- Under inhibitory control of the hypothalamus
- Inhibited by dopamine
- Stimulated by
  - TRH
  - Vasopressin
  - Vasoactive intestinal peptides
  - Endogenous opioids

TRH, thyrotropin-releasing hormone.

Ovarian changes and ovulation

Normal menstrual cycle occurs once in 28 days, although cycle length from 21 to 35 days is considered to be within normal limits. The first day of menstruation is referred to as day 1 of menstrual cycle. Ovulation occurs on day 14.

Menstrual cycle consists of ovarian cycle and endometrial cycle. **Ovarian cycle** includes follicular phase during which ovarian follicles develop and luteal phase during which corpus luteum forms and later regresses. Days 1–14 of the cycle constitute the follicular phase and days 15–28 constitute the luteal phase. **Endometrial cycle** consists of proliferative phase and secretory phase, corresponding to the two phases of the ovarian cycle.

Morphology of the ovary

The ovary has an outer cortex and inner medulla. The cortex consists of specialized stroma in which the primordial follicles are embedded (Fig. 3.6). The development of the ovary is discussed in Chapter 2, *Development of the female genital tract: Normal and abnormal.* The components of the ovary develop from three cellular sources as given in Table 3.1.

Table 3.1 Development of ovarian tissues

Cellular source	Ovarian tissue
Yolk sac	Primordial germ cells
Coelomic epithelial cells	Granulosa cells
Mesenchyme of the gonadal ridge	Ovarian stroma

Primordial germ cells develop into oocytes by meiotic division. Later, they are surrounded by a layer of granulosa cells and are called primordial follicles. In the female foetus, there are about 6–7 million follicles at 20 weeks' gestation, but the majority undergo atresia and only about 1 million are present at birth. Atresia continues throughout reproductive life and only about 400

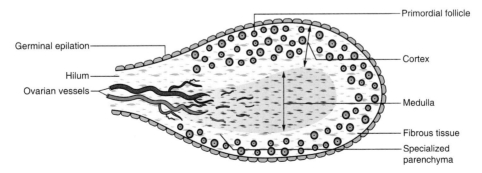

Figure 3.6 Cut section of the ovary showing cortex and medulla. The primordial follicles are located in the cortex. The ovarian vessels enter through the hilum.

primordial follicles ovulate. At menopause, ovary consists mainly of stroma with very few follicles.

Ovarian cycle

Follicular phase

During the follicular phase of the ovarian cycle, ovarian follicular development occurs. The developing follicles secrete oestrogens.

Stages of follicle development The primordial follicle develops into **primary**, **secondary** and **tertiary** follicles as shown in Box 3.7.

Box 3.7 Stages of follicular development

- Primordial follicle
  - Single layer of flattened granulosa cells
- Primary follicle
  - Cuboidal granulosa cells
  - Increase in the number of granulosa cells
  - Pseudostratification
  - Formation of zona pellucida
- Secondary follicle
  - Preantral follicle
  - Increase in the number of granulosa cells
  - Stromal differentiation into theca cells
  - Formation of theca externa and theca interna
- Tertiary follicle
  - Antral follicle
  - Collection of fluid in the follicle
  - Rapid increase in follicular size
  - Formation of cumulus oophorus
  - Formation of corona radiata
  - Formation of Graafian follicle

- The **primordial follicle** consists of the oocyte surrounded by a layer of flattened granulosa cells (Fig. 3.7).
- The granulosa cells increase in number, become cuboidal and arrange themselves in a pseudostratified layer around the oocyte to form the **primary follicle**. A hyaline membrane called **zona pellucida** is formed around the ovum.
- With increasing FSH levels during the follicular phase, the oocyte grows further, granulosa cells multiply and the stroma surrounding the follicle differentiates into theca cells. The layer adjacent to the granulosa cells is called theca interna and the outer layer is called theca externa. At this stage the follicle is known as **secondary follicle** or **preantral follicle**.
- As the FSH levels increase further, fluid collects in the follicle, between the granulosa cells, and

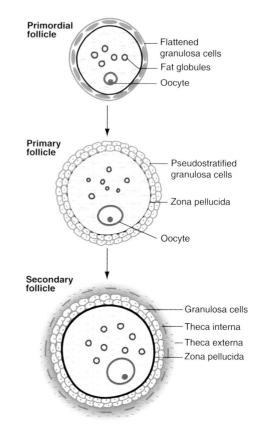

Figure 3.7 Development of secondary follicle from primordial follicle. The flattened granulosa cells become pseudostratified and the layer of theca cells appears.

this is known as the antrum. The follicle is now called the **tertiary** or **antral follicle**. Of the recruited follicles in a given cycle, only about four or five follicles attain this stage.
- FSH levels decline in the late follicular phase, but the dominant follicle continues to grow since it has more FSH receptors. The antral fluid increases, and the follicle grows to a size of more than 1 cm. The granulosa cells surrounding the oocyte are now called **corona radiata** and the cells around the antrum are called **mural granulosa cells**. The mass of cells formed by the ovum and the granulosa cells surrounding it is called **cumulus oophorus**. The follicle is now known as **Graafian follicle** (Fig. 3.8).

Luteal phase

The luteal phase of the ovarian cycle is the period that extends from the time of formation of corpus luteum to the onset of menses (or luteolysis), usually 14 days in length.

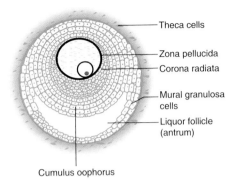

— Theca cells

— Zona pellucida
— Corona radiata

— Mural granulosa cells

— Liquor follicle (antrum)

Cumulus oophorus

Figure 3.8 The mature Graafian follicle. It has a cumulus oophorus that contains the ovum with zona pellucida and corona radiata around it. Liquor folliculi is abundant. Theca cells are seen surrounding the follicle.

Formation of corpus luteum Once the ovum is discharged, the Graafian follicle collapses. The granulosa and theca cells become yellow due to deposition of lipids and lutein pigment, and this process is called **luteinization**. The remaining shell of the Graafian follicle is converted into the corpus luteum. The corpus luteum secretes oestrogen, inhibin A and large amounts of progesterone. Neovascularization of the corpus luteum ensures entry of the secreted hormones into the circulation. High levels of progesterone, which is characteristic of the luteal phase of menstrual cycle, prepare the endometrium for nidation. The corpus luteum attains a size of about 2 cm by day 21 when the hormone production is also at its peak. If pregnancy fails to occur, the corpus luteum degenerates.

Luteolysis This refers to the degeneration of the corpus luteum, which takes place in the late luteal phase unless pregnancy occurs. The blood supply to the corpus luteum decreases, hormone production ceases, the cells become fibrotic and the resulting structure is called **corpus albicans** (Fig. 3.9). In case of pregnancy, human chorionic gonadotropin (hCG) secreted by the trophoblasts prevents luteolysis and the corpus luteum continues to function till the placenta takes over the hormone production at 10–12 weeks' gestation.

Ovulation

Ovulation is the process of release of an oocyte from the ovarian follicle. As mentioned earlier, it occurs on day 14 of the menstrual cycle. The process is triggered by the midcycle LH surge. At this stage, the first meiotic division of the oocyte is completed and the first polar body is extruded. The oocyte is now haploid. The second meiotic division takes place only after fertilization, after which the second polar body is extruded.

The LH surge also initiates an inflammatory reaction in the part of the follicle close to the ovarian cortex (Box 3.8). Prostaglandins (PGs)

Box 3.8 Ovulation

- Triggered by LH surge
- LH surge causes
  - Completion of first meiotic division
  - Extrusion of first polar body
  - Inflammatory reaction in the follicle
  - Release of PG and cytokines
  - Perforation of follicular wall
  - Ovulation
  - Pick-up of oocyte by fimbriae

LH, luteinizing hormone; *PG*, prostaglandin.

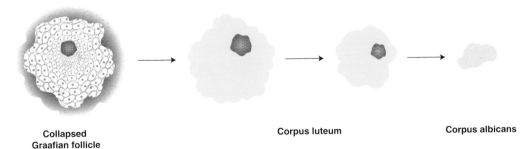

Collapsed Graafian follicle

Corpus luteum

Corpus albicans

Figure 3.9 Formation of the corpus luteum and luteolysis. After ovulation, the collapsed Graafian follicle is converted into the corpus luteum. Lipid deposition occurs and the granulosa and theca cells become yellow. Degeneration of the corpus luteum (luteolysis) takes place in the late luteal phase. The cells become fibrotic and the resulting structure is called corpus albicans.

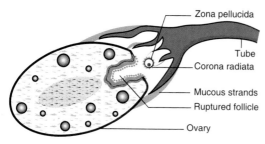

Figure 3.10 Diagrammatic representation of ovulation. The ovum is extruded through an area of weakening and lysis on the follicle close to the ovarian cortex. Mucous strands form between the fimbriae and the follicle to facilitate passage of oocyte into the tube.

and cytokines are released. These cause weakening and lysis of the wall of the follicle at this point, and the oocyte is extruded through this opening. The cytokines also have a chemotactic effect due to which the fimbriae of the fallopian tube are drawn close to the rupturing follicle. Mucous strands also form between the follicle and the fimbriae to facilitate the passage of oocyte into the fallopian tube (Fig. 3.10).

Ovarian hormones

The ovary, during menstrual cycle, secretes steroid hormones, peptides and other substances that have endocrine and local regulatory (autocrine) functions.

Steroid hormones of the ovary

The predominant steroid hormones produced by the ovary are oestrogens, progesterone and androgens. These sex steroids play a major role in preparing the endometrium for implantation and act on other organ systems in the body. **Oestrogen** is the predominant hormone produced during the follicular phase. **Progesterone** is the hormone of the luteal phase, although oestrogen is also produced during this phase. **Androgens** synthesized by the ovary are androstenedione and testosterone, which are aromatized into oestrogen but small amounts are released into the circulation.

Steroid biosynthesis

All steroid hormones are synthesized from acetate, which is converted into cholesterol. In the ovary, cholesterol is converted into pregnenolone and then the steroidogenesis proceeds along two pathways: Δ_4 and Δ_5 pathways (Fig. 3.11).

Oestrogens are formed by aromatization of androgens by the enzyme aromatase in the ovary. This enzyme is not present in the adrenal glands but present in adipose tissue in the body. Hence, in adrenal hyperplasia and adrenal tumours, excess oestrogens are not produced in the adrenal glands. In obese women, adrenal and ovarian androgens may be converted to oestrogens by the excess adipose tissue leading to a hyperoestrogenic state.

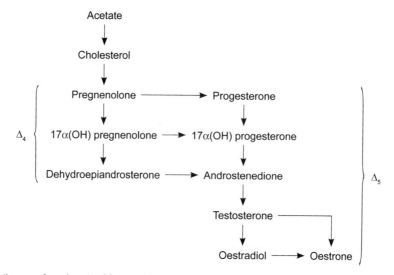

Figure 3.11 Pathways of ovarian steroidogenesis.

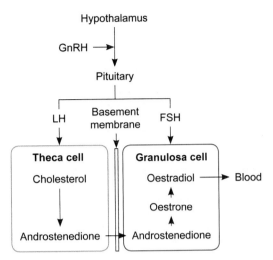

Figure 3.12 Two-cell two-gonadotropin theory. *FSH*, follicle-stimulating hormone; *GnRH*, gonadotropin-releasing hormone; *LH*, luteinizing hormone.

Two-cell two-gonadotropin theory

The synthesis of steroid hormones is compartmentalized to the two different cells of the ovary (granulosa and theca cells) and is regulated by the two gonadotropins (FSH and LH) (Fig. 3.12).

- The granulosa cells have FSH receptors and the theca cells have LH receptors.
- Theca cells have the enzymes for androgen biosynthesis from cholesterol, whereas the granulosa cells lack these. Granulosa cells have aromatase, which is required for conversion of androgens to oestrogens.
- In response to LH stimulation, theca cells synthesize androgens (androstenedione and testosterone). The androgen is transported to granulosa cells.
- Under the effect of FSH, aromatization of androgens to oestrogens takes place in the granulosa cells (Table 3.2).

Table 3.2 **Steroid hormone synthesis by granulosa and theca cells**

Granulosa cells	Theca cells
Have FSH receptors	Have LH receptors
Have aromatase	Do not have aromatase
Cannot synthesize androgens	Can synthesize androgens

FSH, follicle-stimulating hormone; *LH*, luteinizing hormone.

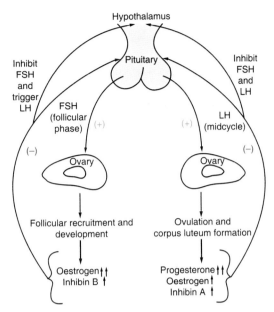

Figure 3.13 Sequence of hormonal changes during menstrual cycle. FSH induces follicular recruitment and secretion of oestrogen and inhibin B by the granulosa cells. High levels of oestrogen inhibit FSH and trigger LH surge. Ovulation follows the LH surge and is followed by secretion of progesterone and inhibin A by the ovary. These inhibit secretion of FSH and LH. *FSH*, follicle-stimulating hormone; *LH*, luteinizing hormone.

Sequence of hormonal changes during menstrual cycle

This is pictorially represented in Fig. 3.13.

- Under the effect of tonic secretion of LH throughout the follicular phase of the cycle, the theca cells synthesize androstenedione.
- This is transferred to granulosa cells where FSH-stimulated aromatase action induces oestrogen secretion.
- This exerts a negative feedback on the pituitary and hypothalamus, thereby reducing FSH levels. The selection of dominant follicle has already occurred before decline in FSH levels. This follicle continues to grow and secretes oestrogen to cause the preovulatory oestrogen peak.
- High levels of oestrogen trigger LH surge.
- LH surge triggers ovulation.
- Theca cells of the corpus luteum secrete progesterone, leading to peak levels during the postovulatory phase.

- The luteinized granulosa cells of the corpus luteum secrete oestrogens, leading to the second oestrogen peak.
- Oestrogen and progesterone levels decrease with the demise of the corpus luteum in the late luteal phase.
- Menstruation occurs.

Oestrogens

Oestrogens are steroid hormones. There are three main oestrogens: oestradiol, oestrone and oestriol. Oestradiol is the main form of oestrogen secreted by the ovary. Oestrone is predominantly produced in the adipose tissue by conversion of androstenedione and only small amounts of oestrone are produced by the ovary. Oestradiol and oestrone are found in the ratio of 1:2. Oestradiol and oestrone are converted to oestriol by the liver (Box 3.9). Level of oestriol is high in pregnancy due to production by foetal liver. Oestrogens are bound to albumin and sex hormone–binding globulin (SHBG) in the circulation and only the unbound fraction is biologically active. Level of oestradiol is low during menstruation but starts rising from the 7th or 8th day to reach a peak on the 12th day. The level falls briefly after ovulation and starts rising again 24 hours later due to production from the corpus luteum and there is a second peak during the luteal phase (Fig. 3.14).

The rise in oestrogen levels during the follicular phase is used for monitoring follicular growth and timing of administration of hCG during ovulation induction.

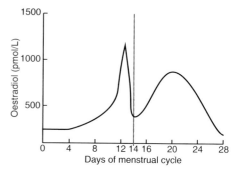

Figure 3.14 Oestrogen levels during menstrual cycle. Level of oestrogen begins to rise from day 7 or 8 and reaches a peak on day 12. The level falls briefly after ovulation but begins to rise again to reach a second peak during the luteal phase.

Progesterone

Progesterone is also a steroid hormone synthesized by the corpus luteum and adrenal glands. It is produced predominantly in the luteal phase, and levels are therefore low in anovulatory cycles (Box 3.10).

Box 3.10 Progesterone

- Steroid hormone
- Site of production
  - Ovary
  - Adrenal glands
- Synthesized by theca cells
- High levels in luteal phase
- Low levels indicate anovulation
- Prepares endometrium for implantation

Level of progesterone is very low in follicular phase, but starts rising immediately after ovulation, to reach peak levels by day 22. Thereafter, the levels decline with failing corpus luteum function (Fig. 3.15). If pregnancy occurs, progesterone levels remain high. Progesterone is also bound to albumin and globulin in the circulation.

Measurement of midluteal progesterone is used as a test for ovulation.

The normal levels of oestrogen and progesterone during menstrual cycle are shown in Table 3.3.

Effects of oestrogens and progesterone on target tissues

Oestrogens and progesterone act by binding to receptors on the cells in the target tissues.

Box 3.9 Oestrogens

- Steroid hormones
- Oestradiol, oestrone and oestriol
- Site of production
  - Ovary
    - Mainly oestradiol
    - Small amount of oestrone
  - Adipose tissue
    - Oestrone
  - Foetal liver
    - Oestriol
- Synthesized by granulosa cells
- Predominant hormone of follicular phase
- Inhibit FSH
- Trigger LH surge

FSH, follicle-stimulating hormone; *LH*, luteinizing hormone.

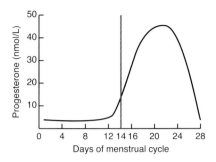

Figure 3.15 Progesterone levels during menstrual cycle. Progesterone level is low during follicular phase but starts rising immediately after ovulation and reaches a peak on day 22. The level falls after that.

Table 3.3 Normal levels of oestrogen and progesterone during menstrual cycle

	Follicular phase	Ovulation phase	Luteal phase
Oestradiol (pg/mL)	30–200	200–600	30–200
Progesterone (ng/mL)	0.06–3		4.5–20

There are two types of oestrogen receptors (ER): ERα and ERβ. These are expressed to varying extents in various tissues. ERα is more abundantly expressed in the female reproductive tract, breast, hypothalamus and vascular endothelium. ERβ is expressed more in ovary and bone. Many tissues express both the receptors. Apart from their action on the reproductive tract (Table 3.4), they act on different organ systems in the body (Table 3.5). Oestrogens are essential for the development of secondary sexual characteristics at puberty.

Table 3.4 Action of oestrogens and progesterone on the reproductive system

	Oestrogen	Progesterone
Uterus	Myohyperplasia	• Myohyperplasia • Increased contractility
Endometrium	• Growth and vascularization • Proliferative change	• Glandular secretion • Secretory endometrium
Cervix	• Increases secretions • Mucus thin, elastic	• Reduces secretions • Mucus thick, nonelastic
Vagina	• Superficial keratinized cells • Deposition of glycogen	Intermediate cells
Breasts	Growth of stroma and duct	Growth of alveoli

Table 3.5 Action of oestrogens and progesterone on other organ systems

System	Oestrogen	Progesterone
Cardiovascular	• Vasodilatation • Water and salt retention	Water and salt retention
Hypothalamus/pituitary	• Inhibits FSH • Triggers LH surge	Modulates GnRH pulse amplitude and frequency
Skeletal	• Increases osteoblastic activity • Reduces osteoclastic activity • Prevents osteoporosis • Fusion of epiphysis	Increases osteoblastic activity
Carbohydrate metabolism	Slight decrease in fasting glucose	Decreases glucose tolerance
Lipid metabolism	• Increases triglycerides • Increases HDL • Decreases LDL, triglycerides	• Slight decrease in HDL • Decreases LDL
Coagulation	• Increases factors II,VII, IX, X, XII • Decreases proteins C and S, antithrombin III	
Neurological	Beneficial effect on cognition	• Thermogenic action • Causes depression
Pregnancy		Maintenance of pregnancy

FSH, follicle-stimulating hormone; *GnRH*, gonadotropin-releasing hormone; *HDL*, high-density lipoprotein; *LDL*, low-density lipoprotein; *LH*, luteinizing hormone.

Regulation of ovarian function by growth factors

Apart from the pituitary gonadotropins, there are other substances/growth factors that play a major role in the control of ovarian function (Box 3.11).

Insulin-like growth factors (IGF)

These are of two types: IGF-I and IGF-II. They bind to IGF receptors on the granulosa and theca cells and stimulate gonadotropin-induced steroidogenesis. **Transforming growth factors** (TGF) and **epidermal growth factor** (EGF) bind to the respective receptors and regulate granulosa cell proliferation and differentiation. **Interleukin-1** is a cytokine with antigonadotropic activity and controls luteinization of granulosa cells.

Inhibin, activin and follistatin

These peptides play a role in regulation of ovarian FSH secretion and ovarian steroidogenesis. Two types of inhibin, **inhibin A** and **inhibin B**, are produced by the granulosa cells. Inhibin B is produced predominantly in the follicular phase and inhibin A in the luteal phase. They inhibit FSH release and stimulate local androgen production in the ovary. **Activin** opposes inhibin action, stimulates FSH release and increases aromatase activity and progesterone production. **Follistatin** binds activin and, therefore, reduces activin-induced increase in FSH release (Box 3.12).

Endometrial changes in menstrual cycle

The endometrium is divided into superficial functional layer and deep basal layer as shown in Box 3.13. The functional layer is very responsive to oestrogens and progesterone and undergoes cyclic changes according to the phase of the menstrual cycle. The basal layer does not undergo changes and serves as a source for endometrial regeneration. The endometrial cycle is divided into phases: **proliferative phase** (corresponding to the follicular phase of the ovarian cycle) and **secretory phase** (corresponding to the luteal phase of the ovarian cycle).

Proliferative phase

Proliferative phase extends from day 1 to 14 in a 28-day cycle. The duration of follicular phase may vary depending on the cycle length.

During menstruation the entire functional layer is shed. Under the influence of oestrogens, regeneration of the lining cells, glands and stroma takes place and proceeds rapidly. There is a high level of mitotic activity. The glands become elongated and the lining cells are low columnar. The endometrium is only 1–2 mm thick. By late

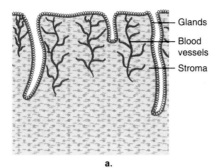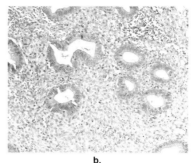

Glands
Blood vessels
Stroma

a.   b.

Figure 3.16 Endometrial changes in proliferative phase. a. A diagrammatic representation. The glands are elongated and lined by columnar cells. Blood vessels are prominent with dilated capillaries. b. Image showing histology of proliferative endometrium under magnification. The glands are lined by columnar cells.

follicular phase, the lining cells undergo pseudostratification and the glands appear tubular and dilated (Box 3.14; Fig. 3.16a and b).

Box 3.14 **Proliferative phase**

- Day 1 to ovulation (day 14)
- Effect of oestrogen
- Endometrial changes
  - Glands: Elongation and dilatation
  - Lining cells: Columnar and pseudostratified
  - Thickness: Increases from 1 to 12 mm

The blood vessels become prominent and capillaries are dilated. The increase in vascularity sometimes leads to oozing of blood into the cavity during ovulation, causing midcycle spotting. Stroma is dense and compact and the endometrial thickness increases to 12 mm just before ovulation.

Secretory phase

Secretory phase extends from day 15 to 28 in a 28-day cycle. The duration of secretory phase is constant and does not vary even if the cycle length varies.

Progesterone acts on the endometrium only if it is already primed with oestrogen. Secretory changes take place under the influence of progesterone (Box 3.15). This is the period of preparation for implantation of the embryo. The first sign of secretory change is the appearance of secretions in the form of subnuclear vacuoles in the cells lining the glands. This is considered to be an indication of ovulation. With further stimulation by progesterone, the vacuoles move towards the lumen and the secretions are emptied into

Box 3.15 **Secretory phase**

- Days: 15–28
- Effect of progesterone
- Endometrial changes
  - Glands: Secretion
  - Stroma
    - Oedema
    - Leucocytic infiltration
  - Arteries: Elongated and coiled

the glands (Fig. 3.17a and b). The glands become tortuous and cork-screw shaped, and the stroma becomes oedematous. The spiral arteries elongate and have a coiled appearance. By day 21 of the cycle, the division of compact and spongy layer becomes distinct. The stroma is infiltrated with leucocytes towards the late secretory phase. The glands become saw-toothed. This is followed by menstruation.

Endometrial dating

The histological changes in the endometrium correlate with the phase and day of the menstrual cycle. Endometrial biopsy and histological evaluation has been used for 'dating' the endometrium in women with infertility and diagnosis of luteal phase defect.

Menstruation

With the demise of the corpus luteum, the levels of oestrogen and progesterone fall. There is local production of $PGF_{2\alpha}$ causing vasospasm of the spiral arteries, endometrial ischaemia and tissue destruction. The endometrium breaks down and the functional layer is shed and expelled by

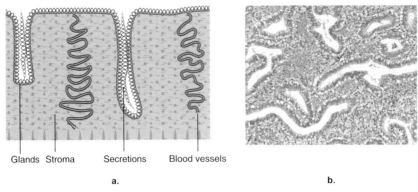

Glands Stroma   Secretions   Blood vessels

a.   b.

Figure 3.17 Endometrial changes during secretory phase. a. A diagrammatic representation. The glands are tortuous and cork-screw shaped. The spiral arteries are coiled. The stroma is infiltrated with leucocytes. b. Image showing histology of early secretory endometrium under magnification. The cells show subnuclear vacuolation.

myometrial contraction. The degeneration and shedding proceed rapidly during the first 2 days. The vasoconstriction and myometrial contractility are regulated by PGs $F_{2\alpha}$, E_2, I_2 and thromboxane. $PGF_{2\alpha}$ and thromboxane are vasoconstrictors and PGE_2 and PGI_2 are vasodilators. A fine balance is maintained in the production of these PGs so that normal menstrual bleeding occurs but is controlled. Endometrial degradation, haemorrhage, uterine contraction and vasoconstriction are regulated by cytokines, growth factors, platelet plugs, fibrinolytics, matrix metalloproteinases, endothelins and several other substances. Imbalance or abnormality in the production of PGs and other substances leads to abnormal uterine bleeding.

The composite events of hormone production by the pituitary and ovary, and ovarian and endometrial changes in menstrual cycle are depicted in Fig. 3.18.

Implantation

Fertilization takes place in the fallopian tube. The fertilized oocyte enters the uterus on day 3, at the morula stage. Implantation takes place on day 4, at the blastocyst stage. The trophectoderm of the blastocyst adheres to the prepared endometrium. This is facilitated by endometrial integrins, adhesion proteins, osteopontin and several other substances produced by the endometrium. Continued progesterone secretion by the corpus luteum plays a major role in the production of these regulators.

Decidualization

Decidua is the specialized endometrium of pregnancy. This transformation is dependent on oestrogens, progesterone and stimuli by the blastocyst. Secretory changes in the endometrium persist and become more pronounced. The glands become crenated. The lining cells are irregular. The characteristic decidual cells appear in the stroma. These are stromal cells that enlarge, become polygonal or stellate with vesicular nuclei and clear cytoplasm, and are surrounded by lymphocytes. The decidua produces cytokines and growth factors to promote placental growth.

Changes in cervical mucus

As the oestrogen levels rise during the follicular phase, the cervical mucus becomes thin and elastic, and can be stretched to 8–10 cm (Fig. 3.19). This phenomenon is called **spinnbarkeit**. The quantity of mucus also increases close to ovulation. This copious flow of thin cervical mucus at ovulation is known as **ovulation cascade**. The thin mucus facilitates sperm movement through the mucus. The sodium chloride in the mucus crystallizes in a characteristic fernlike pattern when allowed to dry on a glass slide (Fig. 3.20). After ovulation, when progesterone levels rise, the mucus becomes thick and nonelastic and the ferning disappears.

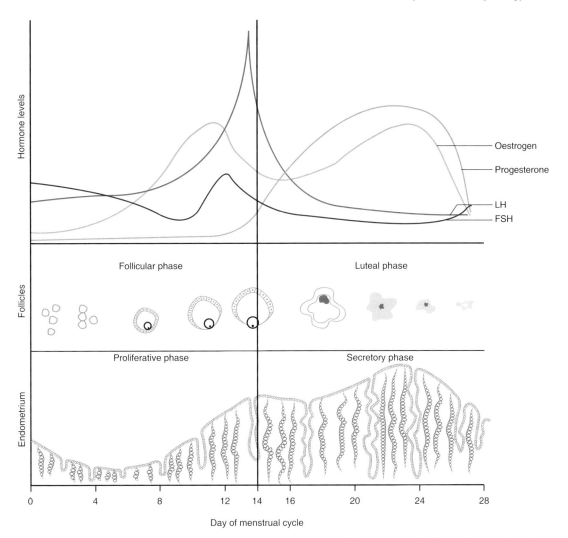

Figure 3.18 The synchronization between secretion of various hormones during menstrual cycle, and the associated ovarian and endometrial changes. *FSH*, follicle-stimulating hormone; *LH*, luteinizing hormone.

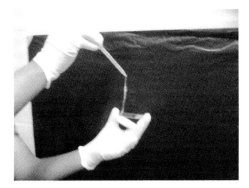

Figure 3.19 Spinnbarkeit. The cervical mucus is placed on a slide, covered with a coverslip and drawn into a thread.

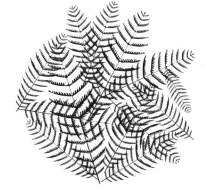

Figure 3.20 Fern pattern of cervical mucus in the preovulatory phase.

Key points

- Reproductive physiology is controlled by various hormones and is dependent on normal functioning of the hypothalamic–pituitary–ovarian axis.

- The hypothalamus controls pituitary function through secretion of gonadotropin-releasing hormone (GnRH) and neurotransmitters such as dopamine. The secretion of these is controlled by hormonal feedback and impulses from other parts of the brain.

- The anterior pituitary secretes gonadotropins and prolactin, whereas the posterior pituitary secretes oxytocin and vasopressin. Secretion of these hormones is controlled by hormonal feedback and the hypothalamus.

- Normal menstrual cycle occurs once in 28 days, although cycle length from 21 to 35 days is considered normal. Menstrual cycle consists of ovarian and endometrial cycles.

- Ovarian cycle is divided into follicular phase (days 1–14) and luteal phase (days 15–28). Oestrogen secretion starts in the follicular phase and continues in the luteal phase, but progesterone is produced only in the luteal phase.

- Follicle-stimulating hormone (FSH) levels start rising by later luteal phase. This is responsible for recruitment of follicles, follicular growth and increase in luteinizing hormone (LH) receptors in the granulosa cells. The level decreases by day 6 of the cycle and peaks again before ovulation.

- Recruitment of the follicles takes place during the luteal phase of the previous cycle. Of the recruited follicles, four or five develop into tertiary follicles and one dominant follicle develops into Graafian follicle. The granulosa cells secrete oestrogen.

- Ovulation is triggered by LH surge.

- The corpus luteum secretes large amounts of progesterone in addition to oestrogen and inhibin A.

- There are three main types of oestrogens, namely oestradiol, oestrone and oestriol. Oestradiol is the main form of oestrogen secreted by the ovary. It is bound to albumin and sex hormone–binding globulin (SHBG) and only the free form is biologically active.

- Oestrogen triggers LH surge and inhibits FSH secretion.

- Progesterone prepares the endometrium for implantation.

- Oestrogen and progesterone have physiological actions on the reproductive organs, other systems and metabolism.

- The corpus luteum degenerates by the late luteal phase and hormone production ceases. This leads to a fall in the level of ovarian hormones and menstruation.

- Endometrial cycle is divided into proliferative phase and secretory phase. The superficial functional layer of the endometrium undergoes proliferative changes under the influence of oestrogen. Secretory changes occur after ovulation and the endometrium is prepared for implantation.

- The functional layer is shed during menstruation.

- The fertilized oocyte enters the uterine cavity on day 3 and implantation takes place on day 4, at the blastocyst stage.

- The endometrium undergoes decidualization under the influence of oestrogens and progesterone.

- The cervical mucus also undergoes changes to facilitate sperm movement during the time of ovulation.

Self-assessment

Case-based questions

Case 1

Miss GF, 28, presented with a history of scanty menstruation for 3 years. Further questioning revealed that her menarche was at 14 years of age, and menstrual cycles were regular for 5 years after menarche, but had become progressively infrequent. For the past 3 years she had no spontaneous menstruation, only withdrawal bleeding after administration of hormones.

1. What hormonal assays will you order?
2. If serum FSH and LH are low, what is the diagnosis?
3. If serum FSH is grossly elevated, what is the diagnosis?

Case 2

Mrs KC, 25, married for 3 years, came with an inability to conceive. Her husband was a small-time farmer, and they lived in a village nearby. She wanted to know about fertile period and advice on how to detect ovulation.

1. What is the fertile period?
2. How can she determine time of ovulation?
3. Are there more accurate methods of prediction of ovulation?

Answers

Case 1

1. Serum FSH and LH, prolactin and thyroid-stimulating hormone.

2. Probable hypothalamic dysfunction.
3. Probable premature ovarian insufficiency.

Case 2

1. It is usually the day of ovulation and a few days preceding and after ovulation.
2. Testing the cervical mucus for spinnbarkeit and checking basal body temperature to look for rise in temperature at ovulation are methods that can be used in a village setting.
3. Urinary LH measurement kits and measurement of serum LH to look for LH surge are more sensitive but expensive methods.

Long-answer question

1. Describe the physiology of menstrual cycle.

Short-answer questions

1. Follicle-stimulating hormone
2. Graafian follicle
3. Hormonal changes in menstruation
4. Physiological actions of oestrogens
5. Physiological actions of progesterone
6. Endometrial changes in menstrual cycle
7. Diagnosis of ovulation

Gynaecological Evaluation

Box 4.4 History of chief complaints

- Duration
- Associated symptoms
- Related symptoms
- General symptoms
  - Recent weight loss/weight gain
  - Fever/fatigue
  - Appetite
- Bladder and bowel symptoms

can help in making a diagnosis of ovulatory or anovulatory bleeding and conditions such as myomas, endometriosis or cervical cancer.

Often, a list of differential diagnosis can be arrived at after a detailed history regarding the presenting illness. General symptoms such as weight gain, weight loss, fever and appetite need attention. Loss of appetite, weight and fever in a young woman indicate infection, but in an older woman, malignancy must be considered. Weight gain is common in polycystic ovarian syndrome (PCOS) and other obesity-related anovulatory disorders.

Since gynaecological diseases can affect the urinary system and bowel, specific symptoms related to these organs should be asked for. Urinary symptoms are common in pelvic organ prolapse, myomas and pelvic masses. Constipation may be related to enterocele, but diarrhoea and tenesmus are usually seen in pelvic abscess.

Menstrual history

Age at menarche and characteristics of the menstrual cycles such as duration, regularity, volume and frequency of menstrual cycles should be noted. Early menarche and late menopause are risk factors for endometrial cancer. Characteristics of normal menstrual cycle are listed in Box 4.5.

Box 4.5 Normal menstruation

- Cycle length: 28 days (21–35 days)
- Mean menstrual blood loss: 30–40 mL
- Duration: 2–8 days

The volume of flow is assessed by the number of pads or tampons used, whether the pads are fully or partially soaked, and the presence of clots. Pictorial blood loss assessment chart

Pads		1	2	3	4	5	6	7	8
(light)	× 1	//	/	/					
(moderate)	× 5	////	//	//					
(heavy)	× 20	///	/						
		87	31	11					
Tampons									
(light)	× 1	/							
(moderate)	× 5	//							
(heavy)	× 15	//// /							
Daily points:		101							

Total score =

Figure 4.1 Pictorial blood loss assessment chart. It is used to assess the volume of menstrual blood loss. The chart has diagrams of pads and tampons. Pads that are lightly, moderately and heavily soaked are given scores of 1, 5 and 20, respectively, and tampons that are lightly, moderately and heavily soaked are given the scores of 1, 5 and 15, respectively. The number of pads/tampons used each day is marked and the total score calculated.

(Fig. 4.1) may also be used. The chart consists of diagrams representing pads and tampons that are soaked lightly, moderately or heavily. The score is calculated by multiplying the number of pads by a factor of 1, 5 or 20 for lightly, moderately and heavily soaked pads, respectively, and a factor of 1, 5 and 15 for lightly, moderately and heavily soaked tampons, respectively. Clots are assigned a score of 1 for the size of 1 penny, 5 for 50 pennies and 5 for flooding. A total score of 100 or more indicates excessive bleeding. Menstrual blood is normally fluid in nature since the clots are lysed by fibrinolytics. The presence of clots indicates larger-than-normal volume of blood.

Midcycle pain and/or spotting and spasmodic dysmenorrhoea indicate ovulatory cycles. Date of last menstrual period (LMP) is essential to rule out pregnancy. Radiological procedures and teratogenic drugs should be avoided in the postovulatory phase of the menstrual cycle. Previous menstrual period (PMP) allows calculation of menstrual interval.

Gynaecological history

Past history of gynaecological problems is important (Box 4.6). Many gynaecological conditions such as myomas, ovarian cysts, endometriosis and pelvic infections recur. In some women, the present problem may be the result of a previous gynaecological condition. Chronic pelvic or abdominal pain may result from pelvic inflammatory disease or previous pelvic surgeries. History of lower genital tract infections may be indicative of sexually transmitted diseases. Previous gynaecological surgeries, major and minor, abdominal and vaginal, may give a clue to the diagnosis. The operative notes should be reviewed.

Box 4.6 Past gynaecological history

- Vaginal infections
- Pelvic pain
- History of known recurrent conditions
  - Myomas
  - Endometriosis
  - Pelvic organ prolapse
  - Benign ovarian tumours
- Prior gynaecological surgery

Obstetric history

Age at marriage is important when dealing with patients with infertility. Evaluation of infertility may be required earlier in older women and those who are married for long duration.

Parity, number of miscarriages, terminations of pregnancies, and molar and ectopic pregnancies should be noted (Box 4.7). Women with endometriosis and endometrial carcinomas are usually nulliparous, but women with cervical cancer, adenomyosis, pelvic organ prolapse and stress urinary incontinence are often multiparous.

Box 4.7 Obstetric history and gynaecological illness

- Nulliparity
  - Endometriosis
  - Endometrial cancer
  - Breast cancer
- Multiparity
  - Adenomyosis
  - Cervical cancer
  - Ovarian cancer
  - Pelvic organ prolapse
- Recent delivery/miscarriage
  - Sepsis
  - Retained products of conception
- Molar pregnancy
  - Gestational trophoblastic neoplasia

Interval between pregnancies, type of delivery and duration of second stage may bear a causal relationship to pelvic organ prolapse.

History of bleeding following recent miscarriage suggests postabortal complications such as infection or retained products of conception. Fever or foul-smelling discharge suggests post-delivery/postabortal sepsis.

Details of contraception

Abnormal uterine bleeding may be related to intrauterine contraceptive device (IUCD; Box 4.8). Use of combined pill for 5 years or more protects against ovarian and endometrial cancer. Tubal sterilization may increase the risk of ovarian cancer. Levonorgestrel intrauterine system (LNG-IUS) causes amenorrhoea. Unless specifically asked for, women may not discuss the details of contraception. Depot medroxyprogesterone (Depo-Provera) injections can be associated with irregular bleeding or amenorrhoea. History of tubal ligation should also be obtained.

Box 4.8 Contraceptive history

- Combined OC pills
  - Protect against ovarian cancer
  - Protect against endometrial cancer
  - May increase the risk of cervical cancer
- IUCD
  - Causes heavy menstrual bleeding and dysmenorrhoea
- LNG-IUS
  - Causes amenorrhoea
- Depo-Provera
  - Causes amenorrhoea, irregular bleeding
- Tubal ligation
  - Protects against endometrial cancer

IUCD, intrauterine contraceptive device; LNG-IUS, levonorgestrel intrauterine system; OC, oral contraceptive.

Sexual history

Women are often hesitant to talk about sexual problems such as vaginismus, lack of orgasm, dyspareunia and vaginal dryness (Box 4.9). They may complain of nonspecific symptoms till they are asked specifically about the sexual symptoms. Vaginismus may be due to tight introitus or the result of psychological factors. Deep dyspareunia is usually a symptom of deep infiltrating endometriosis. Superficial dyspareunia is usually due to local painful lesions. Vaginal dryness is a problem of postmenopausal oestrogen deficiency.

Box 4.9 Sexual history

- Vaginismus
- Sexual satisfaction/orgasm
- Lax introitus
- Dyspareunia
  - Superficial
  - Deep
- Vaginal dryness

Menopausal history

In perimenopausal or postmenopausal women, it is important to know the age at menopause and symptoms of menopause such as hot flushes, mood swings, urogenital symptoms and sleep disturbances (Box 4.10). Bleeding in a postmenopausal woman may be the result of hormone therapy. Details regarding lifestyle, dietary calcium intake, duration of exposure to sunlight, family history of osteoporosis and ischaemic heart disease are also mandatory for ordering appropriate investigations and making decisions regarding treatment.

Box 4.10 Menopausal history

- Age at menopause
- Menopausal symptoms
  - Vasomotor symptoms
  - Mood changes
  - Dyspareunia/vaginal dryness
  - Urinary symptoms
- Family history
  - Osteoporosis
  - Coronary heart disease/diabetes/hypertension
- Calcium supplements
- Dietary calcium
- Lifestyle and sunlight exposure

History of medications

The patient may be on medications for medical illnesses, oestrogen replacement therapy or drugs for the treatment of other gynaecological problems (Box 4.11). Some drugs have interactions with anaesthetic agents. Drugs used to treat common neurological disorders such as epilepsy can interfere with the action of sex

---

Box 4.11 History of medications

- Medications for
  - Diabetes
  - Hypertension
  - Cardiac disease
  - Thyroid dysfunction
  - Anticoagulants
  - Other medical disorders
- Oestrogen therapy
- Progestogens
- Combined OC pills
- NSAIDs and corticosteroids
- Medication for other gynaecological conditions
- Drugs that can cause amenorrhoea/galactorrhoea

NSAID, nonsteroidal anti-inflammatory drug; *OC*, oral contraceptive.

---

steroid hormones. Drugs such as oestrogens and aspirin must be discontinued prior to hospitalization for surgery, and oral anticoagulants must be changed to heparin. Failure of prior medical treatment of the patient's problem necessitates increase in dose or changeover to other drugs or other modalities of treatment.

History of smoking, alcohol and substance abuse

Information regarding smoking, alcohol use and substance abuse should be asked for.

Past medical and surgical history

Many medical disorders are associated with increased risk of gynaecological problems. Previous surgery may have a bearing on diagnosis and management of the present problem.

- Medical disorders such as diabetes, hypertension, obesity and cardiovascular disease are common in older women.
- Obese, diabetic women are at an increased risk for endometrial cancer. In young girls with obesity and irregular periods, PCOS and metabolic syndrome must be ruled out.
- Women with thyroid dysfunction may present with menstrual disorders, weight gain and/or infertility.
- Hormones must be prescribed with caution in women with diabetes, hypertension and obesity.

- Adolescents with coagulation disorders and thrombocytopaenia can present with abnormal uterine bleeding.
- Gastrointestinal conditions such as irritable bowel syndrome and Crohn disease may present as chronic pelvic pain.
- Women with genital tuberculosis may have a past history of pulmonary tuberculosis.
- Previous abdominal or pelvic surgery increases the risk of adhesions and chronic pelvic pain. In women with Müllerian anomalies, history of surgery for renal or ureteric anomalies may be present since the two systems are closely associated developmentally. Surgery for inguinal hernia during childhood should arouse a suspicion of androgen insensitivity with inguinal testes.

Family history

Endometrial, breast and ovarian cancers have a familial predisposition. Women with sporadic colorectal cancer and hereditary nonpolyposis colorectal cancer (HNPCC) are also at an increased risk for endometrial cancer. Breast–ovarian cancer syndromes occur in women who are *BRCA* mutation carriers (Box 4.12). Family history of diabetes, hypertension and ischaemic heart disease is important in the evaluation and screening of older, postmenopausal women.

Box 4.12 Family history

- Familial cancers
  - Ovarian
  - Endometrial
  - Breast
- Chromosomal disorders
  - Androgen insensitivity
  - Turner syndrome
  - Noonan syndrome
- Medical disorders
  - Diabetes
  - Hypertension
  - Coronary heart disease
  - Dyslipidaemia
  - Infectious diseases
  - Tuberculosis and STD

STD, sexually transmitted disease.

Androgen-insensitivity syndrome and other chromosomal aberrations causing amenorrhoea are also familial.

Occupational and social history

Occupation of the woman and her husband gives an idea about the socioeconomic status. Multiple sexual partners of the patient or spouse increase the risk of sexually transmitted diseases and human papillomavirus (HPV) infection, which is a causative agent for cervical cancer.

Symptoms pertaining to other systems

Review of other systems is mandatory before arriving at a diagnosis.

- Cardiovascular and respiratory diseases have a bearing on anaesthesia and surgery.
- Hypothalamic/pituitary problems can give rise to menstrual disorders and infertility. Menstrual abnormalities can occur due to thyroid or adrenal disorders.
- Neuromuscular diseases can lead to pelvic organ prolapse.
- Gastrointestinal diseases can present with chronic pelvic/abdominal pain. Gastrointestinal and urinary tract may be affected by pelvic diseases such as endometriosis or malignancy. Reproductive and urinary systems are closely associated developmentally; therefore, developmental anomalies can affect both the systems.
- Often women with depression, anxiety and other mental illnesses present with gynaecological symptoms such as chronic pelvic pain, chronic vaginal discharge and dyspareunia.

Physical examination

A thorough physical examination is an integral and essential part of medical practice. A diagnosis should not be arrived at or investigations ordered before completing the physical examination. Adequate privacy should be ensured. It is advisable to have a chaperone while performing a gynaecological examination so that the intentions of the gynaecologist are not misunderstood.

General examination

This begins with an examination of the patient's height, weight and gait (Fig. 4.2). Body mass index should be calculated. The rest of the

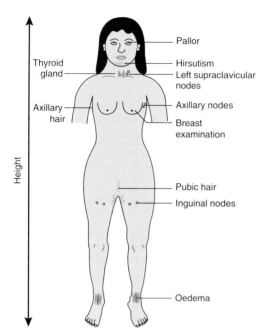

Figure 4.2 Diagrammatic representation of details to be noted on general examination.

Labels on Figure 4.2:
- Pallor
- Thyroid gland
- Hirsutism
- Left supraclavicular nodes
- Axillary hair
- Axillary nodes
- Breast examination
- Height
- Pubic hair
- Inguinal nodes
- Oedema

Box 4.13 General examination

- Height
- Weight
- BMI
- BP, pulse, respiratory rate
- Gait
- Pallor
- Oedema
- Lymph nodes
  - Cervical
  - Left supraclavicular
  - Inguinal
  - Axillary
- Hirsutism: Ferriman–Gallwey score
- Secondary sexual characteristics
  - Breast
  - Axillary hair
  - Pubic hair
- Examination of the thyroid

BMI, body mass index.

general examination should proceed as given in Box 4.13.

Examination of the breast

This is an integral part of gynaecological examination. Breast examination should be performed in all women. In girls presenting with primary amenorrhoea, breast development should be staged according to Tanner staging (*see* Chapter 18, *Primary amenorrhoea*). In women with secondary amenorrhoea, galactorrhoea should be looked for. Hirsutism should be scored according to the Ferriman–Gallwey scoring system (*see* Chapter 20, *Hirsutism and virilization*). Women should be taught to perform self-breast examination and advised to do it postmenstrually every month (Fig. 4.3). Systematic method of clinical breast examination is given in Box 4.14. Clinical examination should be carried out with the pads of three middle fingers, with the patient in sitting and supine positions (Fig. 4.4). Any dimpling of skin, oedema or erythema should be noted. Breasts should be palpated systematically for lumps, and, if present, the size, location, mobility and consistency should be noted. Nipple discharge should be looked for, and axillary and supraclavicular nodes should be palpated.

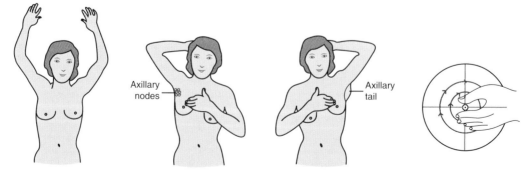

Labels on Figure 4.3:
- Axillary nodes
- Axillary tail

Figure 4.3 Technique of self-breast examination. Breast should be examined with the pad of the three middle fingers, proceeding in a clockwise, circular fashion.

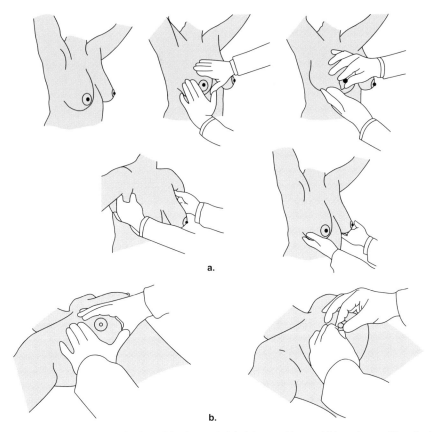

a.

b.

Figure 4.4 Technique of physical examination of the breast in (a) sitting position and (b) supine position. Pad of three fingers should be used, and examination should include axillary tail and axillary nodes.

Box 4.14 Clinical breast examination

- Position
  - Sitting with arms raised
  - Supine
- Extent
  - Midsternum to posterior axillary line
  - Costal margin to clavicle
- Inspection
  - Dimpling of skin
  - Erythema, oedema
  - Nipple retraction
  - Nipple eczema
- Palpation
  - Nipple discharge
  - Palpable mass/cyst
  - Fixity
  - Tissue thickening
- Lymph nodes
  - Axillary
  - Supraclavicular

Examination of other systems

Cardiovascular and respiratory systems should be examined in the usual way. Spine must be examined especially in older women to rule out vertebral fractures. In women with suspected Turner syndrome, peripheral pulses must be checked and coarctation of aorta ruled out.

Examination of the abdomen

Examination of the abdomen by inspection, palpation, percussion and auscultation is mandatory.

Inspection may reveal distension due to ascites or mass, scars of previous surgery, displacement of the umbilicus or visible peristalsis (Box 4.15). Striae gravidarum and linea nigra are indicators of previous pregnancy.

Box 4.15 Abdominal examination—Inspection

- Distension
- Ascites
- Mass
- Scars of previous surgery
- Displacement of umbilicus
- Striae gravidarum and linea nigra

Palpation should begin with an area where the patient has no pain or tenderness; otherwise, muscle guarding may preclude adequate examination. Enlargement of the liver and spleen must be looked for on palpation.

If a mass is palpated, the quadrant of the abdomen in which it is present should be delineated, its size, shape, margins, surface, consistency and mobility determined (Box 4.16). A mass arising from the pelvis must be distinguished from an abdominal mass. If the lower margin of the mass cannot be palpated and if it is not possible to 'get below' the swelling, it is a pelvic mass (Fig. 4.5). Most midline masses arise from the uterus, and their size can be expressed in terms of the size of gravid uterus in weeks (Fig. 4.6). Adnexal masses are usually found in the iliac fossae but can extend to midline. A fullness or mass in the upper abdomen may be an 'omental cake' due to secondaries in ovarian cancer. Masses arising from the pelvis can usually be moved side to side, but they do not move freely in the vertical axis unless the pedicle is long. The presence of fluid thrill indicates ascites, encysted fluid or a large ovarian cyst.

Box 4.16 Abdominal examination—Palpation

- Area of tenderness
- Hepatomegaly
- Splenomegaly
- Mass
  - Site, extent
  - Size
  - Margins
  - Consistency
  - Mobility
- Mass arising from the pelvis
  - Lower margin cannot be felt
  - Cannot 'get below' the mass
- Fluid thrill
  - Ascites
  - Large ovarian cyst
  - Encysted fluid

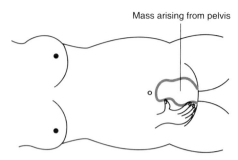

Mass arising from pelvis

Figure 4.5 Abdominal examination—Palpation. In a mass arising from the pelvis, the lower border cannot be palpated. (It is not possible to 'get below' the swelling.)

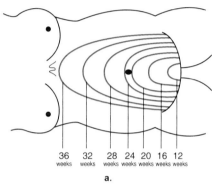

36 weeks 32 weeks 28 weeks 24 weeks 20 weeks 16 weeks 12 weeks

a.

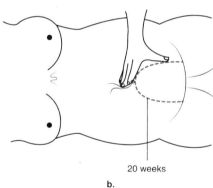

20 weeks

b.

Figure 4.6 Gravid uterus and uterine mass. a. The gravid uterus at various gestational ages. The size of uterus is expressed in terms of gravid uterus in weeks. b. Mass in the lower abdomen corresponding to 20-week gravid uterus.

Percussion should elicit dullness in flanks and resonance anteriorly in ascites. This dullness shifts on turning the patient to side, to the anterior abdomen, and the flank becomes resonant (shifting dullness). On the other hand, flanks are resonant and the central dullness does not shift, in large ovarian cyst (Fig. 4.7).

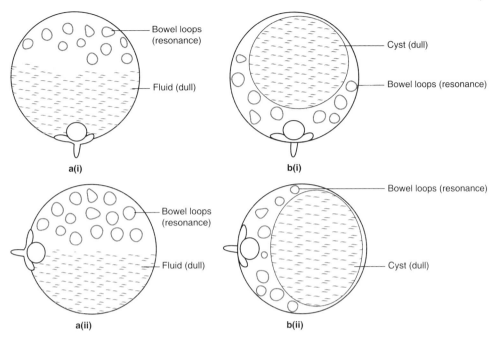

Figure 4.7 Differentiating ascites (**a**) from large ovarian cyst (**b**). a. Shifting dullness is elicited in ascites (**i and ii**). b. The dullness does not shift in ovarian cyst (**i and ii**).

Auscultation is very useful in patients who present with severe abdominal pain; absent bowel sounds may indicate peritonitis and exaggerated bowel sounds intestinal obstruction. Rarely, a bruit may be audible over a highly vascular, tumour-like, large myoma.

Examination of the pelvis

This is usually performed in the dorsal position with the patient's legs flexed at the hip and knee with feet resting on the examination couch or on footrests (Fig. 4.8). The gynaecologist usually stands on the right side of the patient near the foot end. A dorsal lithotomy position with the patient's legs in stirrups is recommended but may be too cumbersome in a busy clinic. The patient should be brought to the edge of the couch to facilitate introduction of speculum. Head end may be elevated by 30 degrees to relax abdominal muscles. If there is difficulty in visualization or examination, a lithotomy position should be used. Proper lighting is mandatory.

In patients with pelvic organ prolapse, examination may have to be performed with the patient standing or squatting if the prolapse

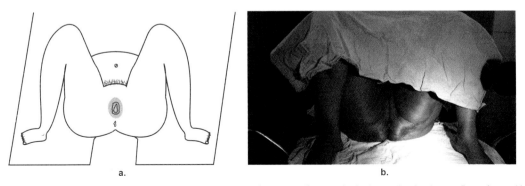

Figure 4.8 Dorsal position of the patient. a. Diagrammatic. b. Image. Gynaecological examination is usually performed in this position.

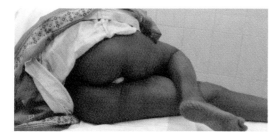

Figure 4.9 Left lateral position of the patient. The left leg is extended and the right leg is flexed at the hip and knee.

cannot be demonstrated in the dorsal position. A left lateral (Sims') position with the left leg extended and right leg flexed at the hip and knee is useful for rectal examination, examination of the perianal area, visualization of anterior vaginal wall after insertion of Sims speculum (especially urinary fistulae) and demonstration of enterocele (Fig. 4.9). The patient should be asked to void before pelvic examination.

Examination of external genitalia

The vulva should be inspected first (Box 4.17). Mons pubis, labia majora and minora, clitoris, perineal body and perianal region should be examined to look for hair distribution, skin lesions, ulcers, pigmentation/depigmentation, scratch marks, swelling or growth. Pelvic organ prolapse should be noted.

Box 4.17 Examination of external genitalia

- Inspection
  - Vulva
  - Hair distribution
  - Skin lesions
    - Pigmentation/depigmentation
    - Ulcer
    - Swelling
    - Growth
  - Introitus
  - Hymen
  - Urethral orifice
  - Cystocele
  - Rectocele
  - Descent of cervix
- Palpation
  - Urethral discharge
  - Bartholin glands
  - Tone of levator ani

Labia minora should be separated to visualize the introitus, hymen and urethral orifice.

The patient should be asked to bear down to look for urethrocele, cystocele and rectocele or descent of the cervix up to the introitus.

Palpation should be performed systematically. Urethra is palpated and 'milked' to express any discharge. Bartholin glands are located lateral to the posterior third of the introitus, deep to the bulbospongiosus muscle. Index finger should be placed within the introitus and thumb on the labium majus to look for enlargement of the gland. Normally, Bartholin glands are not palpable. Tones of the pubovaginalis fibres of the levator ani muscles are tested at the same time, after asking the patient to contract the muscle.

Speculum examination

This should be performed before bimanual pelvic examination. Cusco speculum is usually used (Fig. 4.10). Medium size is suitable for most women, but narrow speculum should be used for older women and young girls who are not sexually active. According to currently available evidence, lubricating the speculum by water-based gel increases the comfort of examination and does not interfere with Papanicolaou smear (Pap smear) or culture of discharge. Labia minora are separated; speculum is introduced with transverse diameter of blades in the anteroposterior position and guided posteriorly towards the rectum in the normal axis of the vagina. The speculum is then rotated 90 degrees so that the transverse diameter lies in the transverse diameter of

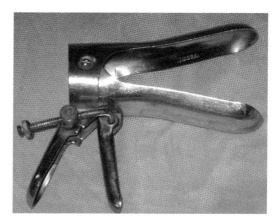

Figure 4.10 Cusco speculum. It is used for visualization of cervix and vagina. The blades can be retained in position with a screw.

the vagina. When the speculum is opened, the cervix should come into view (Fig. 4.11). Vagina and cervix are examined and findings noted (Box 4.18).

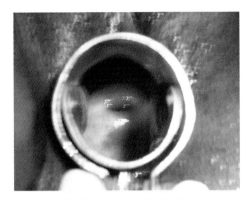

Figure 4.11 Visualization of cervix with Cusco speculum. The anterior and posterior vaginal walls are retracted with the two valves of the speculum, so the entire cervix is clearly seen.

Box 4.18 Speculum examination

Vagina
- Colour
- Dryness/discharge
- Mucosal lesions
- Cysts
- Growth
- Bleeding
- Structural abnormalities

Cervix
- Colour
- External os
- Tears/lacerations
- Squamocolumnar junction/ectropion
- Discharge
- Nabothian follicles/cysts
- Polyp/growth
- Bleeding on touch
- Bleeding through the os

A normal vagina is pink, but can become erythematous and red in case of vaginitis. Vagina is usually moist, but in postmenopausal women, oestrogen deficiency leads to dryness. Discharge is present in case of infection; bleeding may be from the vagina or from the uterine cavity. Mucosal lesions as seen in *Trichomonas vaginalis* vaginitis and *Candida* vaginitis should be noted. Gartner cysts are usually located on the anterolateral walls; growth may arise from the vagina or extend from the cervix. Structural abnormalities can be congenital or acquired.

Prolapse of the anterior and posterior vaginal walls, level of defect and nature of defect can be ascertained on speculum examination.

Cervix is normally dull pink in colour. The external os is round in nulliparous women but transversely slit with an anterior and a posterior lip in multiparous women. Old tears and lacerations are usually the result of childbirth. Discharge indicates cervicitis caused by gonococcal or chlamydial infection but can also be seen in malignancy.

The squamocolumnar junction is visible as an irregular junction between the dull pink squamous epithelium of the portiovaginalis and the bright red columnar epithelium of the endocervix. This is normally located at or around the external os during the reproductive age. In postmenopausal women, it may be within the endocervix. The area between the original and the present squamocolumnar junction is known as **transformation zone**. Most cervical cancers arise in this zone; therefore, this area of ectocervix should be adequately sampled when taking a Pap smear. Polyps and nabothian cysts are usually benign. Nabothian cysts are retention cysts of the endocervical glands. Cervical cancer presents as a cauliflower-like growth, which is friable and bleeds on touch. Uterine bleeding can be seen flowing down through the external os.

A Sims speculum may be used to visualize the anterior vaginal wall in women with lesions on the anterior vaginal wall or urinary fistulae (Fig. 4.12a and b). It is also useful for visualization of enterocele (for details refer to Chapter 24, *Pelvic organ prolapse*). The patient should be in Sims' left lateral position.

Pap smear should be performed before the speculum is withdrawn, and if discharge is present, sample should be taken for microscopic examination (described later in this chapter) and culture.

Bimanual examination

This is also known as 'abdominopelvic examination' or just 'pelvic examination'. The index and middle fingers of the right hand should be inserted into the vagina and the left hand placed on the lower abdomen (Fig. 4.13a and b). The cervix is palpated; tenderness on movement of the cervix is looked for. The fingers in vagina are then placed in the posterior fornix, the uterus is pushed upwards and anteriorly towards the abdominal hand and the uterus is palpated between the two hands. Findings are noted as given in Box 4.19. The vaginal fingers are then moved to the right and left lateral fornices, the

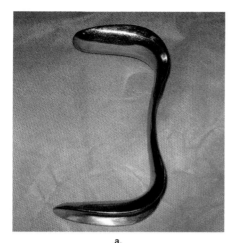

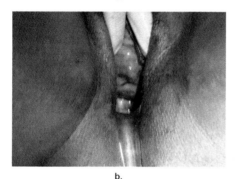

Figure 4.12 Speculum examination with Sims speculum. a. Sims speculum. It may have a single valve or two valves. b. Visualization of the anterior vaginal wall with Sims speculum.

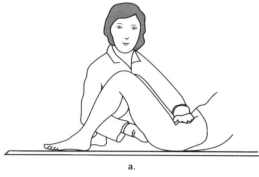

a.

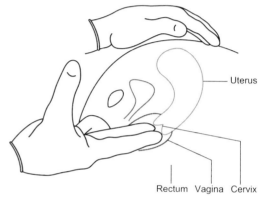

Uterus

Rectum   Vagina   Cervix

b.

Figure 4.13 Bimanual pelvic examination. a. The patient is usually in dorsal position. The gynaecologist stands to the right of the patient. b. The uterus and the adnexa are palpated between the abdominal and vaginal fingers.

Box 4.19 Bimanual examination

- Uterus
  - Anteverted/retroverted/midposition
  - Size—Normal/enlarged
  - Shape—Regular/irregular
  - Consistency—Firm/soft
  - Mobility—Mobile/fixed/restricted
  - Tenderness—Absent/present
- Adnexa
  - Palpable/not palpable
  - If palpable and enlarged
    - Size
    - Shape
    - Unilateral/bilateral
    - Consistency
    - Tenderness
    - Induration/mobility
    - Attachment to the uterus
- Pouch of Douglas
  - Mass
  - Fullness

---

abdominal hand is placed just medial to the right anterosuperior iliac spine and the adnexa are palpated between the two hands.

The normal uterus is anteverted, pear-shaped, firm, mobile, regular and nontender. The uterine axis is tilted forwards in relation to the axis of the vagina, which is termed **anteversion**; when uterine axis is titled posteriorly, it is **retroversion**, and when the uterine axis is in line with that of the vagina, it is said to be in **midposition**. The cervix points backwards or posteriorly when the uterus is anteverted, anteriorly when retroverted and is in the centre when the uterus is in midposition. This finding is important for sounding the uterus, for if the sound is guided anteriorly in a retroverted uterus, the uterus may be perforated.

The uterus is normally firm and about 6 × 4 cm in size. It is soft in pregnancy (Box 4.20). It is uniformly or regularly enlarged in adenomyosis, endometrial polyp, pyometra, haematometra, carcinoma and pregnancy. It is irregularly

Box 4.20 Bimanual examination—Uterus

- Consistency
  - Soft: Pregnancy, pyometra
  - Hard: Malignancy, calcified myomas
- Enlargement
  - Regular: Pregnancy, adenomyosis, pyometra, haematometra, carcinoma
  - Irregular: Myoma, endometrioma
- Mobility
  - Mobile: Myoma, adenomyosis, pregnancy
  - Fixed/restricted: Pelvic inflammatory disease, endometriosis, malignancy

Table 4.1 Differentiating uterine from adnexal mass

	Uterine	Adnexal mass
Location	Central	Lateral
Normal uterus	Not palpable	Palpable
Groove between mass and uterus	Absent	Present
Transmitted mobility	Present	Absent

enlarged when there are myomas. Enlargement can be expressed in weeks in terms of the size compared to that of the gravid uterus. The uterus is normally mobile, but in case of pelvic inflammatory disease, endometriosis or malignancy, it may be fixed. Tenderness indicates infection.

The ovaries are about 3 × 2 cm in size and not usually palpable unless enlarged. A palpable ovary in a postmenopausal woman should be viewed with suspicion. When the ovary slips between the examining fingers, the woman experiences a peculiar unpleasant sensation. Adnexal masses may be ovarian, benign or malignant, paraovarian cysts, hydrosalpinx or a tubo-ovarian mass (Box 4.21). Size, shape, consistency, mobility and tenderness should be noted. Large masses are more likely to be malignant, but some benign tumours such as mucinous cystadenoma can grow to a very large size. Large ovarian masses with long pedicle, which are entirely in the abdomen, may not be palpable on bimanual examination. Hydrosalpinx

Box 4.21 Bimanual examination—Adnexa

- Size
  - Large >10 cm: Malignancy
  - Bilateral: Malignancy
- Shape
  - Retort shaped: Hydrosalpinx
- Mobility
  - Mobile: Benign, noninflammatory
  - Fixed: Endometriosis, PID, malignancy
- Consistency
  - Cystic: Benign
  - Solid: Malignancy
  - Variable consistency: Inflammatory, malignancy
- Tenderness
  - Tender: Inflammatory

PID, pelvic inflammatory disease.

is retort shaped. Inflammatory endometriotic and malignant lesions are fixed. Inflammatory lesions are also tender. Bilateral masses are often malignant. Cystic lesions are benign, but hard masses and masses with varying consistency are likely to be malignant.

Uterine versus adnexal mass A mass arising from the uterus must be differentiated from an ovarian mass. The features are listed in Table 4.1. The uterine mass is centrally located in the normal position of the uterus. The adnexal masses are felt through lateral fornices. Normal uterus can be palpated separate from the mass in an adnexal lesion, and a groove is felt between the mass and the uterus (Fig. 4.14a and b). On moving the mass with the abdominal hand, the uterus moves en masse and the movement is transmitted to the vaginal fingers in case of a uterine mass. But in case of adnexal mass, unless it is adherent to the uterus, the movement is not transmitted.

The posterior fornix should be palpated. Collection of fluid, pus or blood in the pouch of Douglas can be felt as a bulge in the posterior fornix. Nodules can be felt in the pouch in cases of endometriosis and metastatic ovarian tumour. Ovarian mass when fixed posteriorly may be felt through the posterior fornix. Tumours of the rectovaginal septum and posterior rectal wall can also be palpated.

Rectovaginal examination

The gloves are changed, the middle finger is inserted into the rectum after lubrication and the index finger is placed in the vagina (Fig. 4.15). The rectovaginal septum can be palpated between the fingers. Induration of the uterosacral ligaments and the rectovaginal septum can be felt in women with endometriosis. Perineal body can be palpated, and deficient perineum should be looked for.

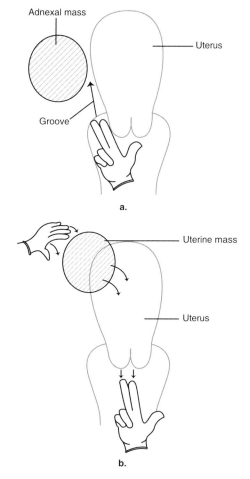

Figure 4.14 Differentiating uterine mass from adnexal mass. a. A groove is felt between the uterus and the adnexal mass. b. When the mass is moved by the abdominal hand, the movements are transmitted to the cervix in case of uterine mass.

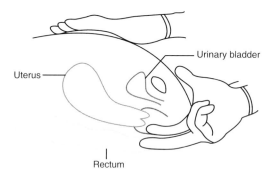

Figure 4.15 Pictorial representation of rectovaginal examination with index finger in the vagina and middle finger in the rectum.

Rectal examination

This is recommended as a routine examination in all women. Retroverted uterus, contents of the pouch of Douglas and intraluminal lesions in the rectum can be evaluated. Parametrial infiltration in cervical cancer, secondary deposits in the pouch of Douglas in case of ovarian malignancy, prolapsed and adherent ovaries in endometriosis, collection of blood in ruptured ectopic pregnancy and pus in the pelvic abscess are best made out on rectal examination (Fig. 4.16). Tone of the rectal sphincter should be assessed, and rectocele should be looked for. Any growth or intraluminal lesion can also be felt during rectal examination. If a posterior vaginal wall defect is found, the patient should be asked to strain and the presence of rectocele should be noted.

Special situations

Children, adolescents and old women present special situations. A speculum examination should not be performed in a child. External genitalia may be examined with the mother's help, but if there is suspicion of a foreign body, examination under anaesthesia is required. All adolescents with gynaecological complaints do not need vaginal examination. If there is excessive bleeding or a pelvic pathology is suspected, pelvic examination may be performed. The procedure should be explained to the patient, and a speculum examination can be omitted if considered unnecessary. Postmenopausal women with prolonged oestrogen deficiency and narrow vagina may find speculum examination uncomfortable. Smallest available speculum should be used with lidocaine jelly as lubricant.

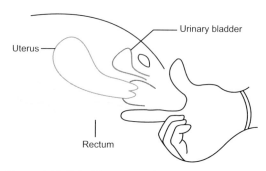

Figure 4.16 Pictorial representation of rectal examination.

Screening/diagnostic procedures performed during gynaecological examination

Routine cervical cytology by Pap smear is usually performed during gynaecological examination. In addition, there are other tests that are feasible (Box 4.22).

Box 4.22 Procedures performed during gynaecological examination

- Cytological screening for cervical cancer
  - Pap smear
  - Liquid-based cytology
- Examination of vaginal discharge
  - Saline preparation
  - KOH preparation
- Endometrial sampling
- Culdocentesis

KOH, potassium hydroxide.

Examination of vaginal discharge

Common causes of vaginal discharge are bacterial vaginosis, *T. vaginalis* vaginitis and *Candida* vaginitis. Cervicitis is caused by *Gonococcus* or *Chlamydia*. They can be diagnosed by examination of the discharge (Table 4.2). Examination of the vaginal discharge is an essential component of gynaecological examination. Diagnosis

Table 4.2 Diagnosis of vaginitis by examination of discharge

	Wet film	KOH preparation	Gram stain
Bacterial vaginosis	Clue cells	Amine (fishy) odour	
T. vaginalis vaginitis	Flagellated organism		
Candida vaginitis		Fungal hyphae, spores	
Gonococcal cervicitis			Gram-negative diplococci

KOH, potassium hydroxide.

of chlamydial infection requires culture of the discharge.

After inspecting the vagina and cervix, a drop of vaginal discharge is placed on a glass slide with a cotton swab, mixed with a drop of saline and covered with a coverslip. Another drop of vaginal secretion is mixed with a drop of potassium hydroxide (KOH) solution. If there is discharge from the cervix, it should be smeared on a glass slide and stained with Gram stain.

A fishy odour on mixing with KOH is suggestive of bacterial vaginosis. When examined under the microscope, clue cells that are epithelial cells with adherent bacteria are seen in bacterial vaginosis. Motile, flagellated organism is seen in *T. vaginalis* vaginitis (Fig. 4.12). KOH lyses epithelial cells, leaving only the hyphae, pseudohyphae and spores in *Candida* infection.

Cytological screening for cervical cancer

This should be performed in all women from 21 years of age. This may be combined with HPV testing in women who are >30 years of age. Current recommendations are discussed in Chapter 28, *Premalignant diseases of the cervix*.

Cytological screening can be performed by either traditional Pap smear or liquid-based cytology.

During the speculum examination, after visualizing the cervix, the screw on the speculum is tightened to keep the blades open, a cytobrush is first introduced into the endocervical canal and rotated to obtain endocervical sample (Fig. 4.17a and b) and a wooden spatula or Ayre spatula is used to scrape the transformation zone of the ectocervix (Fig. 4.18a and b). The spatula should be applied to the ectocervix and rotated by 360 degrees. The cells are smeared on a slide and fixed before drying, using a spray or a 1:1 mixture of 95% ethanol and ether. The smears are stained by Papanicolaou's method and reported using the Bethesda system (*see* Chapter 28, *Premalignant diseases of the cervix*).

For liquid-based cytology, a special broom is used to scrape the endocervix and ectocervix (*see* Chapter 28, *Premalignant diseases of the cervix*). The broom must be rotated similar to the spatula. The broom is then immersed in a liquid medium and swirled vigorously 10 times and discarded. The liquid is sent for cytological analysis.

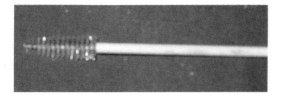

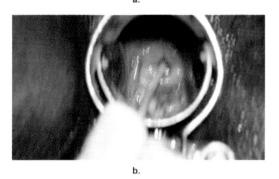

Figure 4.17 Endocervical sampling. a. A cytobrush. b. The endocervical sample—Obtained by rotating the cytobrush within the cervical canal.

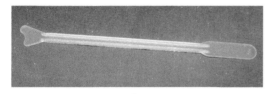

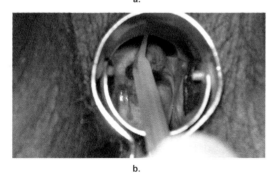

Figure 4.18 Ectocervical sampling. a. Ayre spatula. b. The ectocervical sample is obtained using Ayre spatula.

Endometrial sampling

Endometrial sampling is performed in women with abnormal uterine bleeding. It is used for the confirmation of ovulation, diagnosis of tuberculosis, malignancy and hyperplasia. Sample can be obtained using a brush, cannula or curette. Flexible cannulae such as Pipelle (Fig. 4.19) can be used to aspirate endometrial tissue while

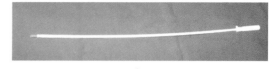

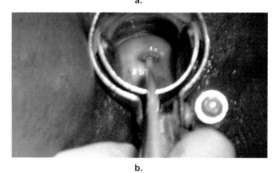

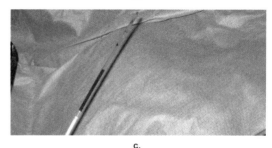

Figure 4.19 Endometrial sampling. a. Pipelle used for endometrial sampling. b. Pipelle introduced into the uterine cavity. c. Sample of endometrium aspirated in the Pipelle.

performing a gynaecological examination. These are 2–4 mm in diameter and can be introduced through the internal os with ease even in postmenopausal women.

The woman is placed in dorsal lithotomy or dorsal position, bivalve speculum is inserted and the cervix is brought into view. The blades are kept open by tightening the screw. In most multiparous women, Pipelle can be inserted into the uterine cavity through the external and internal os and sample aspirated. In nulliparous and postmenopausal women, a tenaculum is used to steady the cervix before introducing the Pipelle. The sample is sent in formalin for histopathological examination.

Culdocentesis/colpocentesis

Aspiration of fluid/pus or blood from the pouch of Douglas or cul-de-sac is termed **culdocentesis** or colpocentesis. The pouch of Douglas is

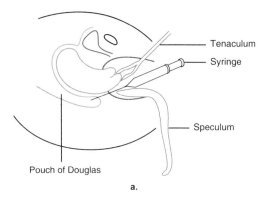

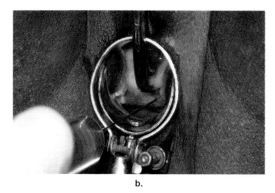

a.   b.

Figure 4.20 Colpocentesis. a. Pictorial representation of colpocentesis. b. Picture showing needle being introduced through the posterior fornix. The posterior lip of the cervix is lifted up and the posterior fornix is visualized.

the most dependent part of the peritoneal cavity. Blood, pus and fluid collect in this area and can be easily aspirated by inserting a needle through the posterior fornix. This was commonly used for diagnosis of ectopic pregnancy and pelvic abscess prior to the availability of transvaginal sonography. It is a useful procedure even now in developing countries where ultrasonography is not readily available. Delay in laparotomy or referral can be avoided.

Fullness is felt on rectal examination when there is a collection of pus or blood in the cul-de-sac. The cervix is visualized using a bivalve speculum, blades are kept open by tightening the screw, cervix is pulled upwards with a single-tooth tenaculum and a long, 20-gauge, needle attached to a 5- or 10-cm^3 syringe is inserted into the pouch of Douglas through the posterior fornix (Fig. 4.20). If pus is obtained, it is sent for culture and a colpotomy or laparotomy is planned. If blood is aspirated, diagnosis of ruptured ectopic pregnancy or tubal abortion is a strong possibility and laparoscopy/laparotomy is considered.

Key points

- Elaborate history of the woman's illness is essential for making the correct diagnosis. The patient should be made comfortable and allowed to describe the symptoms in her own words.

- Age, presenting symptoms, menstrual, gynaecological and obstetric history, details of contraception, smoking, substance abuse, medications and past medical/surgical history should be asked for.

- Different gynaecological disorders are common in different age groups, and this helps in narrowing down the differential diagnosis.

- Common gynaecological complaints are abnormal vaginal bleeding, painful menstruation, vaginal discharge, mass descending per vaginum, abdominal mass, distension and inability to conceive. Women may present to the gynaecologist with symptoms pertaining to the bladder and bowel as well.

- Details of the history of presenting complaint(s) and other associated and related symptoms should be obtained.

- Past gynaecological history is important since some gynaecological conditions such as myomas, endometriosis and benign tumours recur.

- Details of obstetric history are necessary in women with pelvic organ prolapse. Parity must be noted since some diseases are associated with nulliparity, while others are common in multiparous women.

- Details of medications that the patient is taking must be asked for. They give an insight into the patient's medical problems. Some drugs can be responsible for the symptoms, some drugs have significant drug interactions and some drugs have to be modified or stopped preoperatively.

- General examination and examination of the breast and thyroid and other systems are mandatory.

- Abdominal examination should be performed systematically. If a lower abdominal mass is found, it must be ascertained as to whether it is arising from the pelvis or not. Free fluid must be looked for.

- Pelvic examination includes examination of the external genitalia, speculum examination and bimanual examination.

- Pelvic examination should be performed with the patient in dorsal position. Sims' left lateral position may be used for examination of anterior vaginal wall and demonstration of enterocele.

(Continued)

Key points *(Continued)*

- Cervix and vagina are visualized using a Cusco speculum. Presence of discharge, bleeding, growth and prolapse of the vaginal walls or cervix are looked for.
- On bimanual examination, uterine size, position and mobility, and presence of adnexal mass must be ascertained.
- Rectal and rectovaginal examinations are essential to look for collection of fluid, pus or blood in the pouch of Douglas, induration of uterosacral ligaments, para-

metrial infiltration in cervical cancer and evaluation of posterior vaginal wall prolapse.

- Obtaining sample for cervical cytology [Papanicolaou smear (Pap smear)] is an integral part of gynaecological examination. Collection of sample of vaginal discharge for microscopic examination, endometrial sampling with Pipelle in women with perimenopausal or postmenopausal bleeding and culdocentesis when collection of pus or blood is suspected in the pouch of Douglas can be performed during gynaecological examination.

Self-assessment

Case-based questions

Case 1

A lady presents with vaginal discharge to the gynaecological clinic.

1. Give an outline of the history that you will ask for.
2. How will you proceed with the examination?
3. If vaginal discharge is present, how will you proceed?

Case 2

A 50-year-old lady presents with lower abdominal mass.

1. Highlight the important points in history that you will focus on.
2. What will you look for on physical examination?
3. How will you know if it is a mass arising from the pelvis, and if so, whether it is from the uterus or adnexa?

Answers

Case 1

1. (a) Age, duration of the complaint, nature of discharge, associated symptoms such as pruritus, ulcer, dyspareunia, dysuria, abdominal or pelvic pain
   (b) Menstrual history, intermenstrual bleeding, postcoital bleeding
   (a) Obstetric history, recent childbirth/miscarriage to rule out maybe postabortal or postdelivery infection
   (d) Contraception—Barrier/IUCD/combined OC pill
   (e) Past history of similar episodes, chronic pelvic pain to rule out chronic infection
   (f) History of sexually transmitted diseases
   (g) Husband's occupation, history of multiple sexual partners
2. (a) General examination for fever, tachycardia
   (b) Breast examination and system review

(c) Abdominal examination for tenderness, lower abdominal mass
(d) Per speculum examination for vaginal mucosa, type of discharge, colour, odour, mucopus from the cervix, growth
(e) Bimanual examination for uterine tenderness, adnexal mass/tenderness, tenderness on movement of the cervix, fullness in posterior fornix
(f) Rectovaginal and rectal examination for collection in the pouch of Douglas

3. Pap smear
   (a) A drop of discharge should be mixed with saline and examined under the microscope for *T. vaginalis* and clue cells.
   (b) Another drop should be mixed with KOH and examined for hyphae, pseudohyphae and spores and for fishy odour.
   (c) Discharge should be smeared on the slide and stained with Gram stain for gonococci.
   (d) Swab should be sent for *Chlamydia trachomatis*.

Case 2

1. (a) Duration of the complaint, rapidity of growth; associated symptoms such as pain, discomfort, heaviness, vomiting, bowel symptoms, bladder symptoms, loss of appetite and weight
   (b) Menstrual history, menopausal status, heavy menstrual bleeding
   (c) Obstetric history, parity
   (d) Contraception—Combined OC pills
   (e) Past history of gynaecological surgery, abdominal mass
   (f) Family history of breast/ovarian/endometrial/colonic cancer
2. (a) General examination for pallor, lymphadenopathy (supraclavicular, inguinal)
   (b) Breast examination and system review; respiratory system for pleural effusion
   (c) Abdominal examination for ascites, hepatosplenomegaly; location of the mass, size, margins, consistency, mobility, lower border
   (d) Per speculum examination, Pap smear

(e) Bimanual examination for size of uterus, shape, consistency, mobility, transmitted mobility, bilateral or unilateral

(f) Rectovaginal and rectal examination for nodules in the pouch of Douglas

3. (a) Mass arising from the pelvis—Lower border is not palpable and cannot get below the swelling.

(b) Uterine mass and adnexal mass are distinguished on the basis of the following features:

(i) Feeling the mass through lateral fornices or midline

(ii) Uterus palpable separately or not

(iii) Groove between the mass and the uterus

(iv) Transmitted mobility

Long-answer question

1. Describe the gynaecological examination in a parous woman. What simple procedures can be performed during gynaecological examination?

Short-answer questions

1. How will you take a Pap smear?
2. How will you differentiate a uterine mass from an adnexal mass on clinical examination?
3. How will you perform culdocentesis? What are the indications?

5 | Imaging in Gynaecology

Case scenario

Mrs HK, 42, mother of three children, came to the line on a Friday morning and presented a thick file containing details of prior consultations and investigations. She had visited three hospitals already and had received three different opinions. Mrs HK was diagnosed to have a 3 × 2 cm simple cyst in the left ovary on ultrasonography during a master health check-up. She had no symptoms, but on the basis of the findings on sonography, she was advised hysterectomy. She sought second opinion; a computed tomography (CT) scan was performed and the presence of cyst was confirmed. She was advised to return for follow-up after 6 months. Ultrasonography was repeated in the third hospital and laparoscopic surgery was advised. Mrs HK was confused, worried and anxious.

Introduction

There have been tremendous advancements in imaging techniques in the past few decades. Most of the techniques are noninvasive and have greatly increased the accuracy of diagnosis. Some are also used for therapy. Earlier imaging techniques such as plain X-ray and hysterosalpingography (HSG) have been replaced by newer methods. The various techniques have applications that overlap. The clinician must choose the appropriate modality for the patient, keeping in mind the strengths and weaknesses of each modality, contraindications and, of course, the cost.

However, imaging is extremely sensitive and detects many incidental abnormalities such as small uterine myomas, functional ovarian cysts, small insignificant nodes and findings in other organs seen within the region imaged, which are unrelated to the patient's symptoms. Thus, imaging findings should always be interpreted in the light of clinical information. Clinician decision making should always take into account the patient's clinical picture and the imaging findings together. The clinician should be careful in counselling the patients about these incidental lesions.

Ultrasonography

In ultrasonography, high-frequency sound waves are used and they are reflected by the interfaces between tissues of varying density. The reflected sound waves are captured as images. Ultrasound appearance depends on the difference in the density of the tissues imaged. For example, when the difference in the density is high like calcification or bone and surrounding tissues, the sound wave almost completely reflects back and appears white or echogenic with posterior acoustic shadowing. On the other hand, when the difference is low like fluid in the urinary bladder or an ovarian cyst, no sound is reflected back and ultrasonography appearance is black or anechoic with posterior acoustic enhancement.

Ultrasonography has now come to be considered as an extension of the clinician's hand. Transabdominal and transvaginal transducers are commonly used. Transperineal and transrectal techniques are useful for imaging of the pelvic floor muscles and the anal sphincter (Box 5.1).

Box 5.1 Techniques for pelvic ultrasonography

- Transabdominal (curvilinear, 2- to 5-MHz probe)
  - Full bladder required
  - Panoramic view
  - Useful for large masses
  - Ascites
  - Intra-abdominal organs
  - Lymph nodes
- Transvaginal (curvilinear, 7- to 12-MHz probe)
  - Bladder should be empty
  - Most useful in gynaecology
  - Normal-size uterus
    - Endometrial thickness
    - Polyps
    - Growth
  - Normal ovaries, follicles
  - Small masses
  - Pouch of Douglas
- Transperineal
  - Pelvic floor muscles
- Transrectal
  - Puborectalis muscle
  - Anal sphincter
  - Rectovaginal septum

The American Institute of Ultrasound Medicine (AIUM) has developed guidelines (2005) for indications, equipment and documentation for pelvic ultrasonography.

Indications

Indications listed by AIUM include but not necessarily limit to what is given in Box 5.2.

Box 5.2 Indications for ultrasonography (AIUM)

- Pelvic pain
- Postmenopausal bleeding
- Abnormal uterine bleeding
- Dysmenorrhoea
- Abnormal or technically difficult pelvic examination
- Amenorrhoea
- Pelvic infection
- Abnormality noted by other imaging
- Infertility
- Congenital anomalies of the genital tract
- Delayed/precocious puberty
- Postoperative pain/bleeding/infection
- Localization of IUCD
- Screening for cancer in high-risk women
- Urinary incontinence/POP
- Preoperative for guidance

AIUM, American Institute of Ultrasound Medicine; *IUCD*, intrauterine contraceptive device; *POP*, pelvic organ prolapse.

Guidelines also describe the specifications of examination of each organ in the pelvis (Box 5.3). All findings should be documented.

Box 5.3 Examination of pelvic organs

- Uterus
  - Size, shape, orientation
  - Endometrium
  - Myometrium
  - Cervix
- Adnexa
  - Ovaries—Size in three dimensions
  - Dilated tubes
  - Mass—Size
  - Sonographic characteristics
- Cul-de-sac
  - Fluid
  - Mass—Size, position, shape
  - Sonographic characteristics

Normal ultrasonography findings

It is important to know the normal sonographic features in order to diagnose abnormalities.

Uterus

The normal features of uterus are listed in Box 5.4. Uterine length is measured from fundus to cervix, depth from anterior to posterior wall (Fig. 5.1a) and width in the coronal view (Box 5.4).

The endometrium is well demarcated from the myometrium. The endometrium undergoes changes during the menstrual cycle and so does the ultrasound appearance. Normal endometrium appears as a thin echogenic stripe in the early proliferative phase. In the late proliferative phase, endometrium appears trilaminar, which is composed of a central thin echogenic stripe, middle hypoechoic band and outer echogenic stripe (Fig. 5.1b). Endometrium is thickest in the secretory phase (8–10 mm) and appears homogeneously echogenic. It is normal to have small amount of fluid in the endometrial cavity in the menstrual and early proliferative phases of the menstrual cycle.

Box 5.4 Ultrasonography of normal uterus

- Size: 7.5 × 5.0 × 2.5 cm
- Length: Fundus to cervix
- Depth: Anteroposterior
- Width: Coronal view
- Myometrium
  - Homogeneous
  - Hypoechogenic
- Endometrium
  - Changes during menstrual cycle
  - 1–4 mm after menstruation
  - 8–10 mm at ovulation
  - Trilaminar at ovulation

Adnexa

The ovaries are well demarcated and located above the internal iliac vessels. They undergo cyclic changes during menstrual cycle. Follicles are seen as anechoic structures (Fig. 5.2), and the dominant follicle grows to 18–20 mm in size before ovulation. Normal ovaries are 3 × 2 × 2 cm in size with a volume of 10 cm³, but become much smaller postmenopausally (2 × 1.5 × 1 cm). The fallopian tubes are normally not visible. A small volume of fluid in the cul-de-saac is normal.

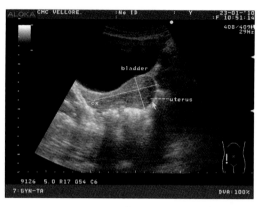

a.

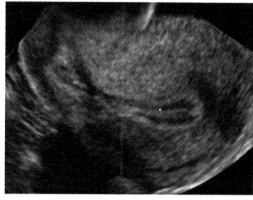

b.

Figure 5.1 Ultrasonographic pictures of normal uterus. a. Sagittal view with lines indicating uterine length and depth. b. Trilaminar endometrium—Linear central echogenic stripe indicating the endometrial canal, the central hypoechoic band corresponds to the functional layer of the endometrium and the outer echogenic layer corresponds to the basal layer.

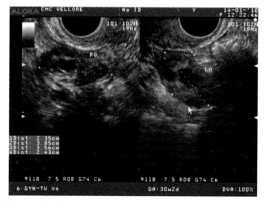

Figure 5.2 Ultrasonographic pictures of normal ovaries with follicles.

Abnormalities diagnosed through ultrasonography

Uterus

Abnormalities of the uterus can be diagnosed on ultrasonography. The characteristic findings are listed in Box 5.5. Ultrasonography is a useful tool to differentiate uterine enlargement due to myoma and adenomyosis (Fig. 5.3a–c). Evaluation of the size, the site and the number of

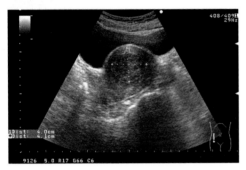

a.

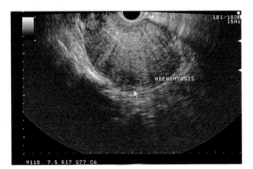

b.

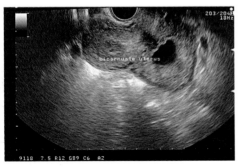

c.

Figure 5.3 Ultrasonographic pictures showing uterine abnormalities. a. Myoma on the anterior wall. b. Adenomyosis—Myometrial thickening at the fundus. c. Bicornuate uterus. Two uterine horns are visible with collection of blood in one.

myomas also helps in making decision regarding the surgery and/or follow-up. If the uterus is large and palpable abdominally, transabdominal scan should be performed first. Ultrasonogram is used for the diagnosis of uterine anomalies as well.

Box 5.5 Uterine abnormalities

- Myomas
  - Irregular uterine contour
  - Hypoechoic/isoechoic/hyperechoic masses
  - Size, number and location
- Adenomyosis
  - Uterine enlargement
  - Asymmetric thickening
  - Heterogeneous echotexture
- Uterine anomalies
  - Bicornuate/septate uterus
  - Haematometra

Endometrium

Endometrial abnormalities are evaluated using transvaginal transducer. The endometrium is usually evaluated in women with infertility, abnormal uterine bleeding, amenorrhoea, postmenopausal bleeding, endometrial carcinoma, and in women on tamoxifen (Fig. 5.4a and b). Conditions where ultrasonography is useful and the related sonographic features are listed in Box 5.6.

Box 5.6 Endometrial abnormalities

- Abnormal uterine bleeding
  - Polyps
    - Focal lesions
    - Hypoechoic/hyperechoic
    - Surrounded by endometrial lining
  - Submucous leiomyoma
- Postmenopausal bleeding
- Endometrial thickness
- Endometrial cancer
  - Myometrial invasion
- Tamoxifen therapy
  - Increase in thickness
  - Subendometrial stromal vacuolation
- Missing IUCD
  - Bright, echogenic
  - Penetration into the myometrium
  - Translocation into the peritoneal cavity
- Infertility
  - Endometrial thickness
  - Uterine anomalies

IUCD, intrauterine contraceptive device.

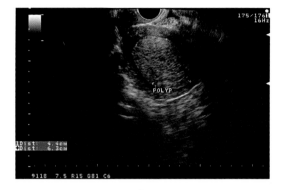

a.

b.

Figure 5.4 Ultrasonographic picture showing imaging of the endometrial cavity. a. Endometrial polyp. b. Intrauterine device (copper T) in the uterine cavity.

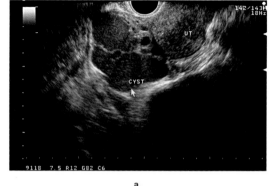

a.

b.

Figure 5.5 Ultrasonographic pictures of ovarian lesions. a. Ovarian endometrioma. The cyst reveals middle-level uniform internal echoes giving it a ground-glass appearance. b. Multiloculated cyst—Several small and large locules with varying echogenicity.

Ovaries

Functional cysts, endometriotic cysts, benign neoplasms and malignant tumours of the ovary are initially evaluated by ultrasonography. It is also useful for follicular monitoring during ovulation induction, diagnosis of endometriosis and functional ovarian cysts associated with abnormal uterine bleeding and gestational trophoblastic tumours (Fig. 5.5a and b). Ultrasonographic features of non-neoplastic conditions of ovary and evaluation of infertility are listed in Box 5.7. Endometriosis presents varied sonographic appearances and can be difficult to diagnose on ultrasonography.

Ultrasonography is extensively used in the management of ovarian neoplasms. It is useful to differentiate between benign and malignant ovarian masses, and detect lymph node enlargement and ascites (Box 5.8; Fig. 5.6a and b). Ultrasonographic features of benign and malignant tumours of the ovary are listed in Box 5.8.

Box 5.7 Ultrasonography—Non-neoplastic ovarian lesions

- Infertility
  - Follicular monitoring
  - Dominant follicle 18–20 mm
- Functional cysts
  - Follicular cyst
    - 3–8 cm, uniloculated
  - Corpus luteum cyst
    - 3–10 cm, uniloculated
  - Theca lutein cyst
    - Large, bilateral, multiloculated
- Endometriotic cyst
  - Fine low- to middle-level internal echoes
  - Ground-glass appearance
  - Hyperechoic foci in the wall
  - Rectovaginal nodules

- Serous cystadenoma
  - Cystic, few thin internal septations
- Mucinous cystadenoma
  - Large, multiloculated, each locule with different echogenicity
- Brenner tumour
  - Small, solid, smooth
- Benign cystic teratoma
  - Complex, solid and cystic lesion, calcification, fat-fluid levels
  - Echogenic internal components
- Malignant tumours
  - Bilateral
  - Solid or mixed solid and cystic
  - Septae >3 mm thick
  - Papillary excrescences
  - Thick cyst wall, >3 mm
  - Ascites, omental thickening
  - Enlarged para-aortic nodes
  - Liver metastasis

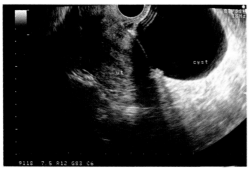

a.

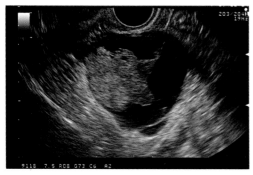

b.

Figure 5.6 Ultrasonographic pictures of simple and complex ovarian mass. a. Uniloculated, uniformly anechoic, thin-walled simple cyst. b. Complex cystic lesion with a large solid component.

Fallopian tubes

Although the normal tube is not visible on ultrasonography, enlarged, thickened and dilated tubes can be clearly seen. Hydrosalpinx is retort shaped and elongated with incomplete septations and is seen adjacent to the ovary.

Acute/chronic pelvic pain

Ultrasonography is commonly used for the evaluation of women with pelvic pain, acute or chronic. Conditions causing acute pelvic pain and their ultrasonographic features are listed in Box 5.9. Pyosalpinx can be made out readily in view of the dilatation and thickening of the walls of the tube. Torsion of ovarian cyst can be diagnosed only if colour Doppler is used. Other conditions that give rise to pelvic pain, such as appendicitis, ureteric stones, diverticulitis and inflammatory bowel disease, are difficult to diagnose by ultrasonography.

Box 5.9 Ultrasonography in acute pelvic pain

- Ectopic pregnancy
  - Absence of gestational sac in the uterus
  - Complex adnexal mass
  - Gestational sac in the tube
  - Foetal pole with/without cardiac activity
  - Blood in peritoneal cavity/cul-de-sac (fluid with internal echoes)
- Torsion of ovarian cyst
  - Adnexal mass
  - Cyst with haemorrhage
- Acute PID
  - Inflamed tubes
  - Free fluid in cul-de-sac (anechoic)
  - Pyosalpinx
    - Pear/retort-shaped tube with anechoic/echogenic fluid
    - Incomplete septae, fluid debris
    - Cogwheel appearance
  - Pus in cul-de-sac (echogenic)
  - Tubo-ovarian abscess
    - Echogenic fluid-filled complex mass

PID, pelvic inflammatory disease.

Gynaecological causes of chronic pelvic pain are endometriosis, chronic pelvic inflammatory disease (PID), ovarian remnant or residual ovary syndrome and pelvic congestion syndrome. Ultrasonography may reveal endometriosis, tubo-ovarian mass, hydrosalpinx or residual/remnant ovary trapped in the pelvis (Figs 5.7 and 5.8; Box 5.10).

- Tubo-ovarian mass
  - Complex mass
  - Ovary and tube adherent, but can be identified
  - Loculated fluid collection around ovary
- Hydrosalpinx
  - Tubular shape
  - Incomplete septae

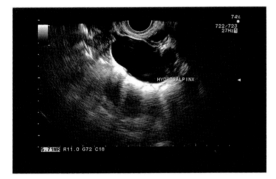

Figure 5.7 Ultrasonographic picture of hydrosalpinx. Elongated, tubular and anechoic lesion in a woman with chronic pelvic pain.

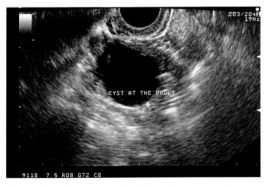

Figure 5.8 Ultrasonographic picture showing ovarian cyst at the vault of the vagina in a woman who had undergone hysterectomy 2 years earlier.

Doppler technology

Blood flow through the organs can be visualized using Doppler technology. Colour flow Doppler displays blood flow in red and blue. Conventionally, red indicates flow towards the transducer and blue away from the transducer.

Flow during systole and diastole are measured and various indices are calculated mechanically.

The **resistance index** and the **pulsatility index** are commonly used. The resistance index is low (<0.4) when there is neovascularization and increase in blood flow as in malignancy, ectopic pregnancy and myomas. High resistance indicates normal tissue or benign disease (Fig. 5.9).

Vascularity can be assessed using colour Doppler. In endometrial cancer, colour flow is increased and the presence of myometrial invasion can be assessed. In ovarian torsion, there is reduction or lack of colour flow. The conditions where colour Doppler test is useful are listed in Box 5.11.

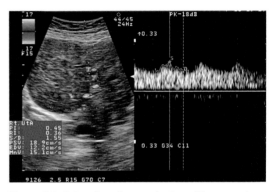

Figure 5.9 Colour Doppler examination of the ovary. There is increased blood flow within this vascular, solid ovarian mass and the Doppler waveform reveals a low-resistance continuous flow pattern with low resistance index of 0.4.

- Torsion of ovarian cyst
- Ectopic pregnancy
- Ovarian malignancy
- Endometrial cancer
- Myoma
- Adenomyosis

Saline infusion sonography

Saline infusion sonography (SIS) is also called **sonohysterography** (SHG; Fig. 5.10). When tubal patency is also assessed by this, it is termed **sonohysterosalpingography** or **sonosalpingography**.

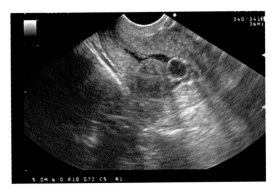

Figure 5.10 Saline infusion sonography. Picture shows endometrial cavity with polyp. Bulb of Foley's catheter is also visible.

- The procedure is usually performed on day 5 or 6 of the cycle. It is an outpatient procedure and is well tolerated.
- After excluding contraindications such as acute PID, haematometra and cervical stenosis and performing a transvaginal ultrasonography, a cannula is inserted into the uterine cavity. Backflow may be prevented by using a catheter with a balloon and inflating the balloon. About 5–30 mL of saline is injected gradually (Box 5.12).
- The endometrial cavity is visualized with the transvaginal transducer. Polyps and submucous myomas are well delineated since they are surrounded by anechoic fluid.
- Tubal patency can be studied by direct visualization of the presence or the absence of fluid spill into the peritoneal cavity using transvaginal ultrasonography or Doppler test.

Box 5.12 Saline infusion sonography (performed on day 5 or 6 of the cycle)

- To visualize
  - Uterine cavity
    - Polyps
    - Submucous myoma
  - Tubes
    - Tubal patency
- Catheter/cannula inserted into the uterus
  - 5–30 mL saline injected
- Contraindications
  - Acute PID
  - Haematometra
  - Cervical stenosis

PID, pelvic inflammatory disease.

Hysterosalpingography

HSG is used in the evaluation of infertility. Uterine anomalies, abnormalities of uterine cavity, tubal occlusion and hydrosalpinx can be visualized.

- HSG must be performed in the follicular phase, after the bleeding stops.
- A cannula is inserted into the uterine cavity and water or oil-soluble radio-opaque dye is injected. Water-soluble dye is better for delineating intraluminal pathology, but oil-soluble dye provides a better-quality image.
- A therapeutic effect has been noted with HSG especially in women with unexplained infertility.
- Since the prevalence of chlamydial infection is high among infertile women, prophylactic doxycycline, 100 mg twice daily, beginning on the day prior to the procedure and continued for 5 days is recommended.
- Tubal spasm may give a false impression of tubal block. This may be relieved by antispasmodics. Abnormalities can be diagnosed. Contraindications and complications are listed in Box 5.13.
- Intrauterine lesions such as polyp, uterine anomalies such as bicornuate uterus, tubal block, hydrosalpinx, beaded appearance in tuberculous salpingitis and intrauterine adhesions can be visualized by hysterosalpingogram (Fig. 5.11a and b).

Selective salpingography

Hysteroscopic tubal cannulation and injection of radio-opaque dye into the tube to selectively visualize tubal pathology is termed **selective salpingography**. Tubal cannulation may also be performed under fluoroscopic guidance. It is performed during the follicular phase; water or oil-soluble dye is used. A guidewire can be introduced to relieve proximal tubal block.

Computed tomography

Computed tomography (CT) scan is an imaging modality that uses X-rays to generate the images. With the current-generation multidetector CT

Box 5.13 **Hysterosalpingography**

- Procedure
  - Performed in follicular phase (days 6–11)
  - Water- or oil-soluble contrast dye
  - Fluoroscopic visualization
  - X-rays for documentation
- Indication
  - Evaluation of
    - Infertility
    - Recurrent pregnancy loss
    - Uterine anomalies
- Therapeutic effect
  - Increase in spontaneous pregnancy rate
- Uterine pathology
  - Polyps
  - Myomas
  - Congenital anomalies
  - Bicornuate, septate, T-shaped, arcuate
  - Intrauterine synechiae
- Tubal pathology
  - Tubal block
  - Hydrosalpinx
  - Diverticuli
- Disadvantages
  - Cannot diagnose peritubal pathology
  - Tubal spasm—False-positive result
- Contraindications
  - Acute PID
  - Bleeding
  - Allergy to iodine
- Complications
  - Infection or flare-up
  - Uterine perforation
  - Vasovagal reaction
  - Intravasation of dye
  - Embolic phenomena—Oil-soluble dye
  - Allergic reaction to dye

PID, pelvic inflammatory disease.

scanner, imaging can be performed in less than a minute. Images are acquired in axial plane. However, current technology allows images to be reconstructed in other planes, most commonly the coronal and the sagittal plane.

The average radiation dose from a CT of the abdomen and pelvis is around 10 mSv, which is approximately equal to 500 chest radiographs. Thus, there must be absolute indications for CT scan that should outweigh its risks. Intravenous nonionic iodinate contrast agent is used for better delineation of anatomy. However, renal failure and allergy to previous IV contrast agents are absolute contraindications for IV contrast injection. Oral and rectal contrast can also be used to improve visualization.

Applications of CT in gynaecology are listed in Box 5.14 (Fig. 5.12). CT scan is an excellent staging investigation for gynaecological cancers

Box 5.14 **Applications of CT in gynaecology**

- Gynaecological malignancies
  - Ascites, omental and peritoneal thickening
  - Retroperitoneal nodes >1.5–2 cm
  - Hydroureteronephrosis
  - Bowel involvement
  - Metastasis in liver and spleen
  - Subdiaphragmatic disease
- Benign disease
  - Intraperitoneal abscess
  - Dermoid cyst
  - Pelvic vein thrombosis

CT, computed tomography.

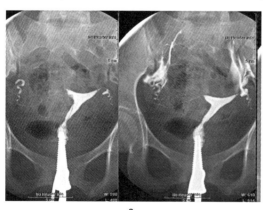

a.

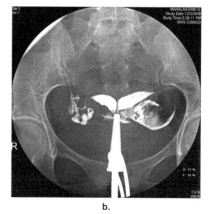

b.

Figure 5.11 Hysterosalpingogram. a. Early and late phases of a hysterosalpingogram showing a normal uterus and fallopian tubes. There is bilateral free peritoneal spill of the contrast material. b. Hysterosalpingogram in a young lady showing two separate uterine horns with a single cervix (bicornuate unicollis). Both tubes are patent with peritoneal spill demonstrated on the left side.

adenopathy and metastases to the liver, adrenal glands, lungs and the bones.

Disadvantages of CT scan are radiation exposure and poor soft tissue resolution in the pelvis. Thus, CT is not useful to assess uterine pathologies or visualizing parametrial infiltration; therefore, its value is limited in local staging of gynaecological malignancies especially in endometrial and cervical cancer and evaluation of uterine anomalies.

Positron emission tomography

Biochemical and metabolic abnormalities precede the anatomical changes in malignancy. Certain radiochemical compounds are taken up by these tissues and metabolized. These compounds can be used as tracers to locate the areas of malignant change or infection. The commonly used tracer is 2-[^{18}F]fluoro-2-deoxy-d-glucose (FDG). Positron emission tomography (PET) along with CT in the form of PET–CT gives the advantage of good two-dimensional anatomical delineation along with metabolic information. PET is useful in staging cancers and detecting early recurrences in cancer. It is being used in follow-up of patients with ovarian cancer and other gynaecological malignancies (Fig. 5.13). The role of PET in early diagnosis of cancers is uncertain.

Magnetic resonance imaging

Magnetic resonance imaging (MRI) is one of the great advancements in imaging technology and involves no ionizing radiation. Patient is placed in a high-strength magnet, commonly 1.5- or 3-T magnets. This magnetic field polarizes the protons in the body. Radio-frequency signals emitted by the depolarizing tissue protons when the magnetic field is switched off temporarily are used to construct the images. The images can be obtained in any desired plane. By varying the time of application of radio-frequency pulses and sampling the emitted signal, T1- and T2-weighted images are obtained.

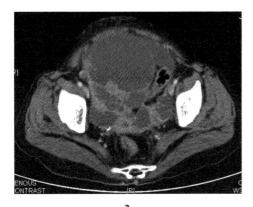

a.

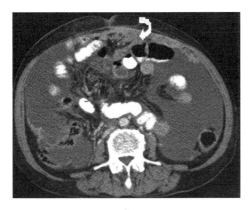

b.

c.

Figure 5.12 CT scan with oral and IV contrast. a. Bilateral cystic and solid masses in the adnexa with enhancement of the solid areas. b. The asterisk (*) denotes the uterus; adjoining cysts show enhancing walls. c. Omental thickening (curved arrow) is referred to as 'omental cake'. *CT*, computed tomography.

and widely used for this purpose. CT can clearly demonstrate ascites, omental caking, ureteric and bowel involvement, retroperitoneal

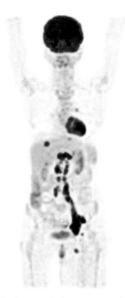

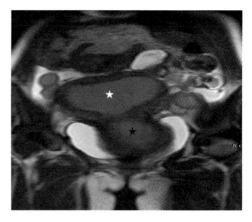

Figure 5.13 Positron emission tomography of the whole body after intravenous FDG in a woman with recurrent ovarian cancer reveals abnormal increased FDG accumulation in the left adnexal mass, multiple left internal iliac, bilateral common iliac, para-aortic and aortocaval nodes, right lobe of liver, pubic bone, left acetabulum and left paravertebral soft tissue. *FDG*, 2-[¹⁸F] fluoro-2-deoxy-D-glucose.

Different tissues appear with different intensity or brightness in T1- and T2-weighted images depending on the density of protons within them (Figs 5.14 and 5.15). Paramagnetic contrast agents such as gadolinium–DTPA are used for better delineation of the tissues.

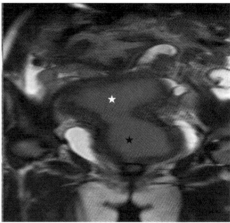

Figure 5.15 MRI showing transverse vaginal septum with haematocolpos (black star) and haematometra (white star). Between the distended vagina and distended uterus is the narrow cervix. *MRI*, magnetic resonance imaging.

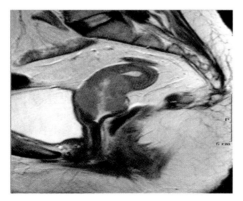

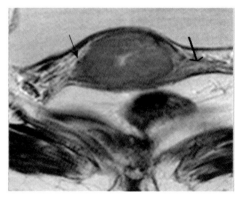

Figure 5.14 Magnetic resonance imaging (MRI). T2 high-resolution sagittal and axial images through the pelvis of a lady with intermittent vaginal bleeding. Cervix is replaced by tumour with breach of endocervical stromal ring and extracervical extension into bilateral parametrium (arrows). MRI can accurately stage cervical cancer.

Applications of MRI in gynaecology are listed in Box 5.15.

Advantages

Overall, superior soft tissue resolution offered by MRI makes it the modality of choice when delineation of accurate anatomy and morphology of the lesion is important. Thus, MRI scores over other modalities such as ultrasonograpy and CT and most commonly used for conditions such as adenomyosis, local staging of gynaecological malignancies, uterine anomalies and endometriosis.

Box 5.15 Applications of MRI in gynaecology

- Myoma
  - Differentiation of myoma from adenomyoma
  - Localization of submucous, intramural and subserous myoma
  - MRI-guided FUS to treat myoma
- Adenomyosis
  - Accurate diagnosis
- Endometriosis
  - Modality of choice in deep pelvic endometriosis
  - Extent of disease and roadmap for surgery
- Congenital uterovaginal anomalies
  - Bicornuate, septate, subseptate
  - Unicornuate, didelphys, rudimentary horn
  - Vaginal anomalies
- Gynaecological cancer
  - Modality of choice for local staging of pelvic cancers
    - Cervical cancer
      - Parametrial infiltration
      - Endocervical extension
    - Endometrial cancer
      - Myometrial invasion
      - Cervical extension
    - Ovarian cancer
      - Modality of choice for characterizing ovarian masses
      - Malignant versus benign masses
      - Ascites
      - Retroperitoneal nodes
      - Bowel, bladder metastasis
      - Liver, omental metastasis
    - Vulval cancer
      - Urethral, vaginal and anal canal involvement
  - Can be used in gynaecological cancers in pregnancy
- Vascular malformation in the pelvis and perineum
  - To assess extent

FUS, focused ultrasound surgery; *MRI*, magnetic resonance imaging.

Disadvantages

MRI may not be available in all centres. High cost of MRI is a disadvantage. MRI is contraindicated in patients with cardiac pacemakers and defibrillating devices. Hip prosthesis and implants used in spine surgeries can cause severe artefacts in the pelvic MR images. Just like CT contrast agents, MRI contrast agents are also contraindicated in renal failure. Lastly, MRI is a noisy procedure and claustrophobia is a relative contraindication for MRI.

Imaging-guided procedures

Diagnostic and therapeutic procedures guided by imaging are becoming popular since they are minimally invasive, avoid unnecessary laparotomy and help in early diagnosis. Procedures commonly performed are enumerated in Box 5.16.

Box 5.16 Imaging-guided procedures

- Ultrasound/CT-guided procedures
  - Aspiration of ascitic fluid
  - Aspiration of pus/blood for the diagnosis of haemoperitoneum/pyoperitoneum
  - Drainage of pus/blood from cul-de-sac
  - Drainage of pus from abdomen
  - FNAC of pelvic/abdominal masses
  - FNAC of lymph nodes for the diagnosis of
    - Malignancy
    - Tuberculosis
  - Guided biopsy from abdominal/pelvic masses
  - Stenting of ureters
- MR-guided procedures
  - MR-guided FUS

CT, computed tomography; *FNAC*, fine-needle aspiration cytology; *FUS*, focused ultrasound surgery; *MR*, magnetic resonance.

Uterine artery embolization

Uterine artery embolization (UAE) is used to reduce the vascularity, which in turn causes necrosis and shrinkage of myomas. This helps in reducing the symptoms such as heavy menstrual bleeding and dysmenorrhoea. Polyvinyl alcohol particles are used to embolize the vessels. Both uterine arteries are super selectively cannulated through bilateral femoral arterial access under fluoroscopic guidance and the particles are injected. The effects and complications of the procedure are listed in Box 5.17. Several pregnancies have been reported in literature after the procedure.

Choice of imaging modality

Familiarizing oneself with the strengths and weaknesses of each modality, their indications and contraindications will help one choose the right modality of imaging. Having said that, the ground rule is that the ultrasonography is the first and initial modality of choice because of its wide applications, nonionizing nature and wide availability. CT is a useful modality for staging cancers and can be a good problem-solving tool in specific situations. MRI is the modality of

> **Box 5.17 Uterine artery embolization**
>
> - Procedure
>   - Polyvinyl alcohol particles
>   - Uterine arteries cannulated through femoral arterial access
>   - Fluoroscopic guidance
> - Results
>   - Reduction in bleeding, pain, size
>   - Relief of pressure symptoms
> - Complications
>   - Postembolization syndrome
>   - Nausea, vomiting
>   - Fever, malaise
>   - Passage of necrotic tissue through vagina
>   - Pain
>   - Infection
>   - Occasional ovarian failure

choice for uterine anomalies, endometriosis and local staging of gynaecological cancers.

Algorithms for choosing the appropriate imaging modality are given in Figs 5.16 and 5.17.

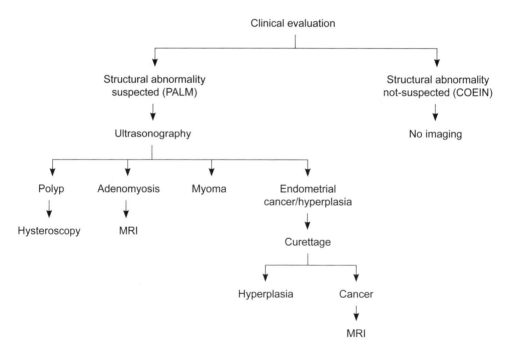

Figure 5.16 Algorithm for imaging in abnormal uterine bleeding. *MRI*, magnetic resonance imaging.

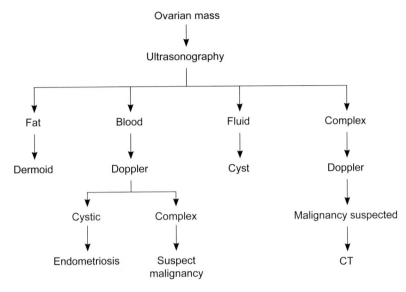

Figure 5.17 Algorithm for imaging in ovarian mass. *CT*, computed tomography.

Key points

- Several imaging modalities are currently available, and these have greatly increased the diagnostic accuracy. They may also detect incidental abnormalities that are not of clinical significance.

- Ultrasonography is the most commonly used imaging modality. The American College of Ultrasound Medicine has developed guidelines for indications, equipment and documentation of pelvic ultrasonography.

- The gynaecologist should be familiar with the appearance of normal uterus and adnexa.

- Ultrasonography may be used in the evaluation of abnormalities of the uterus, endometrium, ovaries and fallopian tubes.

- Ultrasonography can be used to detect gynaecological conditions causing acute or chronic pelvic pain. It is not very useful in conditions such as appendicitis, diverticulitis and inflammatory bowel disease.

- Blood flow through the organs can be visualized by Doppler technology. Resistance index can be used to differentiate benign from malignant lesions, detect myometrial invasion of tumour and diagnose ectopic pregnancy.

- Saline infusion sonography is useful for diagnosis of endometrial lesions such as polyps and submucous myomas.

- Hysterosalpingography is used in the evaluation of infertility and uterine anomalies. Shape of the uterine cavity, uterine anomalies and tubal occlusion can be visualized.

- Computed tomography (CT) with IV contrast is an excellent modality for the diagnosis of intraperitoneal and retroperitoneal spread of ovarian cancer and other malignancies.

- Positron emission tomography (PET) is useful in detecting recurrence of cancer.

- Magnetic resonance imaging (MRI) is superior to the other modalities in the diagnosis of adenomyosis, congenital uterovaginal anomalies, myometrial infiltration in endometrial cancer and parametrial infiltration in cervical cancer. Ultrasound and CT-guided procedures are used for aspiration of ascitic fluid, ovarian cysts and pus, fine-needle aspiration cytology (FNAC) of pelvic and abdominal mass or lymph nodes, and guided biopsy of tumours. Uterine artery embolization is a fluoroscopic-guided procedure used to reduce the vascularity that causes necrosis and shrinkage of myomas.

Self-assessment

Case-based questions

Case 1

A 42-year-old lady was found to have an ovarian cyst of 5 × 6 cm on ultrasonography during master health check-up.

1. What features suggest malignancy?
2. What further tests will you order?

Case 2

A 17-year-old girl presents with recurrent cyclical abdominal pain and history of primary amenorrhoea. Clinical examination revealed a blind vagina about 2 inches deep and a mass above it.

1. What is the diagnosis?
2. What imaging will you order initially?
3. Before deciding on surgical intervention, what imaging will you ask for and why?

Answers

Case 1

1. Bilateral tumours, solid or mixed solid and cystic, septae >3 mm thick, papillary excrescences thick cyst wall >3 mm, ascites, omental thickening, enlarged para-aortic nodes and liver metastasis.

2. If malignancy is suspected, a CT scan to look for disease on the under surface of the diaphragm, lesser sac and other areas in upper abdomen. CA 125 and Doppler studies if the cyst looks benign, to exclude malignancy.

Case 2

1. Outflow obstruction of the genital tract, probably transverse vaginal septum or partial vaginal atresia.
2. Ultrasonography to look for haematocolpos, haematometra and involvement of tubes.
3. MRI to locate the site and extent of vaginal atresia, extent of involvement of tubes (haematosalpinx) and ovarian endometriosis. Also to exclude renal anomalies.

Long-answer questions

1. Discuss the role of ultrasonography in gynaecology.

Short-answer questions

1. Hysterosalpingography
2. Sonohysterography
3. Uterine artery embolization
4. Ultrasonographic features of malignant ovarian tumours
5. Uses of MRI in gynaecology

6

Gynaecological Symptoms and Differential Diagnosis

Case scenario

Mrs VK, 28, recently married, was brought to the emergency room with acute lower abdominal pain. She had vomited once, but had no other symptoms. Examination revealed tenderness in the right iliac fossa, and the surgeons made a diagnosis of acute appendicitis. Laparoscopy was performed and the appendix looked normal, but the right tube was the site of an ectopic pregnancy. Postoperatively, on questioning, the patient gave a history of amenorrhoea for 45 days and spotting on and off for 5 days.

Introduction

Women present to gynaecologists with a symptom or a group of symptoms. The symptoms of different gynaecological and nongynaecological problems overlap. A basic understanding of the pathophysiology of these symptoms leads to a set of possible differential diagnoses. This forms the basis of relevant details in history taking, thorough clinical examination, further evaluation and appropriate investigations so as to arrive at a diagnosis and in turn systematic management of the patient.

Common gynaecological symptoms

The symptoms that the patient presents with give an idea as to where the problem is and what it could be. Attention to the patient's complaints is extremely important. Leading questions pertaining to the symptoms may improve clarity. The common gynaecological symptoms are listed in Box 6.1.

Box 6.1 Common symptoms in gynaecology

- Abnormal uterine bleeding
- Vaginal discharge
- Lower abdominal mass
- Mass descending per vaginum
- Acute/chronic pelvic pain
- Dysmenorrhoea
- Genital ulcer/swelling/pruritus
- Dyspareunia
- Urinary symptoms
- Bowel symptoms

Abnormal uterine bleeding

Normal menstrual cycles vary from 21 to 35 days, duration of bleeding from 2 to 8 days and volume of flow from 30 to 40 mL. Specific terms used to describe abnormal bleeding, pathogenesis and management of abnormal uterine bleeding (AUB) are dealt with in detail in Chapter 7, *Abnormal uterine bleeding*.

Causes

The classification of AUB is given in Box 6.2.

Box 6.2 Classification of abnormal bleeding

PALM
- P—Polyp
- A—Adenomyosis
- L—Leiomyomas
  - Submucosal myoma (LSM)
  - Other (LO)
- M—Malignancy and hyperplasia

COEIN
- C—Coagulopathy
- O—Ovulatory dysfunction
- E—Endometrial
- I—Iatrogenic
- N—Not yet classified

Postmenopausal bleeding

In women with postmenopausal bleeding, a few other conditions should be considered (Box 6.3).

Although cervical cancer usually occurs in the perimenopausal age, it is not uncommon in the postmenopausal woman. Oestrogen deficiency vaginitis (senile vaginitis) presents with scanty bleeding or blood-stained discharge. Speculum examination reveals a thin, dry, erythematous vaginal mucosa. Atrophic endometrium, hyperplasia and polyp are diagnosed by transvaginal ultrasonography (TVS). All women with

---

Box 6.3 Postmenopausal bleeding

- Oestrogen deficiency vaginitis
- Atrophic endometrium
- Endometrial hyperplasia
- Endometrial polyps
- Endometrial cancer
- Cervical cancer
- Granulosa cell tumour of the ovary

---

postmenopausal bleeding, however, should be evaluated by TVS and endometrial sampling to rule out endometrial cancer.

Polyp may be endometrial or cervical. Intrauterine contraceptive device (IUCD)-related bleeding is iatrogenic, and bleeding associated with endometriosis and retained products of conception is unclassified bleeding.

Clinical evaluation

Clinical evaluation in a woman with AUB should be as given in Box 6.4.

It is possible to arrive at a diagnosis in most cases with history and physical examination. If structural abnormalities are suspected, **ultrasonography** is the next step in evaluation. Abdominal and vaginal ultrasonography should be performed. **Pap smear** is mandatory in all, except young girls who are not sexually active. **Endometrial sampling** with Pipelle is required in postmenopausal or perimenopausal women in whom endometrial cancer is suspected. If a cervical growth is seen, it should be **biopsied**.

Women with AUB and no structural anomalies have coagulopathy, AUB-O, AUB-E or iatrogenic causes of bleeding and should be evaluated accordingly

Algorithm for differential diagnosis and investigations of AUB is given in Fig. 6.1. Evaluation of postmenopausal bleeding is discussed in Chapter 30, *Premalignant and malignant diseases of the uterus*.

Box 6.4 Clinical evaluation of abnormal uterine bleeding

- History
  - Type of bleeding
  - Associated symptoms
    - Preceded by amenorrhoea
    - Pelvic pain
    - Dysmenorrhoea—Congestive/spasmodic
    - Dyspareunia
    - Vaginal discharge
- Physical examination
  - Abdominal mass
  - Speculum examination—Polyp, growth
  - Bimanual examination
    - Uterine enlargement—Regular/irregular
    - Adnexal mass—Cystic/solid/mixed; tenderness

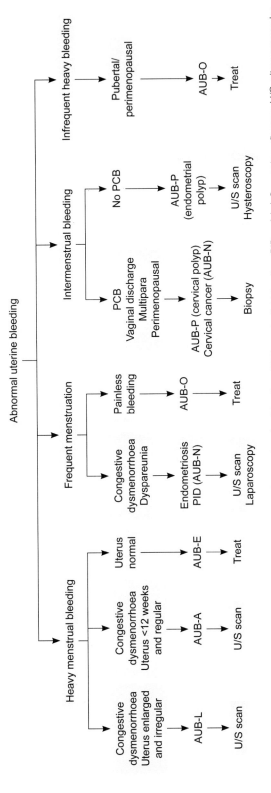

Figure 6.1 Differential diagnosis and investigation of AUB. *AUB*, abnormal uterine bleeding; *PCB*, postcoital bleeding; *PID*, pelvic inflammatory disease; *U/S*, ultrasonography.

Vaginal discharge

Vaginal discharge may be **physiological** or **pathological**. Physiological increase in secretions occurs during ovulation, premenstrually and during pregnancy. The discharge is mucoid, has no odour and is nonirritant. Pathological discharge may be from lesions in the vagina or cervix, or due to pelvic inflammatory disease (PID). The aetiology varies in different age groups. In children, it is commonly due to vulvovaginitis; in women of reproductive age, it is due to vaginitis, cervicitis or PID; and in postmenopausal women, malignancy must be ruled out.

In children

Prepubertal oestrogen deficiency increases the susceptibility of the vagina to infections. This can be nonspecific or due to specific causes (Box 6.5).

Box 6.5 Causes of vaginal discharge in children

- Nonspecific vulvovaginitis
  - Poor hygiene
  - Allergy
  - Foreign body
- Specific vulvovaginitis
  - *Streptococcus*
  - Other bacteria
  - Pinworm
  - *Candida*
  - *Trichomonas*

Clinical evaluation

Examination under good light helps to evaluate the nature of discharge and take a swab for culture and microscopic examination for *Candida* and *Trichomonas*. Presence of pinworms or skin lesions indicating fungal infection should also be looked for. If the discharge is blood-stained or foreign body is suspected, examination under anaesthesia is recommended.

In reproductive years

Causes of vaginal discharge in women of reproductive age are listed in Box 6.6.

Vaginitis is the most common cause of vaginal discharge. *Trichomonas* infection is sexually transmitted, and bacterial vaginosis (BV) is a sexually associated disease. Pruritus is

---

Box 6.6 Causes of vaginal discharge in reproductive years

- Vaginitis
  - Bacterial vaginosis
  - *Trichomonas* vaginitis
  - *Candida* vaginitis
- Cervicitis
  - Gonococcal infection
  - *Chlamydia trachomatis* infection
- Acute pelvic infection
  - Gonococcal infection
  - *C. trachomatis* infection
  - Other aerobic and anaerobic pathogens
- Chronic pelvic infection
  - Tuberculosis
  - Other infections

---

intense in *Candida* and *Trichomonas* infections. Distinguishing features of the three common types of vaginitis, their diagnosis and management are discussed in Chapter 12, *Infections of the lower genital tract*.

Both gonococcal and chlamydial infections are sexually transmitted. They present with mucopurulent discharge. Infections can ascend to cause acute PID. Clinical features of gonococcal and chlamydial cervicitis and their management are discussed in Chapter 12, *Infections of the lower genital tract*.

Acute pelvic infections are most often caused by the same organisms that cause cervicitis. When infection ascends to become PID, women present with other symptoms such as fever, tachycardia, lower abdominal pain and signs of septicaemia. The triad of lower abdominal pain, adnexal tenderness and cervical motion tenderness is said to be diagnostic. The Centers for Disease Control and Prevention (CDC) guidelines for diagnosis of acute PID are given in Chapter 13, *Infections of the upper genital tract*. TVS may reveal inflamed tubes, tubo-ovarian mass, free fluid in the pelvis or pelvic abscess.

Women with genital tuberculosis present with other symptoms such as fever, weight loss, AUB, amenorrhoea or infertility. They may also complain of vaginal discharge.

Clinical evaluation

It is possible to make a diagnosis by history, physical examination and microscopic examination of the discharge after addition of saline and KOH (Box 6.7). Culture is required in some

- History
  - Type of discharge
  - Pruritus
  - Dysuria, spotting
  - Lower abdominal pain
  - Constitutional symptoms
  - Sexual activity, new sexual partner
- Abdominal examination
  - Tenderness, mass
- Speculum examination
  - Discharge—Colour, odour, consistency
  - Nature—Frothy, curdy, homogeneous
  - Mucopus from the cervix
  - Vaginal pH
- Pelvic examination
  - Adnexal mass, tenderness
  - Tenderness on moving the cervix
  - Fullness in the pouch of Douglas

women. Syndromic approach is discussed in Chapter 12, *Infections of the lower genital tract.*

Investigations

After a thorough history and clinical examination, evaluation of the discharge, cultures and Pap smear should be performed. Since women with *Trichomonas* infection, gonorrhoea and chlamydial infections are at a high risk for other sexually transmitted infections, Venereal Disease Research Laboratory (VDRL)

and human immunodeficiency virus (HIV) test should also be ordered (Box 6.8). A simple algorithm for diagnosis of vaginal infections is given in Fig. 6.2.

Box 6.8 Investigations—Examination of the vaginal discharge in women during their reproductive years

- Wet film
  - *Trichomonas* vaginalis
  - Clue cells
  - KOH preparation
  - Whiff test
  - Fungal pseudohyphae/spores
- Gram stain
  - Gram-negative diplococci
  - Neutrophils
- Pap smear
- Serology for syphilis
- HIV serology
- Full blood count
  - If PID is suspected

HIV, human immunodeficiency virus; *PID*, pelvic inflammatory disease.

In postmenopausal women

Women who are postmenopausal have oestrogen deficiency, which causes atrophy and thinning of the epithelium and alters the vaginal pH. This increases the susceptibility to infection by bacteria. But cervical cancer, endometrial

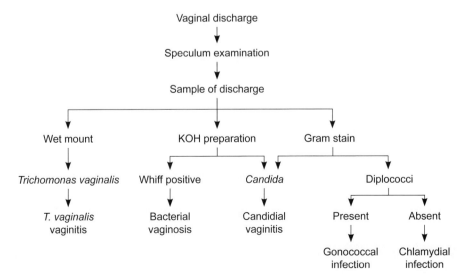

Figure 6.2 Diagnosis of vaginal infections in reproductive age.

Table 6.1   Causes of discharge in postmenopausal women

Condition	Clinical features
Oestrogen deficiency vaginitis	• Purulent discharge • Spotting/bleeding
Cervical cancer	• Foul odour, purulent discharge • Bloodstained discharge • Postcoital bleeding
Pyometra	• Fever, tachycardia • Bloodstained discharge • Enlarged, tender uterus

cancer with pyometra and occasionally cancer of the fallopian tube can present with discharge. Therefore, postmenopausal women with discharge must be evaluated for malignancy.

Causes of discharge in postmenopausal women are listed in Table 6.1.

Clinical evaluation

This is as listed in Box 6.9.

Box 6.9   Clinical evaluation of vaginal discharge in postmenopausal women

- History
  - Type of discharge
  - Bloodstained discharge
  - Postmenopausal bleeding
  - Postcoital bleeding
  - Family history of genital cancers
- Examination
  - Fever, tachycardia
  - Speculum examination
    - Oestrogen deficiency changes
    - Nature of discharge
    - Growth on the ectocervix
  - Bimanual examination
    - Endocervical enlargement
    - Uterine enlargement
    - Uterine tenderness
    - Adnexal mass

Investigations

Appropriate investigations should be ordered after a clinical diagnosis is arrived at (Box 6.10).

Box 6.10   Investigations in postmenopausal women with vaginal discharge

- Pap smear
- Transvaginal ultrasound
  - Endocervical growth
  - Endometrial growth
  - Pyometra
  - Adnexal mass
- Endometrial sampling
- Cervical biopsy

Lower abdominal mass

Lower abdominal mass in women most commonly arises from internal genital organs, although it can arise from bowel, bladder and other organs as well. Most masses arising from genital organs are uterine or ovarian, and occasionally paraovarian, tubal or cervical. The types of tumours vary in different age groups. However, benign ovarian neoplasms can occur at any age.

In adolescents

Below 10 years of age, dysgerminomas, teratomas and granulosa cell tumours can occur. However, their occurrence is rare. During adolescence, with the hormonal changes of puberty, functional ovarian cysts appear. Once menstruation begins, uterovaginal anomalies with outflow obstruction present haematometra or haematocolpos (Box 6.11). Other masses are seen occasionally (Fig. 6.3).

In reproductive years

Pregnancy must always be thought of in all women during their reproductive years presenting with lower abdominal mass. Ectopic pregnancy and vesicular mole are other conditions to be kept in mind. Conditions giving rise to lower abdominal masses in this age group are listed in Box 6.12. Myomas arising from the uterus or cervix are the most common tumours in this age group. When an adnexal mass is seen, functional cysts must be considered first. They can vary in size from 3 to 10 cm. They regress when followed up for 2–3 months. Benign cystic teratoma and serous cystadenoma are the most common neoplastic ovarian masses. Other epithelia tumours such as mucinous, endometrioid and Brenner

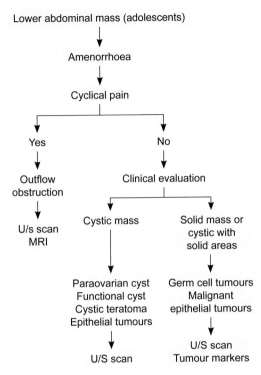

Figure 6.3 Evaluation of lower abdominal mass in adolescents. *MRI*, magnetic resonance imaging; *U/S*, ultrasound.

Box 6.11 **Lower abdominal mass in adolescents**

- Outflow obstruction
  - Haematocolpos
  - Haematometra
  - Haematosalpinx
- Paraovarian cyst
- Ovarian masses
  - Benign
    - Follicular cyst
    - Benign cystic teratoma
    - Serous/mucinous cystadenoma
    - Other epithelial tumours
  - Malignant
    - Germ cell tumours
      o Dysgerminoma
      o Malignant teratoma
      o Embryonal carcinoma
      o Other germ cell tumours
  - Epithelial tumours

Box 6.12 **Lower abdominal masses in reproductive years**

- Pregnancy
  - Intrauterine
  - Ectopic
  - Vesicular mole
- Uterine
  - Myoma
  - Adenomyoma
- Cervix
  - Myoma
- Mesonephric remnants
  - Paraovarian/paratubal cysts
- Fallopian tube
  - Hydrosalpinx
  - Tubo-ovarian mass
- Ovary
  - Functional cysts
  - Endometriotic cysts
  - Benign cystic teratoma
  - Serous cystadenoma
  - Mucinous/endometrioid/Brenner tumours
  - Malignant
    - Epithelial tumours
    - Germ cell tumours

tumour are next in the list. Malignant epithelial tumours can occur, though not as commonly as in the older women. Fig. 6.4 gives the algorithm for diagnosis of lower abdominal mass during reproductive years.

In the perimenopausal and postmenopausal years

Lower abdominal masses in this group may still be benign (75%), but malignant tumours of the uterus and ovaries are more common than in younger women (25%). Therefore, as in the case of postmenopausal women with bleeding or discharge, evaluation to rule out malignancy is mandatory. Common causes of lower abdominal mass in this age group are listed in Box 6.13. Benign epithelial tumours and endometriotic cysts do occur in this age group and are usually <5 cm, cystic and uniloculated. Most masses that are >10 cm in size, solid and

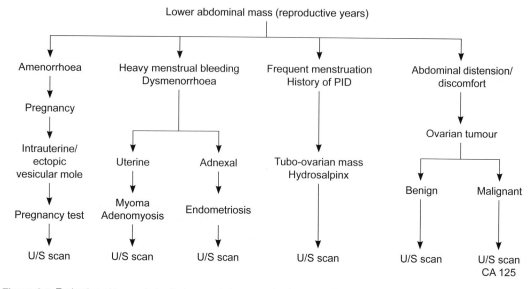

Figure 6.4 Evaluation of lower abdominal mass during reproductive years. *PID*, pelvic inflammatory disease; *U/S*, ultrasound.

Box 6.13 **Common causes of lower abdominal mass in older women**

- Uterine
  - Myoma
  - Adenomyoma
  - Endometrial carcinoma
  - Uterine sarcomas
- Ovarian
  - Benign
    - Epithelial tumours
    - Endometriosis
  - Malignant
    - Epithelial tumours
    - Secondary tumours
    - Stromal and germ cell tumours
- Other tumours
  - Lymphoma
  - Bowel/bladder tumours

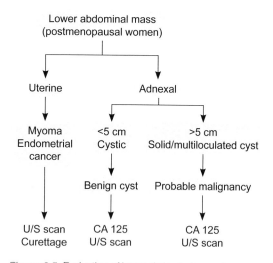

Figure 6.5 Evaluation of lower abdominal mass in postmenopausal women. *U/S*, ultrasound.

associated with ascites are malignant. CA 125 is used as a tumour marker in malignant epithelial tumours. Algorithm for diagnosis of lower abdominal mass in older women is given in Fig. 6.5.

Clinical evaluation

Symptoms

Most uterine and cervical masses are associated with AUB, dysmenorrhoea or pressure symptoms (Box 6.14). Adnexal masses may be asymptomatic or give rise to pain.

Physical examination

General examination for other signs of malignancy and lymphadenopathy, and abdominal and pelvic examination should be performed. It is important to ascertain if the mass is arising from pelvis (*see* Chapter 4, *Gynaecological history and physical examination*). Lower margin of the

- Adolescents
  - Menstrual abnormality/amenorrhoea
  - Cyclic abdominal pain
- Reproductive years
  - Amenorrhoea/abnormal uterine bleeding
  - Congestive/spasmodic dysmenorrhoea
  - Pressure symptoms
    - Urinary retention
    - Difficulty in voiding
  - Lower abdominal pain
  - Dyspareunia/infertility
- Perimenopausal/postmenopausal years
  - Abnormal uterine/postmenopausal bleeding
  - Abdominal distension
  - Loss of appetite/weight

mass is not palpable, and it is not possible to 'get below' the swelling in a mass arising from the pelvis (Box 6.15).

Investigations

Imaging is most important in the evaluation of lower abdominal masses. This may be by ultrasonography, computed tomography (CT) or magnetic resonance imaging (MRI; *see* Chapter 5, *Imaging in gynaecology*). **Doppler flow studies** and calculation of resistance index may be required when there is a suspicious adnexal mass. **Tumour markers** such as CA 125, α-fetoprotein and lactic dehydrogenase are useful in the diagnosis of malignant ovarian tumours.

Algorithms for the evaluation of lower abdominal mass in adolescents, women during their

Box 6.15 Physical examination in lower
         abdominal mass

- General examination
  - Lymphadenopathy
  - Weight loss
- Abdominal examination
  - Location of the mass
  - Size, consistency
  - Mobility, margins
  - Ascites
  - Hepatosplenomegaly
- Pelvic examination
  - Uterus versus adnexal mass
  - Uterus—Size, shape, mobility
  - Adnexal mass—Size, consistency, mobility, tenderness

reproductive years and postmenopausal women are given in Figs 6.3–6.5, respectively.

Mass descending per vaginum

The most common cause of mass descending per vaginum is **pelvic organ prolapse** (POP). This usually occurs in multiparous women, often postmenopausal (*see* Chapter 24, *Pelvic organ prolapse*). Other causes of mass descending per vaginum are congenital hypertrophic elongation of the cervix, polyps arising from the cervix or endometrium, vaginal cysts and chronic inversion of the uterus (Table 6.2).

Table 6.2 Mass descending per vaginum

Condition	Clinical features
Pelvic organ prolapse	• Uterine prolapse • Anterior vaginal wall prolapse • Posterior vaginal wall prolapse • Distance from bladder sulcus to external os normal • Fornices shallow
Congenital elongation of cervix	• Elongation of portiovaginalis of cervix • Distance from bladder sulcus to external os increased • Fornices deep
Polyps	• Pedicle attached to or extending through the os • Cervix in normal position • On traction on polyp, cervix does not move up
Chronic inversion of uterus	• Often has a myoma polyp at fundus • Uterine fundus not palpable • Cervix high up • On traction on inverted fundus, cervix moves up • Uterine sound cannot be passed beyond few centimetres • Vaginal cysts rarely protrude beyond introitus • Gartner cysts are anterolateral

Chronic uterine inversion is rare and difficult to diagnose clinically. Often a myoma polyp attached to the uterine fundus is the cause. Traction due to the polyp leads to partial inversion. Occasionally, complete inversion that occurs after delivery remains untreated. Traction

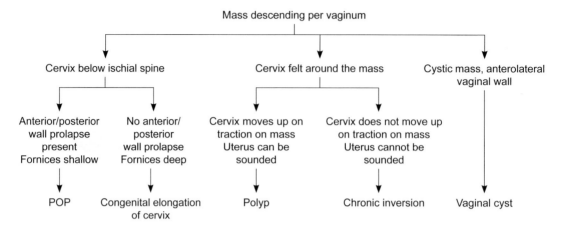

Figure 6.6 Evaluation of mass descending per vaginum. *POP*, pelvic organ prolapse.

on the inverted uterine fundus causes the cervix to go up, but this does not happen with traction on a polyp attached to the fundus.

Investigations

Clinical examination is sufficient for the diagnosis of POP, elongation of the cervix, Gartner cyst and polyps. Diagnosis of inversion requires ultrasonography.

Fig. 6.6 gives the evaluation of mass descending per vaginum.

Acute pelvic/lower abdominal pain

Pain due to gynaecological conditions presents a slower abdominal or pelvic pain. Acute pain often arises from other organs such as bladder, bowel and appendix as well. Gynaecological conditions giving rise to acute abdominal pain are dealt with later in this chapter. Causes of acute lower abdominal pain of gynaecological origin are listed in Table 6.3.

Nongynaecological conditions that cause acute lower abdominal/pelvic pain are listed in Box 6.16.

Clinical evaluation

Some conditions cause predominantly upper abdominal pain but can radiate to lower abdomen and make it difficult to distinguish from pain of gynaecological origin. Location of the pain, radiation, history of amenorrhoea, associated

Table 6.3 Acute lower abdominal pain of gynaecological origin

Condition	Clinical features
Abortion	• Amenorrhoea, uterine enlargement • Positive pregnancy test
Ectopic pregnancy	• Amenorrhoea, tender adnexal mass • Haemoperitoneum, positive pregnancy test
Salpingitis	Fever, systemic signs of sepsis
Pyosalpinx Tubo-ovarian abscess	Adnexal mass, tenderness
Red degeneration of myoma	Irregularly enlarged uterus, history of OC pill use or pregnancy
Endometrioma	Dysmenorrhoea, dyspareunia, adnexal mass
Torsion of ovarian cyst	Adnexal mass, acute pain, tenderness
Rupture of ovarian cyst	Adnexal mass, acute pain

OC, oral contraceptive.

Box 6.16 Nongynaecological causes of acute lower abdominal/pelvic pain

- Acute appendicitis
- Crohn disease
- Cystitis
- Ureteric/renal calculus
- Acute cholecystitis
- Perforated peptic ulcer
- Acute pancreatitis
- Mesenteric lymphadenitis

symptoms such as vomiting and bowel disturbances and urinary symptoms are important clues to diagnosis (Box 6.17).

Investigations

Haemoglobin, full blood count, urine culture and urine pregnancy test should be asked for when appropriate. Abdominal ultrasonography will clinch the diagnosis in most cases, but, occasionally, CT or MRI may be required.

Fig. 6.7 gives the evaluation of women with acute lower abdominal/pelvic pain.

Chronic pelvic pain

Chronic pelvic pain (CPP) is defined as noncyclic pain of at least 6-month duration, unrelated to menstruation, intercourse or pregnancy. It is most common in women between 26 and 30 years of age. It must be differentiated from dysmenorrhoea and dyspareunia.

Several nongynaecological and gynaecological conditions can give rise to CPP. Chronic urinary tract infection, irritable bowel syndrome and urethral syndrome are common. Women with CPP with no clinical findings and not responding to traditional treatment may have psychosomatic disorders such as anxiety or depression. CPP is dealt with in detail in Chapter 16, *Chronic pelvic pain*. Fig. 6.8 gives the algorithm for diagnosis of CPP.

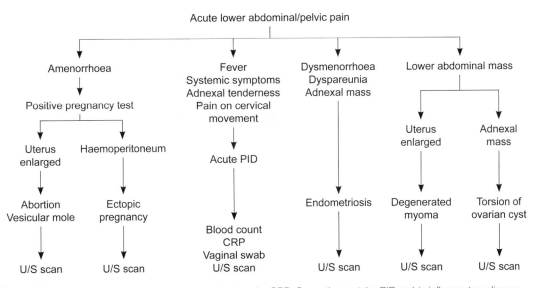

Figure 6.7 Evaluation of acute lower abdominal/pelvic pain. *CRP*, C-reactive protein; *PID*, pelvic inflammatory disease; *U/S*, ultrasound.

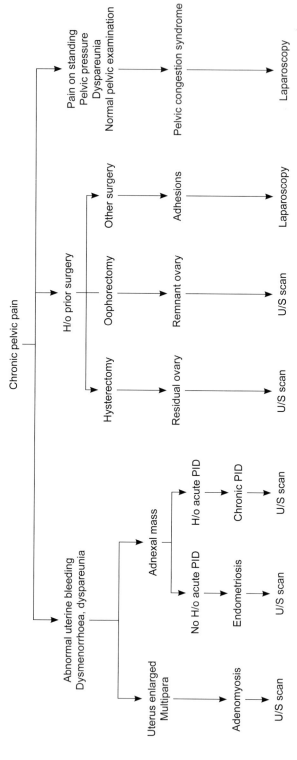

Figure 6.8 Evaluation of chronic pelvic pain. *H/o*, history of; *PID*, pelvic inflammatory disease; *U/S*, ultrasound.

Dysmenorrhoea

Painful menstruation is referred to as dysmenorrhoea (*see* Chapter 8, *Disorders associated with menstrual cycle*). It is one of the most common gynaecological problems. Dysmenorrhoea is of two types. **Spasmodic dysmenorrhoea** is a colicky pain that starts with or just before menstruation and lasts throughout the period of bleeding. **Congestive dysmenorrhea** starts a few days prior to the onset of bleeding and intensifies with menstruation, and the pain is constant. Dysmenorrhoea is also classified as primary and secondary. **Primary dysmenorrhoea** begins a few years after menarche when ovulatory cycles set in. It is due to $PGF_{2\alpha}$ produced in the endometrium during ovulatory cycles. It is common in young nulliparous women and disappears after a few years. But **secondary dysmenorrhoea** starts later and is due to pelvic pathology (Table 6.4). It is most often congestive in nature. Spasmodic secondary dysmenorrhoea is usually due to pathology in the uterine cavity such as IUCD, polyp or submucous myoma.

Clinical evaluation

The first step is to determine whether the dysmenorrhoea is primary or secondary, spasmodic or congestive. Gross pelvic pathologies such as myoma and ovarian masses can be diagnosed on pelvic examination (Box 6.18).

Box 6.18 Clinical evaluation of dysmenorrhoea

- History
  - Type of pain—Spasmodic/congestive
  - Location of pain
  - Age of onset
  - Abnormal uterine bleeding
  - Dyspareunia
  - Gastrointestinal/urological symptoms
  - History of pelvic inflammatory disease/vaginal surgery
- Physical examination
  - Per abdominal examination
    - Mass
    - Tenderness
  - Speculum examination
    - Scarred cervix, pinhole os
  - Pelvic examination
    - Uterine size
    - Adnexal mass
    - Tenderness
  - Per rectal examination
    - Rectovaginal nodules
    - Tenderness

Table 6.4 Causes of secondary dysmenorrhoea

Condition	Clinical features
Endometriosis	• Heavy menstrual bleeding, dyspareunia, infertility • Adnexal mass, in duration of uterosacrals
Adenomyosis	• Perimenopausal multipara, heavy menstrual bleeding • Uterine enlargement <12 weeks
Chronic pelvic infection	• History of pelvic inflammation disease, frequent menstruation • Dyspareunia, adnexal mass
Cervical stenosis	History of vaginal surgery, infertility
Leiomyoma uterus	• Heavy menstrual bleeding, pressure symptoms • Irregular uterine enlargement
Ovarian mass	Abdominal/pelvic mass
Müllerian anomalies	Amenorrhoea, cyclic pain, pelvic mass
Pelvic congestion syndrome	• Pelvic pressure, pain on standing, dyspareunia • Dilated veins at laparoscopy

Investigations

Most women with primary dysmenorrhoea do not need any further investigations. Abdominal ultrasonography and TVS are usually required in secondary dysmenorrhoea. If they are noncontributory, MRI or laparoscopy may be required depending on the clinical diagnosis. Adenomyosis and Müllerian anomalies are best seen on MRI, but diagnosis of pelvic congestion syndrome or minimal endometriosis requires laparoscopy.

Evaluation of dysmenorrhoea is given in Fig. 6.9.

Pruritus vulva

This is a very common symptom in women attending the gynaecological clinic. Most vulvar lesions, benign and malignant, present with pruritus.

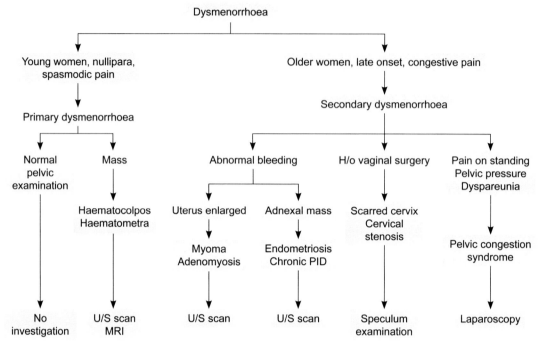

Figure 6.9 Evaluation of dysmenorrhoea. *H/o*, history of; *MRI*, magnetic resonance imaging; *PID*, pelvic inflammatory disease; *U/S*, ultrasound.

In most cases, it is due to **vulvovaginitis**, but dermatitis and inflammatory lesions of the vulva also present with pruritus. **Lichen simplex**, which is usually associated with chronic dermatitis, is a common condition that gives rise to intense pruritus. Some systemic illnesses such as Crohn disease, pyoderma and Behçet's syndrome are associated with vulval lesions and pruritus. **Psoriatic lesions** also occur on the vulva. Common conditions causing pruritus vulva are listed in Box 6.19.

Clinical evaluation

History and physical examination are the mainstay of diagnosis (Box 6.20).

Investigations

In most cases, history and examination are sufficient to make a diagnosis in case of vulvar lesions and pruritus. Microscopic examination of the vaginal discharge or scraping from the skin

---

Box 6.19 Common conditions causing pruritus vulva

- Vulvovaginitis
  - *Candida*
  - Trichomoniasis
  - Gonococcal
  - Bacterial vaginosis
- Dermatitis
  - Seborrhoeic
  - Allergic
  - Primary irritant
  - Atopic
  - Iatrogenic
- Infestation
  - Pediculosis, scabies
- Other conditions
  - Lichen simplex
  - Lichen planus
  - Intertrigo
  - Psoriasis
  - Vulvar cancer
  - Paget disease of the vulva

Box 6.20 Clinical evaluation of pruritus vulva

- History
  - Vaginal discharge
    - Colour, odour, nature of discharge
  - History of allergies
    - Atopy, eczema, asthma, contact dermatitis
  - Allergens
    - Local applications, latex, perfumes
  - Family history
    - Psoriasis, allergies
  - History of systemic illnesses
    - Diabetes, Crohn disease
- Physical examination
  - General examination
    - Psoriasis, seborrhoea, lichen planus
  - Examination of the vulva
    - Skin lesions, pigmentation, excoriation, discharge
  - Speculum examination
    - Discharge
  - Bimanual examination
    - Evidence of pelvic inflammatory disease

lesion is usually performed for diagnosis of candidal infection, trichomoniasis, BV or gonococcal infection. Biopsy may be indicated in women with suspected cancer.

Dyspareunia

Pain before, during or after sexual intercourse is referred to as **dyspareunia**. This is traditionally classified into superficial and deep dyspareunia. Pain that occurs at the introitus during insertion of the penis or in the mid-vagina is **superficial dyspareunia**. This occurs due to painful lesions in the vulva or vagina. **Vaginismus** refers to spasm of the perineal muscles and levator ani. This can also be interpreted as superficial dyspareunia. Conditions that give rise to pain during intercourse can also cause involuntary spasm of the muscles. **Deep dyspareunia** is due to painful lesions in the pouch of Douglas or uterosacrals and is experienced during deep penetration. Causes of vaginismus and dyspareunia are listed in Box 6.21.

Clinical evaluation

History of time of pain in relation to sexual intercourse, fear, spasm of muscles, prior sexual abuse and psychiatric illnesses such as depression and

Box 6.21 Causes of dyspareunia and vaginismus

- Superficial dyspareunia/vaginismus
  - Vaginitis—*Candida*, *Trichomonas*, *Gonococcus*
  - Vulvar skin lesions—Lichen planus, lichen sclerosis and dermatitis
  - Vulvodynia
  - Vulvar vestibulitis
  - Lichen sclerosis
  - Prior episiotomy, surgery
  - Postmenopausal oestrogen deficiency
  - Postradiation scarring
  - Psychogenic—Sexual abuse, lack of sexual interest
- Deep dyspareunia
  - Endometriosis
  - Chronic pelvic inflammatory disease
  - Ovaries prolapsed in the pouch of Douglas
  - Acutely retroverted uterus
  - Adnexal pathology

anxiety can give an indication about the aetiology. Examination should be aimed at ruling out local painful lesions. Pelvic examination may reveal adnexal masses or a fixed, retroverted uterus (Box 6.22).

Investigations

If vulval lesions or vaginitis is found on examination, diagnostic workup should be as for

Box 6.22 Clinical evaluation in dyspareunia

- History
  - Timing of pain in relation to intercourse
  - Vaginal discharge
  - Dyspareunia
  - Menopause
  - Prior surgery/radiation
  - Prior sexual abuse
  - Anxiety, depression
- Physical examination
  - General examination
    - Depression, anxiety
  - Local examination
    - Vulvar lesions, excoriation
  - Speculum examination
    - Spasm of muscles, discharge, scarring, dryness; signs of vaginitis
  - Bimanual examination
    - Retroverted uterus, mobility; adnexal mass, induration of uterosacrals

those disorders. Vaginismus due to anxiety or fear needs consultation with a psychiatrist. Women with deep dyspareunia need a TVS to rule out endometriosis, PID or acutely retroverted uterus.

Urinary symptoms

Dysuria is the most common urinary symptom and is due to infection. Other urological symptoms such as **incontinence** and **painful bladder syndrome** are discussed in Chapter 25, *Urogynaecology*. **Urinary retention** is another common problem with which women can present to a gynaecologist. Since the urinary tract is anatomically closely related to the genital tract, several gynaecological conditions can give rise to retention by causing pressure on the urethra or bladder neck. Gynaecological causes of urinary retention are discussed in Chapter 25, *Urogynaecology*.

Bowel symptoms

Increased frequency of bowel movement is a common symptom in women. The most common cause is irritable bowel syndrome. When the symptom is of recent onset and associated with symptoms and signs of acute infection and tenesmus, pelvic abscess must be thought of. Incontinence of faeces and flatus is a symptom of anal sphincter injury or rectovaginal fistula (*see* Chapter 26, *Urinary tract injuries, urogenital fistulas; anal sphincter injuries and rectovaginal fistulas*). Pain during defaecation can occur in rectovaginal endometriosis.

Key points

- Women consult gynaecologists with some common symptoms. Each of these symptoms is caused by a few conditions. An algorithm for evaluation of these symptoms is useful for arriving at a diagnosis.

- Abnormal vaginal bleeding may be heavy menstrual bleeding, frequent menstruation or intermenstrual bleeding, postcoital bleeding, infrequent cycles or postmenopausal bleeding. A simple algorithm with minimal investigations is given.

- Causes of vaginal discharge vary with the age of the patient. This is a common symptom in reproductive age and is often due to upper or lower genital tract infections. In postmenopausal women, malignancies of the cervix and uterus must be kept in mind.

- Lower abdominal masses can occur in adolescents, women of reproductive age or older women. The conditions are different in the three age groups. Ultrasonography is the mainstay of diagnosis in most cases; other modalities of imaging such as magnetic resonance imaging (MRI) and computed tomography (CT) scan are used in specific situations.

- The most common mass descending per vaginum is pelvic organ prolapse. Other conditions such as elongation of the cervix, chronic inversion and vaginal cysts are uncommon. They can be differentiated by clinical examination.

- The most common causes of acute lower abdominal pain are ectopic pregnancy, twisted ovarian cyst and acute pelvic inflammatory disease (PID). Nongynaecological conditions such as appendicitis may also present with acute pain. History, clinical examination and ultrasonography would clinch the diagnosis in most cases.

- Chronic pelvic pain is a noncyclic pain and can be caused by gynaecological and nongynaecological conditions. Common causes are endometriosis, adenomyosis, chronic PID, postoperative adhesions or pelvic congestion syndrome. Ultrasonography and laparoscopy may be required to establish a diagnosis.

- Dysmenorrhoea may be primary or secondary. Clinical examination reveals the cause of secondary dysmenorrhoea in most cases. Ultrasonography may be required in a few cases.

- Pruritus vulva is a common problem and can be due to a variety of dermatological conditions. But the most common cause is *Trichomonas* or candidal vaginitis.

- Superficial dyspareunia or vaginismus is usually due to local lesions in the vagina or psychogenic. Deep dyspareunia is usually caused by endometriosis, chronic PID or other pathology in the pelvis.

- Causes of acute urinary retention vary with age. Most common causes are retroverted gravid uterus, pelvic haematocele, cervical myoma and procidentia.

Self-assessment

Case-based questions

Case 1

A 30-year-old nulliparous lady presents with dyspareunia.

1. List the differential diagnosis.
2. What details will you focus on in history?
3. What will you look for on clinical examination?
4. How will you evaluate further?

Case 2

A 28-year-old lady, married for 8 months, presents with acute lower abdominal pain.

1. List the differential diagnosis.
2. What details will you focus on in history?
3. How will you proceed to evaluate her?

Answers

Case 1

1. Endometriosis, chronic PID, vaginitis, local vulvar lesions.
2. (a) Menstrual history, history of dysmenorrhoea, infertility, acute/chronic PID, vaginal discharge
   (b) Type of dyspareunia—Superficial/deep
   (c) History of vaginismus, vulvar lesions
3. (a) Abdominal examination—Lower abdominal tenderness, ovarian/tubo-ovarian mass
   (b) Examination of vulva—For painful lesions; vagina—For acute vaginitis
   (c) Bimanual examination—Tenderness on movement of cervix, tenderness in the pouch of Douglas, retroversion of the uterus, mobility of uterus, adnexal mass, tenderness, nodules in POD
   (d) Rectal examination—Induration of uterosacral ligaments
4. (a) Abdominal and transvaginal ultrasonography to look for endometriosis, tubo-ovarian mass
   (b) Laparoscopy, if ultrasonography is inconclusive

Case 2

1. Ectopic pregnancy, acute appendicitis, acute PID, twisted ovarian cyst.
2. Duration of pain, location, radiation, nature of pain, associated vomiting, fever.
   Date of last menstrual period, fainting attacks, vaginal bleeding, vaginal discharge. History of contraception.
3. (a) Abdominal examination for ovarian cyst, location of tenderness, shifting dullness (free fluid)
   (b) Bimanual examination for tenderness, adnexal mass, pain on movement of cervix
   (c) Urine pregnancy test, haemoglobin, blood count
   (d) Abdominal and transvaginal ultrasonography

Long-answer questions

1. Enumerate the causes of mass per abdomen in a 35-year-old woman. Discuss the differential diagnosis and management of myoma uterus.
2. Discuss the differential diagnosis in a woman presenting with postmenopausal bleeding. Classify endometrial hyperplasia. How will you manage endometrial hyperplasia in a 50-year-old woman?

Short-answer questions

1. Causes of postmenopausal bleeding
2. Vaginal discharge in childhood
3. Gynaecological causes of lower abdominal pain in an adolescent
4. Differential diagnosis of acute lower abdominal pain in a 35-year-old multiparous woman
5. List the gynaecological causes of urinary retention.
6. Define vaginismus. What are the causes of vaginismus?
7. Evaluation of deep dyspareunia
8. Differential diagnosis of mass descending per vagina

Section 3

Benign Gynaecology

7 | Abnormal Uterine Bleeding

Case scenario

Miss UD, was studying in class X. She hailed from a village nearby, and her parents were farmers. She had attained menarche at age 12 and ever since had irregular menstrual cycles, once in 2–3 months, bleeding lasting for 15 days. She had not consulted a doctor for this, since her neighbours had reassured her mother that this problem was common in young girls and the menstruation would regularize in a few years. Miss UD had been complaining of feeling tired, weak and unable to concentrate on her studies. She was brought to the hospital with heavy menstrual bleeding for 15 days, following amenorrhoea for 3 months. On examination, she was pale as paper and so weak that she could hardly sit.

Introduction

Menstruation is a cyclic phenomenon that begins at menarche and ends at menopause. The normal menstrual rhythm is regulated by hormones secreted by hypothalamus, pituitary and ovaries. Menstrual disorders are very common and occur at all ages. Heavy menstrual bleeding can lead to anaemia, time off from work and affect quality of life. Several treatment modalities are available now. However, early diagnosis of the cause of bleeding and appropriate management are essential to reduce morbidity.

Abnormal uterine bleeding (AUB) can occur due to abnormal hormone production or organic causes, both genital and extragenital. It can occur at any age, but is common in the prepubertal and postmenopausal women.

The normal menstrual cycle

Although the average duration of menstrual cycle is 28 days, it can vary from 21 to 35 days. The average menstrual flow is about 30 mL, and the duration of bleeding varies from 2 to 8 days. Up to eight fully soaked pads may be used, but usually such heavy flow is limited to 2 days (Box 7.1).

- Cycle length: 28 ± 7 days (21–35 days)
- Mean menstrual blood loss: 30–40 mL
- Duration: 2–8 days
- Product use: 3–6 pads/day

Arrest of bleeding

Arrest of bleeding normally occurs by three mechanisms:

- Haemostasis by platelet plug and clot formation
- Prostaglandin (PG)–mediated vasoconstriction
- Tissue repair

Haemostasis by platelet plug and clot formation

Once the bleeding starts, the coagulation cascade starts functioning in the endometrium and clots form to plug the vessels. Platelet aggregation leads to platelet plug formation. Once the bleeding from the vessels is controlled, fibrinolytic activity begins. Absence of fibrinolysis can lead to intrauterine adhesions and scar formation. Fibrinolysis also makes sure that the menstrual blood is fluid and the flow is smooth.

Prostaglandin-mediated vasoconstriction

Arachidonic acid, a substrate for the synthesis of PGs, and the enzyme PG synthetase are present in the endometrium. Several PGs with vasoconstrictor and vasodilator effects on the endometrium are synthesized by the endometrium and the myometrium under the influence of oestrogens and progesterone. Oestrogens lead to the synthesis of both PGE_2 (vasodilator) and $PGF_{2\alpha}$ (vasoconstrictor) in the ratio of 1:1. In the postovulatory phase, progesterone is released, which leads to production of PGE_2 and $PGF_{2\alpha}$ in the ratio of 1:2 so that the bleeding can be controlled. PGI_2 (vasodilator) and thromboxane A_2 (vasoconstrictor) are also released in the secretory phase. A fine balance is maintained between the various PGs in order to maintain haemostasis (Fig. 7.1).

Tissue repair

Re-epithelialization takes place after the shedding of the endometrium during menstruation. This process starts at the mouth of the basal glands and spreads across the raw surface of

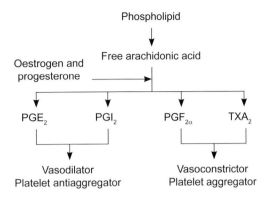

Figure 7.1 Prostaglandin-mediated vasoconstriction. *PG*, prostaglandin; *TX*, thromboxane.

the endometrium. The epidermal growth factor (EGF) and fibroblast growth factor (FGF), which are produced by the endometrium, control this process. Repair of the vessels also takes place under the influence of the vascular endothelial growth factor (VEGF).

Abnormal uterine bleeding

Definition

AUB is defined as any bleeding from the genital tract that is a deviation from the normal in frequency, cyclicity, duration or quantity.

Incidence

AUB is one of the common disorders in gynaecology and accounts for 30–40% of cases in the outpatient clinic. It occurs in about 25–30% of women of reproductive age and 50% of perimenopausal women. In adolescents the prevalence varies with years after menarche, the cycles during the first 2–3 years being predominantly anovulatory (40–60%).

Classification of AUB

The International Federation of Gynecology and Obstetrics (FIGO) has introduced a classification system for AUB in nonpregnant, reproductive-age women in 2011, as given in Box 7.2. The classification system is referred to by the acronym PALM-COEIN.

Box 7.2 FIGO classification of AUB

PALM	COEIN
P—Polyp	C—Coagulopathy
A—Adenomyosis	O—Ovulatory dysfunction
L—Leiomyomas	E—Endometrial
– Submucosal myoma (LSM)	I—Iatrogenic
– Other (LO)	N—Not yet classified
M—Malignancy and hyperplasia	

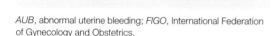

AUB, abnormal uterine bleeding; FIGO, International Federation of Gynecology and Obstetrics.

PALM consists of structural abnormalities, whereas COEIN includes conditions that are unrelated to structural abnormalities.

Leiomyoma is subdivided into patients with at least one submucoasal myoma (LSM) and those with other myomas (LO).

Notation

Abnormal bleeding in each category is represented by AUB followed by a hyphen and the letter that represents the category. (AUB due to polyp would be represented as AUB-P.) If a woman has heavy menstrual bleeding (HMB) due to ovulatory dysfunction and has an intramural myoma, it is represented as AUB-O; L.

Terminology

AUB may be chronic which is more common, or acute.

- **Chronic AUB** refers to abnormal bleeding that persists for >6 months. This occurs at all ages.
- When AUB is of sufficient severity to require immediate intervention to stop the bleeding, it is referred to as **acute AUB**. This is more common in adolescents but can also occur in other age groups.

There are specific terms used to describe the various bleeding patterns that are commonly

encountered (Box 7.3). Terms such as menorrhagia, metrorrhagia and polymenorrhagia are no longer used. Menorrhagia is now referred to as HMB. The term 'dysfunctional uterine bleeding (DUB)' is no longer used. Most women formerly classified as DUB now come under the category of AUB-O.

Box 7.3 Terminology—Type of bleeding

- Heavy menstrual bleeding
  - Regular cycles, prolonged or heavy bleeding
- Irregular bleeding
  - Cycles <21 or >35 days
- Intermenstrual bleeding
  - Small amounts of bleeding in between regular cycles
- Amenorrhoea
  - Absence of menstruation (>90 days)

Key menstrual parameters used in AUB

Certain parameters are used to define the regularity, frequency, duration and volume of bleeding as given in Box 7.4.

Box 7.4 Key menstrual parameters

- Regularity
  - Irregular: Variation >20 days
  - Regular: Variation ± 2–20 days
  - Absent: No bleeding
- Frequency
  - Frequent: <21 days (>4/90 days)
  - Normal: 21–35 days
  - Infrequent: >35 days (1-2/90 days)
- Duration
  - Prolonged: >8 days
  - Normal: 2–8 days
  - Shortened: <2 days
- Volume
  - Heavy: >80 mL
  - Normal: 15–80 mL
  - Light: <15 mL

Aetiology

According to the FIGO classification, aetiological factors can be broadly divided into structural abnormalities of the genital tract (PALM) and those due to nonstructural abnormalities (COEIN).

Structural abnormalities of the genital tract

Polyp

Endometrial polyps are one of the most common causes of AUB. They occur during reproductive age and in postmenopausal women. Majority of these are benign, but they can be, occasionally, malignant. They give rise to HMB, intermenstrual bleeding or postmenopausal bleeding (refer Chapter 10, *Benign diseases of the uterus*).

Cervical polyps that arise from the cervical glands are also benign. They can cause postcoital bleeding or intermenstrual bleeding (refer Chapter 9, *Benign diseases of the vulva, vagina and cervix*).

Adenomyosis

This is usually seen in multiparous women of perimenopausal age group and presents with HMB and dysmenorrhoea. This is discussed in Chapter 10, *Benign diseases of the uterus*.

Leiomyoma

Leiomyomas are the most common causes of AUB in the reproductive age. Myomas can be submucous, intramural or subserous. Intramural myomas are the most common. In the FIGO classification, leiomyomas are subclassified into those with at least one submucous myoma and those that have no submucous component. Myomas can give rise to HMB, intermenstrual bleeding and irregular bleeding. Leiomyomas are discussed further in Chapter 10, *Benign diseases of the uterus*.

Malignancy or hyperplasia

Endometrial hyperplasia, carcinoma and sarcoma usually present with HMB or irregular bleeding, usually in the postmenopausal or perimenopausal age (*see* Chapter 30, *Premalignant and malignant diseases of the uterus*). Cervical cancer occurs at a younger age (mid-forties) and is associated with intermenstrual bleeding. Vaginal cancer is rare but can present with bleeding.

Structural abnormalities causing AUB are summarized in Table 7.1.

Table 7.1 Structural abnormalities of the genital tract causing AUB

Abnormality	Age group	Type of bleeding
Polyp		
Endometrial polyp	Reproductive age	• Heavy menstrual bleeding • Intermenstrual bleeding
	Postmenopausal	Postmenopausal bleeding
Cervical polyp	Reproductive age	• Intermenstrual bleeding • Postcoital bleeding
Adenomyosis	Perimenopausal	Heavy menstrual bleeding
Leiomyoma		
Submucosal	Reproductive age	• Heavy menstrual bleeding • Intermenstrual bleeding
	Postmenopausal	Postmenopausal bleeding
Intramural	Reproductive	• Heavy menstrual bleeding • Irregular bleeding
Malignancy/hyperplasia		
Endometrium	Postmenopausal	Postmenopausal bleeding
	Perimenopausal	• Heavy menstrual bleeding • Irregular bleeding
Cervical	Premenopausal	• Intermenstrual bleeding • Postcoital bleeding

AUB, abnormal uterine bleeding.

Conditions not associated with structural abnormalities

Coagulopathy

The common coagulopathies that present with bleeding are von Willebrand disease and thrombocytopaenia (Box 7.5). They usually present in the peripubertal age. Coagulopathy should be suspected when heavy bleeding occurs at menarche. Family history of bleeding disorders is usually present, and there may be a history of easy bruising or prolonged bleeding from wounds.

Anticoagulants such as warfarin and drugs that impair platelet function and leukaemias are also causes of AUB. Women on anticoagulants may have a valve replacement, history of venous thrombosis or antiphospholipid antibody syndrome.

Advanced liver disease may be associated with a change in levels of coagulation factors leading to HMB.

Ovulatory dysfunction

This is the most common cause of AUB and was formerly classified as 'anovulatory DUB'. This is seen in adolescent girls (<20 years) and peri-menopausal women (>41 years), and accounts for 80% of all cases of AUB-O. Ovulatory dysfunction can present as a wide spectrum of menstrual abnormalities, ranging from infrequent, scanty periods to prolonged and heavy bleeding.

Ovulatory dysfunction results from abnormal functioning of the hypothalamic–pituitary–ovarian axis. This may be associated with polycystic ovarian syndrome (PCOS), obesity, mental stress, anorexia or weight loss.

In normal ovulatory cycles, progesterone controls menstrual bleeding by

- Stabilizing the endometrium through production of key proteins and blocking the production of matrix metalloproteinases that degrade the extravascular and stromal matrix
- Stimulating the production of tissue factor, which participates in extrinsic pathway of coagulation that reduces haemorrhage
- Stimulating production of plasminogen activator inhibitor-1, which blocks fibrinolysis and arrests bleeding
- Increasing the synthesis of vasoconstrictor PGs (PGF$_{2\alpha}$ and thromboxane)

Women with ovulatory dysfunction can have anovulation or oligo-ovulation. In anovulatory cycles, there is no midcycle luteinizing hormone (LH) surge, no ovulation and no progesterone production. Lack of progesterone leads to heavy and prolonged bleeding.

In some women with ovulatory dysfunction, ovarian follicles develop and oestrogen is produced, but dominant follicle may not develop. This leads to insufficient levels of oestrogen and failure to trigger an LH surge. There is no ovulation or progesterone production, but there is persistence of ovarian follicles, leading to the formation of *follicular cysts*, which are commonly seen in association with anovulatory cycles.

The insufficient follicular development results in low oestrogen levels that cannot sustain the endometrium or trigger an LH surge. There is no ovulation or progesterone production, cycles are short and bleeding can be profuse due to lack of PGF$_{2\alpha}$.

In some women with anovulation, oestrogen production continues in the absence of ovulation and the continuous, unopposed oestrogen action on the endometrium causes prolonged periods of amenorrhoea. When the endometrium outgrows its blood supply, bleeding occurs. The bleeding pattern is, therefore, characterized by 2–3 months of amenorrhoea followed by profuse and prolonged bleeding for 20–30 days (formerly called 'metropathia haemorrhagica'). Under unopposed oestrogen stimulation, the endometrium goes through a series of changes (Fig. 7.2). Initially, it shows persistent proliferative changes and then becomes hyperplastic.

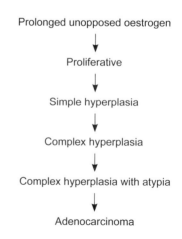

Prolonged unopposed oestrogen
↓
Proliferative
↓
Simple hyperplasia
↓
Complex hyperplasia
↓
Complex hyperplasia with atypia
↓
Adenocarcinoma

Figure 7.2 Unopposed oestrogen action on endometrium.

Occasionally, atypical endometrial hyperplasia and adenocarcinoma can develop.

Characteristic features of ovulatory dysfunction are summarized in Box 7.6.

The endometrium in ovulatory dysfunction with prolonged amenorrhoea usually reveals cystic hyperplasia (simple hyperplasia without atypia, known as the 'Swiss cheese appearance'; Fig. 7.3). Following are the characteristics of cystic hyperplasia:

- Hyperplastic glands and stroma
- Cystic or irregularly dilated glands
- Increase in vascularization
- Thick-walled, tortuous and dilated spiral arterioles and veins

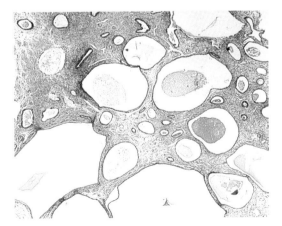

Figure 7.3 Cystic hyperplasia of the endometrium— Cystically dilated glands with densely cellular, compressed stroma, referred to as the 'Swiss cheese appearance'.

- Infarction and thrombosis of blood vessels
- Necrosis of superficial endometrium

The incidence of malignancy is low in simple (cystic) hyperplasia (about 1%), but increases to 29% in complex hyperplasia especially when there is associated atypia. Complex atypical hyperplasia is more common in perimenopausal women with risk factors such as obesity and diabetes. Young girls who are obese with or without other features of polycystic ovarian disease have hyperestrogenism due to conversion of ovarian and adrenal androstenedione to oestrone in the peripheral adipose tissue. They commonly present anovulatory cycles and hyperplastic endometrium.

Endometrial causes

In women with regular ovulatory cycles with no structural uterine abnormalities, HMB is usually due to a primary disorder at the endometrial level. This was formerly known as 'ovulatory DUB'. As described earlier, one of the important mechanisms for the control of bleeding is vasoconstriction brought about by PGs in the endometrium. An alteration in the ratio of $PGE/PGF_{2\alpha}$ occurs in some women despite ovulation and normal progesterone production (Box 7.7). Increase in PGE receptors in the endometrium, reduction in thromboxane production and increase in fibrinolytic activity have also been demonstrated. These changes result in HMB. $PGF_{2\alpha}$ causes uterine cramps, leading to dysmenorrhoea. Histological examination of the endometrium reveals secretory changes, since ovulation and progesterone production are normal. This type of bleeding normally responds to antifibrinolytics and PG synthetase inhibitors.

Chronic inflammation of the endometrium with or without associated pelvic inflammatory disease is an uncommon cause of AUB.

Iatrogenic

Intrauterine contraceptive device is a common cause of AUB. Copper intrauterine devices (IUDs) usually cause HMB, and the levonorgestrel intrauterine system (LNG-IUS) is associated with intermenstrual and irregular bleeding, especially in the first few months after insertion.

Menopausal hormone therapy and oestrogen-progesterone therapy for other conditions can also give rise to irregular bleeding.

Not yet classified

Congenital or acquired arteriovenous malformations in the uterus are rare but can present with HMB. Hypothyroidism and chronic renal disease are other causes.

Clinical evaluation

History and physical examination helps in arriving at a diagnosis regarding the cause of AUB in majority of cases. Clinical evaluation also helps in deciding on further evaluation.

History

History consists of age, parity, age at menarche, detailed menstrual history with special attention to key menstrual parameters and relevant obstetric history (Box 7.8). It is also important to ascertain whether the bleeding is from the genital tract or from the gastrointestinal or urinary tracts. Occasional anovulatory bleeding can occur in all women, more so in adolescent girls. Therefore, the duration of the problem and a 'menstrual diary' indicating the abnormality over the past few months are of help in determining the need for treatment. A pictorial blood loss assessment chart may be used to ascertain the amount of bleeding (*see* Chapter 4, *Gynaecological history and physical examination*). Bleeding disorders and thyroid dysfunction should be looked for in adolescents, but older women are unlikely to have these as the underlying cause for bleeding. Pregnancy must be excluded in women with amenorrhoea.

Physical examination

General and systemic examination will help in assessing the severity of bleeding, need for transfusion and need for hospitalization (Box 7.9). Risk factors for ovulatory dysfunction such as obesity, weight loss and anorexia should be assessed. Speculum examination should be performed to exclude local lesions on the cervix and vagina. Uterine size and contour should be assessed by pelvic examination. Per speculum and bimanual pelvic examination may be omitted in young adolescents who are not sexually active.

Box 7.8 History

- Age
- Age at menarche
- Parity
- Key menstrual parameters
  - Regularity
  - Frequency
  - Duration
  - Volume
- Postcoital bleeding
- Dysmenorrhoea
  - Congestive
  - Spasmodic
- Dyspareunia
- Infertility
- Vaginal discharge
- Recent abortion
- IUCD insertion
- Oral contraceptive/hormone use
- Symptoms of hypothyroidism
- Symptoms of bleeding disorders
- Medications

IUCD, intrauterine contraceptive device.

Box 7.9 Physical Examination

- General
- Pallor
- Thyroid enlargement
- BMI
- Signs of PCOS
  - Hirsutism
  - Acanthosis nigricans
  - Acne
- Speculum examination—Growth
- Bimanual pelvic examination
  - Size and contour of uterus
  - Tenderness
  - Fixity
  - Adnexal mass/tenderness/induration

BMI, body mass index; *PCOS*, polycystic ovarian syndrome.

Investigations

Laboratory tests

Haemoglobin is the first and most important investigation that helps in determining the severity and urgency of the problem. Full blood count, bleeding time (BT), prothrombin time (PT) and partial thromboplastin time (PTT) are indicated in young girls with a history suggestive of bleeding disorders to rule out thrombocytopaenia and von Willebrand disease. Thyroid function tests and thyroid-stimulating hormone (TSH) levels are also indicated in adolescents or in women with a history suggestive of thyroid dysfunction.

Cervical cytology

This should be performed in all women who are sexually active to exclude cervical intraepithelial neoplasia.

Ultrasonography

Transabdominal and transvaginal ultrasonography can help in the diagnosis of small myomas, polyps and adenomyosis.

Indications

- Clinical suspicion of above pelvic pathology such as myoma, polyp or adenomyosis
- When a woman with a normal-sized uterus does not respond to traditional medical treatment, to exclude endometrial polyp (Fig. 7.4)

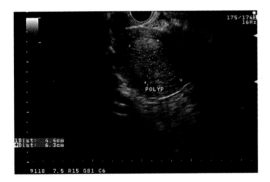

Figure 7.4 Transvaginal ultrasonography showing a large endometrial polyp.

Sonohysterography

In sonohysterography, an ultrasonogram is performed after the introduction of saline into the uterine cavity. It is also helpful in the diagnosis of intracavitary lesions.

Endometrial sampling

Endometrial sampling devices such as the Vabra aspirator and Pipelle (Fig. 7.5) are easier to use and can sample the endometrium adequately. They are more comfortable for the patient, especially perimenopausal women with narrow cervical canal. Hyperplasia and cancer can be diagnosed by endometrial sampling. This is indicated in perimenopausal women.

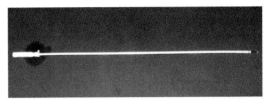

Figure 7.5 Pipelle used for endometrial cytology.

Indications

- Women >45 years (perimenopausal)—To exclude hyperplasia or carcinoma when bleeding is frequent, heavy or prolonged or any AUB associated with risk factors such as obesity and chronic anovulation
- Women of reproductive age—Persistent AUB-O (>6 months), associated with risk factors such as obesity, PCOS or tamoxifen therapy

Hysteroscopy

If transvaginal ultrasonography reveals a polyp, or a submucous myoma, hysteroscopy may be indicated. Endometrial sampling can be performed at the same time.

Management

Management of AUB depends on several factors:

- Age
- Severity of bleeding
- Aetiology
- Desire for fertility
- Contraceptive needs
- Medical comorbidities

General measures

Treatment of anaemia

Oral iron therapy is sufficient for most women and should be prescribed without fail for all those with haemoglobin below 11g%. If blood loss has been heavy and haemoglobin is less than 5 g% or when surgery is planned and haemoglobin is less than 10 g%, packed cells should be transfused.

Lifestyle modification

In women with obesity-related anovulation, weight reduction by diet and exercise is the cornerstone of treatment (Box 7.10). Peripheral oestrogen production in adipose tissue will continue if the body mass index (BMI) is not brought down to near-ideal value.

Box 7.10 General measures

- Treatment of anaemia
  - Oral iron therapy
  - Packed cell transfusion
- Lifestyle modification
  - Weight reduction
  - Diet
  - Exercises

Definitive treatment

This consists of (a) medical management and (b) surgical management.

- Definitive medical or surgical management of AUB should be initiated only after the aetiology is established.
- Endometrial polyps and submucosal myomas should be resected hysteroscopically (*see* Chapter 10, *Benign diseases of the uterus*).
- Intramural myomas that do not respond to medical management have to be removed by myomectomy. Adenomyosis is usually treated with hormones initially (oral or LNG-IUS) but may require hysterectomy. These are discussed further in Chapter 10, *Benign diseases of the uterus*.
- Endometrial cancer and atypical hyperplasia necessitate hysterectomy. Hyperplasia without atypia can be managed medically (*see* Chapter 30, *Premalignant and malignant diseases of the uterus*).
- Women with coagulopathies or on anticoagulants who present with AUB respond to hormonal therapy. When there is a history of venous thrombosis, high-dose progesterone or LNG-IUS should be used.
- Medical treatment is the first line of management for most women with HMB, irregular bleeding or intermenstrual bleeding without any structural abnormalities (AUB-O, AUB-E). Surgical treatment is resorted to only when medical treatment fails.

Medical management

Drugs used in medical management are as listed in Box 7.11.

Box 7.11 Medical management of AUB

- Nonhormonal
  - Antifibrinolytics
  - PG synthetase inhibitors
  - Capillary fragility inhibitors
- Hormonal
  - Progestin only—Oral, injectable and intrauterine systems
  - Oestrogen–progestin combinations
  - Oestrogen-only
- Others
  - Danazol
  - GnRH analogues
  - Ormeloxifene

AUB, abnormal uterine bleeding; *GnRH*, gonadotropin-releasing hormone; *PG*, prostaglandin.

Nonhormonal treatment

Nonhormonal agents are usually used in the management of women with cyclic HMB without structural abnormalities (HMB-E). They can also be used in women with HMB due to other causes to reduce the bleeding.

Antifibrinolytics The fibrinolytic system is active in the endometrium during a normal menstrual cycle. In women with HMB (AUB-E), increased fibrinolytic activity has been demonstrated. Antifibrinolytic agents such as epsilon-aminocaproic acid and tranexamic acid have been used with 50% reduction in blood loss. They are more effective than PG synthetase inhibitors. Tranexamic acid is given in a dose of 1 g thrice daily for the first 3–4 days (time of heavy flow). It is well tolerated and is the first-line treatment in women with cyclic heavy bleeding and normal-sized uterus (AUB-E).

PG synthetase inhibitors Since bleeding in AUB is mediated through PGs, drugs that reduce the synthesis of PG should help in reducing the bleeding. They act by inhibiting cyclooxygenase-mediated conversion of arachidonic acid to PGs and by binding to PG receptors, thereby blocking them. They also relieve dysmenorrhoea.

The drugs in this category are nonsteroidal anti-inflammatory agents such as ibuprofen, naproxen and mefenamic acid. Mefenamic acid, in a dose of 500 mg three times a day, reduces pain and is inexpensive. Side effects are mainly gastrointestinal and are mild with mefenamic acid and related compounds. PG synthetase inhibitors reduce menstrual loss by 25–40% and are used as second-line treatment of AUB-E. They can also be used in combination with tranexamic acid as first-line treatment.

Capillary fragility inhibitors Although drugs such as ethamsylate reduce capillary fragility, they have not been shown to reduce bleeding significantly in women with AUB and are not recommended.

Hormonal treatment

Oral progestins Some of the oral progestins used are as follows:

- Medroxyprogesterone acetate
- Norethisterone
- Norethindrone

These are used to arrest bleeding and regulate the menstrual cycle.

- To arrest bleeding in women who present with acute heavy menstrual bleeding (HMB-O), norethisterone may be used in doses of 10 mg 6 hourly for 24–48 hours (till bleeding stops). The dose is gradually reduced to 10 mg thrice a day, twice a day and continued as once a day for a total of 21 days. After withdrawal bleeding, the same progestogen can be administered in 5- to 10-mg doses from day 5 to 25 for three to six cycles. Medroxyprogesterone acetate (10 mg 6 hourly) or norethindrone (5 mg 6 hourly) may also be used.
- In women who are not currently bleeding and have irregular cycles, oral progestin may be used in 5- to 10-mg daily doses from day 15 to 25. In women in whom the bleeding is not controlled with this regimen and in women with endometrial hyperplasia, the same dose of progestogen should be used cyclically from day 5 to 25. Menstrual loss is reduced by 30% and hyperplasia can be reversed.

Injectable progestogens Injectable progestogens such as depot medroxyprogesterone acetate (150 mg) every 3 months can be used in women with anovulatory cycles or hyperplastic endometrium. Bleeding can be irregular and unpredictable, and some women have amenorrhoea. Due to these reasons, it is not a popular treatment.

Progesterone intrauterine systems The most commonly used progesterone intrauterine system is LNG-IUS. It can reduce the blood loss by 95%, and the system is as effective as endometrial ablation (Fig. 7.6). LNG-IUS delivers 20 μg of levonorgestrel daily to the endometrium where it causes glandular atrophy and stromal decidualization and prevents development of endometrial cancer. It has very little action on the ovary. There are no systemic side effects since very little is absorbed. The results are comparable to endometrial ablation and help to avoid hysterectomy in many women. LNG-IUS is effective in ovulatory dysfunction, AUB-E, adenomyosis, small intramural myomas and coagulopathies. The device has to be changed every 3 years if used for treatment of HMB, and every 5 years if used for contraception only.

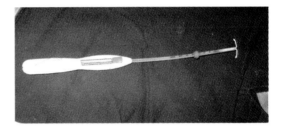

Figure 7.6 Levonorgestrel intrauterine system (LNG-IUS).

Oestrogen–progestin combination This is the first-line treatment in women with HMB, irregular bleeding and intermenstrual bleeding. Cycle control is excellent and bleeding reduces by 60–70%. Endometrial PG production is reduced and periods are pain free. Currently available low-dose preparations contain 20 or 30 μg of ethinyl oestradiol with 50–75 μg of progestogen such as levonorgestrel, norethisterone or other 19 nonsteroids. They are given cyclically from day 5 to 25 and can be used in all age groups. The lower dose of oestrogen makes it safe in the perimenopausal age also. They can be used to treat women with a hyperplastic endometrium as well. Duration of treatment is 3–6 months in most women, except in those with hyperplasia where it should be used for a minimum of 6 months.

They can also be used in acute bleeding, at a dose of one tablet 8 hourly and gradually reduced to one tablet a day over 1 week. Oestrogen–progestin combination pills can be used in cyclic fashion (21-day pills) or as extended-cycle pills, used continuously for 3 months.

Oestrogens Oestrogens alone are seldom used alone in the treatment of AUB-O. Occasionally, young girls with anovulatory bleeding may present with an atrophic endometrium since the endometrium is completely shed during bleeding. An atrophic endometrium does not respond to progestin unless primed with oestrogen. In these situations, to control haemorrhage, conjugated equine oestrogen can be used as 25 mg IV 6 hourly. Alternatively, since parenteral conjugated oestrogen is not available, ethinyl oestradiol can be used, 50 µg daily for 5 days. This should be followed by oestrogen–progestin combination or progestin alone in the usual dose for the rest of the cycle.

Other drugs

Danazol This is an antigonadotropin and can be used in a 100- to 200-mg daily dose in the treatment of AUB-E. Blood loss reduces by 40–50%, but side effects such as weight gain and acne are troublesome. It is not often used in the management of AUB.

GnRH analogues Gonadotropin-releasing hormone (GnRH) analogues cause amenorrhoea by inhibiting pituitary production of gonadotropins. Women can experience troublesome hot flushes, and when used for more than 6 months, they can cause reduction in bone mineral density. They are also very expensive. Currently, they are used only while waiting for surgery or to prepare the endometrium prior to ablative procedures. Injections are given monthly in a dose of 3.6 mg IM.

Ormeloxifene This is a selective oestrogen receptor modulator, used mainly as an oral contraceptive (OC). When used as 60 mg twice weekly for 12 weeks, a substantial reduction in bleeding has been reported. It is marketed as Saheli.

The dosages of various formulations used in medical treatment are given in Table 7.2.

Management of acute bleeding

Acute bleeding is more common in adolescents but also occurs in other age groups. When a patient gets admitted with acute bleeding, the steps of management are as follows:

- History, evaluation of general condition and clinical examination to exclude structural abnormalities and coagulopathies.

Table 7.2 AUB—Drugs used and dosages

Drug	Dosage
Antifibrinolytic: Tranexamic acid	1 g three to four times daily for 3–5 days
PG synthetase inhibitors: Mefenamic acid	500 mg thrice daily for 4–5 days
Capillary fragility inhibitors: Ethamsylate	500 mg four times daily for 4–5 days
Progestins: Norethisterone or medroxyprogesterone	
To arrest haemorrhage	10 mg 6 hourly for 24–48 hours
To regularise cycles	5–10 mg daily from day 5 to 25
Oestrogen–progestin combination pills: Ethinyl oestradiol + norethisterone or norgestrel	20 or 30 µg + 0.5–0.75 mg cyclically from day 5 to 25
Oestrogen-only: Ethinyl oestradiol	50 µg daily for 5 days
Antigonadotropin: Danazol	100–200 mg daily
GnRH analogues	3.6 mg once in 4 weeks
Selective oestrogen receptor modulator: Ormeloxifene	60 mg twice weekly for 12 weeks

AUB, abnormal uterine bleeding; *GnRH*, gonadotropin-releasing hormone; *PG*, prostaglandin.

- Start blood transfusion if haemoglobin is <7 g/dL.
- Begin hormonal treatment:
  - Give oestrogen–progestin combination pill (with 30 µg of ethinyl oestradiol) 8 hourly for 48–72 hours or till the bleeding stops followed by 12 hourly for 5 days and once a day for 2 weeks (total 21 days).
  - Alternatively, high-dose progestin (norethisterone 10 mg 6 hourly) may be started and reduced, after 48 hours, to 10 mg thrice daily for 5 days and to twice daily for 2 weeks.
  - Oestrogen–progestin pill (20 µg ethinyl oestradiol) should be continued cyclically for three to six cycles.

Surgical management

Conservative surgery

Endometrial ablation

It is the elimination of the endometrium by resection or thermal energy. The indications and contraindications of endometrial ablation are listed in Box 7.12.

- Indications
  - AUB-E or AUB-O with
    - Failed medical therapy
    - Young women with a desire to preserve the uterus
    - Poor surgical risk for hysterectomy
- Contraindications
  - Desire for fertility
  - Large uterus (>12 cm cavity length)
  - Endometrial hyperplasia
  - Suspected malignancy of the genital tract
  - Multiple or large myomas
  - Postmenopausal women

AUB, abnormal uterine bleeding.

Endometrial ablation techniques

These are divided into

- Resectoscopic endometrial ablation (first-generation techniques)
- Nonresectoscopic endometrial ablation (second-generation techniques)

The resectoscopic and nonresectoscopic techniques are listed in Box 7.13.

- Resectoscopic (first-generation) ablation techniques
  - Endometrial laser ablation
  - Transcervical endometrial resection
  - Roller ball electrocoagulation
- Nonresectoscopic (second-generation) ablation techniques
  - Thermal balloon ablation
  - Microwave endometrial ablation
  - Radio-frequency–induced ablation
  - Hydrothermablation
  - Cryotherapy
  - Laser interstitial therapy

Preoperative endometrial preparation Since it is easier to resect a thin endometrium, preoperative preparation is advisable prior to resectoscopic ablation. This is achieved with

- GnRH analogues
- Oestrogen–progestin combination pill
- Danazol
- Curettage

Resectoscopic techniques The resectoscopic techniques are performed under anaesthesia and require hysteroscopy. Glycine is used as a distending medium. A roller ball cautery may be used to cauterize the entire endometrium or the endometrium may be resected using a wire loop cautery (Fig. 7.7a and b). The entire endometrium can also be destroyed by laser.

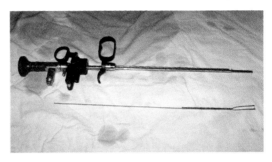

a.

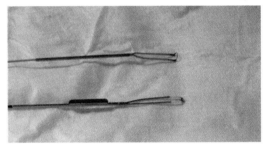

b.

Figure 7.7 Instruments for resectoscopic endometrial ablation. a. Hysteroscope and wire loop electrode. b. Roller ball and wire loop electrodes.

Nonresectoscopic techniques Disadvantages of the resectoscopic techniques (Box 7.14) led to the development of nonresectoscopic destruction techniques. They are also referred to as global ablation since the entire endometrial cavity is usually destroyed. They are easy to learn, are generally performed under mild sedation as outpatient procedure and have fewer complications. Thermal balloon ablation is the most popular technique used currently (Fig. 7.8a–e). Saline is infused through a balloon, warmed to 87°C at pressures of 160–180 mmHg and kept in contact with the endometrium for 8 minutes. On long-term follow-up after endometrial ablation, about 30% women remain amenorrhoeic, 40–50% have reduced bleeding and 10–20% require hysterectomy for continued symptoms.

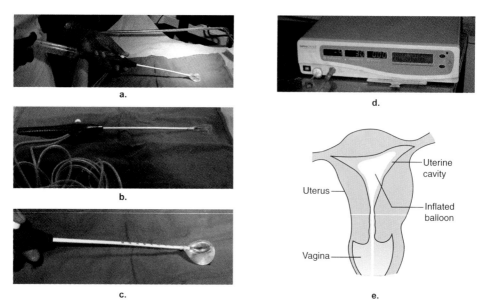

Figure 7.8 Thermal balloon ablation. a. Catheter with balloon deflated. b. Balloon being inflated with saline. c. Balloon filled with saline. d. Monitor with panel displaying pressure, temperature and duration. e. Inflated balloon in uterine cavity.

Box 7.14 Disadvantages of resectoscopic techniques

- Require a skilled operator
- Have a long learning curve
- Require general anaesthesia
- Have a higher risk of complications

Complications

The complications are more with resectoscopic techniques. The efficacy of endometrial ablation is similar to LNG-IUS and complications are more; hence, LNG-IUS has almost replaced endometrial ablation in most centres now. Complications of endometrial ablation are listed in Box 7.15.

Box 7.15 Complications of endometrial ablation

- Uterine perforation
- Fluid overload
- Haemorrhage
- Intrauterine scarring and haematometra
- Pelvic infection

Hysterectomy

With the availability of effective medical therapy, patient satisfaction and excellent control of bleeding with nonresectoscopic ablation techniques and the availability of LNG-IUS that has a high rate of acceptance, hysterectomy is performed only in select cases of AUB. Indications are few (Box 7.16). Hysterectomy may be performed through the abdominal route, the vaginal route or laparoscopically.

Box 7.16 Indications for hysterectomy

- Complex atypical hyperplasia in older women
- Failed medical therapy in perimenopausal women
- Failed endometrial ablation
- Other pelvic pathology that needs concomitant surgery

Summary of management of AUB

Evaluation and management of AUB-O in adolescents, women of reproductive age and perimenopausal women are summarized in the following and shown in Figs 7.9–7.11.

Abnormal uterine bleeding in adolescents

AUB is a common problem in adolescents. Some aetiological factors are different from the other

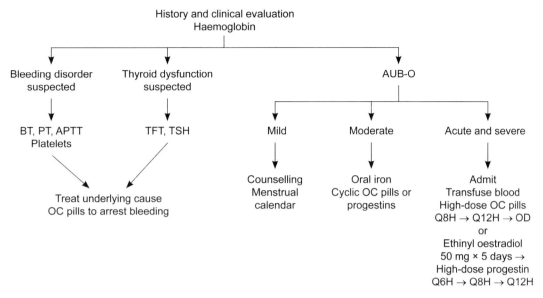

Figure 7.9 Management of abnormal uterine bleeding in adolescent girls. *APTT*, activated partial thromboplastin time; *AUB-O*, abnormal uterine bleeding-ovulatory dysfunction; *BT*, bleeding time; *OC*, oral contraceptive; *PT*, prothrombin time; *TFT*, thyroid function test; *TSH*, thyroid-stimulating hormone.

age groups; therefore, evaluation and management are discussed here.

Due to the immaturity of hypothalamic–pituitary–ovarian axis, the menstrual cycles are anovulatory in the first 2–3 years after menarche. Coagulation disorders, hypothyroidism, anorexia, weight gain with or without PCOS and psychological stress are the other causes of AUB in this age group. Bleeding disorders account for 8–10% of the causes, and the common disorders are Von Willebrand disease, thrombocytopaenia and other platelet disorders. Family history of bleeding disorders and history of excessive bleeding during childhood are usually present.

The adolescent girls may present with HMB, irregular cycles with prolonged intervals and heavy bleeding (AUB-O) or with acute bleeding. History and physical examination are mandatory. Pelvic examination and ultrasonography are not indicated as a routine. Haemoglobin, evaluation for bleeding disorders with BT, PT, PTT, platelet count and serum TSH levels are usually performed.

After evaluation they can be classified as follows:

- **Mild AUB:** Bleeding does not interfere with normal activity; Hb 10–12 g%.
- **Moderate AUB:** Bleeding interferes with normal activity; Hb 8–10 g%.

- **Severe AUB:** Profuse, continuous bleeding is present; Hb <8 g%.

Mild AUB may be managed with reassurance, lifestyle changes if required and cyclic progestin or OC pills.

Moderate AUB requires iron replacement and low-dose OC pills for three to six cycles. If treatment is required for longer duration and if the cycles are irregular, progestin for 7–10 days every month is an accepted treatment.

Girls who present with acute, severe bleeding should be managed as outlined earlier. Priming the endometrium with oestrogen is required before starting high-dose progestins.

Abnormal uterine bleeding in women of reproductive age

Leiomyomas, endometrial polyps and adenomyosis are common in this group. AUB-E is more common and anovulatory dysfunction is less common than in the other age groups. Ultrasonography should be performed if structural abnormality is suspected on examination or if there is no response to hormone therapy. Endometrial sampling is required only in older women (>40 years) and if there are associated high risk factors for hyperplasia/cancer.

Self-assessment

Case-based questions

Case 1

A 15-year-old student was brought to the clinic with bleeding per vaginam for 20 days following a period of 4 months of amenorrhoea. She attained menarche at 12 years of age; prior menstrual cycles were 10–15 days every 2–3 months. She complained of lassitude and weakness, and, on examination, was very pale.

1. What is the diagnosis?
2. What investigations will you order?
3. What is the general management?
4. What medications will you prescribe? Give the dose and duration.

Case 2

A 48-year-old nullipara presents with irregular cycles of 7–8 days every 18–20 days for the past 6 months. Prior cycles were regular. Clinical examination reveals pallor, BMI 32. She is a diabetic and is on metformin. She has been treated with combination pills for 3 months by a local doctor, but bleeding has recurred on stopping the treatment.

1. What is the diagnosis?
2. How will you evaluate clinically?
3. What investigations will you order?
4. How will you manage?

Answers

Case 1

1. AUB-O of adolescence; severe anaemia.
2. Haemoglobin; blood picture; platelet count; TSH.
3. Packed cell transfusion; ferrous sulphate tablets 200 mg daily for 6 months.
4. Medication—Oestrogen–progestin combination pill 8 hourly for 48 hours, 12 hourly for 5 days and once daily for 2 weeks followed by once daily, cyclically for three to six cycles. Alternatively, norethisterone 10 mg 6 hourly for 48 hours followed by 8 hourly for 5 days, 12 hourly for 1 week and once daily for 1 week,

followed by oestrogen–progesterone combination pill for six cycles may be used.

Case 2

1. Perimenopausal AUB-O, obesity, diabetes.
2. Pelvic examination.
3. Pap smear:
   (a) Haemoglobin, blood sugar, lipid profile
   (b) Ultrasonogram for endometrial thickness and to rule out polyp
   (c) Dilatation and curettage to rule out complex hyperplasia/carcinoma
4. Management:
   (a) Lifestyle modification, good control of diabetes
   (b) T ferrous sulphate 200 mg daily for 6 months
   (c) If endometrium is proliferative or shows simple hyperplasia (no carcinoma or complex atypical hyperplasia), a low-dose oestrogen–progestogen combination pill for 6 months
   (d) Can be continued till menopause
   (e) LNG-IUS is another option

Long-answer questions

1. A 45-year-old multipara presents with menstrual cycles once in 60–70 days with profuse bleeding for 10–15 days for the past 6 months. Discuss the diagnosis, evaluation and management.
2. How do you classify abnormal uterine bleeding? Discuss the various options available to manage a 35-year-old patient with AUB-O.
3. What are the causes of heavy menstrual bleeding in a 35-year-old woman? Describe hormonal treatment in AUB.

Short-answer questions

1. Abnormal uterine bleeding in the adolescent
2. Endometrial ablation
3. Medical management of AUB
4. Intermenstrual bleeding

8 | Disorders Associated with Menstrual Cycle

Case scenario

Miss RK 16, a high school student, was brought to the clinic by her parents with painful periods. She had attained menarche 2 years earlier, but the menstruation had become painful since 1 year. In fact, she was so incapacitated by the pain that she was missing classes often. The issue had become embarrassing and worrisome.

Introduction

During the menstrual cycle, women may experience a variety of symptoms. Some are indicative of organic pathology; others may be related to the hormonal changes. These disorders are different from disorders of menstrual cycle such as heavy menstrual bleeding, intermenstrual bleeding or irregular bleeding and physiological phenomena such as midcycle pain. Some disorders associated with menstrual cycle such as primary dysmenorrhoea and menstrual migraine occur during menstruation, and other disorders such as premenstrual syndrome (PMS) and premenstrual dysphoric disorder (PMDD) occur in the luteal phase of the menstrual cycle.

Dysmenorrhoea

Dysmenorrhoea is painful menstruation. This is the most common gynaecological problem for which women seek advice. It is seen in about 50–70% of women in mild-to-severe form. The pain can be of two types: **Spasmodic** or **congestive** (Box 8.1).

Classification

Dysmenorrhoea is classified into primary and secondary dysmenorrhoea.

Box 8.1 Spasmodic and congestive dysmenorrhoea

- Spasmodic dysmenorrhoea
  - Starts with or just before menstruation
  - Colicky pain
  - Suprapubic
- Congestive dysmenorrhoea
  - Starts in luteal phase
  - Increases with menstruation
  - Constant pelvic pain

Primary dysmenorrhoea

Primary dysmenorrhoea is the presence of recurrent, crampy, lower abdominal pain that occurs during menstruation, in the absence of demonstrable disease. It occurs a few years after menarche when ovulatory cycles are established. The pain starts with the onset of menstruation or few hours before and gradually reduces during the next 12–72 hours. The pain is suprapubic and radiates to back and thigh. Associated nausea, vomiting, diarrhoea and syncope are seen in some women (Box 8.2). Women with anxiety and stress are more prone to this disorder. Primary dysmenorrhoea generally disappears after a few years, especially after a vaginal delivery.

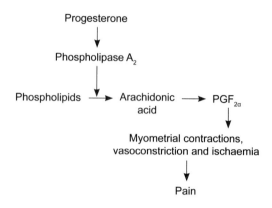

Figure 8.1 Pathogenesis of primary dysmenorrhoea. $PGF_{2\alpha}$, prostaglandin F2 alpha.

Box 8.2 Characteristics of primary dysmenorrhoea

- Occurs at <20 years of age
- Usually spasmodic
- Suprapubic; radiates to back and thigh
- Can be associated with other symptoms
- No pelvic pathology
- Occurs only in ovulatory cycles

Risk factors Primary dysmenorrhoea occurs more often in women with certain risk factors (Box 8.3).

Box 8.3 Risk factors for primary dysmenorrhoea

- Age <20 years
- Body mass index <20 kg/m²
- Nulliparity
- Early menarche
- Heavy menstrual flow
- Increased duration of menstruation
- Anxiety and stress

Pathogenesis Primary dysmenorrhoea is due to increase in level of prostaglandin F2 alpha ($PGF_{2\alpha}$). In ovulatory cycles, progesterone level rises after ovulation. This causes an increase in $PGF_{2\alpha}$ in the endometrium, leading to increase in tone of the myometrium and uterine contraction (Fig. 8.1). The contractions are non-rhythmic, occurring at high frequency. Levels of leukotrienes and vasopressin in the endometrium are also elevated and play a role in primary dysmenorrhoea.

Secondary dysmenorrhoea

Secondary dysmenorrhoea is recurrent, lower abdominal pain associated with menstruation that occurs in women with a pelvic pathology that could account for the symptoms (Box 8.4).

Box 8.4 Secondary dysmenorrhoea

- Secondary to pelvic pathology
- Occurs several years after menarche (>20 years of age)
- Starts 1–2 weeks before menstruation
- Increases with onset of menstruation
- Associated with heaviness in pelvis and backache

Causes of secondary dysmenorrhoea are listed in Box 8.5. Pelvic congestion syndrome is diagnosed when no other pathology is found except for engorged veins in the broad ligament and pelvic walls and a congested uterus.

Box 8.5 Causes of secondary dysmenorrhoea

- Endometriosis
- Adenomyosis
- Chronic pelvic infections
- Cervical stenosis
- Leiomyoma uterus
- Ovarian mass
- Müllerian anomalies
- Pelvic congestion syndrome

Pathogenesis Increase in $PGF_{2\alpha}$ is found in endometriotic lesions and is considered to be the cause of pain. Local congestion and oedema in the pelvis that occurs in normal menstrual cycle is exaggerated in chronic conditions such as pelvic inflammatory disease and leiomyoma. Collection of blood in the uterine cavity with resultant uterine contractions is the cause of pain in cervical stenosis and Müllerian anomalies.

Clinical evaluation

History

History will often be sufficient to arrive at a diagnosis, especially in young girls with primary dysmenorrhoea. In older women and women with secondary dysmenorrhoea, a detailed history should be as given in Box 8.6.

Box 8.6 History in dysmenorrhoea

- Age
  - Age of onset of pain
  - Age at menarche
- Type of pain
  - Spasmodic or congestive
- Location of pain
- Other associated symptoms
  - Gastrointestinal symptoms
  - Syncope
  - Heaviness in pelvis
  - Backache
- Menstrual cycles
  - Duration of flow
  - Amount of flow
  - Regularity
- Parity
- Dyspareunia
- Impact on day-to-day activities

Physical examination

In a young girl with a typical history of primary dysmenorrhoea, if general and abdominal examinations are unremarkable, treatment may be started without pelvic or rectal examination. Older women with primary dysmenorrhoea and women with secondary dysmenorrhoea have to undergo a thorough physical examination as in Box 8.7.

Investigations

Further evaluation (Box 8.8) will depend on provisional diagnosis arrived at after history and clinical examination. Investigations are required also in women who do not respond to

---

Box 8.7 Physical examination in dysmenorrhoea

- General examination
- Per abdominal examination
  - Mass
  - Tenderness
- Pelvic examination
  - Uterine size
  - Adnexal mass
  - Tenderness
- Per rectal examination
  - Rectovaginal nodules
  - Tenderness

Box 8.8 Investigations in dysmenorrhoea

- Ultrasound scan—Abdomen and pelvis
  - Leiomyoma
  - Endometriosis
  - Adenomyosis
  - Ovarian mass
  - Cervical stenosis with haematometra
- Sonosalpingography
  - Intrauterine lesions
  - Müllerian anomalies
- Laparoscopy
  - Endometriosis
  - Chronic pelvic inflammatory disease
  - Pelvic congestion syndrome

---

nonsteroidal anti-inflammatory drugs (NSAIDs) or combined oral contraceptive (COC) pills. Transvaginal ultrasonography is sufficient to make a diagnosis of most pelvic pathology (Fig. 8.2). When a firm diagnosis is not possible, laparoscopy may be performed (Fig. 8.3).

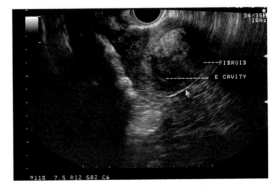

Figure 8.2 Transvaginal ultrasonography showing intramural myoma.

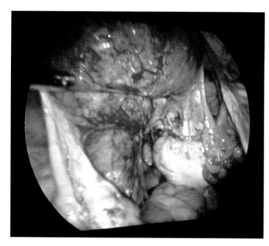

Figure 8.3 Pelvic endometriosis with extensive adhesions.

Management

Primary dysmenorrhoea

- Counselling to alleviate anxiety and lifestyle changes play an important role in management.
- Low-fat diet and supplementation with vitamin E, vitamin D_3, vitamin B_1 and fish oil have been tried in the management of primary dysmenorrhoea, but there are no data to prove their efficacy.

Primary treatment is with medications. Treatment modalities are summarized in Box 8.9.

Medical management

Nonsteroidal anti-inflammatory agents
Since increase in $PGF_{2\alpha}$ is the cause of pain, NSAIDs and prostaglandin (PG) synthetase inhibitors are the mainstay of treatment. The drug should be started at the onset of menses and repeated 6–8 hourly for adequate relief of symptoms. Of the drugs listed in Box 8.9, fenamates have been found to be more effective than ibuprofen and naproxen. All are associated with gastrointestinal side effects. Cyclooxygenase-2 (COX-2) inhibitors are equally effective.

Oestrogen–progestin combinations
COC pills may be the treatment of choice in women who desire contraception. Combination pills containing ethinyl oestradiol 20–30 μg with norgestrel 150 mg can be used monthly or as

---

Box 8.9 Treatment of primary dysmenorrhoea

- Medical management
  - NSAIDs
    - Aspirin: 500 mg thrice daily
    - Mefenamic acid: 500 mg thrice daily
    - Flufenamic acid: 200 mg twice daily
    - Ibuprofen: 400 mg thrice daily
    - Naproxen: 500 mg twice daily
  - COX-2 inhibitors
    - Celecoxib: 200 mg twice daily
    - Etoricoxib: 120 mg twice daily
  - Oestrogen–progestin combinations
    - COC pills one tablet daily, cyclically
    - Oestrogen–progestin patches
  - Progestins
    - Depot medroxyprogesterone injection
    - LNG-IUS
- TENS
- Surgical management
  - LUNA
  - LPSN

COC, combined oral contraceptive; *COX-2*, cyclooxygenase-2; *LNG-IUS*, levonorgestrel intrauterine system; *LPSN*, laparoscopic presacral neurectomy; *LUNA*, laparoscopic uterine nerve ablation; *NSAID*, nonsteroidal anti-inflammatory drug; *TENS*, transcutaneous electrical nerve stimulation.

extended cycles. Combined pills inhibit ovulation; therefore, there is no progesterone production. $PGF_{2\alpha}$ production is reduced.

Oestrogen–progestin transdermal patch, if available, can also be used.

Progestins
Injection depot medroxyprogesterone acetate (DMPA) once in 3 months causes amenorrhoea and alleviates pain.

Levonorgestrel intrauterine system (LNG-IUS) results in 50% reduction in pain and is an option for women desiring contraception and where oestrogen is contraindicated.

Transcutaneous electrical nerve stimulation (TENS)

This relieves pain but is not more effective than mefenamic acid.

Surgical management

Surgical intervention consists of laparoscopic uterine nerve ablation (LUNA) and laparoscopic presacral neurectomy (LPSN). These have been tried but not recommended as routine.

Alternative therapies

Alternative therapies including Chinese herbal medicines and acupuncture have also been tried and found to be useful, but evidence is not sufficient to recommend their routine use.

Secondary dysmenorrhoea

Treatment of secondary dysmenorrhoea consists of treatment of the causative pathology and is dealt with in the respective chapters. NSAIDs are used in addition to specific treatments but are not as effective as in primary amenorrhoea.

Premenstrual syndrome and premenstrual dysphoric disorder

PMS refers to a group of symptoms, both physical and behavioural, that some women experience regularly during the luteal phase and subside when menstruation begins. The symptoms interfere with a woman's ability to function normally. To be considered clinically significant, the symptoms must be present for at least 5 days before menstruation and for three consecutive menstrual cycles. **In the severe form where PMS is associated with at least one affective symptom such as mood swings, irritability or depression, it is called PMDD.** In addition, in some women with psychiatric disorders, worsening of symptoms occurs premenstrually, but they do not come under the category of PMS or PMDD. About 30–80% of menstruating women experience some symptoms of PMS at some time; less than 10% of women have PMDD.

Risk factors

Risk factors for PMS are as shown in Box 8.10.

Box 8.10 Risk factors for PMS

- Family history of PMS
- Past or current mood or anxiety disorder
- History of postpartum depression
- Nulliparity
- Early menarche
- Stress
- Alcohol and caffeine intake

PMS, premenstrual syndrome.

Pathogenesis

PMS and PMDD occur in ovulatory cycles. The disorder was thought to be associated with an increase in progesterone levels in the luteal phase, but there is no evidence to prove this hypothesis. It is now postulated to be due to changes in sex steroid hormones that occur in ovulatory cycles, which cause alterations in neurohormones and neurotransmitters. Adrenergic, serotonergic, opioid and γ-aminobutyric acid pathways are involved (Fig. 8.4). There is a genetic predisposition, and sociocultural influences also play a role. Deficiency of vitamin B_6 and calcium has also been implicated.

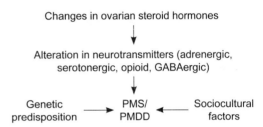

Figure 8.4 Pathogenesis of PMS and PMDD. *GABA*, γ-aminobutyric acid; *PMDD*, premenstrual dysphoric disorder; *PMS*, premenstrual syndrome.

Symptoms

Symptoms of PMS are listed in Box 8.11.

Box 8.11 Symptoms of PMS

- Somatic symptoms
  - Fluid retention, feeling of bloating
  - Breast pain or tenderness
  - Headache
  - Change in bowel habits
  - Increased appetite
- Affective symptoms
  - Mood disturbances
  - Irritability
  - Tension
  - Depression and crying spells
  - Anxiety and anger
  - Insomnia

PMS, premenstrual syndrome.

Diagnosis

- Diagnosis of PMS is made if a woman has one to four symptoms, which may be physical, behavioural, affective or psychological.

- A diagnosis of PMDD is made if a woman has >5 symptoms as described in Box 8.11 and one of them is an affective symptom.

Diagnosis of PMS is by a process of exclusion. There are no laboratory tests to confirm the diagnosis. A daily symptom diary for a minimum of 2 months is essential to confirm the premenstrual timing, severity and nature of symptoms. Diseases to be excluded are as listed in Box 8.12.

Box 8.12   Diseases to be excluded before diagnosing PMS

- Psychiatric illnesses
- Thyroid dysfunction
- Menopausal transition
- Substance abuse

PMS, premenstrual syndrome.

Management

Management of PMS depends on severity of symptoms

Mild symptoms

- **General supportive therapy** is the first line of treatment and may suffice in mild cases.
- **Lifestyle changes** such as diet, exercises, calcium supplements and vitamin B$_6$ are useful.
- Potassium-sparing **diuretics**, such as spironolactone, are used when fluid retention is the main problem.
- **Danazol** and **bromocriptine** relieve premenstrual mastalgia.
- **Alternative therapies**, especially oil of evening primrose, have been used with variable results. They are used in women with mastalgia, fluid retention and behavioural symptoms. Women with PMDD should be referred to a specialist for counselling and psychoactive drug therapy.

Moderate-to-severe symptoms

- **Selective serotonin reuptake inhibitors** (SSRIs) are the psychoactive drugs of choice in women with behavioural and affective symptoms. Several randomized trials have demonstrated their excellent efficacy with minimum side effects. The drugs used are fluoxetine, sertraline, paroxetine and citalopram. They can be administered throughout the cycle or only in the luteal phase. Treatment must be prolonged.
- **COC pills** have shown mixed results and may be useful in women with breast pain, bloating and acne. They act by inhibiting ovulation. Pills containing the progestin drospirenone have been found to be more effective.
- Gonadotropin-releasing hormone (GnRH) agonists with add-back therapy using OC pills (OCPs) may be useful in women who do not respond to SSRIs or OCPs.

Various medications used in treatment of PMS are listed in Table 8.1.

Table 8.1   Medical management of PMS

Therapy	Dose	Indications
Lifestyle modification		All
Diet and exercises		All
Calcium supplements	1 g daily	All
Vitamin B$_6$	200 mg daily	All
Spironolactone	100 mg daily	• Fluid retention • Weight gain
Danazol	200 mg daily	Mastalgia
Bromocriptine	2.5 mg daily	Mastalgia
OC pills (ethinyl oestradiol 20 µg + drospirenone 3 mg)	1 daily	• Mastalgia • Acne • Bloating
SSRIs		
Fluoxetine	20 mg daily	Affective symptoms
Paroxetine	12.5 mg daily	Affective symptoms
Sertraline	25–100 mg daily	Affective symptoms
Citalopram	10 mg daily	Affective symptoms
GnRH agonists	3.75 mg monthly	Not responding to SSRIs and OC pills

GnRH, gonadotropin-releasing hormone; *OC*, oral contraceptive; *PMS*, premenstrual syndrome; *SSRI*, selective serotonin reuptake inhibitor.

Menstrual migraine

Migraine can be triggered by a decline in serum oestrogen levels, and it is referred to as oestrogen-associated migraine. This occurs in association with menstruation (menstrual migraine) or when oestrogen is withdrawn as in the use of cyclic OCPs.

Menstrual migraine is usually more severe and lasts longer than nonmenstrual migraine. It does not respond well to treatment.

Menstrual migraine is of two types:

- *Pure menstrual migraine:* This refers to attacks of migraine that occur only perimenstrually (2 days before to 3 days after the onset of menstruation). At least two-thirds of menstrual cycles are associated with migraine.
- *Menstrually related migraine:* This refers to attacks of migraine that occur regularly during perimenstrual period but occur at other times as well.

Pathogenesis

The fall in oestrogen levels is associated with a fall in serotonin levels. This causes release of vasodilator substances leading to migraine. Other chemical mediators such as nitric oxide, magnesium and PGs also play a role.

Treatment

Treatment consists of abortive therapy with usual migraine-specific drugs and prophylactic therapy (Box 8.13).

Catamenial seizures

Seizures that cluster around menstrual cycle are called catamenial seizures. The pathophysiology is hormone mediated. Oestrogen and progesterone modulate cortical excitability. In ovulatory cycles, seizures occur premenstrually,

---

Box 8.13 Menstrual migraine

- Two clinical types
  - Pure menstrual migraine
    - Attacks of migraine only perimenstrually
  - Menstrually related migraine
    - Attacks of migraine perimenstrually and at other times
- Pathophysiology
  - Decline in oestrogen levels
  - Decline in serotonin
  - Release of vasodilators
- Treatment
  - Abortive therapy
    - Migraine specific—Triptans and ergots
    - Migraine nonspecific—NSAIDs and narcotics
  - Prophylactic therapy
    - Short term—NSAIDs, triptans and oestradiol patches
    - Long term—COC pills
      - GnRH analogues
      - Selective oestrogen receptor modulators
      - Progestins
      - β-Blockers
      - Antidepressants
      - Calcium channel blockers

COC, combined oral contraceptive; *GnRH*, gonadotropin-releasing hormone; *NSAID*, nonsteroidal anti-inflammatory drug.

---

probably due to progesterone withdrawal, and at midcycle, they are triggered by oestrogen surge. In anovulatory cycles, seizures are dispersed throughout the cycle since the oestrogen level remains relatively high.

Treatment is with anticonvulsants as in other patients with seizure disorders. Depot medroxyprogesterone and antioestrogens have been tried with varying results.

Key points

- Women experience a variety of symptoms during menstrual cycle. While some are indicative of organic pathology, others are due to hormonal changes of menstrual cycle.
- Dysmenorrhoea is the most common disorder associated with menstruation. This may be spasmodic or congestive in nature.
- Dysmenorrhoea is classified into primary and secondary. Primary dysmenorrhoea occurs in younger women, is usually spasmodic and is not associated with pelvic pathology. It is due to excess of prostaglandin F2 alpha ($PGF_{2\alpha}$). Secondary dysmenorrhoea is usually secondary to some pelvic pathology and occurs several years after menarche. Endometriosis, chronic pelvic infection, leiomyoma and adenomyosis are common conditions that cause secondary dysmenorrhoea. Local congestion in the pelvis and increase in $PGF_{2\alpha}$ are implicated in the pathogenesis.
- A detailed history regarding the nature of pain, menstrual cycle and other associated symptoms is mandatory. On clinical evaluation, pelvic mass and tenderness should be looked for. Ultrasonography and occasionally laparoscopy may be required in women with secondary dysmenorrhoea.

(Continued)

Key points *(Continued)*

- Primary dysmenorrhoea usually responds to nonsteroidal anti-inflammatory drugs (NSAIDs) or combined oral contraceptive (COC) pills. Treatment of secondary dysmenorrhoea consists of treatment of the causative pelvic pathology.

- Premenstrual syndrome (PMS) is a group of symptoms that women experience regularly during the late luteal phase. When it is severe, it is referred to as premenstrual dysphoric disorder (PMDD). Other psychiatric illnesses, thyroid dysfunction and substance abuse must be excluded before making a diagnosis of PMS or PMDD.

- Treatment of PMDD is by lifestyle modification, calcium and vitamin supplements, danazol, COC pills or selective serotonin reuptake inhibitors (SSRIs).

- Menstrual migraine and catamenial seizures are other less frequent disorders associated with menstrual cycle.

Self-assessment

Case-based questions

Case 1

A 16-year-old high school student presents with lower abdominal cramping pain during menstruation.

1. What details would you ask for in history?
2. What is the next step in evaluation?
3. How will you manage?

Case 2

A 39-year-old mother of two children presents with pain during menstruation for the past 1 year.

1. What details would you ask for in history?
2. What is the next step in evaluation?
3. If there is a suprapubic mass corresponding to the size of 18 weeks' gravid uterus, what investigation will you order?
4. What is the management?

Answers

Case 1

1. (a) Age at menarche
   (b) Menstrual cycles—Duration and regularity
   (c) Time of onset of pain in relation to menstruation
   (d) Type of pain—Spasmodic or congestive
   (e) Other associated symptoms
   (f) Duration of pain
   (g) History suggestive of stress and anxiety
2. If history is suggestive of primary dysmenorrhoea, general examination and abdominal examination.

3. (a) Reassurance
   (b) T mefenamic acid 500 mg 6 hourly, starting at the onset of menstruation, for 3–5 days, to be taken every month

Case 2

1. (a) Menstrual cycles—Duration and regularity
   (b) Heavy menstrual bleeding
   (c) Other associated symptoms—Dyspareunia and heaviness in the pelvis
   (d) Type of pain—Spasmodic or congestive
   (e) History suggestive of pelvic inflammatory disease
2. Clinical examination including abdominal and pelvic examination—Uterine or adnexal mass, tenderness and fixity.
3. Ultrasonogram of abdomen and pelvis.
4. Diagnosis could be leiomyoma of the uterus or endometriosis (chocolate cyst). Management is surgical. NSAIDs may be used initially to relieve pain.

Long-answer question

1. What is dysmenorrhoea? How do you classify dysmenorrhoea? Discuss the aetiology, pathogenesis and management of primary dysmenorrhoea.

Short-answer questions

1. Premenstrual syndrome
2. Congestive dysmenorrhoea
3. Spasmodic dysmenorrhoea
4. Menstrual migraine

9

Benign Diseases of the Vulva, Vagina and Cervix

Case scenario

Mrs AK, 30, was a mother of two children. She noticed pain, discharge and a small swelling in the vulva 2 days ago along with malaise and a feeling of ill health. She was too embarrassed to go to a doctor and therefore tried some home remedies. She developed fever on the next day, and the swelling became larger and more painful. She found it difficult to walk. She felt that she may have contracted a sexually transmitted disease and came to the hospital.

Introduction

Women with lesions in the vulva, vagina and cervix may not seek medical help immediately due to social inhibition and embarrassment. The most common condition that affects the lower genital tract is infection. Other benign diseases of the structures of the vulva, vulvar skin, hair follicles and sebaceous glands can give rise to discharge, swelling, pruritus ulcer or pain.

Benign diseases of the vulva

Diseases of the vulva may involve the structures in the vulva or the vulval skin. Most of the lesions arise from the vulval skin and are dermatological problems, but women visit the gynaecologist for treatment. Infections of the lower genital tract including sexually transmitted infections also present with vulval lesions. The spectrum of vulval disease is so wide that management may require a multidisciplinary approach, involving a gynaecologist, dermatologist, venereologist and physician.

Classification and terminology

Several terms were used in the past to describe vulvar lesions. A morphology-based classification of vulvar lesions was developed by the International Society for the Study of Vulval Disease (ISSVD) in 2011. This has been incorporated in the International Federation of Cervical Pathology and Colposcopy (IFCPC, 2012) classification and terminology. This terminology should be followed for diagnosis, treatment and research purposes. The terminology includes several sections given as follows:

- Structures of the vulva
- Normal findings
- Abnormal findings
  - Morphological types and their definition
  - Lesion colour
  - Secondary morphology
- Suspicion of malignancy

Structures in the vulva Anatomically, the vulva extends from genitocrural folds laterally to mons pubis anteriorly and anus posteriorly. The anatomical structures in the vulva are listed in Box 9.1.

The **normal findings** in the vulva include micropapillomatosis, sebaceous glands and vestibular redness. It is important to be aware of normal findings and not mistake them for vulvar lesions.

Box 9.1　Structures in the vulva

- Labia majora
- Labia minora
- Interlabial sulci
- Clitoris
- Vestibule
- Hymen
- Fourchette
- External urethral meatus
- Vaginal orifice
- Bartholin glands
- Skene ducts

Characteristics of vulvar lesions

Vulvar lesions are characterized by morphological type, colour, size, location and secondary morphological changes, when present. Lesions may be examined with naked eye, using magnifying lens or using a colposcope.

- The morphological types are defined in Table 9.1.
- **The colour of the lesion** may be
  - Red
  - White
  - Dark
  - Skin coloured

Table 9.1　Morphological types of vulvar lesions

Morphological type	Definition
Macule	Small (<1 cm) area of colour change; no elevation and nonpalpable
Patch	Large (>1 cm) area of colour change; no elevation and nonpalpable
Papule	Small (<1 cm) palpable lesion
Nodule	Large (>1 cm) palpable lesion; usually dome shaped; margins may be distinct (sharp) or slope shouldered
Plaque	Large (>1 cm) flat-topped and palpable lesion
Vesicle	Small (<1 cm) fluid-filled blister; clear fluid
Bulla	Large (>1 cm) fluid-filled blister; clear fluid
Pustule	Small or large pus-filled blister; white or yellow fluid
Ulcer	Deep defect into or through the dermis; the base may be red or covered by yellow, blue or black crust. Ulcers heal with scarring
Cyst	Small or large nodule with epithelial-lined central cavity containing solid, semisolid or fluid-filled material

Secondary morphological changes may be seen. These are lichenification, excoriation, scarring, erosion, fissure, bleeding and pigmentation.

Categorization of vulvar lesions

After clinical examination, vulvar lesions may be grouped under the categories listed in Box 9.2. Since the morphological characteristics of some

Box 9.2　Categorization of vulvar lesions

- Red patches and plaques
- Red papules and nodules
- White patches and plaques
- White papules and nodules
- Yellow papules and pustules
- Brown or black papules, patches and plaques
- Skin-coloured papules, nodules and plaques
- Vesicles and bullae
- Erosions
- Ulcers

lesions overlap, same condition may be listed under more than one category.

Common conditions under the different categories are discussed in the chapter. Uncommon and rare conditions and premalignant and malignant lesions are not included.

Red patches and plaques

The common conditions that present as red patches and plaques are listed in Box 9.3.

Candidiasis Candidiasis of the vulva is usually associated with vaginal candidiasis. The skin is excoriated due to pruritus, and vaginal discharge is usually seen. Treatment is discussed in Chapter 12, *Infections of the lower genital tract.*

Dermatitis Dermatitis of vulval skin is common (Box 9.4). It can be atopic, allergic, seborrhoeic or primary irritant dermatitis. It is one of the common conditions affecting the vulva (Fig. 9.1).

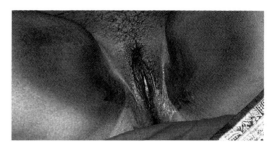

Figure 9.1 Primary irritant dermatitis involving the vulva and medial aspect of thighs caused by use of a local disinfectant.

Lichen simplex or neurodermatitis It presents as thickened patches on vulval skin that are itchy. It is a localized atopic dermatitis. The itch–scratch cycle is responsible, and the pruritus is worse at night.

Lichen planus It is characterized by purplish, polygonal, intensely pruritic papules like in other parts of the body. Erosive lichen planus is painful.

Psoriasis Psoriasis in the genital area is very common and presents with pruritus and pain. The lesions appear as discrete plaques with silvery scales or as inflamed, beefy red areas. Psoriatic lesions in other parts of the body such as the scalp and the extensor aspects of limbs and nail pitting are often present in addition.

Red papules and nodules

Common conditions presenting as red papules and nodules are listed in Box 9.5.

Folliculitis It is a common condition affecting the hairy areas. The infection is usually staphylococcal or fungal. The tip of the papules is covered by pustules.

Haemangiomas They are seen in the neonatal period and usually resolve before 10 years of age. **Cherry angiomas** contain capillaries and blood vessels and may increase during pregnancy.

Furuncles They are collection of pus around the follicles. They are tender, red nodules. Underlying pus may be visible. The organism involved is usually *Staphylococcus aureus*. Systemic symptoms such as fever and malaise may be present.

Hidradenitis suppurativa They are recurrent pustules that are very painful and tender, and occur in vulva, axilla, under the breasts and groin. They may occur in clusters. The pustules enlarge to become abscesses, rupture and drain pus. The condition is chronic, and recurrent lesions lead to scarring. The bacterial cultures are usually negative, but secondary infections can occur.

Bartholin gland abscess The Bartholin glands are located at 5 and 7 o'clock positions at the entrance to the vagina. The glands are 0.5 cm in size, and the ducts, which are 2–2.5 cm in length, open in the groove between the hymen and the labia minora.

When the ducts are obstructed, Bartholin cyst develops. Infection of the cyst gives rise to abscesses. These are located in the posterior part of the labium majus and give the inroitus a typical 'S'-shaped appearance (Fig. 9.2). Bartholin cyst and abscess are discussed in detail in Chapter 12, *Infections of the lower genital tract.*

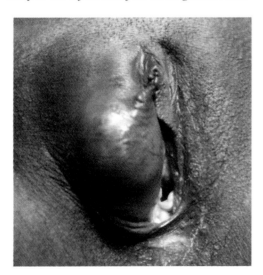

Figure 9.2 Bartholin gland cyst located in the right labia giving the introitus an 'S'-shaped appearance.

Urethral caruncle and urethral prolapse They generally occur in older postmenopausal women. They are usually asymptomatic but may give rise to dysuria.

White patches and papules

Common white patches and papules are listed in Box 9.6.

Box 9.6 White patches and papules of vulva

- Vitiligo
- Postinflammatory hypopigmentation
- Vulvar warts
- Intertrigo
- Lichen sclerosus

Lichen planus and lichen simplex They can also present as white lesions.

White patches or vitiligo They can affect the genital area, especially the periorificial area (Fig. 9.3). They are considered to be an autoimmune disease.

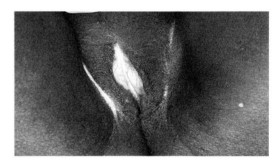

Figure 9.3 Vitiligo presenting as hypopigmented lesion around the introitus.

Postinflammatory hypopigmented lesions They are seen following treatment in women with lichen sclerosus, discoid lupus and other chronic skin lesions.

Intertrigo It is a nonspecific inflammatory lesion usually seen in labiocrural folds due to sweating and friction. It is common in obesity and diabetes. Bacteria and fungi multiply in the moist areas and cause irritation, itching and foul odour. The skin appears inflamed and macerated.

Lichen sclerosus Lichen sclerosus is one of the vulvar dermatoses that has a predilection for genital skin (Fig. 9.4). Clinical features are given in Box 9.7.

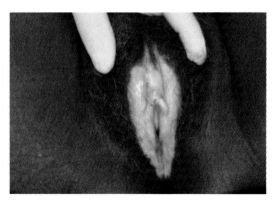

Figure 9.4 Lichen sclerosus of the vulva in a postmenopausal woman. The lesions are thin and white.

Vulvar warts   These are known as condyloma acuminate and are caused by human papillomavirus (HPV) infection. They can occur on the vulva, perianal area or perineum. The lesions may be red, brown or white, depending on the extent of keratinization. The warts may be small papillomas or large and cauliflower-shaped masses. HPV infections can be associated with vulvar and cervical intraepithelial neoplasia or invasive cancer.

White papules and nodules

Molluscum contagiosum, caused by poxvirus infection, usually presents as white papules. They are red when inflamed. The lesions have central umbilication. They are asymptomatic but can be occasionally associated with pruritus.

Yellow papules and pustules

Many red or white lesions such as folliculitis, furunculosis, hidradenitis and molluscum contagiosum, when infected, present as yellow pustules. The other yellow lesions are pustular psoriasis and pyogenic granuloma.

Brown and black macules, papules, patches and plaques

Hyperpigmented lesions They are most often postinflammatory. **Acanthosis nigricans** and pigmented **vulvar melanocytic nevi** are occasionally seen. **Vulvar melanosis** is a large, hyperpigmented patch in the vulva, usually asymptomatic. It must be differentiated from a melanoma by biopsy.

Endometriosis Endometriosis of the vulva is uncommon. The endometriotic deposits are seen on the episiotomy scar or labia majora as bluish black swelling that increase in size and become painful during menstruation.

Skin-coloured papules, nodules and plaques

The common skin-coloured lesions are cysts and benign tumours of the vulva as listed in Box 9.8. Vulvar warts, molluscum contagiosum and lichen simplex can present as skin-coloured papules as well but are not included in the list since they have been discussed earlier.

Bartholin cysts They are unilateral cysts that develop due to occlusion of the duct. The cyst is located in the posterior aspect of the vulva, and the labium minus overlies the middle of the swelling. The cyst is painless, although the woman may be aware of a swelling. Treatment is by marsupialization or excision. Bartholin abscess is formed when the cyst is infected.

Mucous cysts They result from occlusion of the ducts of the mucous glands of the vestibule.

Inclusion cysts and sebaceous cysts They are the most common cysts of the vulva. They are difficult to distinguish on gross examination. The cysts are nontender. Inclusion cysts can be multiple. The contents are white or yellow. They are asymptomatic unless infected and can be left alone.

Lymphangiomas They are rare.

Fibromas, fibromyomas, angiofibromas and lipomas They are benign solid tumours that are generally asymptomatic (Figs 9.5–9.7). They need excision only if large.

Hidradenomas They arise from the apocrine glands of the vulva. They are small, capsulated tumours that occur exclusively in white women and can be mistaken for adenocarcinoma on histological examination. But the tumours are benign.

Bullous lesions

These are common lesions that appear as blisters on the vulval skin and are listed in Box 9.9.

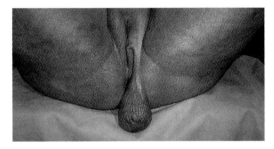

Figure 9.5 Fibroma of the vulva with a long pedicle.

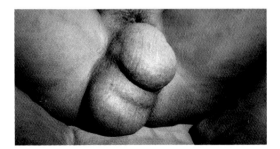

Figure 9.6 Large lipoma of the vulva.

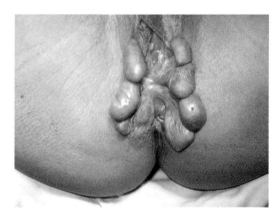

Figure 9.7 Multiple angiofibroma of the vulva.

Opinion of a dermatologist must be obtained for diagnosis and treatment.

Box 9.9 Bullous lesions

- Erythema multiforme
- Bullous pemphigoid
- Cicatricial pemphigoid
- Pemphigus vulgaris
- Epidermolysis bullosa

Vesicles

Genital herpes Genital herpes caused by herpes simplex virus presents as painful vesicles. They break down and form multiple painful ulcers. The lesions can be recurrent.

Intertrigo It is a nonspecific inflammatory lesion usually seen in labiocrural folds due to sweating and friction. It is common in obesity and diabetes. Bacteria and fungi multiply in the moist areas and cause irritation, itching and foul odour. The skin appears inflamed and macerated.

Ulcerative lesions Aphthous ulcers and Behçet's disease are the common ulcerative lesions.

Aphthous ulcers They are similar to the aphthous ulcers that occur in the oral mucosa. The lesions are painful and tend to recur. Aetiology is unknown.

Behçet's disease It is a systemic illness. Ocular manifestations are common. Vulval ulcers are very painful and last for a week.

Congenital malformations

Diagnosis and management of ambiguous genitalia and labial adhesions have been dealt with in Chapter 17, *Paediatric and adolescent gynaecology*. Congenital labial hyperplasia involves the labia minora and usually manifests at puberty. It is a benign condition that does not require any treatment.

Atrophic changes

Genital atrophy occurs due to oestrogen deficiency at menopause. If it is associated with dyspareunia, local or systemic oestrogen therapy is required.

Vulval manifestations of systemic disease

Several systemic diseases such as Crohn disease, Behçet's syndrome and pyoderma gangrenosum can present with vulval lesions. They require multidisciplinary approach to diagnosis and management.

Ulcers of the vulva are generally caused by infections and will be discussed in Chapter 12, *Infections of the lower genital tract*.

Clinical features

Symptoms

The symptoms of vulval lesions are listed in Box 9.10. Pruritus is the most common and significant symptom. Infections, especially vulvovaginitis, are the most common cause of pruritus and should be ruled out.

Box 9.10 Symptoms of vulval diseases

- Pruritus
- Pain
- Dyspareunia
- Swelling
- Ulcer
- Discolouration
- Discharge

Signs

The morphological features of the lesions have already been described.

Clinical evaluation

History

History may be difficult to obtain unless privacy is ensured and leading questions are asked. A detailed history regarding use of systemic medications, topical applications, allergies, past and family history is important (Box 9.11).

Box 9.11 History in vulval diseases

- Predominant symptom
- Duration
- Allergies
  - Atopy
  - Eczema
  - Asthma
  - Allergy to drugs
  - Contact dermatitis
- Allergens
  - Perfumes
  - Local applications
  - Synthetic undergarments
  - Latex and rubber
- Family history
  - Psoriasis
- Past history
  - Seborrhoeic dermatitis
  - Systemic illnesses
  - Anxiety and depression
  - Diabetes

Physical examination

Physical examination should include general examination for other skin lesions, systemic illnesses and local examination under good lighting with the help of a magnifying loop (Box 9.12). The entire vulva including clitoris, labia majora and minora, introitus, perineum and perianal area is inspected.

Investigations

Clinical diagnosis is possible in many situations. Colposcopy of the vulva is useful for identification of vulvar intraepithelial neoplasia. A biopsy is required in some cases (Box 9.13). It can be performed under local anaesthesia in the outpatient clinic.

- General and systemic examination
  - Obesity
  - Psoriasis
  - Seborrhoea
  - Lichen planus
  - Signs of Behçet's syndrome
  - Erythema multiforme
- Examination of the vulva
  - Vulval hair
  - Characteristics of the lesion
    - Colour
      - Red
      - White
      - Black or brown
      - Yellow
    - Location
    - Size, number
    - Nature
      - Macule
      - Papule
      - Plaque
      - Nodule
      - Cyst
      - Ulcer
    - Thickness and keratinization
    - Excoriation
    - Discharge
- Per speculum examination
  - Discharge
- Per vaginal examination

Box 9.13 **Indications for biopsy in vulval diseases**

- Difficulty in establishing the diagnosis
- Lesions that do not respond to the treatment
- When malignancy is suspected
- All pigmented and blistering lesions

Management

Management of vulvar lesions may be by medical treatment, surgical excision or simple observation.

Infected lesions require systemic antibiotics. Vitiligo, hyperpigmentation, hypopigmentation, vulvar nevi and other asymptomatic lesions can be observed without any active intervention.

Management of the various categories of lesions is listed in Boxes 9.14–9.18.

Box 9.14 **Management of red patches and plaques**

• Lichen planus	Clobetasol ointment
• Lichen simplex	Clobetasol ointment
• Psoriasis	Clobetasol
	Coal tar
	Tacalcitol
	Calcitriol
	Systemic therapy
• Irritant dermatitis	Avoid allergen
	Topical steroids
• Atopic dermatitis	Topical steroids
• Allergic dermatitis	Avoid allergen
	Topical steroids

Box 9.15 **Management of red papules and plaques**

• Folliculitis	Antibiotics
• Angiomas/haemangiomas	Observation
	Laser excision
• Furunculosis	Antibiotics
• Hidradenitis suppurativa	Antibiotics
• Bartholin abscess	Incision and drainage
	Antibiotics

Box 9.16 **Management of lichen sclerosus**

- Local hygiene
- Topical steroids
  - 0.05% clobetasol daily for 4 weeks
  - Alternate nights for 4 weeks
  - Twice weekly for 4 weeks
- Intralesional infiltration of steroids
- Topical oestrogen
- Topical retinoids
- Tacrolimus

Box 9.17 **Management of bullous lesions**

• Erythema multiforme	Treat the underlying cause
• Bullous pemphigoid	Topical steroid
• Cicatricial pemphigoid	Topical steroid
• Pemphigus vulgaris	Topical steroid
• Epidermolysis bullosa	No known treatment
• Pigmentary changes	No treatment indicated

Box 9.18 Management of cysts and tumours

• Bartholin gland cyst	Excision if required
• Skene duct cyst	Excision
• Mucous cysts	Excision
• Inclusion cyst	Incision and drainage
	Excision if required
• Sebaceous cyst	Observation
	Excision if required
• Fibroma	Excision if large
• Lipoma	Excision if large
• Lymphangioma	Laser therapy
• Hidradenoma	Excision
• Endometriosis	Excision

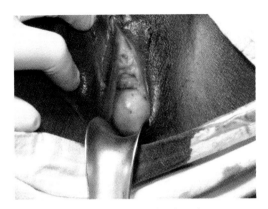

Figure 9.8 Gartner duct cyst arising from the anterolateral wall of the vagina and protruding at the introitus.

Benign diseases of the vagina

Benign diseases of the vagina are less common than those of the vulva. These are listed in Box 9.19.

Box 9.19 Benign diseases of the vagina

- Urethral diverticulum
- Inclusion cysts
- Dysontogenetic cysts
- Atrophic changes
- Lesions due to in utero exposure to diethylstilbestrol

Urethral diverticulum

This usually arises from the posterior wall of the urethra and projects into the anterior vaginal wall. It can be asymptomatic, but most women present with chronic symptoms of lower urinary tract infection, postvoid dribbling, dyspareunia or haematuria. Clinically, they can be mistaken for Gartner duct cysts or Skene duct cysts. Diagnosis is confirmed by cystourethrography or cystourethroscopy. Treatment is by excision.

Inclusion cysts

These are the most common cysts in the vagina. They may be seen in posterior or lateral vaginal walls. They usually result from birth trauma or previous surgery. Majority are asymptomatic. Only symptomatic and large ones need to be excised.

Dysontogenetic cysts

Cysts that have an embryonic origin are referred to as dysontogenetic cysts. The most common are **Gartner duct cysts** (Fig. 9.8). They arise from the remnants of mesonephric duct and are seen in the anterior and lateral wall, generally in the lower one-third. Rarely, cysts may arise from mesonephric elements or urogenital sinus. They can be differentiated histologically by the lining epithelium. Majority of these cysts are asymptomatic. Some women present with vaginal mass, pain, urinary symptoms or dyspareunia. Symptomatic cysts must be excised.

Atrophic changes

Atrophic changes occur in postmenopausal women due to oestrogen deficiency. The epithelium is thin and dry, making it prone to trauma and infection. In women who present with dyspareunia and recurrent infections, local oestrogen therapy is required.

Lesions due to exposure to diethylstilbestrol

Benign lesions of the uterus, cervix and vagina are seen in children and women exposed to diethylstilbestrol in utero. The hormone was used in the past to prevent miscarriage. Abnormalities occur at the junction of Müllerian ducts and sinovaginal bulbs leading to characteristic lesions described as vaginal adenosis. A ridge can be palpated between the cervix and the vagina, which is referred to as a collar or 'cock's comb cervix'.

Benign diseases of the cervix

Apart from the infections and premalignant changes, benign cervical lesions are also common (Box 9.20).

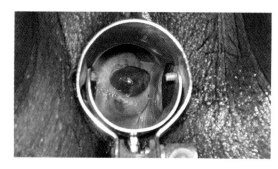

a.

Box 9.20 Benign lesions of the cervix

- Ectropion
- Cervicitis
- Polyps
- Warts
- Nabothian cysts
- Myomas
- Microglandular hyperplasia
- Cervical stenosis

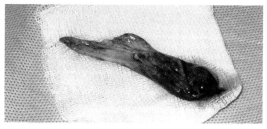

b.

Ectropion

Ectropion is the eversion of the cervix. This occurs in multiparous women or in women taking combined oral contraceptive (OC) pills. The endocervical epithelium is exposed and appears red in colour. There may be excessive mucoid discharge. The condition was earlier referred to as 'erosion', which is a misnomer. Ectropion does not require any treatment. Cryocautery or electrocautery may be used if the discharge is excessive and troublesome.

Cervicitis

Acute cervicitis is the inflammation of cervix. The usual organisms are *Chlamydia trachomatis*, *Neisseria gonorrhoeae*, *Trichomonas vaginalis*, herpes simplex virus and *Mycoplasma genitalium*. Mucopurulent discharge is the presenting symptom. Intermenstrual or postcoital bleeding may also occur. Associated urethritis causes dysuria.

Management consists of identifying the cause and appropriate medical therapy (*see* Chapter 12, *Infections of the lower genital tract*).

Polyps

Endocervical and ectocervical polyps are the most common benign lesions of the cervix. They

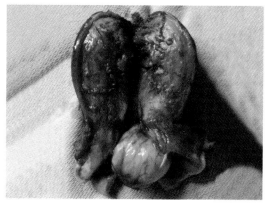

c.

Figure 9.9 Benign endocervical polyp. a. Polyp seen at the external os. b. Same polyp after polypectomy showing a pedicle. c. Cut section of the uterus showing polyp arising from the upper part of the endocervical canal near the internal os.

are generally seen in women in their forties and fifties. They are seen as reddish, smooth lesions protruding through the external os (Fig. 9.9).

They can cause contact bleeding and vaginal discharge. Malignant change is extremely rare. Endocervical polyps must be differentiated from endometrial polyps. Endometrial polyps have a long pedicle and the base is not accessible. Even when found incidentally, polypectomy is advisable since they can produce symptoms later. Polypectomy is an outpatient procedure. Histologically, most are adenomatous polyps.

Warts

These are caused by HPV. They are asymptomatic but may be associated with cervical intraepithelial neoplasia. Evaluation by colposcopy and appropriate treatment are indicated (*see* Chapter 28, *Premalignant diseases of the cervix*).

Nabothian cysts

During the reproductive years, the columnar epithelium of the cervix is replaced by squamous epithelium. The metaplastic squamous epithelium occludes the mouth of some of the glands, while the crypts are still lined by columnar, mucus-secreting epithelium. Retention cysts thus formed are called nabothian cysts and are normally seen in the adult cervix (Fig. 9.10). They can be left alone.

Myomas

Myomas of the cervix are similar to those seen in the uterus but arising from the smooth muscle tissue in the wall of the cervix. They are usually small and can be left alone. Management of large cervical myomas is discussed in detail in Chapter 10, *Benign diseases of the uterus*.

Terms such as 'chronic cervicitis' and 'cervical erosion' are not used now.

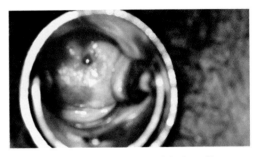

Figure 9.10 Nabothian cyst at 11 o'clock position.

Microglandular hyperplasia

This is usually seen in women using OC pills or depot preparations of medroxyprogesterone acetate. This can also occur in pregnancy and postpartum. It is an exaggerated epithelial response to hormones. Clinically, it can present as small, 1- to 2-cm polyps. On cytology and histology, it can be mistaken for a malignancy, but the condition is entirely benign. No treatment is required.

Cervical stenosis

Cervical stenosis usually occurs following surgeries such as conization, amputation of the cervix, trachelectomy and radiation. Rarely, it is congenital. Collection of blood in the uterine cavity leads to haematometra. In postmenopausal women, hydrometra develops. Cervix may not dilate in labour, leading to cervical dystocia. Treatment is by cervical dilatation.

Key points

- Standardized nomenclature recommended by the International Society for the Study of Vulval Disease is used to describe benign diseases of the vulva.
- Vulvar lesions are classified according to morphological features such as colour, morphological type, size and location.
- Dermatitis, vitiligo, folliculitis, lichen simplex and lichen sclerosus are the common vulvar lesions.
- The most common tumour is Bartholin gland cyst. It is located in the posterior part of the labium majus. It is asymptomatic unless infected.
- Predominant symptom of vulvar lesions is pruritus. Pain, dyspareunia, swelling, ulcer, discharge and discolouration are the other symptoms.
- Diagnosis of vulvar lesions is possible by clinical examination in most. Biopsy is required in a few

- women, when malignancy is suspected or when diagnosis is difficult.
- Management includes lifestyle modification, weight reduction, local hygiene, control of diabetes and treatment of other systemic illnesses. Topical medications are effective in most cases. Surgical excision may be required especially in case of tumours, cysts and hamartomas.
- Benign lesions of the vagina are less common. Inclusion cysts and dysontogenetic cysts occur in the reproductive age, and atrophic changes are seen in postmenopausal women.
- Nabothian cysts are common benign lesions of the cervix. Cervicitis, mucous polyps and myomas are other benign lesions of the cervix.

Self-assessment

Case-based questions

Case 1

A 30-year-old lady, mother of two children, presents with painful swelling in the vulva of 3 days' duration.

1. What findings would you expect in a Bartholin abscess?
2. How would you manage?
3. If the woman complains of four similar episodes in the past, how will you manage?

Case 2

A 35-year-old obese lady presents with pruritus in the genitocrural areas bilaterally. On examination, the area is moist with scratch marks, skin maceration and foul odour. The patient is a diabetic.

1. What is the diagnosis likely to be?
2. What is the management?

Answers

Case 1

1. (a) Swelling in the posterior part of the labium majus
   (b) 'S'-shaped introitus
   (c) Tenderness, oedema, cellulitis and erythema

2. Marsupialization, no need for antibiotics.
3. Excision after the infection subsides.

Case 2

1. Intertrigo.
2. (a) Weight reduction
   (b) Control of diabetes
   (c) Local hygiene
   (d) Avoidance of tight clothing
   (e) Local miconazole ointment

Long-answer question

1. Discuss the classification, clinical features and management of non-neoplastic lesions of the vulva.

Short-answer questions

1. Bartholin cyst
2. Vulvar dermatitis
3. Gartner duct cyst
4. Nabothian cyst

10 | Benign Diseases of the Uterus

Case scenario

Mrs VK, 39, a housewife, mother of two children, came to the outpatient clinic 1 day, looking quite distressed. She had consulted a local general practitioner for irregular menstrual cycles. She had been treated with oral contraceptive pills for nearly 2 years, but the problem persisted. After an ultrasonogram, she had been advised hysterectomy. She felt she was too young to undergo hysterectomy, her husband was worried about the complications of surgery and the family was also facing financial difficulties. She wanted to know what her problem was, whether hysterectomy was the only solution to her problem or whether there was an alternative.

Introduction

Benign diseases of the uterus are very common. The predominant symptom is abnormal uterine bleeding. They are the most common indication for hysterectomy. New modalities of conservative treatment are currently available, and this has reduced the hysterectomy rates. They are asymptomatic in many women and are diagnosed more often now due to the availability of imaging techniques. These asymptomatic lesions picked up on imaging give rise to management dilemmas.

The uterine wall consists of three layers—endometrium (which is lined by epithelium and contains glands and stroma), the myometrium (which is made of smooth muscle) and serosa (which is peritoneum). Benign lesions arise from the endometrium (polyp) or myometrium (myoma). In addition, extension of endometrial glands and stroma into the myometrium also occurs, leading to adenomyosis. The benign diseases of the uterus are listed in Box 10.1.

Box 10.1 Benign diseases of the uterus

- Endometrial polyps
- Adenomyosis
- Myomas

Endometrial polyps

Endometrial polyps are localized outgrowths of the endometrium and contain an inner core of blood vessels surrounded by endometrial glands and stroma. They are seen in women of all ages, but peak incidence is between 40 and 49 years. Incidence is high in women treated with tamoxifen. Endometrial polyps may be single or multiple. Salient features of endometrial polyps are given in Box 10.2.

Box 10.2	Salient features of endometrial polyps
• Age	All age groups (peak: 40–49 years)
• Size	Few millimetres to several centimetres
• Number	Single or multiple
• Types	Pedunculated (common)
	Sessile
• Symptoms	Asymptomatic
	Abnormal uterine bleeding
	Heavy menstrual bleeding
	Intermenstrual bleeding
	Postmenopausal bleeding
• Signs	Uterus normal or uniformly enlarged
	Polyp protruding through external os (occasional)

Pathology

Grossly, polyps may be pedunculated or sessile (Fig. 10.1a). On cut section of the uterus, polyps appear grey or reddish brown (Fig. 10.1b). The endometrial lining of the polyp may be proliferative, show cystic hyperplasia or undergo squamous metaplasia especially at the tip. The endometrium of the uterus may be hyperplastic, and this may account for the heavy menstrual bleeding. Malignant changes occur in 0.5% of polyps.

Endometrial polyps express oestrogen and progesterone receptors. Progesterone reduces proliferative activity in polyps and may cause regression.

Endometrial polyps are benign in 95% of cases. Risk of malignancy is higher in larger polyps (>1.5 cm) and in women on tamoxifen.

Clinical features

Endometrial polyps are often asymptomatic. Intermenstrual bleeding and heavy menstrual bleeding are the usual symptoms. Postmenopausal bleeding can also occur. Uterus is usually normal in size. Occasionally, endometrial polyp with long pedicle may protrude through the external os and be visible on speculum examination. Diagnosis by clinical examination is often difficult.

Diagnosis

Some polyps are incidentally found during evaluation for infertility. Endometrial polyps must be ruled out in women with abnormal uterine bleeding who do not respond to traditional treatments. Diagnosis is usually by transvaginal ultrasonography or hysteroscopy (Fig. 10.2a and b) usually performed during evaluation of refractory bleeding, infertility or other gynaecological indications (Box 10.3). Polyps can also be seen on saline infusion sonography (Fig. 10.2c). This

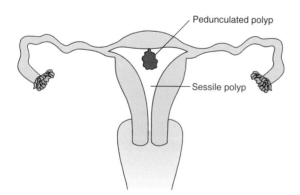

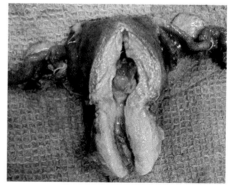

a.

b.

Figure 10.1 Endometrial polyps. a. Pedunculated and sessile. b. Cut section of the uterus showing pedunculated endometrial polyp.

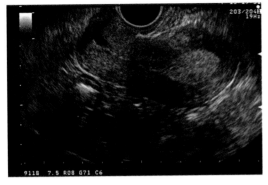

a.

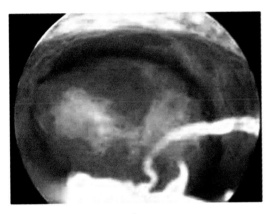

b.

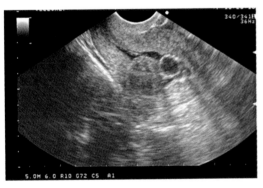

c.

Figure 10.2 Diagnosis of endometrial polyp. a. Transvaginal ultrasonography of the uterus. Endometrial polyp is visible in the uterine cavity. b. Endometrial polyp as visualized on hysteroscopy. c. Sonohysterography revealing endometrial polyp. The bulb of Foley catheter is seen as a perfect circle.

is performed when the diagnosis is not certain on ultrasonography.

Box 10.3 **Diagnosis of endometrial polyps**

- Transvaginal ultrasonography
- Saline infusion sonography
- Hysteroscopy

Management

- Asymptomatic polyps can be left alone except in situations listed as follows:
  - Polyp >1.5 cm in diameter
  - Associated with infertility
  - Postmenopausal women
  - Multiple polyps
- Symptomatic polyps must be removed.

Endometrial polyps are managed by **hysteroscopic polypectomy**. Curettage of the endometrium must be performed to rule out associated hyperplasia.

- In women on tamoxifen therapy, levonorgestrel intrauterine system (LNG-IUS) has been used to prevent progression to malignancy. Data are insufficient to recommend this as routine practice.

Adenomyosis

Adenomyosis is defined as the presence of endometrial tissue in the myometrium at least one low-power field (2.5 mm) from the basal layer of the endometrium. Endometrial glands and stroma must be present.

Incidence

Incidence of adenomyosis varies; incidence of asymptomatic disease found in hysterectomy specimens may be up to 60%, but clinical diagnosis is made only in about 8–10% of symptomatic women. Adenomyosis occurs often in association with uterine myoma and endometriosis.

Pathogenesis

The exact pathogenesis of adenomyosis is not known. Oestrogen and progesterone, pituitary hormones such as prolactin and growth factors may play a role. Oestrogen receptor mutations in the adenomyomatous areas and gene polymorphisms have been postulated. Adenomyosis may occur by

- Invagination of basal endometrium into the myometrium
- Metaplasia of Müllerian rests in the myometrium

The basal layer of the endometrium including glands and stroma infiltrates into the myometrium (Fig. 10.3). The surrounding myometrial tissue undergoes hypertrophy and hyperplasia giving rise to uterine enlargement.

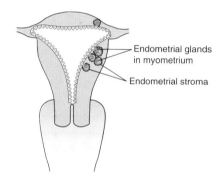

Endometrial glands in myometrium

Endometrial stroma

Figure 10.3 Pathogenesis of adenomyosis represented diagrammatically. The basal layer of the endometrium is seen to infiltrate into the myometrium.

Pathology

Adenomyosis is of two types: (a) Diffuse and (b) localized.

Diffuse adenomyosis involves anterior and posterior uterine walls and causes uniform uterine enlargement (Fig. 10.4a). The myometrium is thickened and reveals haemorrhagic foci of adenomyosis (Fig. 10.4b and c). This is the most common form. **Localized adenomyosis** is called **adenomyoma**, and grossly may mimic leiomyoma, but there is no capsule or a distinct plane of dissection (Fig. 10.5). Occasionally, it protrudes into the uterine cavity as submucous adenomyoma or adenomyomatous polyp.

Microscopically, islands of endometrial glands and stroma are seen in the myometrium (Fig. 10.6). These areas of endometrium may reveal proliferative, hyperplastic or secretory changes. Some of them undergo cyclic changes during menstrual cycle, resulting in areas of haemorrhage. Local prostaglandin production and bleeding are responsible for dysmenorrhoea experienced by these patients.

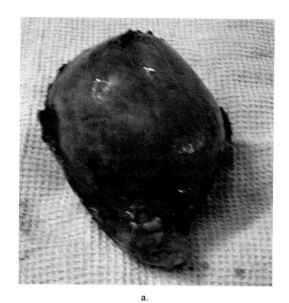

a.

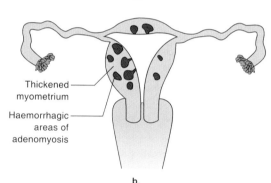

Thickened myometrium

Haemorrhagic areas of adenomyosis

b.

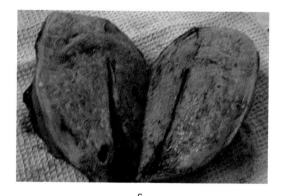

c.

Figure 10.4 Diffuse adenomyosis. a. Uterus with diffuse adenomyosis. Uterus is uniformly enlarged to about 12 weeks' size. b. Diagrammatic representation of diffuse adenomyosis showing diffuse thickening of myometrium and haemorrhagic foci of adenomyosis. c. Cut section of the uterus showing diffuse adenomyosis with areas of haemorrhage and thickened myometrium.

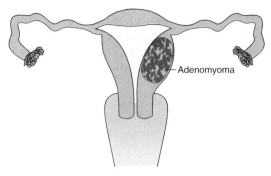

Figure 10.5 Localized adenomyosis (adenomyoma).

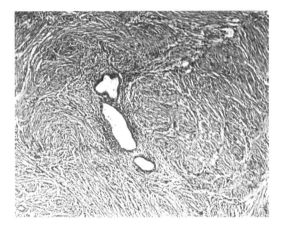

Figure 10.6 Histological photomicrograph of adenomyosis showing endometrial glands and stroma within the myometrium.

Risk factors

Risk factors are listed in Box 10.4.

Box 10.4 Risk factors for adenomyosis

- Multiparity
- Previous uterine surgery and trauma
  - Dilatation and curettage
  - Induced abortion

Clinical features

Symptoms

Adenomyosis is commonly seen in multiparous women of age 40–50 years, but can occur in younger women as well. It does not occur before menarche and regresses after menopause. It is more common in multiparous women. Dysmenorrhoea and heavy menstrual bleeding are the most common symptoms. Dysmenorrhoea is usually of congestive type and increases with increasing duration of disease and depth of infiltration of the myometrium. Chronic pelvic pain is a less common symptom.

Signs

Uterus is uniformly enlarged and usually just palpable abdominally (<14 weeks' size). Rarely, localized adenomyoma can occur and is difficult to distinguish clinically from intramural myoma. Clinical features are listed in Box 10.5.

Box 10.5 Clinical features of adenomyosis

• Age	Most common in 40–50 years
• Parity	Multipara
• Symptoms	Asymptomatic
	Secondary dysmenorrhoea
	Heavy menstrual bleeding
	Chronic pelvic pain
• Signs	Uterus uniformly enlarged
	<14 weeks' size

Adenomyosis may coexist with other pelvic pathology that may be responsible for the symptoms (Box 10.6). Uterine myoma is also an important differential diagnosis since it causes similar symptoms and uterine enlargement.

Box 10.6 Other pelvic pathology associated with adenomyosis

- Leiomyoma
- Endometrial hyperplasia
- Endometrial polyp
- Endometriosis
- Endometrial carcinoma

Diagnosis

Adenomyosis has to be distinguished from leiomyoma of the uterus and other pelvic conditions causing heavy menstrual bleeding and dysmenorrhoea. Decision regarding medical or surgical management depends on the diagnosis. Therefore, when adenomyosis is clinically suspected, ultrasonography is required to rule out other conditions (Box 10.7; Fig. 10.7a). Magnetic resonance imaging (MRI) is useful for confirmation of diagnosis (Fig. 10.7b) but is required only in situations where conservative surgical or medical management is preferred as in a young woman with infertility.

Box 10.7 Investigations in adenomyosis

- Transvaginal ultrasonography
  - Asymmetrical thickening of uterine walls
  - Myometrial cysts
  - Loss of clear endomyometrial border
  - Localized lesions
- Doppler sonography—To differentiate from myoma
- Magnetic resonance imaging—Only when required
- Image-directed needle biopsy—Rarely used

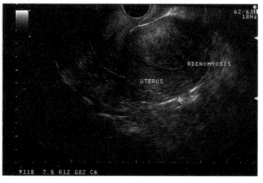

a.

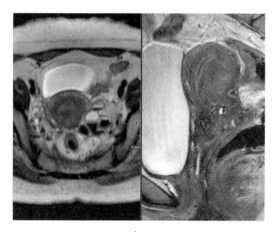

b.

Figure 10.7 Diagnosis of adenomyosis. **a.** Transvaginal ultrasonography of the uterus showing adenomyosis and thickening of anterior wall. **b.** Magnetic resonance imaging—Thick posterior wall and area of adenomyosis are clearly visualized. There is no distinct plane between the area of adenomyosis and the myometrium unlike in a myoma.

Management

Treatment may be medical or surgical. Coexisting conditions such as myomas should also be kept in mind when management decisions are made.

Medical management

Medical treatment is based on hormone dependency of the disease and its similarity to endometriosis. The endometriotic tissue in the myometrium is not as responsive to hormonal therapy as in endometriosis. Most women undergo hysterectomy after a short trial with medical therapy, since it is a disease seen predominantly in perimenopausal women. Moreover, adenomyosis is often associated with other pelvic pathology such as leiomyoma necessitating surgical intervention. But younger women and those who wish to conceive require medical or conservative surgical therapy. Methods of medical management are listed in Box 10.8.

Box 10.8 Medical management of adenomyosis

- NSAIDs
- Combined oral contraceptive pills
- Danazol
- GnRH analogues
- Aromatase inhibitors
- LNG-IUS
- Danazol-loaded IUS

GnRH, gonadotropin-releasing hormone; *LNG-IUS*, levonorgestrel intrauterine system; *NSAID*, nonsteroidal anti-inflammatory drug.

Nonsteroidal anti-inflammatory drugs (NSAIDs) These have been used to treat dysmenorrhoea and heavy menstrual bleeding, but the response is temporary and not adequate. They are generally used while awaiting surgery or when diagnosis is in doubt.

Combined oral contraceptive pills Although they are effective in the treatment of endometriosis, they have not been found useful in adenomyosis.

Danazol Androgen, oestrogen and progesterone receptors are present in the adenomyomatous lesions. Adenomyomas may reduce in size, uterine endometrium undergoes atrophy and heavy menstrual bleeding reduces, but symptoms recur immediately after stopping treatment.

Gonadotropin-releasing hormone (GnRH) analogues The GnRH analogues cause reduction in uterine size and volume and alleviation of symptoms in adenomyosis. They can be used prior to conservative surgery to reduce the size of adenomyoma and vascularity. But symptoms recur after discontinuation of the therapy. Long-term use of GnRH analogues is associated with side effects.

Aromatase inhibitors Aromatase inhibitors such as anastrozole have been used in some studies in women after conservative surgery. They are not used in routine practice.

Levonorgestrel intrauterine system Although this was originally introduced as a method of contraception, it has been found to be useful in several gynaecological conditions. Small trials have shown that the endometrium undergoes decidualization and later atrophy under the continuous effect of progesterone. Menstrual flow decreases, adenomyotic deposits reduce in size and uterine size decreases. Dysmenorrhoea improves due to reduction in local prostaglandin production. LNG-IUS has been found to be useful in women with endometriosis, but large randomized studies are not available to support its use in adenomyosis.

Danazol-loaded intrauterine devices These have been found to reduce pain and bleeding in women with adenomyosis, but they are still at experimental stage.

Surgical management

Surgical management may be hysterectomy or conservative surgery as given in Box 10.9.

Box 10.9 Surgical management in adenomyosis

- Definitive surgery
  - Hysterectomy
- Conservative surgery
  - Resection of adenomyoma
  - Myometrial reduction
  - Hysteroscopic resection

Hysterectomy This is the treatment of choice in most women for reasons listed in Box 10.10.

Ovaries may be retained unless there is associated endometriosis or the woman is close to menopause. Hysterectomy may be abdominal, vaginal or laparoscopic.

Box 10.10 Justifications for hysterectomy in adenomyosis

- Perimenopausal age
- Poor response to medical therapy
- Associated pelvic pathology common

Conservative surgery This is indicated in younger women who wish to preserve the uterus.

- *Resection of adenomyoma*: Localized adenomyoma may be resected by adenomyomectomy. Unlike in a leiomyoma, plane of dissection is difficult since there is no capsule.
- *Myometrial reduction*: Women who have diffuse adenomyosis involving anterior and/or posterior walls of uterus can be managed by partial resection of the uterine walls to reduce the volume of the disease. Heavy menstrual bleeding and dysmenorrhoea reduce significantly after this procedure.
- *Hysteroscopic endometrial resection*: For submucosal adenomyosis or polypoidal lesions, this is recommended. But failure rates are high due to associated myometrial disease. Preoperative diagnosis is difficult since the polyps are often diagnosed as myomatous polyps.

Newer interventional techniques Preoperative diagnosis of adenomyosis is now made more often with transvaginal ultrasonogram and MRI. This has led to the development of some new interventional techniques that are still experimental (Box 10.11). Experience with these modalities is limited since they are not widely used.

Box 10.11 Newer interventional techniques in adenomyosis

- Endometrial ablation
- UAE
- MRgFUS

MRgFUS, magnetic resonance–guided focused ultrasound surgery; *UAE*, uterine artery embolization.

Leiomyoma uterus (myomas)

Definition

Uterine leiomyomas are benign tumours that arise from the smooth muscle cells of the uterus but contain varying amounts of fibrous tissue. They vary in size from small 'seedling' myomas to large ones of several centimetres in size. They may be single, but often are multiple.

Prevalence

Leiomyomas are the most common tumours in women. They occur at all ages except in prepubertal girls, but are most common in the reproductive age. About 30–50% of women in perimenopausal age have leiomyomas.

Pathogenesis

There are several factors that contribute to the pathogenesis of myomas. Each myoma develops from a single muscle cell.

- Multiple chromosomal abnormalities have been demonstrated in the myomas by cytogenetic analysis. These may be translocations, rearrangements or deletions.
- A familial predisposition has been identified.
- Abnormalities in angiogenic growth factors such as transforming growth factor beta (TGF-β), epidermal growth factor (EGF), insulin-like growth factor (IGF), granulocyte-macrophage colony-stimulating growth factor (GM-CSF) and angiogenic growth factor have been implicated. Elevated levels of these cytokines may stimulate mitotic activity and formation of myoma.
- It is well accepted that growth of leiomyoma is dependent on sex steroids. Oestrogen receptors are found in myomas, and oestrogens stimulate their growth. In addition, aromatase enzyme that converts androgens to oestrogens is also found in myoma cells.
- Effect of progesterone on myoma is variable and not well understood. Progesterone receptors are also upregulated in myomas, but progesterone may increase or decrease the size of myomas.

Pathology

Gross and microscopic features are given in Box 10.12. The tumours are round or oval, firm and pearly white. They are usually multiple (Fig. 10.8), but occasionally solitary. A layer of connective tissue separates the myomas from the myometrium and forms the 'pseudocapsule'. This allows easy enucleation of myomas during myomectomy. Cut surface of the myoma is white and glistening (Fig. 10.9a), and has a characteristic 'whorled' appearance (Fig. 10.9b). On microscopic examination, interlacing smooth muscle bundles with a swirled pattern can be seen. Variable amount of fibrous tissue is also present (Fig. 10.10).

Box 10.12 Gross and microscopic appearance of myomas

- Gross appearance
  - Round or oval
  - Firm
  - Pseudocapsule
  - Cut surface
    - Whorled appearance
    - White, glistening
- Microscopic appearance
  - Interlacing smooth muscle bundles
  - Smooth muscle cell proliferation
  - Variable amount of fibrous tissue

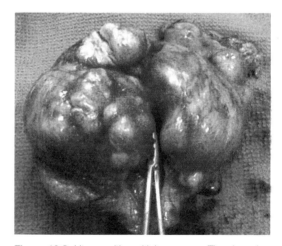

Figure 10.8 Uterus with multiple myomas. The clamp is placed in the endometrial cavity. Subserosal, intramural and submucosal myomas are seen.

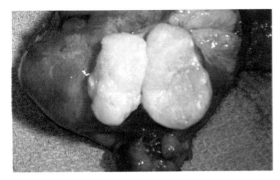

a.

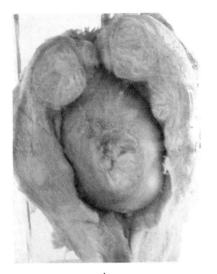

b.

Figure 10.9 Hysterectomy specimen. a. Cut section, white and glistening. b. Cut section with characteristic whorled appearance.

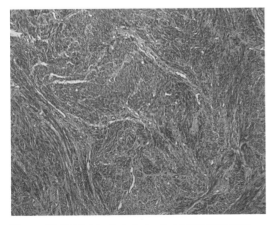

Figure 10.10 Histological photomicrograph of myoma. Note the smooth muscle bundles.

Anatomical classification

According to their relative anatomical relationship and position and location within the layers of the uterus, myomas are classified into subgroups (Box 10.13). Symptoms and treatment are dictated by the location of the myoma.

Box 10.13 Anatomical classification of myomas

- Myomas in the body of the uterus
  - Subserosal
  - Intramural
  - Submucosal
- Cervical myomas
  - Anterior
  - Posterior
  - Central
- Broad-ligament myomas
  - True: Arising from smooth muscle in broad ligament
  - Pseudo: Arising from the uterus and projecting into broad ligament

Myomas are further subclassified as given in Box 10.14 and Fig. 10.11a and b.

Box 10.14 Subclassification of uterine myoma

- SM—Submucosal
  - 0: Pedunculated, lies entirely within the uterine cavity
  - 1: <50% intramural
  - 2: >50% intramural
- O—Other
  - 3: Contacts endometrium; 100% intramural
  - 4: Intramural
  - 5: Subserosal >50% intramural
  - 6: Subserosal <50% intramural
  - 7: Subserosal pedunculated
  - 8: Other (cervical, broad ligament)

Hybrid or transmural leiomyomas These are leiomyomas that extend from endometrium to serosa. To denote these myomas, two numbers separated by a hyphen are used. The first number denotes relationship to endometrium, and the second number denotes relationship to peritoneal cavity.

Hybrid myomas 2–5 indicate submucosal myoma, which is >50% intramural and extends subserosally.

Myomas in the body of the uterus

Subserosal myomas They project into the peritoneal cavity from the surface of the uterus. They can be sessile or pedunculated. Subserosal myomas are usually asymptomatic. Large pedunculated ones can undergo torsion. They can become attached to other intra-abdominal structures. Occasionally, a subserosal myoma can become adherent to the omentum, receive its blood supply from omental vessels and detach itself from the uterus—Called parasitic myoma.

Intramural myomas They lie within the myometrium and are the most common. The surrounding connective tissue gets compressed, forming a **pseudocapsule** separating it from the myometrium. Intramural myomas give rise to a variety of symptoms.

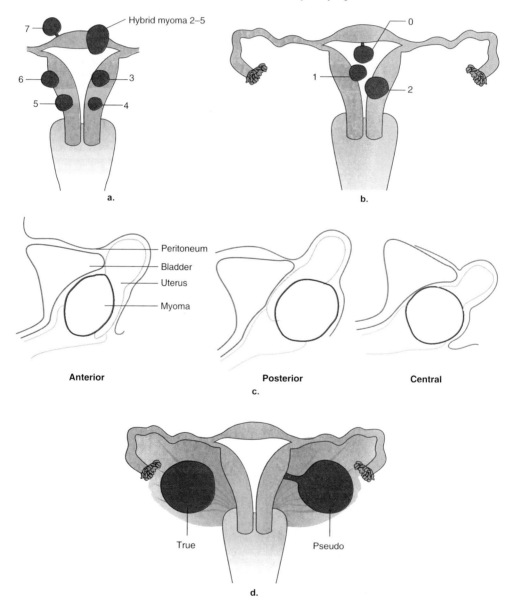

Figure 10.11 Pictorial representation of anatomical locations and classification of myomas. a. Submucosal and intramural myomas (refer Box 10.14). b. Subserosal and intramural myomas (Box 10.14). c. Types of cervical myomas. d. Broad-ligament myomas.

Submucosal myomas They are the least common, accounting for 5–10% of all myomas arising from the uterine body. They project into the uterine cavity and may be partly in the myometrium (Fig. 10.12). They give rise to a variety of symptoms; predominantly bleeding submucosal myomas may become pedunculated and protrude through the cervical os (Fig. 10.13). They are subdivided into three types depending on the extent to which they project into the uterine cavity.

Cervical myomas

They arise from the smooth muscle tissue in the cervix and are classified depending on their location into anterior, posterior and central cervical myomas (Fig. 10.11c). They press on the urinary bladder and urethra and displace the urethrovesical junction, giving rise to frequency of micturition and urinary retention. They also displace and compress the ureters.

Broad-ligament myomas

They are located between the layers of the broad ligament (Fig. 10.11d). The **true broad-ligament myomas** arise from the smooth muscle tissues in the round ligament, ovarian ligament or perivascular connective tissue and have no attachment to the uterus. They displace the ureters medially (Fig. 10.14a and b).

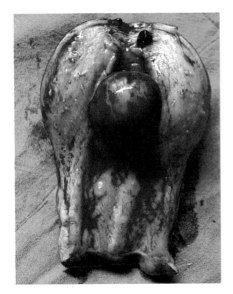

Figure 10.12 Cut section of the uterus showing submucosal myoma.

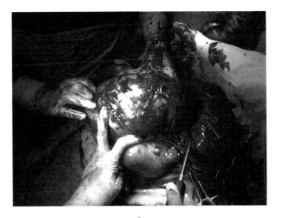

a.

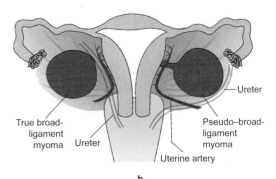

b.

Figure 10.14 Broad ligament myoma. a. Left broad-ligament myoma. b. True broad-ligament myoma displaces the ureter medially, but the pseudo–broad-ligament myoma displaces the ureter laterally.

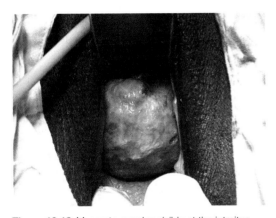

Figure 10.13 Myomatous polyp visible at the introitus.

The **pseudo** or **false broad-ligament myomas** are subserosal myomas arising from the lateral wall of the uterus and protruding between the layers of the broad ligament. They displace the ureters laterally as they grow and have a pedicle attached to the uterus. Broad-ligament myomas can be mistaken for adnexal masses on pelvic examination and imaging.

Degenerative changes in myomas

Vascular supply of the myoma is from (a) the small arteries that penetrate the pseudocapsule and (b) a large single vessel providing the major blood supply. The vascularity in the periphery of the myoma is increased, but the centre of the myoma has less blood supply. The tumour out-grows its blood supply and degenerative changes appear (Box 10.15). The most common is hyaline degeneration (Fig. 10.15).

Box 10.15 Degenerative changes in myomas

- Hyaline
  - Most common
  - Homogeneous appearance
  - Loss of whorled pattern
- Cystic
  - Localized liquefaction
  - Cystic spaces
- Myxomatous
  - Mucus-like fluid-filled spaces
- Fatty
  - Yellowish discolouration
- Calcific
  - Deposition of calcium salts
  - Long-standing myoma
  - Radio-opaque deposits
  - Honeycomb appearance
- Red
  - Occurs in pregnancy, oral contraceptive pills
  - Rapid growth, thrombosis, haemorrhage, disco-louration

Red or **carneous degeneration** is a unique phenomenon that occurs in 5–10% of pregnant women with myomas and has been reported with the use of oestrogen–progesterone oral con-traceptive (OC) pills and GnRH therapy and after uterine artery embolization. There is thrombosis and infarction of the myoma with peritoneal irri-tation giving rise to pain, fever and constitutional symptoms. Leucocytosis may be present. The condition is self-limiting and should be man-aged conservatively with analgesics and rest.

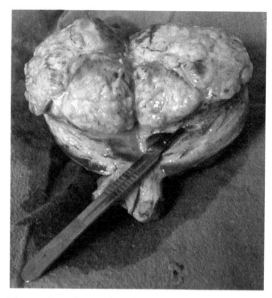

Figure 10.15 Cut section of the uterus with myoma showing hyaline degeneration in the myoma.

Complications

Torsion This occurs with subserosal peduncu-lated myomas. The patient presents with acute pain. Other conditions that give rise to acute abdomen should be considered because torsion is a rare complication.

Infection Submucosal myomas are prone to infection and ulceration. Infection of intramural myomas can occur in the puerperium or post-abortion period.

Malignancy Malignant tumour of the uterine smooth muscle is leiomyosarcoma. Malignancy arising in a leiomyoma is rare and occurs in sixth and seventh decades. The cytogenetic profile is different from benign leiomyoma; therefore, it is now believed that most leiomyosarcomas arise de novo. Only about 0.5% of myomas undergo malig-nant change, mainly in the older women. Increase in size of the myoma, which was considered to be a sign of malignancy, is significant only in the older, postmenopausal women. Histologically, malignant lesions have 10 or more mitotic figures per high-power field. When the mitotic figures are 5–10 per high-power field, they are called **smooth muscle tumours of uncertain malignant poten-tial** (STUMP). Benign myomas have <5 mitotic figures per high-power field.

Risk factors

Factors that increase the risk of development of leiomyoma are listed in Box 10.16.

Box 10.16 Risk factors of myomas

- Increasing age
- Early menarche
- Low parity
- Obesity
- High-fat diet
- Family history
- African-American race

Clinical features

Symptoms

About 50% of myomas are asymptomatic and found incidentally. Even large myomas can be silent. Myomas can give rise to a variety of symptoms depending on their location, size and number (Box 10.17).

Box 10.17 Symptoms of myomas

- Menstrual symptoms
  - Heavy menstrual bleeding
  - Intermenstrual bleeding
- Dysmenorrhoea
- Pelvic pain/discomfort
- Abdominal mass/distension
- Pressure symptoms
  - Urinary symptoms
    - Frequency
    - Difficulty in voiding
    - Retention
  - Rectal symptoms
    - Constipation
    - Difficulty in evacuation
- Subfertility
- Adverse pregnancy outcomes

Menstrual symptoms About 30–40% of women with myomas have abnormal uterine bleeding, which may be prolonged, heavy or intermenstrual. The amount of blood loss can be significant, causing anaemia. Menstrual abnormality is usually seen in submucosal and intramural myomas, but can be associated with subserosal myomas as well. Causes for abnormal bleeding are listed in Box 10.18.

Box 10.18 Causes for abnormal bleeding in myomas

- Increase in endometrial surface area
- Increase in vascularity of the uterus
- Interference with normal uterine contractility
- Ulceration of submucosal myomas
- Stasis and dilatation of venous plexuses
- Associated anovulation
- Associated endometrial hyperplasia
- Dysregulation of angiogenic factors

Dysmenorrhoea Secondary dysmenorrhoea of congestive nature is the usual symptom due to increase in vascularity of the uterus and venous stasis. Uterus may attempt to expel a large submucosal myoma, causing spasmodic dysmenorrhoea.

Pelvic pain/discomfort Even large and multiple myomas may be painless. A feeling of dragging or discomfort may be experienced when the myoma is large. Pelvic pain or pressure may occur during and between menstrual periods. Acute pain can occur with torsion of the myoma and with red degeneration.

Abdominal mass Large myomas, the size of 20 weeks' gravid uterus or more, may be felt as an abdominal mass by the patient, especially if the woman is thin.

Pressure symptoms include the following:
Urinary symptoms Myomas can compress the surrounding structures and give rise to symptoms. Those on the anterior wall and cervical myomas are in close proximity to the urinary bladder. Large myomas on the uterine body, broad-ligament myomas and cervical myomas can compress the ureters, causing hydroureteronephrosis (Box 10.19; Fig. 10.16).

Box 10.19 Effects of compression of urinary tract

- Increase in frequency
  - Change in bladder dynamics
  - Change in bladder capacity
- Urinary retention and difficulty in initiation
  - Pressure on urethrovesical junction
  - Compression of urethra
- Hydroureteronephrosis
  - Compression of ureters

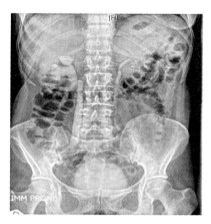

Figure 10.16 Intravenous urogram. There is dilatation of right ureter and renal pelvis. Hydroureteronephrosis—Caused by pressure on the pelvic ureter by myoma.

Rectal symptoms They are seen less frequently. Large myomas on the posterior wall and posterior cervical myomas can compress the rectum and interfere with complete evacuation.

Subfertility Clear association between myoma and subfertility has not been proved. But it has been found that in women with no other demonstrable cause for infertility, removal of the myoma improves pregnancy rates. There are several ways in which myomas are thought to interfere with conception (Box 10.20).

Box 10.20 Mechanism of subfertility in myomas

- Impaired gamete transport
  - Tubal occlusion
    - Impaired tubal motility
    - Impaired tubal function
  - Impaired uterine contractility
- Interference with implantation
  - Submucosal myoma
    - Atrophy
    - Ulceration
  - Endometrial changes
    - Thinning
    - Poor vascularization
  - Distortion of cavity
- Displacement of cervix from vaginal pool of semen

Adverse pregnancy outcomes Pregnancy can be adversely affected by the presence of leiomyoma (Box 10.21).

Box 10.21 Effect of leiomyoma on pregnancy

- Spontaneous miscarriage
- Preterm labour
- Abnormal foetal lie/malpresentations
- Dysfunctional labour
- Placental abruption
- Intrauterine growth restriction
- Operative delivery
- Postpartum haemorrhage

The endometrial changes and changes in vascularity account for the increase in spontaneous miscarriage. If the myoma underlies the site of placental implantation, abruption and intrauterine growth restriction can occur. But it is important to note that in most cases, pregnancy and labour progress without any complications.

Changes in myomas due to pregnancy

Pregnancy can cause changes in the leiomyoma. It was believed that myomas always increase in size during pregnancy. But recent research has shown that they remain the same in most cases, but may marginally increase in size in others. **Red degeneration** can occur in pregnancy as previously discussed. Torsion of a pedunculated myoma and infection of submucosal myoma can occur in the postpartum period.

Other associated features

Heavy menstrual bleeding causes anaemia. **Polycythaemia, hypercalcaemia and hyperprolactinaemia** may be associated with uterine leiomyomas.

Physical examination

Enlargement of the uterus can be diagnosed clinically in most women with myomas. A thorough physical examination with attention to details listed in Box 10.22 will help in making a clinical diagnosis.

- **Broad-ligament myomas** are felt in the region of the adnexa and have to be differentiated from ovarian masses.
- **Submucosal myomas** cause a uniform enlargement of the uterus.
- **Cervical myomas** can be felt on pelvic examination and cause stretching and thinning of cervical lips. They also push the uterus up into the abdomen and give rise to the typical

Box 10.22 Physical examination in myomas

- General examination
  - Anaemia
- Abdominal examination
  - Mass arising from the pelvis
  - Midline mass
  - Firm
  - Irregular
- Speculum examination
  - Displacement of the cervix
  - Myoma, polyp
- Pelvic examination
  - Uterus irregularly enlarged
  - Movement of mass transmitted to the cervix
  - Uterus not separately made out

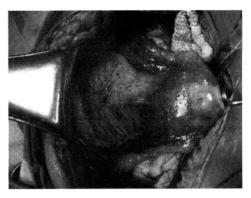

a.

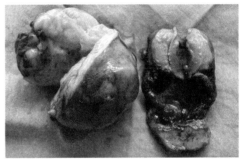

b.

'lantern on St. Paul's cathedral' appearance (Figs 10.17 and 10.18a and b).

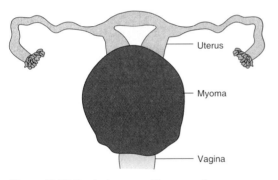

Figure 10.18 Central cervical myoma. **a.** The uterovesical peritoneum is pulled upwards. Uterus is pushed up. **b.** The cervical myoma has been enucleated. The cavity of myoma can be seen below the uterus.

Figure 10.17 Cervical myoma. Diagrammatic representation of central cervical myoma with uterus pushed up and perched on top—'Lantern on St. Paul's cathedral'.

Investigations

It is important to confirm the diagnosis and exclude ovarian mass and adenomyosis by ultrasonogram. Haemoglobin estimation should always be performed to assess the severity of heavy menstrual bleeding and correct anaemia. Other investigations will depend on the symptoms, clinical findings, age of the patient and the type of management planned. Investigations also contribute to management decisions (Box 10.23).

Imaging

Ultrasonography is not always necessary for diagnosis, especially when the uterus is

Box 10.23 Investigations in myomas

- Haemoglobin
- Ultrasound scan (abdominal and transvaginal)
  - Location of myomas
  - Number
  - Size
  - Adnexal masses
  - Adenomyosis
  - Hydroureteronephrosis
- Saline infusion sonography
  - Submucosal myomas
- Hysteroscopy
  - Submucosal myoma
    - Type
    - Resectability
    - Endometrial sampling
- Laparoscopy
  - Uterus <12 weeks' size
  - Evaluation of pelvic pain
  - Subfertility
  - Exclude ovarian mass

grossly enlarged. It is indicated in the following situations:

- When diagnosis is in doubt
- For initial evaluation and follow-up during medical management
- Before planning myomectomy/hysteroscopic resection
- In women with infertility

On ultrasonography, the myomas appear as solid, hypoechoic masses with a whorled appearance. They may distort the uterine contour and displace the endometrial stripe. Posterior acoustic shadowing is usually seen. Doppler imaging shows vascularity in the periphery of the tumour and a relatively avascular centre (Fig. 10.19a–d).

Management

Management depends on several factors. Age of the woman, severity of symptoms and location of the myoma are important considerations.

Asymptomatic myomas

As mentioned earlier, >50% of myomata are asymptomatic. It was believed that surgical intervention was required for all myomas >12 weeks' size. However, intervention on the basis of size of myoma alone is not advised now since

- Surgery for larger myomas is not associated with increase in morbidity.
- They do not necessarily produce symptoms in the future.
- Risk of malignant change is extremely low.

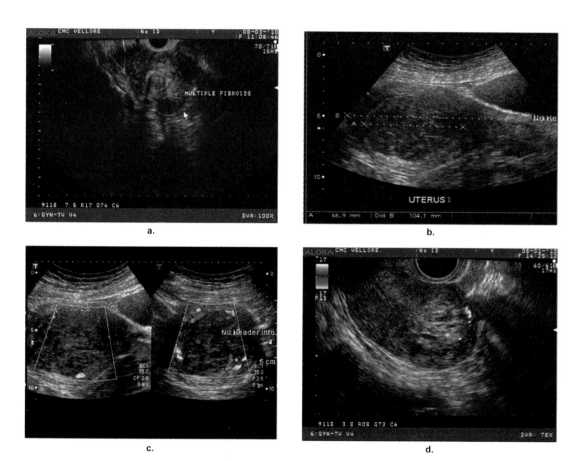

a.

b.

c.

d.

Figure 10.19 Ultrasonographic appearance of myoma. a. Uterus with multiple rounded myomas. b. Single intramural myoma. Myoma is well demarcated from surrounding myometrium. c. Intramural myoma with blood vessels in the periphery and few in the substance of the tumour. d. Blood vessels are mainly at the periphery of the myoma.

There is no definite size above which surgery is recommended, and each case has to be judged individually. Women who are perimenopausal can be counselled that the myomas will not increase in size after menopause, and in fact may reduce in size marginally. Therefore, asymptomatic myomas are managed as shown in Box 10.24.

Box 10.24 Management of asymptomatic myomas

- Initial assessment of size, number and location by ultrasonography
- Counselling
- Annual assessment
  - Symptoms
  - Ultrasonography
- Interfere when required

Symptomatic myomas

Management of symptomatic myomas will depend on age of the woman, size, number and location of the myoma and associated infertility.

Medical management

The objectives of medical management are to alleviate the symptoms and decrease the size of myoma. It can also be used preoperatively to reduce the size to facilitate endoscopic surgery. There is no drug available that will reduce the size of myomas and alleviate symptoms without side effects. Therefore, medical treatment of myomas is far from satisfactory and is used only for short periods of time. Indications for medical treatment are listed in Box 10.25.

Box 10.25 Indications for medical management of myomas

- Young women attempting conception
- Small symptomatic myomas at any age
- Control bleeding while waiting for surgery
- Control bleeding while anaemia is being corrected
- Women approaching menopause
- Shrink the myoma preoperatively

Drugs used for medical treatment are listed in Box 10.26.

Nonsteroidal anti-inflammatory drugs

Mefenamic acid reduces bleeding and pain and can be used in small myomas with heavy menstrual bleeding. There is no reduction in size of

Box 10.26 Drugs used in the medical management of myomas

- Nonsteroidal anti-inflammatory drugs
- Combination oral contraceptive pills
- Progestins
  - Oral
  - LNG-IUS
- GnRH agonists
- Antigonadotropins
  - Danazol
  - Gestrinone
- Antiprogestogens
  - Mifepristone
- Selective oestrogen receptor modulators
  - Raloxifene
  - Ormeloxifene
- Selective progesterone receptor modulators
  - Ulipristal
- GnRH antagonists
- Aromatase inhibitors
  - Anastrozole
- Cabergoline

GnRH, gonadotropin-releasing hormone; *LNG-IUS*, levonorgestrel intrauterine system.

myomas, and the response may be limited to a few cycles.

Combination oral contraceptive pills

Low-dose oestrogen–progesterone combination pills have been used in medical treatment of myomas. Theoretically, since myomas have oestrogen receptors, growth of myomas is a possibility when OC pills are used. However, clinically, many women with heavy menstrual bleeding and small myomas respond well to OC pills. Correction of anaemia by oral iron therapy is important.

Oral progestins

Progestins can be used alone in the management of heavy bleeding associated with myomas. Larger myomas and submucosal myomas do not respond to hormone therapy. OC pills are, however, the first line of hormonal therapy.

Levonorgestrel intrauterine system

This can be used when the myomas are small and the endometrial cavity is not distorted or enlarged. Randomized trials have shown that there is significant reduction in bleeding and dysmenorrhea with LNG-IUS. The device may be expelled if the uterus is large or cavity is distorted.

GnRH agonists

There is sufficient evidence available from randomized trials to prove the beneficial effect of GnRH agonists in reducing the size of the myomas, size of uterus, anaemia, heavy menstrual bleeding and other symptoms. After the initial stimulation, they suppress the gonadotropin production by the pituitary gland and induce a state of pseudomenopause. Any of the currently available preparations may be used. But due to the adverse effects, use of GnRH agonists has to be limited to 3–6 months. When the medication is stopped, the myomas bounce back to their original size within weeks. Hence, they are used

- While waiting for surgery to improve the haemoglobin levels
- To shrink the tumour to enable endoscopic surgery

The cost is prohibitive, and this makes it an unsuitable choice of treatment in developing countries.

Add-back therapy with OC pills is used to minimize adverse effects such as bone loss and menopausal symptoms. The advantages and disadvantages of GnRH agonists are listed in Box 10.27.

GnRH agonists are often used preoperatively, as mentioned earlier. The advantages and disadvantages of preoperative therapy are listed in Box 10.28.

Other drugs

Other drugs used in the medical management of myomas are listed in Table 10.1.

Surgical management of myomas

Surgery is the mainstay of treatment in women with myomas. In younger women, myoma alone can be removed by myomectomy. In older women, hysterectomy is the treatment of choice (Box 10.29).

Hysterectomy

- Hysterectomy is the treatment of choice in women with symptomatic myomas in the perimenopausal age.
- If the uterus is <14 weeks' size, vaginal hysterectomy can be performed.
- Laparoscopic hysterectomy is an alternative to open abdominal hysterectomy.

Box 10.27 Advantages and disadvantages of GnRH agonists

- Advantages
  - Reduction in size of myoma (30–60%)
  - Reduction in size of uterus
  - Correction of anaemia
  - Amenorrhoea
  - Relief from heavy bleeding, pelvic pain and other symptoms
- Disadvantages
  - Reduction in bone mineral density
  - Menopausal symptoms
    - Hot flushes
    - Vaginal dryness
    - Mood disturbances
  - High cost

GnRH, gonadotropin-releasing hormone.

Box 10.28 Advantages and disadvantages of preoperative therapy with GnRH agonists

- Advantages
  - Increase feasibility of vaginal hysterectomy
  - Increase feasibility of endoscopic surgery
  - Reduce blood loss
- Disadvantages
  - Plane of surgery more difficult
  - Increase in recurrence after myomectomy

GnRH, gonadotropin-releasing hormone.

Box 10.29 Surgical management of myomas

- Definitive surgery
  - Hysterectomy
    - Abdominal — Large myomas (>14 weeks); Broad-ligament myomas; Cervical myomas
    - Vaginal — Uterus <14 weeks
    - Laparoscopic — Same as abdominal
- Conservative surgery
  - Myomectomy
    - Open — Myomas >10 cm; Number >5
    - Laparoscopic — Myomas <10 cm; Number <5
    - Hysteroscopic — Submucosal types 0 and I

- The large myomas must be morcellated to facilitate removal. **Morcellation** is contraindicated

Table 10.1 Action, dosage and side effects of drugs used in medical management of myomas

Drug	Category	Action	Dosage	Adverse effects
Danazol	Antigonadotropin	Reduction in bleeding	400 mg/day	• Acne, weight gain • Hirsutism, hot flushes
Gestrinone	Antigonadotropin	Decreases size and bleeding	2.5 mg three times per week	• Acne, hirsutism • Seborrhoea
Mifepristone	Antiprogestogen	• Reduction in size • Reduction in bleeding	5–10 mg/day	Endometrial hyperplasia
Ulipristal	Selective progesterone receptor modulator	• Reduction in size • Reduction in bleeding	5–10 mg/day for 13 weeks	
Raloxifene	SERM	Small reduction in size	60–180 mg/day	Venous thrombosis
Ormeloxifene	SERM	Reduction in bleeding	60 mg/week	Nausea, headache
Cetrorelix	GnRh antagonist	• Rapid effect • Reduction in size and bleeding	0.25 mg/day	Allergic reaction
Anastrozole	Aromatase inhibitor	Small reduction in size and bleeding	1 mg/day	• Hot flushes • Vaginal dryness

GnRH, gonadotropin-releasing hormone; SERM, selective oestrogen receptor modulator.

if malignancy is suspected. It should be performed only after preoperative counselling.
• Intraoperative blood loss is more with large and multiple myomas.
• Cervical myomas push up the bladder and displace the ureters laterally. Clamping the uterine arteries may be difficult. Myomas may have to be enucleated to facilitate this.
• Broad-ligament myomas displace the ureters and care should be taken to avoid injury to these.

Myomectomy

Myomectomy should be considered in younger women with symptomatic myomas, especially if fertility is desired.

• This may be by laparotomy or laparoscopy for intramural and subserosal myomas. Intraoperative bleeding can be reduced by injecting vasopressin or using tourniquets/myomectomy clamp to occlude uterine vessels.
• Since there is a pseudocapsule, myomas can be enucleated unlike adenomyomas.
• Myomas of any size or number can be removed by open myomectomy, but laparoscopic myomectomy has its limitations.
• Pedunculated subserosal myomas and intramural myomas <5 cm in diameter and <3 in number are ideal for laparoscopic approach; however, myomas <10 cm in diameter and <5 in number are acceptable. Operating time

and blood loss increase when the size and the number increase.
• Myomectomy is associated with more complications than hysterectomy (Box 10.30). Complication rates are similar with laparoscopic and open myomectomy.

Box 10.30 Complications of myomectomy

• Immediate
  – Haemorrhage
  – Infection
  – Postoperative fever
  – Risk of hysterectomy
• Long-term
  – Adhesions
  – Recurrence
  – Scar rupture in labour

Preoperative preparation with oral iron therapy is mandatory. Counselling is important especially regarding complications and the occasional need for hysterectomy if the myomas are too many in number or if there is uncontrolled bleeding.

Hysteroscopic myomectomy is usually performed when the myoma is submucosal and type 0 or 1. Type II lesions may be removed by a two-stage procedure. The size of the myoma should be preferably <4 cm. Associated adenomyosis or other myomas necessitating treatment are contra-indications to hysteroscopic procedure.

Newer methods of treatment

Several operative and nonoperative methods are now being tried (Box 10.31).

Myolysis is the reduction in the size of myomas using thermal electrodes, cryoprobe, laser or radio-frequency probes. They are still being evaluated. Ligating the uterine artery achieves the same results as uterine artery embolization. Magnetic resonance–guided focused ultrasound surgery reduces the size of myomas and relieves symptoms but is expensive.

Box 10.31   Newer methods of treatment of myomas

- Laparoscopic myolysis
  - Thermal myolysis
  - Cryomyolysis
  - Laser myolysis
  - Radio-frequency myolysis
- Laparoscopic uterine artery ligation
- UAE
- MRgFUS

MRgFUS, magnetic resonance–guided focused ultrasound surgery; *UAE*, uterine artery embolization.

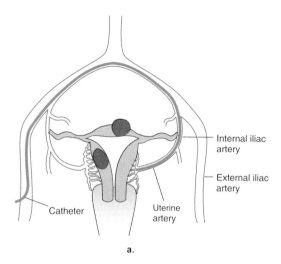

Internal iliac artery
External iliac artery
Catheter
Uterine artery

a.

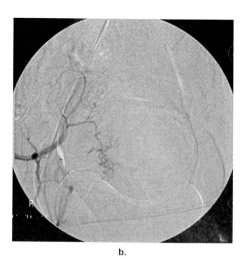

b.

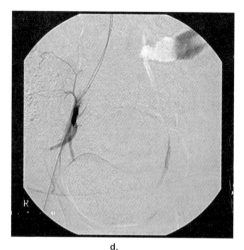

d.

Figure 10.20 Uterine artery embolization. **a.** Diagrammatic representation of uterine artery embolization. Catheter is introduced through the femoral vessel and negotiated into the uterine artery. **b.** Pre-embolization picture. Selective uterine artery catheterization shows the vessels supplying the myoma. **c.** Postembolization picture. Nonpacification of vessels is visible.

Uterine artery embolization

The procedure consists of occlusion of both uterine arteries with emboli causing ischaemic necrosis of the myomas. The procedure is performed under radiological guidance, accessing the uterine arteries through femoral artery. Polyvinyl alcohol (PVA) particles are used as emboli (Fig. 10.20a–c). Embolization results in reduction in size of myomas and relief from symptoms (Box 10.32).

Currently, the procedure is expensive and not readily available. Ovarian failure is another known complication. Although pregnancies have been reported following the procedure, currently it is not recommended in young, infertile women.

Box 10.32 Uterine artery embolization

- Outcomes
  - Reduction in size of myomas
  - Reduction in size of uterus
  - Decrease in menstrual blood loss
  - Relief from other symptoms
- Complications
  - Pain
  - Infection
  - Expulsion of myoma
  - Postembolization syndrome
  - Amenorrhoea
  - Ovarian failure
  - Recurrence

Key points

- Benign diseases of the uterus include endometrial polyp, adenomyosis and leiomyoma. Leiomyoma is the most common condition for which women seek a gynaecologist's opinion.

- Endometrial polyps are localized outgrowths of the endometrium. They occur in all age groups, may be asymptomatic and can be single or multiple. They can cause heavy menstrual bleeding and intermenstrual bleeding.

- Endometrial polyps should be ruled out in all women who present with abnormal uterine bleeding, not responding to medical management.

- Polyps are diagnosed by ultrasonography, saline infusion sonography or hysteroscopy. They can be removed by hysteroscopic polypectomy.

- Adenomyosis is the presence of endometrial tissue in the myometrium at least one high-power field (2.5 mm) from the basal layer. It is most often diffuse, but the localized form called adenomyoma is also known.

  - Adenomyosis occurs commonly in multiparous women in the perimenopausal age. The most common symptoms are heavy menstrual bleeding and congestive dysmenorrhoea.

  - The uterus is uniformly enlarged, but is usually less than the size of a 14 weeks' gravid uterus. Ultrasonogram is used to differentiate adenomyosis from leiomyoma. Occasionally, magnetic resonance imaging (MRI) is used.

  - Adenomyosis does not respond well to medical treatment. Nonsteroidal anti-inflammatory drugs (NSAIDs), combined oral contraceptives (COCs), gonadotropin-releasing hormone (GnRH) analogues and danazol can be tried. Most women require hysterectomy.

- Leiomyomas of the uterus arise from the smooth muscle of the uterus but also contain fibrous tissue.

  - They are classified into subserosal, intramural and submucosal myomas. They may also arise from the smooth muscle tissue in the broad ligament or cervix.

  - They can undergo degenerative changes. Hyaline degeneration is the most common. Malignant change occurs in 0.5% of tumours.

  - They can be asymptomatic or give rise to a variety of symptoms. Abnormal uterine bleeding and dysmenorrhoea are the most common symptoms. They can also cause pelvic discomfort, urinary symptoms and abdominal distension.

  - They usually cause irregular uterine enlargement. In case of submucosal myomas, uterus can be uniformly enlarged.

- Ultrasonography helps in excluding an ovarian mass or adenomyosis. The size, location and number of myomas can also be determined.

- Asymptomatic myomas can be observed. Symptomatic myomas are managed medically or surgically.

- Medical management of myomas is indicated in perimenopausal women and in younger women attempting conception or awaiting surgery. Drugs commonly used for medical treatment include COCs, danazol and GnRH analogues. Other drugs include raloxifene, ormeloxifene, anastrozole, mifepristone and ulipristal.

- Surgical treatment of myomas may be conservative, by myomectomy. This can be performed by laparoscopic, hysteroscopic or open method depending on the size and location of the myomas.

- Hysterectomy is indicated in women with large, multiple myomas and those who do not respond to medical management.

- Uterine artery embolization is a new technique used to treat myomas in young women. The procedure is expensive and has its complications.

Self-assessment

Case-based questions

Case 1

A 30-year-old lady presents with irregular menstrual cycles. She has been treated with combination oral contraceptive pills for three cycles with no response.

1. What diagnosis will you consider?
2. What investigation will you order?
3. What is the management?

Case 2

A 40-year-old lady comes for routine gynaecological check-up. On examination, the uterus is irregularly enlarged to about 12 weeks' size.

1. What is your management?
2. How will you counsel the woman?

Case 3

A 32-year-old lady, mother of one child, presents with heavy menstrual bleeding. Her haemoglobin is 6 g%. On evaluation, the uterus is irregularly enlarged to 18 weeks' size.

1. What investigation will you order?
2. What is the management?
3. How will you counsel this woman?

Answers

Case 1

1. Endometrial polyp—Irregular cycles not responding to hormone therapy; endometrial polyp must be considered.
2. Transvaginal ultrasound.
3. Hysteroscopic polypectomy and endometrial curettage.

Case 2

1. Observation.
2. (a) Myoma is not a malignant condition.
   (b) Chances of malignant transformation are extremely low (<1%).

(c) Annual ultrasound examination is all that is required.
(d) Medical treatment can be tried if symptoms occur.
(e) Surgery can be resorted to if there is no response to medical management.

Case 3

1. Abdominal and transvaginal ultrasound.
2. Correction of anaemia, myomectomy—Open or laparoscopic depending on the size and number of myomas.
3. Counsel regarding risk of
   (a) Haemorrhage and need for transfusion
   (b) Hysterectomy
   (c) Postoperative adhesions
   (d) Recurrence

Long-answer questions

1. What are the types of myomas? Give clinical features of submucosal myomas, diagnosis by recent methods and conservative treatment in a patient of 25 years of age with infertility.
2. What are the symptoms of leiomyoma uterus? Describe the pathogenesis of the symptoms. Discuss the medical management of myomas.
3. What is adenomyosis? Discuss the signs, symptoms, diagnosis and management of adenomyosis in a 40-year-old multiparous woman.

Short-answer questions

1. Red degeneration of myoma
2. Submucosal myomas
3. Complications of myomas
4. Differential diagnosis of myomatous polyp
5. Endometrial polyp
6. Adenomyosis
7. Adenomyoma
8. Use of GnRH analogues in the management of myoma

11 Benign Diseases of the Ovary and Fallopian Tube

Case scenario

Miss BL, 19, a college student, developed severe, acute lower abdominal pain while attending a lecture demonstration session. She also vomited once. She had noticed mild lower abdominal distension during the past 6 months but had put it down to general weight gain. Her teachers rushed her to the emergency department at the hospital.

Introduction

Benign diseases of the ovary, fallopian tube and paraovarian cysts give rise to an adnexal mass, which can be felt on pelvic examination or, when large, palpated abdominally. They are usually asymptomatic unless complications such as torsion occur. Adnexal mass can be due to benign, malignant or borderline malignant lesions. It is critical to determine whether the clinical features are suggestive of benign pathology or suspicious of malignant disease. Further evaluation and referral to specialized oncology centre depends on this distinction.

Infections involving fallopian tubes and ovary are discussed in Chapter 13, *Infections of the upper genital tract*. Other benign conditions that cause ovarian enlargement or adnexal mass are dealt with in this chapter.

Benign diseases of the ovary

Ovarian enlargement can occur due to hormonal stimulation, neoplasm or other benign conditions. The cut-off for diagnosis of ovarian enlargement varies with the menopausal status of the woman. The postmenopausal ovary undergoes atrophy and is smaller. Dimensions of a normal ovary are given in Box 11.1.

Benign conditions causing ovarian enlargement may be functional cysts or benign neoplasms. These are listed in Box 11.2.

Functional cysts

Functional cysts are usually associated with abnormal gonadotropin or ovarian hormone production.

- Premenopausal ovary
  - Size: 3 × 2 × 2 cm³
  - Volume: 10 cm³
  - Upper limit of normal: 18 cm³
- Postmenopausal ovary
  - Size: 2 × 1.5 × 1 cm³
  - Volume: 3 cm³
  - Upper limit of normal: 8 cm³

Box 11.2 Benign conditions causing ovarian enlargement

- Functional cysts
  - Follicular cysts
  - Corpus luteum cysts
  - Theca lutein cysts
- Benign neoplasms
  - Epithelial cell tumours
  - Germ cell tumours
  - Stromal tumours
- Others
  - Endometrioma
  - PCOS
  - OHSS

OHSS, ovarian hyperstimulation syndrome; *PCOS*, polycystic ovarian syndrome.

Follicular cysts

These are the most common functional cysts. They may be caused by temporary variations in gonadotropin levels. A normal follicle can develop into a cyst when it fails to rupture or undergo atresia. The size of the follicle should be greater than 3 cm to be called a follicular cyst (Fig. 11.1). Follicular cysts may produce oestrogen. They are usually found in adolescents and in early reproductive years but can occur in perimenopausal women with an ovulatory cycle as well. Progestin-only pills, levonorgestrel intrauterine system (LNG-IUS) and tamoxifen are also associated with follicular cysts. The characteristics of follicular cysts are given in Box 11.3.

Corpus luteum cysts

Bleeding into the corpus luteum after ovulation leads to formation of corpus luteum cysts (Fig. 11.2). Size of the cyst varies from 3 to 10 cm. The cysts may produce progesterone and cause delay in menstruation or amenorrhoea.

Box 11.3 Characteristics of follicular cysts

- Size: >3 and <8 cm
- Occur in
  - Adolescents
  - Reproductive age groups
  - Anovulatory cycles
  - Progestin-only pills/LNG-IUS
  - Tamoxifen
- Thin-walled, unilocular, filled with straw-coloured fluid
- Usually asymptomatic
- Occasionally rupture
- Diagnosis incidental
- Regress spontaneously in 4–6 weeks

LNG-IUS, levonorgestrel intrauterine system.

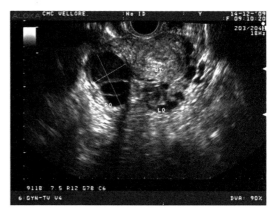

Figure 11.1 Ultrasonographic picture showing normal uterus, left ovary with multiple follicles and right ovary with follicular cyst. Dimensions of the follicular cyst are marked (5.3 × 3.6 cm).

Grossly, they are pink or haemorrhagic cysts. The cut section is typically yellowish orange due to the luteinization of lining cells, and the cysts are filled with blood clots. They are usually associated with dull, unilateral pelvic pain. Rupture with haemoperitoneum is more common and occurs between days 20 and 26 of the cycle. The condition can mimic a ruptured ectopic pregnancy. Urine β-human chorionic gonadotropin (hCG) level and transvaginal ultrasonography are useful in making a diagnosis. Unruptured cysts can be observed but those that undergo rupture should be removed laparoscopically, leaving behind normal ovarian tissue. Features of corpus luteum cysts are summarized in Box 11.4.

- Size: 3–10 cm
- Occur in reproductive age group
- Symptoms
  - Dull ache or unilateral pelvic pain
  - Delayed menses or amenorrhoea
- Cut section: Yellowish orange filled with blood clots
- Can rupture causing haemoperitoneum
- Regress spontaneously, if unruptured
- Can be observed
- Laparoscopic cystectomy in case of rupture

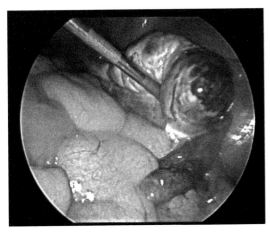

Figure 11.2 Corpus luteum cyst seen at laparoscopy. The ovary is otherwise normal. Fallopian tube is also seen.

Theca lutein cysts

They are least common and are usually the result of stimulation by excessive endogenous or exogenous gonadotropin. They are most often seen in association with molar pregnancy and choriocarcinoma, which produce hCG. They are also seen in other conditions where hCG is produced in excess, for example, multiple pregnancy, gestational/pregestational diabetes and Rh isoimmunization. When they occur due to exogenous administration of gonadotropins for ovulation induction, the condition is called **ovarian hyperstimulation syndrome** (OHSS).

Theca lutein cysts are bilateral, usually 10–15 cm in size, multicystic with a honeycomb appearance and greyish blue in colour. The cysts are filled with straw-coloured fluid or blood. Smaller cysts are asymptomatic, but large ones can produce discomfort, pain and feeling of pressure. They should be looked for while doing ultrasonogram in all patients with molar pregnancy or choriocarcinoma (Fig. 11.3). They occasionally undergo torsion or rupture. The cysts usually regress when the gonadotropin levels decline. Management is conservative. Combined oral contraceptive pills have been used to reduce pituitary gonadotropin production and thereby reduce the size of the cyst. Further evaluation is required only if the cysts persist for 6 months or longer or increase in size. Characteristic features of theca lutein cysts are summarized in Box 11.5.

Box 11.5 Features of theca lutein cysts

- Occur due to excessive gonadotropin
- Occur with molar pregnancy/choriocarcinoma
- Size: 10–15 cm
- Bilateral, multicystic
- Appearance
  - Greyish blue
  - Honeycombed
- Filled with straw-coloured fluid
- Smaller cysts: Asymptomatic
- Large cysts: Dull ache, discomfort
- Occasionally undergo torsion, rupture
- Management: Conservative

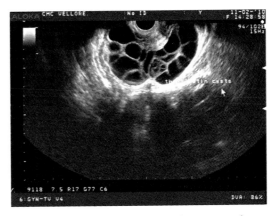

Figure 11.3 Ultrasonographic picture in a woman after evacuation of hydatidiform mole, showing bilateral theca lutein cyst. The cysts are multiloculated and have the characteristic honeycomb appearance.

Benign ovarian neoplasms

Benign ovarian neoplasms can arise from the ovarian surface epithelium, germ cells or stromal cells (Box 11.6).

- Epithelial tumours
  - Serous cystadenoma
  - Mucinous cystadenoma
  - Endometrioid cystadenoma
  - Mesonephroid (clear cell) tumours
  - Brenner tumours
  - Mixed epithelial tumours
- Germ cell tumours
  - Benign cystic teratoma
- Stromal tumours
  - Fibroma
  - Thecoma
  - Cystadenofibroma

Benign epithelial tumours

About 60% of all ovarian tumours are epithelial in origin. They are classified according to the histological cell type. Epithelial tumours can be benign, malignant or borderline. It is crucial to categorize them for decision regarding management. Benign lesions can occur at all ages, although individual types cluster around certain age groups.

Serous cystadenoma This is the most common benign epithelial tumour and is bilateral in up to 20% of the cases. Other characteristics are as in Box 11.7 (Fig. 11.4a–c).

Box 11.7 Serous cystadenoma

- 30% of all ovarian tumours
- Most common in reproductive years
- Bilateral in 20% of the cases
- Multiloculated or uniloculated
- Possibility of presence of papillary projections
- Lined by columnar/cuboidal epithelium
- Filled with thin, clear, yellowish fluid

Mucinous cystadenoma It is the second most common epithelial tumour, usually multilocular, filled with mucinous fluid, and can be very large (Box 11.8; Fig. 11.5a–c).

The surface is smooth, and cut section reveals multiple locules. They can rupture, resulting in a condition called **pseudomyxoma peritonei**. The seedling growths following rupture continue to secrete mucin, causing dense bowel adhesions and ureteric obstruction.

Endometrioid cystadenoma Benign endometrioid cystadenoma is difficult to distinguish

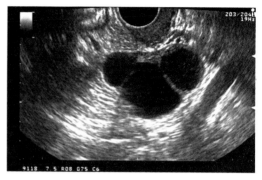

a.

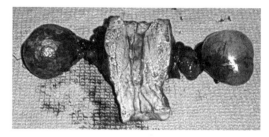

b.

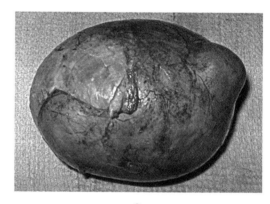

c.

Figure 11.4 Serous cystadenoma. a. Ultrasonographic picture showing simple, anechoic, multiloculated cyst. b. Specimen of uterus with bilateral serous cystadenoma. c. Specimen of a large serous cystadenoma.

Box 11.8 Mucinous cystadenoma

- 15–25% of all epithelial tumours
- Most common in age group of 30–50 years
- Bilateral in 5% of the cases
- Usually multiloculated
- Can be very large in size—Up to 30 cm
- Cyst wall smooth; papillary projection rare
- Lined by columnar mucin-secreting epithelium
- Filled with thick, mucinous fluid

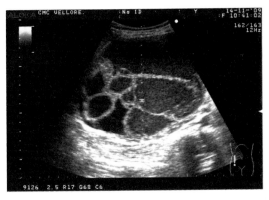

a.

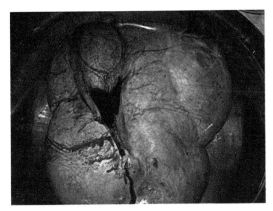

b.

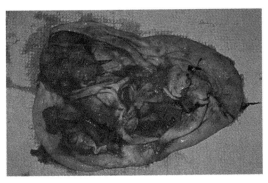

c.

Figure 11.5 Mucinous cystadenoma. **a.** Ultrasonographic picture showing a multiloculated cyst with low- to middle-level echoes indicating mucinous material. **b.** Specimen of a mucinous cyst. **c.** The same cyst showing several small locules filled with mucin.

from endometrioma. The lining cells resemble those of the endometrium. Only 5% of benign epithelial lesions are endometrioid.

Mesonephroid (clear cell) tumours These are rare tumours, lined by clear cells with abundant glycogen, called hobnail cells, and are most often malignant.

Brenner (transitional cell) tumours These are rare tumours, usually small, solid and diagnosed incidentally. They are usually benign and may secrete oestrogen. They are composed of transitional cells and fibrous stroma (Box 11.9).

Box 11.9 Brenner tumour

- Forms 2–3% of epithelial tumours
- Small (<5 cm)
- Solid, smooth, grey-white
- Associated with serous/mucinous tumours
- Most common in age 50–70 years
- Composed of transitional cells and fibrous stroma
- Cells having 'coffee bean' nucleus
- Usually benign, may secrete oestrogen

Benign germ cell tumours

Benign (mature) cystic teratoma It is the most common germ cell tumour. It is commonly known as **dermoid cyst**. It is a cystic tumour that contains elements from all three germ cell layers, namely the ectoderm, the endoderm and the mesoderm (Box 11.10). The ectodermal elements are predominant and are located in a solid area known as **Rokitansky protuberance**. Rarely, single tissue may predominate (monodermal teratoma), giving rise to carcinoid or struma ovarii. The malignant or immature teratoma is usually solid with cystic areas. Benign teratomas are filled with fat, float freely and are often found in the pouch of Douglas or anterior to the uterus.

Box 11.10 Components of benign cystic teratoma

- Ectoderm
  - Skin, hair and teeth
  - Sebaceous material
  - Nervous tissue
- Endoderm
  - Thyroid
  - Bronchus
  - Intestine
- Mesoderm
  - Bone
  - Smooth muscle

They are usually filled with thick, sebaceous material and hair, and contain teeth or cartilage. Although predominantly asymptomatic, a feeling of pressure or dull ache can occur.

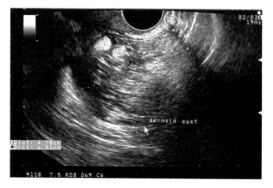

a.

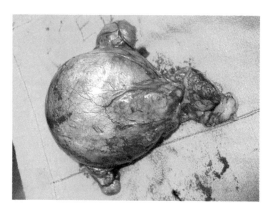

b.

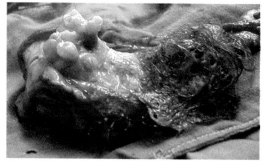

c.

Figure 11.6 Benign cystic teratoma. a. Ultrasonographic picture showing a large cystic teratoma. The echogenic areas indicate teeth or bone. b. Specimen of a benign cystic teratoma. c. Cut section of cystic teratoma showing sebaceous material, hair and teeth.

Ultrasonographic features of cystic teratoma are fat–fluid or hair–fluid levels, presence of hair and hyperechoic mural nodule with teeth or bone.

Characteristics of benign cystic teratoma are given in Box 11.11 (Fig. 11.6a–c).

Box 11.11 Benign cystic teratoma
• Accounts for 40% of all ovarian tumours
• All ages, mostly young, median 30 years
• Bilateral in 10–12%
• Usually unilocular
• Few centimetres to 25 cm in size
• Torsion: 10%; rarely rupture, infection
• Mostly asymptomatic
• Ultrasound
– Cystic/solid
– Mural nodule with teeth/bone
– Hair
– Fat–fluid/hair–fluid levels

Benign stromal tumours

Fibroma These are the most common benign solid tumours (Fig. 11.7a and b). They are slow growing and can become as large as 30 cm. They occur mostly in the postmenopausal age and arise from ovarian stroma. Small tumours are asymptomatic, but large ones can present with abdominal mass, feeling of pressure or ascites. The combination of ovarian fibroma, ascites and hydrothorax is called **Meigs syndrome**.

Thecomas These are common sex cord-stromal tumours, produce oestrogens and occur before the age 30 years. Endometrial hyperplasia and carcinoma can occur due to excess oestrogen. The tumours are solid.

Adenofibroma/cystadenofibroma It contains fibrous and epithelial components. Usually seen in postmenopausal women, it is asymptomatic unless large.

Other tumours

Endometrioma, polycystic ovarian syndrome (PCOS) and OHSS are dealt with in Chapter 15, *Endometriosis*; Chapter 19, *Secondary amenorrhoea and polycystic ovarian syndrome*; and Chapter 22, *Infertility*, respectively.

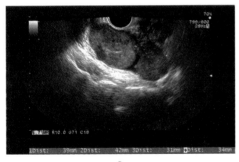

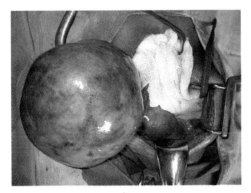

Figure 11.7 Ovarian fibroma. a. Ultrasonographic picture showing solid adnexal mass. b. Normal uterus and a large, smooth, solid ovarian mass.

Benign diseases of the fallopian tube

Benign lesions of the fallopian tube are rare and only two types are known—Leiomyomas and adenomatoid tumours (Box 11.12). Inflammatory masses such as hydrosalpinx and tubo-ovarian masses are discussed in Chapter 13, *Infections of the upper genital tract.*

Box 11.12 Benign diseases of the fallopian tube

- Leiomyomas
  - Coexist with uterine leiomyomas
  - Arise from muscle cells in the tubal wall
  - Asymptomatic
  - Can cause tubal occlusion
- Adenomatoid tumours
  - Small, circumscribed
  - Subserosal
  - Arise from mesothelium
  - Asymptomatic

Paraovarian cysts

Paraovarian cysts (Box 11.13) are benign cysts that originate from mesonephric or paramesonephric tissues (Fig. 11.8). They are usually discovered incidentally. Their clinical significance is that they may be mistaken for ovarian cysts and, when large, can present as an abdominal mass.

Box 11.13 Paraovarian cysts

- Vary from small to 15 cm in size
- Filled with clear fluid
- Ovary visualized separately
- Tube may be stretched over the cyst
- Asymptomatic
- Can be mistaken for ovarian cyst clinically

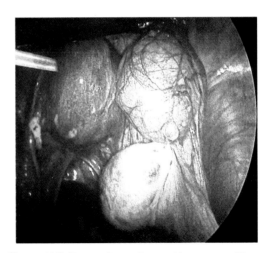

Figure 11.8 Paraovarian cyst seen at laparoscopy. The normal ovary and uterus are also seen.

Clinical features

Since benign lesions of the fallopian tube are extremely rare, the discussion will focus on benign diseases of the ovary.

Evaluation of women who present with adnexal mass should be systematic and thorough in order to exclude ovarian malignancy.

Symptoms

- Most benign lesions of the ovary are asymptomatic. They are diagnosed during ultrasound scanning, especially transvaginal ultrasound for other indications.

- Symptoms such as weight loss and anorexia should arouse suspicion of malignancy.
- Pain is predominantly a dull ache or feeling of heaviness, especially seen with large tumours. Acute pain indicates torsion, rupture, haemorrhage or infection.
- Menstrual disturbances are usually seen with functional cysts. History of amenorrhoea and recent molar pregnancy must be noted.
- Dysmenorrhoea and dyspareunia are suggestive of endometrioma.
- Symptoms of hyperthyroidism or carcinoid are rare but may be found in women with monodermal teratoma.

Symptoms are listed in Box 11.14.

Box 11.14 Symptoms of benign ovarian lesions

- Asymptomatic
- Pain
  - Dull ache
  - Acute severe pain
    - Torsion
    - Rupture
    - Haemorrhage
    - Infection
- Abdominal mass
- Menstrual disturbances
  - Delayed menses
  - Amenorrhoea
  - Anovulatory cycles
- Dysmenorrhoea, dyspareunia
- Pressure symptoms

Physical examination

Physical examination must be systematic when a woman presents with symptoms or when referred with incidental finding of an ovarian mass on clinical examination or ultrasound scan. The aim is to rule out the possibility of malignancy and decide on the treatment (Box 11.15).

- Large masses may be palpable abdominally and are usually located in the iliac fossa, mostly cystic and mobile (Fig. 11.9). Mucinous cysts can be very large and can present with abdominal mass. Other large tumours can also be palpable per abdomen.
- Smaller ones are usually felt on pelvic examination. They are usually felt through the lateral fornix, cystic, mobile and nontender. Some are bilateral, but most benign cysts are unilateral.

Box 11.15 Physical examination in benign ovarian lesions

- General examination
  - Signs of PCOS
  - Hydrothorax
  - Lymphadenopathy
- Abdominal examination
  - Mass
    - Location and size
    - Consistency and surface
    - Mobility
    - Arising from pelvis/abdomen
  - Ascites
- Per speculum examination
- Pelvic examination
  - Mass felt through lateral fornix
  - Mass in the pouch of Douglas
  - Unilateral/bilateral
  - Mobility and consistency
  - Tenderness

PCOS, polycystic ovarian syndrome.

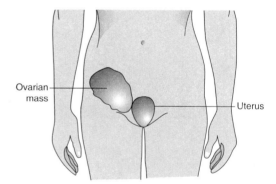

Figure 11.9 Diagrammatic representation of ovarian cyst on abdominal examination. The mass arises from the pelvis and is in the iliac fossa.

Clinical signs suggestive of benign lesion are as listed in Box 11.16.

Box 11.16 Clinical signs of benign ovarian enlargement

- No weight loss/anorexia
- Age: Young/reproductive
- Size: <7–8 cm
- Mobile
- Cystic
- Regular and smooth
- No ascites
- No lymphadenopathy

Investigations

Investigations are aimed at ruling out malignancy and making a provisional diagnosis of the nature of the cyst.

Ultrasonography

Ultrasonography is the first step in the evaluation of adnexal mass. Typical features of dermoid cyst, endometrioma and PCOS, when present, are diagnostic.

Ultrasonographic features suggestive of benign ovarian lesions are listed in Box 11.17 (Fig. 11.10).

Box 11.17 Ultrasonographic features of benign ovarian lesions

- Size: <8 cm, ovarian volume <10 cm^3
- Cystic lesions
- No solid areas
- No papillary excrescences
- Thin-walled (<3 mm)
- Uniloculated
- If multiloculated, thin septae (<2 mm)
- Unilateral
- No ascites/retroperitoneal nodes
- No metastasis

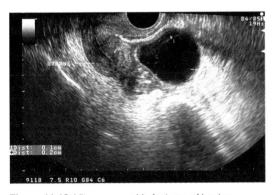

Figure 11.10 Ultrasonographic features of benign ovarian mass. Unilateral, anechoic cyst with no solid areas or papillary excrescences. Thickness of cyst wall is 2 mm and septal thickness is 1 mm. There is no ascites.

Tumour markers

CA 125 is a tumour marker for epithelial ovarian cancer. Level of 35 units/mL is used as cut-off for diagnosis of malignancy. But this marker is elevated in several benign gynaecological conditions such as endometriosis, pelvic inflammatory disease, abdominal or genital tuberculosis, leiomyomas and pregnancy. Since all these conditions are encountered in the premenopausal women, the test is not as useful as in the postmenopausal women. A cut-off of 200 units/mL is therefore used in premenopausal women. Other markers for germ cell tumours are measured when a solid tumour is detected in a young girl. β-hCG serves as a marker and helps in diagnosing ectopic pregnancy (Box 11.18).

Box 11.18 Other investigations in benign ovarian lesions

- Tumour markers
  - CA 125
    - Epithelial tumours
  - α-Fetoprotein
    - Germ cell tumour
  - β-hCG
    - Theca lutein cysts
    - Suspected ectopic pregnancy
- Doppler studies—Resistance index
- Other imaging modalities
  - CT/MRI
    - If malignancy suspected

CT, computerized tomography; *hCG*, human chorionic gonadotropin; *MRI*, magnetic resonance imaging.

Doppler flow studies

Due to the neovascularization in malignant tissue, the resistance to blood flow is low in malignant tumours (Fig. 11.11). A low resistance index of <0.40 is suggestive of malignancy, but cut-off values have been different in the various studies. The test cannot be used alone but along with morphological features on ultrasonogram. Doppler studies may enhance the diagnostic accuracy.

Several scoring systems using features on sonographic morphology, CA 125 levels and menopausal status have been developed with varying sensitivity for diagnosing malignancy.

Other imaging modalities

Computerized tomography and magnetic resonance imaging are useful when malignancy is suspected. Involvement of surrounding structures, metastasis to liver, subdiaphragmatic space, peritoneal and omental deposits, para-aortic lymphadenopathy and hydronephrosis can be assessed

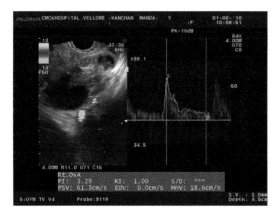

Figure 11.11 Blood flow in the cyst by Doppler study. The vessels are in the periphery and the resistance index is high (RI = 1).

more accurately by these imaging modalities (*see* Chapter 5, *Imaging in gynaecology*).

Management

Management of non-neoplastic ovarian and paraovarian lesions

If clinical diagnosis is functional cyst in a young girl or woman in early reproductive age with anovulatory cycles, observation is sufficient. Combined oral contraceptive pills may be used for 3–6 months. Theca lutein cysts are associated with high gonadotropin levels and resolve when the underlying condition producing hCG is treated.

Women with PCOS and endometrioma are managed accordingly (Box 11.19).

Management of asymptomatic cysts

Management of women with asymptomatic benign neoplastic lesions depends on several factors, the most important being exclusion of malignancy with reasonable certainty (Box 11.20). Further management in premenopausal and postmenopausal women is given in Figs 11.12 and 11.13.

Management of symptomatic cysts

Symptoms are usually due to large size or some complication such as torsion. They need surgical intervention.

> **Box 11.19 Management of non-neoplastic ovarian lesions and paraovarian cysts**
>
> - Follicular/corpus luteum cysts
>   - Observation
>   - Combined OC pills—Three to six cycles
> - Theca lutein cysts
>   - Evacuation of molar pregnancy
>   - Chemotherapy if required
> - Endometrioma
>   - Laparoscopic cystectomy
>   - Medical therapy
> - Polycystic ovarian syndrome
>   - Combined OC pills
>   - Other medical therapies
> - Paraovarian cysts
>   - If small—Observation
>   - If large—Laparoscopic cystectomy
>
> *OC*, oral contraceptive.

> **Box 11.20 Asymptomatic benign neoplastic lesions**
>
> Management depends on
> - Age
> - Menopausal status
> - Size of mass
> - Sonographic morphology
> - Tumour marker levels

Surgical management

Ultrasound-guided aspiration

This has been studied in a limited number of trials. The cyst fluid reaccumulates rapidly, and no advantage over cystectomy has been found. This procedure is of limited use and is restricted to pregnant women with large simple cysts where aspiration helps in postponing surgery to until after delivery.

Laparoscopic surgery

This is the treatment of choice for all benign lesions. Laparoscopy can be performed to rule out malignancy when in doubt and for therapeutic procedures (Box 11.21).

Diagnostic laparoscopy

When the cyst morphology is suspicious, tumour is solid or CA 125 levels are borderline, diagnostic

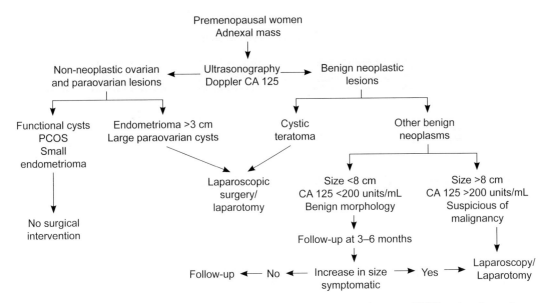

Figure 11.12 Management of benign ovarian neoplastic lesions in premenopausal women. *PCOS*, polycystic ovarian syndrome.

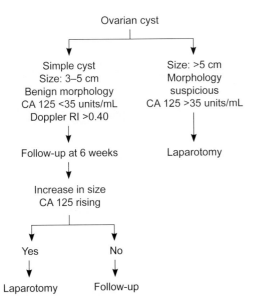

Figure 11.13 Management of benign ovarian neoplastic lesions in postmenopausal women. *RI*, resistance index.

Box 11.21 Laparoscopy in benign ovarian lesions

- Diagnostic
  - Exclude malignancy
- Therapeutic
  - Cyst aspiration
  - Cystectomy
  - Oophorectomy/salpingo-oophorectomy

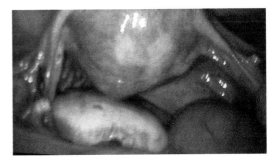

Figure 11.14 Laparoscopic evaluation of benign cyst. Cyst is unilateral with no papillary excrescences, adhesions or ascites. There are no metastatic deposits.

laparoscopy is used to exclude malignancy (Fig. 11.14). Inspection of the tumour, assessment of morphology, adhesions, infiltration of other structures, contralateral ovarian status, peritoneal washing for cytology and evaluation of other organs are mandatory. If found to be malignant, conversion to laparotomy is recommended. Preoperative counselling is mandatory.

Cyst aspiration

This has the disadvantages of spill of tumour if malignant and reaccumulation of fluid. It may be performed under ultrasonographic guidance or at laparoscopy if probability of malignancy is low. Aspiration may also be performed prior to cystectomy to reduce the tumour size.

Ovarian cystectomy

This is the procedure of choice in premenopausal women especially when reproductive function is desired. Normal ovarian tissue should be left behind. Most benign neoplasms can be managed by cystectomy.

Oophorectomy/salpingo-oophorectomy

The entire ovary with the tumour may have to be removed if the woman is perimenopausal or when the entire ovary is replaced by tumour with very little or no visible normal ovarian tissue. The tube may have to be removed if adherent to the tumour or stretched over it.

Laparotomy

Laparotomy is required when malignancy is suspected, when the tumour is large and multiloculated (Fig. 11.15) or when the tumour is solid. Postmenopausal women with ovarian mass requiring surgery are better managed by laparotomy. Thorough assessment including peritoneal washing for cell cytology is required. Tumour tissue must be sent for frozen section even in young girls where malignant or borderline tumours are suspected. Oophorectomy, salpingo-oophorectomy or hysterectomy with bilateral salpingo-oophorectomy is performed depending on the age, menopausal status and histology.

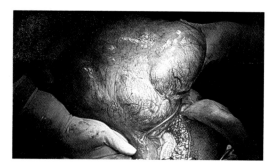

Figure 11.15 A large mucinous cyst being removed by laparotomy.

Complications of benign neoplastic lesions

The complications that can occur with benign ovarian neoplasms are listed in Table 11.1. They can occur at anytime, but certain conditions can predispose to complications.

Table 11.1 Complications of benign ovarian neoplasms

Complication	Predisposing condition
Torsion	• Cysts >6 cm • Dermoid cyst • Long pedicle • Postnatal • Second trimester of pregnancy
Rupture	• Labour • Rapid growth
Infection	Postnatal
Malignancy	Older age

Torsion

- Torsion is the most common complication of ovarian cyst (Fig. 11.16).
  - Cystic teratomas are filled with fat, are heavy and undergo torsion more often than other tumours.
  - When the ovary enlarges to >6 cm, it rises into the abdomen and is more prone to torsion.
  - During second trimester when the ovary becomes an abdominal organ and during puerperium before involution of the uterus, the cysts move freely in the abdomen and can undergo torsion.
  - Long utero-ovarian ligaments also predispose to torsion.
- With torsion of the pedicle, the veins are compressed but arterial flow into the ovary may continue; therefore, the ovary may be congested and oedematous, but infarction does not occur immediately. Hence, it is possible to salvage the ovary by detorsion if surgery is undertaken early.
- The woman usually presents with acute lower abdominal pain, which may be intermittent initially; nausea and vomiting may be present. The cyst is tender and signs of acute abdomen are usually present.

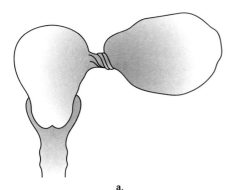

a.

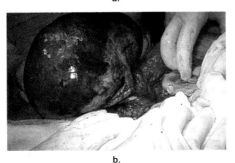

b.

Figure 11.16 Torsion of ovarian cyst. a. Diagrammatic representation of torsion of ovarian pedicle. b. Ovarian torsion. The twisted pedicle can be seen. Ovary is haemorrhagic and partly gangrenous.

- Ultrasonography may reveal an ovarian mass with disruption of vascular flow.
- Admission and emergency laparoscopy/laparotomy are required.
  - The ovary should be untwisted, ovarian cyst should be excised and the normal ovarian tissue should be salvaged. Oophoropexy should be performed to prevent recurrence.
  - If gangrenous, the ovary should be removed.

Rupture, infection and haemorrhage

Rupture of ovarian cyst can occur in labour. Rupture of dermoid cyst can give rise to peritonitis, and rupture of mucinous cyst may later give rise to pseudomyxoma peritonei. Laparotomy and excision of cyst and peritoneal toilet are indicated.

Women with infected cysts present with fever and pain. White cell counts are elevated. Antibiotics and emergency laparotomy and oophorectomy are indicated.

Haemorrhage into the cyst is associated with acute pain. It can usually be managed conservatively. Laparotomy may be required if symptoms persist.

Key points

- Most benign lesions of the ovary are diagnosed incidentally. If they are large, they have suspicious features or the woman is older, malignancy must be ruled out by thorough evaluation.
- Benign ovarian lesions include functional cysts, neoplasms and other conditions such as endometriosis, polycystic ovarian syndrome (PCOS) and ovarian hyperstimulation syndrome (OHSS).
- Functional cysts are due to abnormal gonadotropin or ovarian hormone production. Follicular cysts are the most common functional cysts and occur in adolescents and perimenopausal women with anovulatory cycles.
- Corpus luteum cysts occur in women of reproductive age and can rupture.
- Theca lutein cysts are seen in association with hydatidiform mole in response to high levels of human chorionic gonadotropin (hCG).
- Benign ovarian neoplasms may be epithelial, germ cell or stromal tumours.
- Serous cystadenoma is the most common epithelial tumour, and dermoid cyst is the most common germ cell tumour.

- Paraovarian cysts are common, but benign lesions of the fallopian tube are rare.
- Most women with benign ovarian lesions are asymptomatic. Some present with dull ache or acute pain due to complications such as torsion. Abdominal mass or menstrual disturbances are also seen. Physical examination may reveal an abdominal or pelvic mass.
- Fixity, solid mass, large size, presence of ascites or lymphadenopathy suggests malignancy.
- Ultrasonography is the most important mode of evaluation. Features suggestive of malignancy are large multiloculated cysts with solid areas, papillary excrescences, thick septae, ascites, lymphadenopathy and metastasis.
- Tumour markers such as CA 125, α-fetoprotein and hCG may be used when in doubt. Doppler studies to look for resistance index in the vessels lack sensitivity.
- Functional cysts do not require intervention and can be observed.

(Continued)

Key points *(Continued)*

- Cystic teratomas are managed by laparoscopic ovarian cystectomy.
- Epithelial cysts <6–8 cm can be observed. If the cyst is large or enlarges during observation, laparoscopic cystectomy is indicated.

- If malignancy is suspected, laparotomy is indicated.
- Torsion is the most common complication of benign ovarian lesions. Rupture and haemorrhage also occur but are uncommon.

Self-assessment

Case-based questions

Case 1

A 28-year-old lady, mother of two children, presents with dull ache in the lower abdomen of 3 months' duration and lower abdominal distension of 5 months' duration. She has no menstrual irregularity. On evaluation, she has a cystic mass up to the umbilicus.

1. What is your provisional diagnosis?
2. What clinical features will you look for?
3. What is the next step in the evaluation?
4. What is the management?

Case 2

A 19-year-old girl presents with acute abdominal pain of 6 hours' duration. She has no other associated symptoms. On clinical evaluation, she has a tender abdomen and a mass in the left iliac fossa.

1. What is your diagnosis?
2. How will you confirm the diagnosis?
3. What type of cyst is usually present with this complication?
4. What is the management?

Answers

Case 1

1. Ovarian cyst.
2. (a) General examination—Weight loss
   (b) Abdominal examination—Mass arising from pelvis, size, mobility, consistency, margins, ascites, hepatomegaly
   (c) Pelvic examination—Size, bilateral/unilateral, mobility, consistency

3. (a) Ultrasonogram (abdominal and transvaginal) confirms clinical findings, solid areas, papillary excrescences, morphology of the other ovary, ascites, retroperitoneal nodes, Doppler flow study.
   (b) CA 125 level.
4. If simple cyst, laparoscopic cystectomy.

   If suspicious of malignancy, laparotomy.

Case 2

1. Twisted ovarian cyst.
2. (a) Clinical examination
   (i) *Abdominal examination:* Tender abdominal mass may be palpable.
   (ii) *Pelvic examination:* Tender adnexal mass.
   (b) Ultrasonography
3. Benign cystic teratoma.
4. Emergency laparoscopy, detorsion, ovarian cystectomy and oophoropexy.

   If ovary is gangrenous, oophorectomy.

Long-answer question

1. A 38-year-old lady is found to have an ovarian cyst during routine pelvic examination. How will you evaluate her? How will you decide on the management?

Short-answer questions

1. Dermoid cyst
2. Functional cysts of the ovary
3. Torsion of ovarian cyst
4. Benign epithelial tumours of the ovary
5. Theca lutein cysts

12 | Infections of the Lower Genital Tract

Case scenario

Mrs PV, 19, came to the clinic with vaginal discharge, intense pruritus, dysuria and soreness of the vulva. She was married recently to a 25-year-old lorry driver who travelled a lot and spent several nights in other towns. Mrs PV had suffered similar episodes in the past and had been given some tablets in the primary health centre, but this one was particularly severe, so she came to the tertiary centre for opinion and treatment.

Introduction

The female genital tract is a continuous, open pathway from the exterior to peritoneal cavity. Infections of the genital tract are, therefore, common. Infections may involve any or multiple parts of the genital tract and can spread from the vagina to fallopian tube, ovary and peritoneum. For purposes of simplification, genital tract infections are classified as lower genital tract infections and upper genital tract infections.

Definition

Lower genital tract infections are infections of the vulva, vagina and cervix. They are also referred to as reproductive tract infections (RTIs). Some of the infections such as trichomoniasis, chlamydial, human papillomavirus (HPV)

and gonococcal infections, syphilis, chancroid, lymphogranuloma venereum (LGV) and granuloma inguinale are **sexually transmitted infections** (STIs).

Prevalence

Prevalence of lower genital tract infections in India varies widely depending on whether the diagnosis is based on symptoms alone (11–72%), on clinical examination (17–40%) or on laboratory confirmation (38%).

Complications and sequelae

Infections of the lower genital tract most often present as vaginal discharge and/or pruritus, which are among the most common conditions seen in a gynaecological clinic. The infections must be recognized and treated without delay because untreated infections can lead to complications and sequelae (Box 12.1). Many of the lower genital tract infections are sexually transmitted.

Box 12.1　Complications and sequelae of lower genital tract infections

- Acute/chronic pelvic inflammatory disease
- Infertility/subfertility
- Postoperative infection
- Obstetric complications
  - Prelabour rupture of membranes
  - Preterm labour
  - Chorioamnionitis
  - Postabortal sepsis
  - Postcaesarean section sepsis

There are several defence mechanisms in place to prevent lower genital infections (Box 12.2).

Box 12.2　Defence mechanisms in lower genital tract

- Vulva
  - Stratified squamous epithelium lining the vulva
  - Acidic secretion of the apocrine sweat glands
- Vagina
  - Acidic pH of vagina
  - Production of substances by normal bacterial flora
    - Lactic acid and hydrogen peroxide
    - Bacteriocins—Acidocin and lactacin
  - Squamous epithelial lining of mucosa
- Cervix
  - Mucous plug
  - Squamous epithelial lining of ectocervix

Infections of the vulva

Infections can affect the vulvar skin or structures in the vulva such as Bartholin, sebaceous and sweat glands. Benign lesions of the vulva are discussed in Chapter 9, *Benign diseases of the vulva, vagina and cervix.* Vulval infections may be **primary**, involving the vulval skin, **or secondary** to vaginitis (Box 12.3).

Viral infections

Molluscum contagiosum

This is a chronic condition characterized by dome-shaped, often umbilicated papular lesions.

It is caused by poxvirus. In children, it may be present in other parts of the body, but in adults, it is limited to vulvar skin. The disease is asymptomatic and mildly contagious, and spreads by contact. Treatment is by cryotherapy or excision.

Box 12.3　Infections of the vulva

- Viral infections
  - Molluscum contagiosum
  - Condyloma acuminata
  - Genital herpes
- Infestations
  - Pediculosis
  - Scabies
- Infections of the vulval structures
  - Hair follicles
  - Bartholin glands
- Genital ulcers
  - Syphilis
  - Chancroid
  - Lymphogranuloma venereum
  - Donovanosis
  - Genital herpes
- Secondary infections
  - Vulvovaginitis
    - Candidiasis
    - Trichomoniasis
    - Gonococcal infections
    - Bacterial vaginosis

Condyloma acuminata or genital warts

These are caused by HPV. There are more than 70 serotypes identified, but the benign lesions are usually caused by types 6 and 11. Infection by high-risk serotypes (16, 18, 31 and 33) can lead to intraepithelial and invasive cancers of the lower genital tract. The virus infects the vulva, vagina, perianal region and cervix (Fig. 12.1). The disease is sexually transmitted and the lesions are seen more in the moist areas (Box 12.4).

Treatment is surgical or with topical applications. Larger lesions (>2–3 cm) are treated surgically (Box 12.5).

Since **genital herpes** (herpes simplex infection) presents with ulcers, it is discussed with other genital ulcers.

Infestations

Pediculosis

Pediculosis is caused by crab louse and **scabies** is caused by *Sarcoptes scabiei*. Both present with intense pruritus and can be transmitted

- Peak age
  - 15–25 years
- Sites
  - Vulva, vagina, perianal and cervix
- Gross appearance
  - Soft, sessile or pedunculated, warty
- Symptoms
  - Asymptomatic/pruritus/pain
- HPV serotypes
  - 6 and 11
- Predisposing factors
  - Immunosuppression
  - Diabetes
  - Pregnancy

HPV, human papillomavirus.

- Topical
  - Patient administered
    - Podophyllotoxin
    - Imiquimod
  - Provider administered
    - Podophyllin resin
    - Trichloroacetic acid
- Surgical
  - Cryotherapy
  - Electrocautery
  - Laser therapy
  - Excision
  - LEEP

LEEP, loop electroexcision procedure.

sexually or through nonsexual contact. Patients, partners and other contacts should be treated concurrently with single application of permethrin cream or lindane. Concurrent treatment is essential to prevent reinfection.

Infections of other structures in the vulva

Bartholin adenitis and abscess

Bartholin glands are located bilaterally at the base of the labia minora and are not palpable unless enlarged. They drain through the ducts that are 2–2.5 cm long and open into the vestibule at 5 and 7 o'clock positions. Infection of the glands leads to adenitis or abscess formation.

- When the ducts are occluded due to oedema, inflammation or trauma, Bartholin cysts develop. Infection of the cyst gives rise to Bartholin abscess. The most common organism isolated is *Escherichia coli*. Infections may be polymicrobial, and the organisms include *Staphylococcus, Streptococcus, Bacteroides, Neisseria gonorrhoeae* and *Chlamydia trachomatis*.
- Bartholin abscesses are located in the posterior part of the labium majus and are usually unilateral. The introitus, therefore, has a typical 'S'-shaped appearance (Fig. 12.2).
- Patient presents with acute pain, dyspareunia and pain during walking. Local examination reveals oedema, erythema, cellulitis and tenderness.

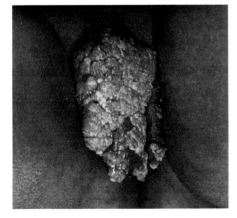

Figure 12.1 A large warty lesion in the vulva— Condyloma acuminata.

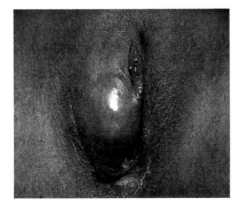

Figure 12.2 Painful, cystic lesion occupying the posterior part of right labium majus. Skin over the lesion is red and shiny—The Bartholin abscess.

- Incision and drainage with placement of a rubber or glove drain is recommended. Alternatively, incision and marsupialization can also be performed.
- Antibiotics are indicated only in immunocompromised women, in recurrent abscesses or when there is associated cellulitis or systemic infection.
- Excision is not usually recommended in the presence of active infection. Recurrent infection necessitates excision of the gland.

Infections of the hair follicles

Infection of the hair follicles of the vulva presents like folliculitis in other parts of the body. Staphylococcal infection is most common. The lesions are painful and multiple, and may be recurrent. Treatment is with oral cloxacillin or erythromycin.

Genital ulcers

Infections that cause genital ulcers are genital herpes and other STIs as seen in Table 12.1. Two or more infections can coexist in these women. Infection with human immunodeficiency virus (HIV) coexists with other STIs and should be looked for. Syphilis should always be excluded in all women presenting with genital ulcers. Since tests requiring sophisticated equipment may not be available in all centres, clinical diagnosis is important (see Table 12.1).

Genital herpes

It is the most common disease presenting as ulcer, caused by herpes simplex virus (HSV).

Both the types, HSV1 and HSV2, can cause genital disease. Genital herpes is sexually transmitted and contagious, and can be asymptomatic. The vesicles are painful and break down to form ulcers. Ulcers may be seen on vaginal wall and cervix as well. Fever, malaise and painful inguinal lymphadenopathy are common. Patients experience vulvar pain even before lesions develop. Recurrent infections are common, especially with HSV2. These are less severe.

Diagnosis of genital herpes is as shown in Box 12.6.

Box 12.6 Diagnosis of genital herpes

- Clinical
- Viral culture
- Serology for HSV-specific antibodies
- Polymerase chain reaction
- ELISA

ELISA, enzyme-linked immunosorbent assay; *HSV*, herpes simplex virus.

Current recommendations for treatment of genital herpes are given in Box 12.7. Oral analgesics, topical and anaesthetic ointments should be used for pain relief. Treatment for initial episode and recurrence, and suppression therapy for a woman with six or more episodes in a year are listed. Suppressive therapy is given for 6 months. The patient should be counselled regarding abstinence from onset of prodromal symptoms to complete recovery.

Syphilis

Syphilis is the second most common cause of genital ulcer. It is caused by *Treponema*

Table 12.1 Clinical features of genital ulcers

	Herpes	Syphilis	Chancroid	LGV	Donovanosis
Genital lesion	Vesicle	Papule	Papule	Papule/vesicle	Papule
Number	Multiple	Single	Multiple	Single	Single/multiple
Size	1–2 mm	0.5–1 cm	0.5–2 cm	0.2–1 cm	Variable
Margin	Erythematous	Punched out	Undermined	Elevated	Elevated
Depth	Superficial	Deep	Deep	Superficial	Elevated
Induration	Absent	Present	Absent	Occasional	Present
Pain	++	–	+++		–
Nodes	Bilateral Tender	Bilateral Nontender	Unilateral Tender Suppurate	Unilateral Tender Suppurate (bubo)	Pseudobubo

LGV, lymphogranuloma venereum.

Box 12.7 CDC-recommended treatment of genital herpes

Box 12.7 CDC-recommended treatment of genital herpes

- Initial episode
  - Acyclovir 400 mg thrice daily for 7–10 days
  - (or) Valacyclovir 1000 mg twice daily for 7–10 days
  - (or) Famciclovir 250 mg thrice daily for 7–10 days
- Recurrent episodes
  - Acyclovir 400 mg thrice daily for 5 days
  - (or) Valacyclovir 1000 mg daily for 5 days
  - (or) Famciclovir 125 mg twice daily for 5 days
- Daily suppressive therapy
  - Acyclovir 400 mg twice daily
  - (or) Valacyclovir 500 mg daily
  - (or) Famciclovir 250 mg twice daily

CDC, Centers for Disease Control and Prevention.

pallidum, and the disease has primary, secondary, latent and tertiary stages. The ulcer is painless, indurated and associated with inguinal lymphadenopathy. After the ulcer heals, the patient remains asymptomatic for a few weeks to months and then goes on to secondary stage with skin and mucosal involvement with lymphadenopathy. The tertiary stage ensues years later with cardiac and/or central nervous system involvement.

Diagnosis of syphilis It is by various tests as outlined in Box 12.8.

Box 12.8 Diagnosis of syphilis

- Dark-field examination of smear
- Direct fluorescent antibody test
- VDRL
- Rapid plasma reagin
- Microhaemagglutination
- FTA-ABS test

FTA-ABS, fluorescent treponemal antibody absorption; *VDRL*, Venereal Disease Research Laboratory.

Treatment of syphilis It is with benzathine penicillin G 2.4 million units intramuscular single dose for primary, secondary and early latent syphilis and three doses at weekly interval for late latent, tertiary and cardiovascular syphilis. Penicillin-sensitive patients may be treated with doxycycline 100 mg orally, twice daily for 2–4 weeks.

Chancroid, lymphogranuloma venereum and granuloma inguinale

Other sexually transmitted genital ulcers such as chancroid, LGV and granuloma inguinale (donovanosis) are uncommon causes of genital ulcerative disease at present. **Chancroid** presents as multiple ulcers that are extremely painful with tender inguinal nodes. The nodes may become fluctuant. The organism causing the infection is *Haemophilus ducreyi*. Treatment is with single oral dose of azithromycin 1 g. Large inguinal nodes matted together forming a bubo with a small superficial papule or vesicle that is almost painless and transient are usually LGV. It is a chronic infection of the lymphatic tissue caused by *C. trachomatis*. Doxycycline 100 mg daily orally for 21 days is the recommended treatment. **Granuloma inguinale** is caused by Gram-negative intracellular bacilli—*Calymmatobacterium granulomatis*. The ulcers are painless and beefy red, bleed on touch and coalesce to form a large lesion. Inguinal nodes are enlarged if secondarily infected, forming pseudoadenopathy. Smear from the ulcer shows pathognomonic Donovan bodies, which are clusters of bacilli within large mononuclear cells. Treatment is with oral doxycycline 100 mg twice daily for 21 days.

Treatment [Centers for Disease Control and Prevention (CDC) recommendation] is listed in Box 12.9.

Box 12.9 Treatment of other genital ulcers

- Chancroid
  - Azithromycin 1 g oral single dose
  - (or) Ceftriaxone 250 mg IM single dose
  - (or) Ciprofloxacin 500 mg twice daily for 3 days
- LGV
  - Doxycycline 100 mg twice daily for 21 days
  - (or) Azithromycin 1 g once a week for 3 weeks
  - (or) Ciprofloxacin 750 mg twice daily for 3 weeks
- Granuloma inguinale
  - Same as for LGV

IM, intramuscular; *LGV*, lymphogranuloma venereum.

Secondary infection of the vulva—Vulvovaginitis

Any discharge from the vagina or cervix can lead to secondary erythema, excoriation and infection of skin of the vulva. The term vulvovaginitis is used when the infection involves the vagina and vulva as in candidial vulvovaginitis. Vaginal discharge and pruritus vulva are the common symptoms. The discharge may be from the cervix or vagina, but it causes irritation of the vulval skin and pruritus. Treatment is that of the primary infection of the vagina or cervix, local hygiene and topical applications—Antifungal cream or mild corticosteroids if there is secondary eczema.

Infections of the vagina

Normal vaginal secretions

Normal secretion or discharge from the vagina is white and odourless and collects in the dependent part of the vagina (posterior fornix). It consists of secretions from sweat, sebaceous and Bartholin glands in the vulva, transudates from vaginal epithelium and secretions from cervical glands. The components of normal vaginal secretions are listed in Box 12.10.

The vaginal epithelium is sensitive to hormonal changes during menstrual cycle. Under the influence of oestrogen, maturation and keratinization of cells take place and these cells are seen in the desquamative tissue. In the presence of progesterone, intermediate cells are seen, and when both hormones are absent as in postmenopausal state, the parabasal cells predominate. The superficial cells produce glycogen under the effect of oestrogen, which is converted to lactic acid by lactobacilli. The pH of vagina is, therefore, acidic. Lactobacilli also produce hydrogen peroxide, and this along with the acidic pH protects against bacterial infections. In the postmenopausal and prepubertal states, due to the absence of oestrogen, the glycogen content is low, pH is alkaline and epithelium is nonkeratinized and thin, and, therefore, susceptibility to infection is greater.

Normal secretions increase during the following physiological conditions:

- Ovulation
- Premenstrual state
- Pregnancy

Vaginal infections

Infections of the vagina in childhood and adolescence are discussed in Chapter 17, *Paediatric*

Box 12.10 Normal vaginal secretions

- Characteristics
  - White, odourless
- Components
  - Secretions from glands of vulva
  - Transudate from vaginal wall
  - Secretions from cervical glands
  - Tubal and endometrial fluids
- Normal flora
  - Aerobic bacteria
    - Lactobacilli
    - *Streptococcus* and *Staphylococcus*
    - *Gardnerella vaginalis*
  - Anaerobic bacteria
    - *Peptococcus*, *Peptostreptococcus* and *Bacteroides*
- Normal pH
  - 3.8–4.5
- Microscopy
  - Desquamated epithelial cells
  - Few white blood cells
  - Lactobacilli

---

and adolescent gynaecology. The common conditions giving rise to vaginal infections and discharge are as follows:

- Bacterial vaginosis
- Trichomonal vaginitis
- Candidal vaginitis

The symptom common to all types of vaginitis is vaginal discharge. The distinguishing features are given in Table 12.2.

Bacterial vaginosis

This is the most common vaginal infection caused by a shift in the composition of the normal bacterial flora. There is an increase in anaerobic bacteria including *Gardnerella vaginalis*, *Prevotella* and *Mobiluncus* species and a decrease in lactobacilli. No single infectious agent has been identified. Multiple sexual partners are a risk factor. Hence, it is not a sexually transmitted disease, but a sexually associated disease. Discharge with fishy odour is characteristic. There are four criteria for diagnosis of bacterial vaginosis (Box 12.11). Three out of four of the **Amsel criteria** should be present for making a diagnosis. Clue cells that are seen in bacterial vaginosis are epithelial cells with adherent bacteria on the surface (Fig. 12.3).

Table 12.2 Distinguishing features of vaginitis

	Bacterial vaginosis	Trichomoniasis	Candidiasis
Discharge	• White, thin, homogeneous • Foul odour	• Yellow, frothy • Foul odour	• Thick, curdy • No odour
Other symptoms		Pruritus, dysuria	Pruritus, dysuria
Signs	No erythema	Strawberry vagina	Erythema ++
pH	>4.5	>4.5	<4.5
Diagnosis	• Wet mount • Clue cells • Amine odour with KOH	• Wet mount • Motile organisms	• KOH • Pseudohyphae or spores

KOH, potassium hydroxide.

Box 12.11 Criteria for diagnosis of bacterial vaginosis

- Homogeneous vaginal discharge
- Vaginal pH >4.5
- Amine-like odour on addition of KOH (whiff test)
- Clue cells on wet smear

KOH, potassium hydroxide.

Bacterial vaginosis increases the risk for pelvic inflammatory disease, postoperative and post-abortal infections, and obstetric complications such as preterm labour and prelabour rupture of membranes. Recurrent infections are common.

Trichomonal vaginitis

This infection is caused by the protozoan *Trichomonas vaginalis*. It is a highly contagious **sexually transmitted** disease. The vagina is usually inflamed and oedematous with typical 'strawberry' appearance. There may be associated soreness of the vulva, perineum and thighs. Dysuria and dyspareunia may also be present. The discharge is malodorous, greenish and frothy. 'Strawberry vagina' is characteristic of *Trichomonas* infection. Diagnosis is by examination of saline preparation of the discharge, which reveals motile flagellated organisms (Fig. 12.4). Culture, nucleic acid amplification test and *Trichomonas* rapid test are not readily available and not practical for routine use. The organism can also be identified on Pap smear. The infection can coexist with bacterial vaginosis. In pregnant women, it can cause prelabour rupture of membranes and preterm labour. Clinical features, diagnosis and treatment of trichomonal vaginitis are summarized in Box 12.12.

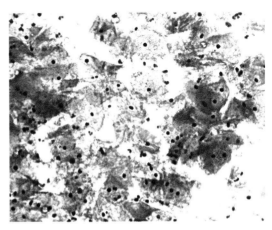

Figure 12.3 Photomicrograph of a Pap smear in a woman with bacterial vaginosis showing clue cells. Bacteria adherent to the cells make the cytoplasm appear 'fuzzy'.

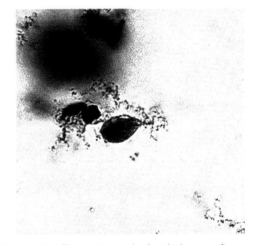

Figure 12.4 Photomicrograph of vaginal smear after Giemsa stain showing flagellated organism—*T. vaginalis*.

- Sexually transmitted
- Caused by *Trichomonas vaginalis*
- Symptoms
  - Vaginal discharge
  - Pruritus
  - Dysuria, dyspareunia
- Signs
  - Inflamed, oedematous vulva
  - Foul, greenish, frothy discharge
  - Strawberry vagina
- Diagnosis
  - Saline preparation—Flagellated organism
  - Culture
  - Nucleic acid amplification test
  - *Trichomonas* rapid test
  - Pap smear
- Complications in pregnancy
  - PPROM
  - Preterm labour

PPROM, preterm prelabour rupture of membranes.

Candidal vaginitis

Candida albicans is a part of the normal vaginal flora in 25% of women and causes 90% of candidal vaginitis. Other species of *Candida* are responsible for 10% of infections. The fungi multiply and grow rapidly when concentration of lactobacilli decreases. Risk factors for candidal infection are as given in Box 12.13. Candidal infection is not sexually transmitted.

- Pregnancy
- Oral contraceptive use
- Menstruation
- Antibiotic use
- Obesity
- Diabetes
- Debilitating illness
- Immunosuppression
  - Corticosteroids
  - Immunosuppressive drugs
  - HIV infection

HIV, human immunodeficiency virus.

Discharge and pruritus are the predominant symptoms. The vulval skin is usually involved as well with erythema, excoriation, oedema and dysuria. The discharge is curdy (Fig. 12.5)

and tends to adhere to the vaginal wall forming plaques.

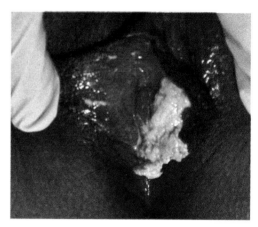

Figure 12.5 Thick, curdy white discharge from the vagina seen at the introitus—Severe candidal vaginitis.

In contrast to other types of vaginitis where pH is elevated, in candidal infection, pH is <4.5. Potassium hydroxide (KOH) must be added to the discharge to lyse the cells and visualize the hyphae, pseudohyphae and spores (Fig. 12.6). A sample may be sent for culture when clinical suspicion is high but smear is negative. However, the treatment can be initiated on the basis of clinical diagnosis.

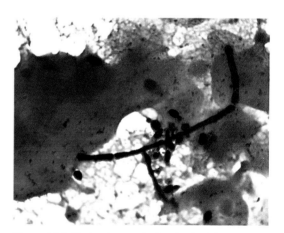

Figure 12.6 Photomicrograph showing budding oval yeast with pseudohyphae—*Candida albicans*.

Recurrent candidal infection About 3–5% of women develop recurrent infections (>4 infections in a year). Culture is required to confirm the diagnosis, identify the fungal species and determine sensitivity.

Management of vaginitis

Male partner must be treated simultaneously in *Trichomonas* infection, and patients should be instructed to avoid intercourse till treatment is completed. Treatment of male partner is not required in candidal vaginitis and bacterial vaginosis. Treatment of vaginitis (CDC recommendation, 2010) is outlined in Tables 12.3 and 12.4.

Cervicitis

The **ectocervix** is susceptible to the infections that cause vaginitis and to HSV, HPV and *Mycoplasma*, since, like the vagina, ectocervix is also lined by squamous epithelium.

C. trachomatis and *N. gonorrhoeae* are the two organisms that infect the **endocervix** that is lined by columnar epithelium. Both are STIs. Many women with gonococcal and chlamydial infection are asymptomatic. In others, infection by these organisms gives rise to mucopurulent cervicitis with a greenish yellow discharge referred to as **mucopus**.

The cervix should be examined with a speculum; the vaginal secretions should be removed with a swab and a cotton swab introduced into the endocervix to obtain a sample of mucopus. Characteristics of cervicitis are listed in Box 12.14.

Box 12.14 Characteristics of mucopurulent cervicitis

- Caused by *Neisseria gonorrhoeae* and *Candida trachomatis*
- Sexually transmitted
- Definitive diagnostic criteria
  - Ectopy of glandular epithelium
  - Friable epithelium
  - Bleeds on touch
  - Gross visualization of mucopus on cotton swab
  - Ten or more neutrophils on Gram-stained smear
- Possibility of PID due to ascending infection
- Coexistence of *C. trachomatis* and *N. gonorrhoeae*
- Syphilis and HIV ruled out

HIV, human immunodeficiency virus; *PID*, pelvic inflammatory disease.

Table 12.3 Treatment of bacterial vaginosis and trichomonal vaginitis

Disease	Drug and dose	Route	Duration
Bacterial vaginosis	Metronidazole 400 mg twice daily	Oral	7 days
	(or) 0.75% metronidazole gel	Intravaginal	5 days
	(or) 2% clindamycin cream	Intravaginal	7 days
	(or) Clindamycin 300 mg twice daily	Oral	7 days
Trichomonal vaginitis	Metronidazole 2 g single dose	Oral	
	(or) Metronidazole 400 mg twice daily	Oral	7 days
	(or) Tinidazole 2 g single dose	Oral	

Table 12.4 Treatment of candidal vaginitis

Disease	Drug and dose	Duration
Uncomplicated		
Intravaginal azoles	2% Butaconazole cream	4 days
	(or) Clotrimazole 200 mg twice daily	3 days
	(or) 1% clotrimazole cream	7–14 days
	(or) Miconazole 100 mg/200 mg/1200 mg	7/3/1 days
	(or) 2% miconazole cream	7 days
	(or) 0.4%/0.8% terconazole cream	7/3 days
	(or) Terconazole 80 mg once daily	3 days
	(or) Nystatin 100,000 units once daily	14 days
Oral	Fluconazole 150 mg single dose	
Complicated	Intravaginal azole	7–14 days
	(or) Oral fluconazole 150 mg	Two doses 72 hours apart
Recurrent	Oral fluconazole 150 mg	Every 3 days for 9 days Weekly for 6 months thereafter

Gonococcal infection

N. gonorrhoeae is a Gram-negative diplococcus (Fig. 12.7). It infects columnar and transitional epithelium causing cervicitis, cystitis and urethritis. Risk factors are listed in Box 12.15.

> **Box 12.15 Risk factors for *Neisseria gonorrhoeae* infection**
>
> - Age <25 years
> - Multiple sexual partners
> - Prior gonococcal infection
> - Commercial sex workers
> - Drug use

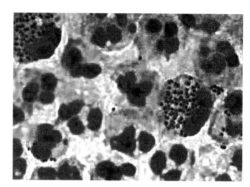

Figure 12.7 Photomicrograph of vaginal discharge after Gram staining showing Gram-negative intracellular diplococci within the polymorphs—*Neisseria gonorrhoeae*.

Clinical features, diagnosis and treatment (CDC recommendation) are outlined in Box 12.16. Sexual partners should be treated. **Since the gonococcal and chlamydial infections often coexist and it is difficult to rule out *C. trachomatis* infection, azithromycin 1 g single dose or doxycycline 100 mg twice daily for 7 days should be added to any of the treatment regimens for gonorrhoea.**

> **Box 12.16 Clinical features, diagnosis and treatment of gonorrhoea**
>
> - Infects cervix, bladder and urethra
> - Symptoms
>   - Vaginal discharge
>   - Dysuria
> - Diagnosis
>   - Gram staining
>   - Intracellular Gram-negative diplococci
>   - Culture
>   - Nucleic acid amplification techniques
>   - DNA probe
> - Treatment
>   - Ceftriaxone 125 mg IM single dose
>   (**plus**) Azithromycin 1 g oral single dose
>   (or) Doxycycline 100 mg oral twice daily **for 7 days**
>   *Alternative regimens*
>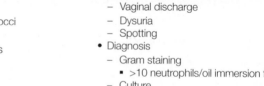
>   Cefixime 400 mg oral single dose or suspension
>   (or) Ceftizoxime 500 mg IM } with azithromycin
>   (or) Cefoxitin 2 g IM
>   (or) Cefotaxime 500 mg IM

IM, intramuscular.

C. trachomatis infection

C. trachomatis is an obligatory intracellular organism. It infects the columnar epithelium but can give rise to an ascending infection leading to pelvic inflammatory disease and, in pregnant women, can cause prelabour rupture of membranes and preterm labour. Clinical features, diagnosis and treatment of *C. trachomatis* infection (CDC recommendation) are outlined in Box 12.17.

As already mentioned, gonococcal infection often coexists; hence, dual therapy is indicated.

> **Box 12.17 Clinical features, diagnosis and treatment of *Chlamydia trachomatis* infection**
>
> - Symptoms
>   - Vaginal discharge
>   - Dysuria
>   - Spotting
> - Diagnosis
>   - Gram staining
>   - >10 neutrophils/oil immersion field
>   - Culture
>   - Nucleic acid amplification techniques
>   - DNA probe
> - Treatment
>   - Azithromycin 1 g oral single dose
>   - (or) Doxycycline 100 mg oral twice daily **for 7 days**
>   - *Alternative regimens*
>   - Erythromycin base 500 mg oral four times daily **for 7 days**
>   - (or) Erythromycin ethylsuccinate 800 mg oral qid **for 7 days**
>   - (or) Ofloxacin 300 mg twice daily oral **for 7 days**

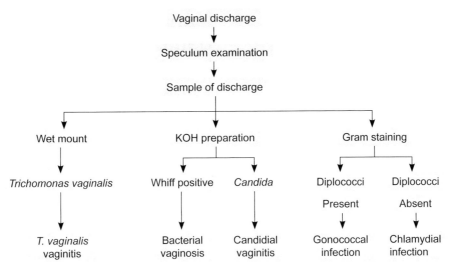

Figure 12.8 Evaluation of vaginal discharge. *KOH*, potassium hydroxide.

Expedited partner therapy (EPT)

This is recommended in gonococcal and chlamydial infections to avoid delay in treatment of sexual partners. The prescription for sexual partner is given without clinical examination.

Fig. 12.8 gives a simple algorithm for management of women with vaginal discharge.

Evaluation and management of reproductive tract infections

Several RTIs are also STIs. The STIs have more severe health consequences. Therefore, they have been identified as a public health problem and strategies for prevention and control of infections have been instituted by National AIDS Control Organisation (NACO), Ministry of Health and Family Welfare, Government of India.

Women with RTIs may present with vaginal discharge, associated abdominal pain or genital ulcer. Lower abdominal pain and constitutional symptoms suggest upper genital tract involvement (pelvic inflammatory disease).

History

History is important for risk assessment for STIs and clinical diagnosis (Box 12.18).

Box 12.18 History

- Age (<21 years)
- Symptoms
  - Vaginal discharge
    - Type of discharge
    - Duration
    - Pruritus
    - Dysuria, dyspareunia
  - Ulcer
  - Lower abdominal pain
  - Constitutional symptoms
- Sexual activity
  - New sexual partner
  - Multiple partners
- Marital status
- Symptoms of STI in the sexual partner
- Contraception
- Recent miscarriage, childbirth
- Previous episodes

STI, sexually transmitted infection.

Physical examination

A diagnosis regarding the nature of infection can be arrived at in most cases by physical examination. It should be performed under good light (Box 12.19). Fever, tachycardia, abdominal or pelvic tenderness, pelvic mass, fullness in the pouch of Douglas and pain on movements of the cervix indicate upper genital tract infection (*see* Chapter 13, *Infections of the upper genital tract*).

- General examination
  - Fever, tachycardia
- Abdominal examination
  - Tenderness, mass
- Inspection of vulva
  - Soreness, oedema, erythema
  - Discharge
    - Colour, odour, consistency
    - Frothy, curdy, homogeneous nature
  - Genital ulcer
    - Size, number
    - Other features
- Examination of the groin
  - Inguinal swelling
- Speculum examination
  - Mucopus from the cervix
  - Vaginal pH
  - Strawberry vagina
  - Pap smear
  - Saline/KOH preparation/Gram stain
  - Swab for culture
- Pelvic examination
  - Tenderness on moving the cervix
  - Fullness in POD
  - Adnexal mass
  - Tenderness in lateral fornices

KOH, potassium hydroxide; *POD*, pouch of Douglas.

Investigations

Examination of the discharge as a wet film or after addition of KOH is the first step (Box 12.20).

Box 12.20 Investigations

- Wet film
  - *T. vaginalis*
  - Clue cells
- KOH preparation
  - Whiff test
  - Fungal pseudohyphae/spores
- Gram staining
  - Gram-negative diplococci
  - Neutrophils
- Dark-field microscopy (syphilis)
- Pap smear
- VDRL
- HIV serology
- Full blood count
  - If PID is suspected

HIV, human immunodeficiency virus; *KOH*, potassium hydroxide; *PID*, pelvic inflammatory disease; *VDRL*, Venereal Disease Research Laboratory.

Management of lower genital (reproductive) tract infections

- *Aetiology-based management*: When facilities for laboratory tests for confirmation of diagnosis are available, appropriate tests should be performed, causative organism should be identified and the infections should be treated as discussed earlier in the chapter.
- *Syndromic case management (SCM)*: In low-resource settings, identifying the cause of infection by laboratory tests can be difficult and expensive. More than one sexually transmitted disease may be present at a time. Since early diagnosis and treatment without delay are crucial in the control of lower genital tract infection, NACO has introduced SCM (Box 12.21). This approach has the disadvantages of overtreatment and emergence of drug resistance. Therefore, this treatment should be restricted to peripheral hospitals with no facilities for examination and confirmation of diagnosis. NACO guidelines have been published by the Ministry of Health and Family Welfare, Government of India, for syndromic management of RTIs and STIs in 2011. **Syndromic management is a scientifically proven approach and covers most common organisms causing a particular syndrome.**

Box 12.21 Syndromic approach in lower genital tract infections

- Based on
  - Set of easily elicited symptoms
  - Set of easily recognized signs
  - Well-defined, limited number of causes
- Enables diagnosis and treatment at first contact
- Reduces secondary cases/infections
- To be used in low-resource settings
- Includes
  - Treatment of patients and partners
  - Patient education and counselling
  - Promotion of condom use
  - Referral to higher centre as required

Clinical examination and syndromic diagnosis

Clinical signs indicative of specific syndromic diagnosis are listed in Table 12.5. The health

Table 12.5 Clinical signs and syndromic diagnosis in reproductive tract infections

Signs	Possible syndromic diagnosis
• Discharge and redness of vulva (common signs of vaginitis) • Discharge is white and curd-like	VD
Ulcers, sores and blisters	GUD, herpetic/non-herpetic
Swelling or lumps in the groin	IB
If cervix bleeds easily on touch or the discharge appears mucopurulent with discolouration	CD
If examined after childbirth, abortion or miscarriage, look for bleeding, tissue fragments; check if the cervix is normal	Complications of abortion; refer to higher centre
Tumours or other abnormal tissues on cervix	Carcinoma, refer to higher centre

CD, cervical discharge; GUD, genital ulcer disease; IB, inguinal bubo; VD, vaginal discharge.

workers and accredited social health activists (ASHA) identify the symptoms and refer the patients to primary health centres (PHCs) and community health centres (CHCs) for SCM. Specialists and trained physicians at designated STI/RTI clinics in district hospitals and medical college hospitals also provide these services. At these centres, the syndromic approach is enhanced by laboratory facilities.

Seven kits, colour coded specifically for each syndromic diagnosis, are supplied free to the PHCs, CHCs and district hospitals. Once syndromic diagnosis is made, the kits are used for treatment as given in Table 12.6.

Counselling and treatment of partners

Counselling regarding safe sex, use of condom and early recognition of symptoms is mandatory. Sexual partner(s) must be traced, evaluated and treated. This is essential because infections of the lower genital tract may lead to pelvic inflammatory disease since the female genital tract is a continuous open pathway from exterior to peritoneal cavity.

Table 12.6 Colour-coded STI drug kits according to syndrome

Kit	Colour	Composition	Syndrome
1	Grey	Tab. azithromycin 1 g stat + Tab. cefixime 400 mg stat	UD, CD
2	Green	Tab. secnidazole 2 g stat + Cap. fluconazole 150 mg stat	VD
3	White	Inj. benzathine penicillin 2.4 mega units IM stat + Tab. azithromycin 1 g stat	Genital ulcer—Nonherpetic
4	Blue	Cap. doxycycline 100 mg BD for 15 days + Tab. azithromycin 1 g stat	Genital ulcer, allergic to penicillin
5	Red	Tab. acyclovir 400 mg TDS for 7 days	Genital ulcer disease, herpetic
6	Yellow	Tab. cefixime 400 mg stat + Tab. metronidazole 400 mg BD for 14 days + Cap. doxycycline100 mg BD for 14 days	Lower abdominal pain
7	Black	Cap. doxycycline 100 mg BD for 21 days + Tab. azithromycin 1 g stat	Inguinal bubo

CD, cervical discharge; IM, intramuscular; STI, sexually transmitted infection; UD, urethral discharge; VD, vaginal discharge.

Key points

• Infections of the lower genital tract are those that involve the vulva, vagina and cervix. They present with vaginal discharge and/or pruritus.

• There are several defence mechanisms such as acidic separations of the vulva, acidic pH of the vagina and mucous plug of the cervix that protect the women from infection.

• Infections of the vulva affect structures of the vulva such as Bartholin glands or the vulval skin. They may be primary or secondary to vaginitis.

(Continued)

Key points *(Continued)*

- Primary infections of the vulva are viral infections, genital ulcers, infestations and infection of the vulvar structures.

- Condyloma acuminata and herpes simplex are the common viral infections of the vulva. Bartholin adenitis and abscess are common in women younger than 30 years. They present with pain and swelling in the vulva. They are treated with antibiotics and incisional drainage/marsupialization. Recurrent abscess is treated by excision of the gland.

- Causes of genital ulcers are herpes infection, syphilis, chancroid, lymphogranuloma venereum and donovanosis.

- Genital herpes is the most common cause of genital ulcer and is caused by herpes simplex virus. It presents with painful ulcers. Treatment is as recommended by the Centers for Disease Control and Prevention with acyclovir or valacyclovir.

- Infections of the vagina are bacterial vaginosis, trichomonal vaginitis and candidal vaginitis. The three conditions are distinguished by their clinical features and by examination of the smear.

- Bacterial vaginosis and trichomonal vaginitis are treated with metronidazole. Candidal vaginitis is treated with intravaginal azole or oral fluconazole.

- Cervicitis is usually caused by *Chlamydia trachomatis* and *Neisseria gonorrhoeae*. Both are sexually transmitted infections.

- Diagnosis of gonorrhoea is by Gram staining and culture of the discharge or by nucleic acid amplification techniques (NAAT). Treatment is with cefixime, ceftriaxone, ciprofloxacin, azithromycin or doxycycline.

- Chlamydial infection is diagnosed by clinical features or culture of the discharge. NAAT may also be used. Treatment is with azithromycin, doxycycline or ofloxacin.

- Evaluation of a woman with vaginal discharge consists of history, physical examination and examination of the discharge as a wet film, potassium hydroxide (KOH) preparation, Gram staining and Pap smear.

- Since early diagnosis and management are crucial in preventing sequelae, the World Health Organization and National AIDS Control Organisation (NACO) have recommended syndromic approach for low-resource settings. This is a scientifically proven approach to treatment of reproductive tract infections.

- Counselling and treatment of partners regarding safe sex and use of condoms is mandatory. Sexual partners must be evaluated and treated.

Self-assessment

Case-based questions

Case 1

A 28-year-old lady, mother of two children, presents with a history of white discharge and intense pruritus.

1. What details would you ask for in history?
2. What examination and investigations will you perform?
3. If a diagnosis of *T. vaginalis* vaginitis is made, how will you manage?
4. If a diagnosis of candidal vaginitis is made, how will you manage?

Case 2

A 30-year-old lady, mother of three children, presents with pain in the vulva and multiple ulcers that are very painful.

1. What details would you like to know in history?
2. What will you look for and what investigation will you do?
3. How will you manage?

Answers

Case 1

1. (a) Nature of discharge—Colour, odour
   (b) Associated symptoms—Dysuria, abdominal pain, fever

   (c) Contraception, menstrual irregularity
2. (a) External genitalia—For ulcer, excoriation
   (b) Per speculum examination—For nature of discharge (frothy, curdy, mucoid)
   (c) Swab from endocervix—To look for mucopus
   (d) Look for erythema, oedema, strawberry vagina
   (e) Pelvic examination—For uterine/adnexal tenderness, mass
   (f) Examination of discharge—Wet film and KOH preparation
3. Tab. metronidazole 2 g oral single dose for the patient and the sexual partner.
   (*Or*) Tab. metronidazole 400 mg twice daily for 7 days for the patient and the sexual partner.
4. (a) Intravaginal miconazole 100 mg daily for 7 days or 200 mg daily for 3 days
   (b) Estimation of blood sugar to exclude diabetes

Case 2

1. History of fever, malaise, time of onset of pain, past history of similar illness.
2. (a) Vesicles and ulcers on the vulva, vagina and cervix
   (b) Number of ulcers, nature of ulcer(s), depth, base, margin, induration
   (c) Inguinal lymphadenopathy
   (d) Swab from the ulcer for culture, serology for syphilis, HSV2

3. **(a)** Acyclovir 400 mg thrice daily for 7–10 days
   (*Or*) valacyclovir 1000 mg twice daily for 7–10
   days
   (b) Counsel regarding recurrences

Long-answer question

1. Discuss the differential diagnosis and management of
   genital ulcers in females.

Short-answer questions

1. *Trichomonas vaginalis*—Diagnosis and treatment
2. Bacterial vaginosis
3. Mucopurulent cervicitis
4. Vaginal candidiasis
5. Bartholin abscess

13 | Infections of the Upper Genital Tract

Case scenario

Mrs PL, 27, was the mother of two children. Her husband was a construction worker and gave a history of multiple sexual partners. Mrs PL had been treated in the past for vaginal discharge. She had complained of fever, malaise, nausea and vomiting 2 days ago. Her husband had given her some native medicines. She developed abdominal pain, diarrhoea, tenesmus and high fever, and was brought to the hospital by her neighbours. On examination, she was dehydrated, toxic and febrile, and had abdominal tenderness. She was immediately hospitalized for further evaluation and management.

Introduction

Infections can spread from the vagina and cervix to the upper genital tract. Infection of the internal genital organs can also occur in the puerperium, following abortion and pelvic surgery and after instrumentation of the uterus. Haematogenous, lymphatic and direct spread of infection from other organs is also possible. Potential consequences of delay in diagnosis and treatment of upper genital tract infection are significant.

Definition

Infections of the upper genital tract include infections involving the endometrium, myometrium, tubes, ovaries, uterine serosa, broad ligaments and pelvic peritoneum. Ascending infection from the lower genital tract is the most common cause. **When infection is not associated with pregnancy, pelvic surgery or instrumentation, it is also known as pelvic inflammatory disease (PID).** This can be acute *or* chronic.

Prevalence

Incidence of lower genital tract infections varies with the population, and data are not easily available. The World Health Organization (WHO) estimates that 1 million women suffer from PID every year globally. Prevalence of upper genital tract infections is about 3–10% in India. Almost 85% are spontaneous or sexually transmitted infections; 15% occur after gynaecological procedures.

Aetiology

PID is caused by organisms ascending from the endocervix and vagina and is, therefore, a **polymicrobial infection**. Gonococcal and chlamydial infections are the most common, but numerous other aerobic and anaerobic organisms have been implicated (Box 13.1). Infections with different organisms can coexist with gonococcal infection. Concurrent bacterial vaginosis is also common in women with PID.

Postoperative, postabortal and puerperal pelvic infection and cellulitis are usually caused by other aerobic and anaerobic pathogenic organisms.

Box 13.1 Organisms causing pelvic infection

Aerobic
- *Neisseria gonorrhoeae*
- *Chlamydia trachomatis*
- *Ureaplasma urealyticum*
- *Mycoplasma genitalium*
- *Gardnerella vaginalis*
- *Streptococcus pyogenes*
- *Staphylococcus* spp.
- *Escherichia coli*
- *Mycoplasma hominis*
- *Mycobacterium tuberculosis*

Anaerobic
- *Bacteroides*
- *Peptostreptococcus*
- *Clostridium*
- *Fusobacterium*

Risk factors

Risk assessment based on known risk factors is essential for prevention and management of PID. The risk factors are listed in Box 13.2. Oral contraceptives and condoms decrease the risk of PID, but intrauterine contraceptive device (IUCD) is associated with an increased risk in the first 3 weeks after insertion, probably due to introduction of organisms during insertion.

Contraception and risk of PID

Barrier contraception protects against PID. Oral contraceptives increase the risk of chlamydial and gonococcal cervicitis but decrease the risk of PID.

Box 13.2 Risk factors for PID

- Young age
- Low socioeconomic status
- Multiple sex partners
- Unmarried/widowed women
- Past history of STI
- Vaginal douching
- IUCD for 3 weeks after insertion
- Smoking
- Substance abuse

IUCD, intrauterine contraceptive device; *PID*, pelvic inflammatory disease; *STI*, sexually transmitted infection.

Currently available intrauterine devices do not increase the risk except in the first 3 weeks after insertion. Tubal ligation is protective (Box 13.3).

Box 13.3 Contraception and risk of PID

- Barrier contraception
  - Protective
- Oral contraceptives
  - Increase risk of cervicitis
  - Decrease risk of PID
- IUCD
  - Increases risk for 3 weeks after insertion
  - No increase after 3 weeks
- Tubal ligation
  - Protective

IUCD, intrauterine contraceptive device; *PID*, pelvic inflammatory disease.

Pathogenesis

The normal vagina is colonized by lactobacilli and other potentially pathogenic bacteria. The endocervical canal functions as a barrier and prevents entry of these organisms into the upper genital tract. This barrier breaks down when there is endocervical infection. The pathogenic bacteria ascend through the endocervical canal and infect the endometrium, tubes, ovarian cortex, pelvic and general peritoneum. The resulting PID may be acute or chronic.

As already mentioned, *Neisseria gonorrhoeae* and *Chlamydia trachomatis* are the most common causes of PID. In gonococcal infection, the organisms ascend from the cervix to the tubes and adhere to the nonciliated mucus-secreting cells. An acute inflammatory reaction ensues, causing tissue damage (Box 13.4). The repair that follows results in scarring and tubal adhesions.

In chlamydial infection, the organism ascends from the cervix and colonizes the fallopian tubes. Inflammatory reaction and tissue destruction occur. Chlamydial infection can give rise to atypical *or* silent PID. Recurrent chlamydial infections are common. The woman is asymptomatic but suffers tubal damage with resultant infertility and ectopic pregnancy. When infection is not adequately treated, unrecognized and/or recurrent chronic PID ensues.

Box 13.4 Pathogenesis of PID

- *Neisseria gonorrhoeae* and *Chlamydia trachomatis* most common
- Infection ascending from the cervix
- Colonization of tubes
- Cell/complement-mediated inflammation, fibrosis and scarring

PID, pelvic inflammatory disease.

Pathology

Acute PID

In acute PID, the tubes that are colonized by the organisms become oedematous and filled with inflammatory exudate. Purulent fluid can be seen to discharge from the fimbrial ends of the tubes. The tube distends with pus, the fimbrial end closes due to inflammation and scarring, and a **pyosalpinx** is formed (Box 13.5). It is typically retort shaped. The ovary gets adherent to the tube to form a **tubo-ovarian** mass *or* pelvic abscess. **Pelvic abscess** usually collects in the pouch of Douglas. Infection may spread to the peritoneal cavity causing pelvic and/or general peritonitis.

Box 13.5 Pathology of acute PID

- Inflamed, fluid-filled tubes
- Pyosalpinx
- Tubo-ovarian abscess
- Pelvic abscess
- Pelvic/general peritonitis

PID, pelvic inflammatory disease.

Fitz-Hugh–Curtis syndrome Inflammation of the liver capsule can occur with chlamydial and gonococcal infection, and the patient presents with right-sided upper abdominal pain and liver tenderness. This is referred to as Fitz-Hugh–Curtis syndrome.

Tubo-ovarian abscess Tubo-ovarian abscess is a collection of pus in an inflammatory mass formed by the tube, ovary and adjacent pelvic organs. An adnexal mass is usually palpable.

Chronic PID

In women who are inadequately treated, are untreated *or* have recurrent infections, chronic PID ensues. The pus in the pyosalpinx becomes a sterile fluid and a **hydrosalpinx** is thus formed (Box 13.6). The uterus, ovaries, tubes and other pelvic structures may adhere together to form a frozen pelvis.

Box 13.6 Pathology of chronic PID

- Hydrosalpinx
- Tubo-ovarian mass
- Chronic pyosalpinx
- Frozen pelvis

PID, pelvic inflammatory disease.

Complications and sequelae of PID

Although some women are asymptomatic and have a silent infection, the disease may run a catastrophic course in others. Rupture of a **tubo-ovarian abscess** is a life-threatening complication (Box 13.7). Even those who have a mild *or* moderate infection can have sequelae due to scarring and adhesions. These long-term sequelae affect fertility and quality of life.

Box 13.7 Complications and sequelae of PID

- Complications
  - Pelvic peritonitis
  - General peritonitis
  - Rupture of tubo-ovarian abscess
  - Septicaemia
  - Subdiaphragmatic/perinephric abscess
  - Septic thrombophlebitis
- Sequelae
  - Ectopic pregnancy
  - Infertility
  - Chronic pelvic pain

PID, pelvic inflammatory disease.

Acute pelvic inflammatory disease

Clinical features

Symptoms

Symptoms of PID vary greatly. Some women are asymptomatic, but others present with severe pain and symptoms of peritonitis (Box 13.8). Women may have high fever, tachycardia and other signs of septicaemia. Lower abdominal pain is the predominant symptom, and the pain is dull and constant. Majority of women with PID have associated endocervicitis, giving rise to vaginal or cervical discharge. Fever, nausea and vomiting, which are systemic manifestations of infection, may also be present. Vaginal bleeding can occur due to endometritis. Pelvic abscess causes diarrhoea and tenesmus.

Box 13.8 Symptoms of acute PID

- Bilateral lower abdominal pain
- Abnormal vaginal or cervical discharge
- Fever >38°C
- Abnormal vaginal bleeding
- Deep dyspareunia
- Nausea and vomiting
- Diarrhoea and tenesmus
- Right upper abdominal pain (perihepatitis)

PID, pelvic inflammatory disease.

Signs

Clinical signs depend on the extent of infection (Box 13.9).

Triad of lower abdominal pain, adnexal tenderness and cervical motion tenderness is considered to be the most important clinical

---

Box 13.9 Signs of acute PID

- Bilateral lower abdominal tenderness
- Liver tenderness
- Vaginal discharge
- Mucopurulent discharge from the cervix
- Adnexal mass/tenderness
- Cervical motion tenderness
- Fullness in the pouch of Douglas
- Signs of peritonitis

PID, pelvic inflammatory disease.

---

feature for the diagnosis of PID. The sensitivity, specificity and positive predictive value of clinical symptoms and signs are low.

Pelvic abscess should be suspected when the patient has symptoms of acute PID along with tenesmus and diarrhoea. Pelvic examination reveals bogginess and fullness in the posterior fornix and induration. A collection between the rectum and the uterus can be felt on rectal examination.

Differential diagnosis

The symptoms and signs of PID can mimic those of several gynaecological and nongynaecological conditions (Box 13.10).

Box 13.10 Differential diagnosis of acute PID

- Gynaecological conditions
  - Ectopic pregnancy
  - Torsion/rupture of ovarian cyst
  - Endometriosis
- Nongynaecological conditions
  - Acute appendicitis
  - Diverticulitis
  - Irritable bowel syndrome
  - Inflammatory bowel disease
  - Urinary tract infection
  - Functional pain

PID, pelvic inflammatory disease.

Investigations

Based on history and physical examination, a clinical diagnosis of acute PID can be made. **Empirical treatment is recommended when the level of suspicion is high since withholding treatment has potential serious consequences.**

Investigations are aimed at excluding other conditions and confirming the diagnosis (Box 13.11). The tests are not highly sensitive or specific but help exclude other conditions. Leucocytosis, elevated sedimentation rate and C-reactive protein are usually seen but are nonspecific and unreliable indicators of the disease. Endocervical sample should be evaluated for chlamydial and gonococcal infections (*see* Chapter 12, *Infections of the lower genital tract*). Serological tests for HIV and syphilis should be performed since these infections may coexist. Transvaginal ultrasonogram and CT scan may help exclude ectopic pregnancy, appendicitis

- Blood tests
  - Total count, ESR
  - C-reactive protein
- Endocervical discharge
  - Pus cells
  - NAAT for *Chlamydia* and *Gonococcus*
- Vaginal discharge
  - Saline preparation/pH for BV
- Urine culture to exclude UTI
- Serology for HIV and syphilis
- Transvaginal ultrasonography
  - Inflamed tubes
  - Free peritoneal fluid
  - Tubo-ovarian mass
  - Pelvic abscess
  - Excludes
    - Ectopic pregnancy
    - Appendicitis

BV, bacterial vaginosis; *ESR*, erythrocyte sedimentation rate; *NAAT*, nucleic acid amplification technique; *PID*, pelvic inflammatory disease; *UTI*, urinary tract infection.

and perihepatitis. Ultrasonography may reveal a pyosalpinx (Fig. 13.1), tubo-ovarian mass (Fig. 13.2) or pelvic abscess (Fig. 13.3). Laparoscopy is considered the gold standard but is not performed as a routine. It is reserved for patients who do not respond to initial

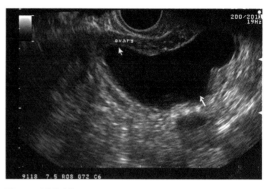

Figure 13.2 Ultrasonogram showing tubo-ovarian mass. The ovary (arrow) is seen adherent to the pyosalpinx (arrow) forming a complex mass.

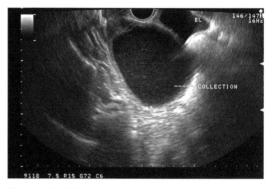

Figure 13.3 Ultrasonogram showing pelvic abscess.

therapy. Presence of dilated hyperaemic tubes, pyosalpinx or tubo-ovarian mass at laparoscopy confirms the diagnosis of acute PID. Other conditions such as appendicitis and ectopic pregnancy can be excluded. Pus can be obtained for culture (Box 13.12). Routine use of hysteroscopy or endometrial biopsy is not recommended.

- To confirm acute PID
  - Dilated hyperaemic tubes
  - Pyosalpinx
  - Tubo-ovarian mass
- To obtain pus for microbiology
- To exclude
  - Appendicitis
  - Ectopic pregnancy

PID, pelvic inflammatory disease.

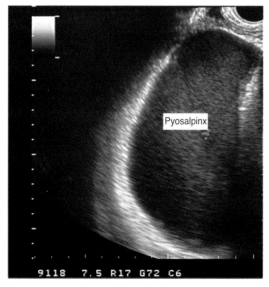

Figure 13.1 Ultrasonogram revealing pyosalpinx. It is elongated and filled with echogenic pus.

CDC guidelines for diagnosis of acute PID

The goal of treatment in acute PID is to reduce the risk of complications, sequelae and chronic PID. Therefore, the Centers for Disease Control and Prevention (CDC) has laid down guidelines (2015; Box 13.13) for diagnosis and clinical criteria for initiating empirical therapy.

Empirical treatment can be initiated in young women and those at risk for sexually transmitted infections when the minimum criteria are present and no other cause for illness is identified.

Box 13.13 CDC guidelines (2015) for diagnosis of acute PID and clinical criteria for initiating therapy

- Minimum criteria
  - Uterine tenderness
  - Adnexal tenderness
  - Cervical motion tenderness
- Additional criteria for diagnosis
  - Oral temperature >38°C
  - Abnormal cervical mucopurulent discharge or cervical friability
  - Vaginal discharge: WBCs on microscopy
  - Laboratory documentation of cervical infection with *Neisseria gonorrhoeae* or *Chlamydia trachomatis*
  - Elevated ESR
  - Elevated C-reactive protein
- Definitive criteria for diagnosis of PID
  - Endometrial biopsy
    - Histopathological evidence of endometritis
  - Transvaginal ultrasonogram/MRI
    - Thickened tubes
    - Fluid-filled tubes
    - Tubo-ovarian mass
  - Doppler studies suggestive of pelvic infection
  - Laparoscopy
    - Tubal erythema, oedema, adhesions
    - Pyosalpinx/tubo-ovarian mass
    - Purulent exudates in POD

CDC, Centers for Disease Control and Prevention; *ESR*, erythrocyte sedimentation rate; *MRI*, magnetic resonance imaging; *PID*, pelvic inflammatory disease; *POD*, pouch of Douglas; *WBC*, white blood cell.

Management

Management of acute PID has several aspects (Box 13.14).

Box 13.14 Management of acute PID

- Assessment of need for hospitalization
- Antimicrobial therapy
- Treatment of partners
- Counselling
- Assessment of response to therapy
- Decision regarding surgical intervention
- Follow-up for sequelae

PID, pelvic inflammatory disease.

Outpatient treatment

As has been repeatedly emphasized in this chapter, treatment must be initiated early to avoid complications and sequelae. A high index of suspicion is required. When one *or* more of the minimum criteria are present, outpatient treatment is started. In the absence of severe infection (tubo-ovarian abscess), the outcome with outpatient treatment is as good as with admission and intravenous antibiotics. Only 15% of women require hospitalization. ***The drugs used should cover gonococcal and chlamydial infections*** (Table 13.1). It is preferable to use drugs that cover anaerobes as well. Metronidazole should be included in women with postoperative or post-instrumentation sepsis. The patient should be reassessed after 48–72 hours, and if response is inadequate, hospitalization and parenteral therapy are required.

Table 13.1 Drugs used and dosages in mild to moderate acute PID

Drug	Dose	Duration
Ceftriaxone	250 mg IM single dose	
(or) Cefoxitin	2 g IM single dose (*plus* probenecid)	
(or) Other third-generation cephalosporins	IM single dose	
With doxycycline	100 mg oral twice daily	14 days
With or *without* metronidazole	400 mg oral twice daily	14 days

IM, intramuscularly; *PID*, pelvic inflammatory disease.

Inpatient treatment

Admission to hospital is indicated in some situations (Box 13.15). The decision should be made based on clinical judgement.

Table 13.2 CDC recommendation for inpatient treatment of acute PID

Drug	Dose	Duration
Regimen A*		
Cefotetan (or)	2 g IV Q12H	Till complete clinical resolution
Cefoxitin	2 g IV Q6H	Till complete clinical resolution
(plus) Doxycycline	100 mg IV Q12H Followed by 100 mg oral Q12H	24–48 hours 14 days
Regimen B#		
Clindamycin	900 mg IV Q8H Followed by 450 mg oral Q6H	Till complete clinical resolution 14 days
(plus) Gentamicin	Loading dose of 2 mg/kg IV or IM Followed by 1.5 mg/kg Q8H (or) Single daily dosing 3–5 mg/kg IV	Till complete clinical resolution

*Regimen A, intravenous therapy is discontinued 24 hours after the patient becomes afebrile. Treatment with doxycycline (100 mg twice daily oral) should continue to complete 14 days. #Regimen B, intravenous therapy is discontinued 24 hours after the patient becomes afebrile. Clindamycin 450 mg oral four times daily should continue to complete a total of 14 days. Alternatively, treatment with doxycycline 100 mg oral twice daily should be started and continued for 14 days. *CDC*, Centers for Disease Control and Prevention; *IM*, intramuscularly; *IV*, intravenously; *PID*, pelvic inflammatory disease.

Box 13.15 Indications for hospitalization

- Not able to rule out surgical emergency (e.g. acute appendicitis)
- No response to outpatient oral treatment
- Presence of tubo-ovarian or pelvic abscess
- Clinically severe disease with nausea, vomiting and high fever
- Oral therapy not tolerated
- PID in pregnancy

PID, pelvic inflammatory disease.

Once hospitalized, intravenous antibiotics should be started. The first-line therapies as recommended by CDC (2015) are given in Table 13.2. Parenteral therapy should be continued until 24 hours after the patient clinically improves. Doxycycline should be continued for 14 days.

Alternative regimens

Alternative regimens (CDC recommendation) are given in Table 13.3. Data on cure rates with these regimens are limited.

Surgical intervention

If recognized and treated early, surgical intervention is rarely required. Indications for

Table 13.3 Alternative regimens for inpatient treatment of acute PID

Drug	Dose	Duration
Ampicillin/ sulbactam	3 g IV Q6H	Till complete clinical resolution
(plus) Doxycycline	100 mg oral or IV Q12H Followed by 100 mg oral Q12H	24–48 hours 14 days
(or) Azithromycin	500 mg IV daily for two doses Followed by 250 mg oral daily	7 days
With or *without* Metronidazole	500 mg oral Q8H	14 days

Parenteral therapy can be discontinued 24 hours after the patient improves clinically and oral preparation of the same drug continued for 14 days. *IV*, intravenously; *PID*, pelvic inflammatory disease.

surgical intervention are listed in Box 13.16. Aspiration *or* drainage of pus can be performed by ultrasound-guided procedure and has excellent results with very few complications. **Pelvic abscess** that is easily palpated through posterior fornix can be drained vaginally by simple colpotomy by making an incision on the posterior vaginal fornix. A drain is left for 24–48 hours.

Laparoscopy *or* laparotomy is required when the pus cannot be easily drained due to locules or adhesions. Drainage of pus and irrigation of the peritoneal cavity is recommended. Removal of the affected ovary and tube (salpingo-oophorectomy) is occasionally required.

Box 13.16 Indications for surgical intervention in acute PID

- Ultrasound-guided aspiration
  - Pelvic abscess
  - Tubo-ovarian abscess
    - Large size (>9 cm)
    - No response to antibiotic therapy
    - Suspected rupture
  - Subdiaphragmatic collection
- Posterior colpotomy
  - Pelvic abscess
- Laparoscopic aspiration/drainage/adhesiolysis
  - Tubo-ovarian abscess/pelvic abscess
- Laparotomy
  - Tubo-ovarian abscess
  - Rupture of tubo-ovarian abscess
  - Multiple intra-abdominal collections

PID, pelvic inflammatory disease.

Management of sexual partners

Since most pelvic infections are sexually transmitted, sexual partner must be traced and screened (Box 13.17).

Box 13.17 Management of sexual partners in acute PID

- Contact partners within 6 months of onset of disease.
- Screen for gonococcal/chlamydial infection.
- If screening not possible, start empirical treatment.
- Avoid intercourse till the partner completes treatment.

PID, pelvic inflammatory disease.

Counselling

Women should be counselled regarding practice of safe sex, prevention of reinfection and possible sequelae (Box 13.18).

Follow-up

Follow-up after 6–8 weeks to ensure adequate response to therapy, compliance and counselling is mandatory.

Box 13.18 Counselling in acute PID

- Early treatment reduces the risk of sequelae but does not eliminate it.
- Barrier contraception reduces risk.
- Recurrence of infection increases the risk of infertility.
- Sexual partner must be treated.

PID, pelvic inflammatory disease.

Postoperative/postinstrumentation infections

These can occur following minor and major surgical procedures. Minor procedures include dilatation and curettage, insertion of intrauterine device, hysterosalpingography and sonosalpingography. Collection of pus in the pelvis and pelvic and general peritonitis can occur following major surgeries including hysterectomy. Pelvic abscess is more common following vaginal hysterectomy and other vaginal surgical procedures. It presents 1–2 weeks after surgery.

The patient presents with fever, abdominal/pelvic pain, vaginal discharge that may be malodorous and tenesmus. Examination reveals abdominal tenderness with or without rebound tenderness and a mass at the vaginal vault or pouch of Douglas.

Treatment is with antibiotics to cover Gram-positive, Gram-negative and anaerobic organisms. Oral amoxicillin with clavulanic acid along with metronidazole can be used in mild cases. If abscess is formed, ultrasound-guided aspiration or surgical drainage through colpotomy or laparotomy is necessary. Parenteral antibiotics should be administered in severe infection with peritonitis (Box 13.19).

Chronic pelvic inflammatory disease

Chronic PID is usually due to inadequate treatment of acute PID *or* reinfection. Due to chronic inflammatory reaction, women develop pelvic adhesions, tubo-ovarian masses *or* hydrosalpinx (Fig. 13.4).

Clinical features

Symptoms

The symptoms of chronic PID are listed in Box 13.20.

- Occur following
  - Minor procedures
  - Major surgeries
    - Vaginal
    - Abdominal
- Clinical features
  - Fever
  - Abdominal/pelvic pain
  - Malodorous vaginal discharge
  - Tenesmus
  - Abdominal tenderness
  - Pelvic mass
- Treatment
  - Mild cases
    - Oral antibiotics
  - Severe infection
    - Parenteral antibiotics
  - Pelvic abscess
    - Ultrasound-guided aspiration
    - Drainage
      - Colpotomy
      - Laparotomy

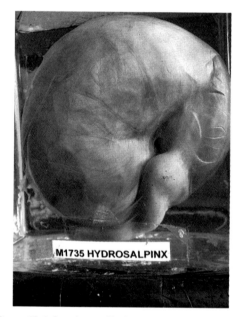

Figure 13.4 Specimen of hydrosalpinx.

Signs

Physical examination may reveal tenderness or mass in the pelvis (Box 13.21). Vaginal or cervical discharge may not be present in chronic PID.

Box 13.20 Symptoms of chronic PID

- History of previous infection
- Lower abdominal pain
- Deep dyspareunia
- Congestive dysmenorrhoea
- Menstrual abnormalities
  - Heavy menstrual bleeding
  - Frequent menstruation
- Low backache
- Chronic pelvic pain
- Infertility

PID, pelvic inflammatory disease.

Box 13.21 Signs of chronic PID

- Abdominal examination
  - Tenderness
  - Mass arising from pelvis
- Per speculum examination
  - Vaginal/cervical discharge may be present
- Pelvic examination
  - Fixed, retroverted, tender uterus
  - Adnexal tenderness
  - Pelvic mass
    - Hydrosalpinx
    - Tubo-ovarian mass
  - Frozen pelvis

PID, pelvic inflammatory disease.

Differential diagnosis

Clinically, chronic PID can be misdiagnosed as endometriosis or other conditions causing chronic pelvic pain (Box 13.22).

Box 13.22 Differential diagnosis of chronic PID

- Endometriosis
- Chronic ectopic pregnancy

PID, pelvic inflammatory disease.

Investigations

Ultrasonography may reveal a hydrosalpinx (Fig. 13.5) *or* tubo-ovarian mass. Ovarian endometrioma can also be identified. Laparoscopy is often required when women present with chronic pelvic pain, dysmenorrhoea and/or dyspareunia to establish the diagnosis and rule out endometriosis (Fig. 13.6a and b).

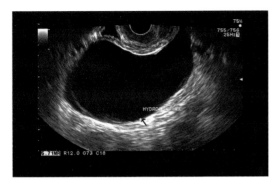

Figure 13.5 Ultrasonogram showing hydrosalpinx.

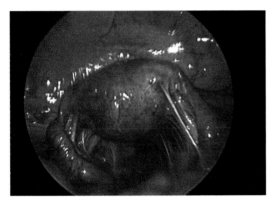

a.

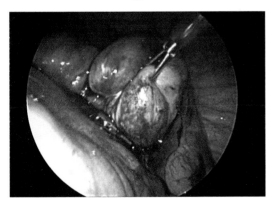

b.

Figure 13.6 Laparoscopy showing (a) pelvic adhesions and (b) tubo-ovarian mass.

Management

If symptoms are mild and there are no large pelvic masses, reassurance and analgesics may be all that is required.

Treatment of women with severe symptoms or pelvic masses is mainly surgical (Box 13.23). The damaged tube and ovary may have to be removed in most situations. Occasionally, in case of frozen pelvis *or* badly damaged adnexa, hysterectomy and bilateral salpingo-oophorectomy (Fig. 13.7) will have to be performed.

Box 13.23 Management of chronic PID

- Laparoscopy
  - Adhesiolysis
  - Salpingo-oophorectomy
- Laparotomy
  - Adhesiolysis
  - Salpingo-oophorectomy
  - Hysterectomy with bilateral salpingo-oophorectomy

PID, pelvic inflammatory disease.

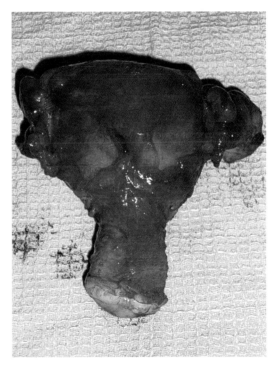

Figure 13.7 Bilateral tubo-ovarian masses.

Key points

- Infections of the upper genital tract include infections of the uterus, tubes, ovaries, broad ligaments and pelvic peritoneum. When the infection is not associated with pregnancy or pelvic surgery, it is also known as pelvic inflammatory disease (PID).

- PID is caused by aerobic and/or anaerobic organisms. The most important aerobic organisms are *Neisseria gonorrhoeae* and *Chlamydia trachomatis*. Other organisms such as *Gardnerella vaginalis*, streptococci, staphylococci, *Escherichia coli* and *Mycoplasma* may also be involved. Anaerobic organisms are *Bacteroides*, *Peptostreptococcus* and *Clostridia*. The infection ascends from the cervix, colonizes the tubes and causes chronic inflammation, fibrosis and scarring.

- PID may be acute or chronic. In acute PID, the tube distends with pus, the fimbrial end closes and a pyosalpinx is formed. Spread of infection causes pelvic/general peritonitis. Chronic PID presents with hydrosalpinx, tubo-ovarian mass or frozen pelvis.

- Risk factors for PID are multiple sexual partners, poor socioeconomic status, young age, past history of sexually transmitted infections, smoking and substance abuse.

- Complications of PID include peritonitis, septicaemia, intra-abdominal abscesses and septic

thrombophlebitis. Sequelae are ectopic pregnancies, infertility and chronic pelvic pain.

- Acute PID presents with high fever, lower abdominal pain and symptoms of sepsis. Vaginal discharge, abdominal tenderness, adnexal mass/tenderness and pelvic abscesses may be present.
  - Triad of lower abdominal pain, adnexal tenderness and cervical motion tenderness is considered to be the most important clinical feature.
  - Treatment is according to the guidelines by the Centers for Disease Control and Prevention. Partners should be treated.
  - Surgical intervention is required when there is pelvic abscess, subdiaphragmatic collection or multiple intra-abdominal abscess.

- Chronic PID presents as lower abdominal pain, deep dyspareunia, congestive dysmenorrhoea, menstrual abnormalities, chronic pelvic pain or infertility. Physical examination reveals adnexal tenderness, mass or frozen pelvis.

- Management is by laparoscopic surgery or laparotomy. Adhesiolysis or salpingo-oophorectomy may be required. Rarely, hysterectomy may be indicated.

Self-assessment

Case-based questions

Case 1

A 27-year-old nulliparous lady presents with fever, lower abdominal pain, vomiting and discharge per vaginum. She also complains of vaginal bleeding for 1 day. Her last menstrual period was 30 days earlier, and she was not on any contraception.

1. What do you want to look for on clinical examination to help you make a diagnosis?
2. What conditions would you think of?
3. What investigations would you order?
4. If the diagnosis is acute PID, how will you manage?

Case 2

A 34-year-old lady, mother of two children, presents with lower abdominal pain of 5-day duration. She has chronic backache and dyspareunia. The patient gives a history of similar abdominal pain in the past. Her menstrual cycles are 3–5 days every 18–20 days.

1. What conditions will you consider in the differential diagnosis?
2. What will you look for on examination?
3. What investigation will you order?
4. If the woman has chronic PID, how will you manage?

Answers

Case 1

1. (a) Temperature, pulse, pallor, blood pressure—To look for septicaemia
   (b) Abdominal tenderness, mass, rebound tenderness, shifting dullness, rigidity—For acute PID, ectopic pregnancy peritonitis; per speculum examination—For mucopurulent discharge from endocervix, vaginal discharge, bleeding; pelvic examination—For adnexal tenderness, unilateral/bilateral tenderness, pain on movement of cervix, adnexal mass, fullness in the pouch of Douglas, uterine size, mobility

2. (a) Acute PID
   (b) Ectopic pregnancy

3. (a) Complete blood count, Hb
   (b) Gram stain of cervical discharge for gonococci
   (c) Sample for NAAT, if available
   (d) Vaginal discharge for whiff test and clue cells
   (e) Serum β-hCG
   (f) Transvaginal ultrasonography if in doubt or hCG equivocal

4. (a) If the temperature is high, the patient looks toxic or has peritonitis, admit and start on IV antibiotics.

(b) If the fever is mild and patient is otherwise well, start on outpatient regimen of antibiotics; review after 48 hours.

(c) Trace sexual partner and treat.

(d) Counsel regarding the use of condom/OC pills.

Case 2

1. Chronic PID, endometriosis.

2. (a) Abdominal tenderness, mass arising from pelvis

(b) Pelvic examination—For fixed, retroverted uterus, adnexal mass/tenderness, frozen pelvis

(c) Per rectal examination—For induration of uterosacral ligaments

3. Transvaginal ultrasonogram, MRI/CT if required.

4. (a) NSAIDs for analgesia

(b) Antibiotics for outpatient treatment

(c) Review after 3–4 weeks. If still symptomatic, do laparoscopy, release of adhesions. Unilateral salpingo-oophorectomy, if required

Long-answer question

1. Discuss aetiopathogenesis, diagnosis and management of acute pelvic inflammatory disease.

Short-answer questions

1. Definition and management of chronic pelvic inflammatory disease
2. Differential diagnosis of acute pelvic inflammatory disease
3. Aetiology of pelvic inflammatory disease
4. Pelvic abscess
5. Organisms that cause pelvic inflammatory disease
6. Hydrosalpinx
7. CDC guidelines for management of acute pelvic infection

14 | Tuberculosis of the Female Genital Tract

Case scenario

Miss KU, 16, was from Bihar. She was attending the village school until a year ago but discontinued since she was feeling tired and lethargic. She had lost 9 kg of weight; her periods had become scanty and stopped 6 months ago. She also had low-grade fever. She was so weak that she could hardly walk and was brought in a wheelchair to the clinic.

Introduction

Tuberculosis (TB) of the genital tract is a common cause of tubal infertility and menstrual abnormalities in the developing world. The incidence has decreased with the use of effective diagnostic and therapeutic methods and neonatal immunization. But recently, with increase in HIV infections, there is a resurgence of TB in some populations. Early diagnosis, detection of smear-negative cases and diagnosis and management of multidrug-resistant TB are the current global priorities.

Incidence

The prevalence of genital TB is about 5–10% in infertile women worldwide and about 18% in India. In general gynaecological population, the prevalence is 1–2% according to various studies. The estimated number of cases of genital TB globally is 8–10 million. But the reported incidence varies depending on the sensitivity of the tests used for diagnosis.

Aetiology and pathogenesis

Genital TB is caused by *Mycobacterium tuberculosis* or *Mycobacterium bovis*. It is almost always secondary. The disease spreads from lungs through bloodstream or adjacent organs by contiguity (Table 14.1). The primary lesion is often inactive and heals when genital lesions manifest. Infection by *M. bovis* is almost always from the gastrointestinal tract. Rarely, primary lesion in the vulva or cervix has been described and is thought to be sexually transmitted.

Table 14.1 Mode of spread of genital TB

Route of spread	Site of infection
Lymphatic	Pulmonary
Haematogenous	Miliary
Direct	Abdominal

TB, tuberculosis.

The **fallopian tubes** are affected in most women. Infection spreads to the endometrium and ovaries from the tubes (Box 14.1).

Box 14.1 Involvement of genital tract

- Tubes: 75–100%
- Endometrium: 30–80%
- Ovaries: 9–11%

Pathology

Macroscopic appearance

Fallopian tube

The fallopian tubes are involved in almost all cases of genital TB. Tubal pathology has been classified into exosalpingitis, endosalpingitis and interstitial salpingitis given in Box 14.2. Direct spread from the adjacent organs causes exosalpingitis, but haematogenous spread usually affects the mucosa or muscularis causing endosalpingitis or interstitial salpingitis. Tuberculous salpingitis grossly resembles pelvic inflammatory disease (PID; Fig. 14.1). In the

Box 14.2 Tubal pathology in genital TB

- Endosalpingitis
  - Involves predominantly mucosa and muscle layer
  - Oedematous, thickened tubes
  - Granulomatous lesions/caseation in the tubal wall
  - Pyosalpinx
  - May have peritubal adhesions
- Exosalpingitis
  - Involves predominantly serosa
  - Tubercles on the tubal surface
  - Dense peritubal adhesions
- Interstitial salpingitis
  - Involves predominantly the tubal wall
  - Thickened tubes
  - May form peritubal adhesions

TB, tuberculosis.

early stages of infection, the tubes are inflamed and congested, but later become thick and rigid. With progressive tubal damage, the tubes become hard, beaded and calcified. Tubercles are usually seen on the peritoneal surface of the tubes and mesosalpinx. Adhesions develop between the tubes and the ovaries, leading to the formation of tubo-ovarian masses. Presence of tubercles and caseation may clinch the diagnosis, but often microscopic examination is required.

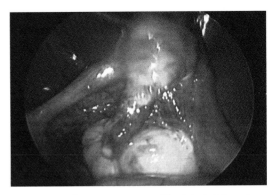

Figure 14.1 Gross appearance of the tube in tuberculous salpingitis. The tube is oedematous and tubercles can be seen on the surface. There are peritubal adhesions.

Endometrium

The endometrium is infected in 30–80% of cases and may be studded with tubercles. Since the endometrium is shed every month, the infection does not spread to the myometrium or progress rapidly. Destruction of endometrial lining and ulceration can lead to intrauterine adhesions similar to Asherman syndrome and result in secondary amenorrhoea.

Cervix, vagina and vulva

Lesions in the lower genital tract may be primary or secondary. The lesions may be ulcerative or proliferative in growth and mimic cervical cancer, and a biopsy is required to confirm the diagnosis. Tuberculous lesions of vulva and vagina are rare. They are usually ulcers and must be distinguished from malignant lesions by biopsy.

Ovary

The tunica albuginea prevents extension of infection to ovarian stroma. The infection is, therefore, limited to the surface and appears as tubercles. Caseating foci in the stroma can occasionally be seen as a result of haematogenous spread.

Tuberculous peritonitis

Genital TB is often associated with peritonitis. This may be wet or dry (Box 14.3).

Box 14.3 Tuberculous peritonitis

- Wet
  - Straw-coloured ascitic fluid
  - Tubercles on the surface of viscera
  - Minimal adhesions
  - Can be mistaken for ovarian cancer
  - Histology typical of TB
- Dry
  - No ascites
  - Dense adhesions
  - Pyosalpinx/tubo-ovarian mass
  - Mimics chronic PID

PID, pelvic inflammatory disease; *TB*, tuberculosis.

Microscopic appearance

Microscopically, the lesions reveal granulomatous inflammation, Langhans giant cells, epithelioid cells and caseation-like tuberculous lesions elsewhere in the body (Fig. 14.2). Acid-fast bacilli (AFB) may be found on histopathology sections.

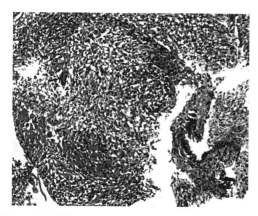

Figure 14.2 Microscopic appearance of tuberculous endometritis showing epithelioid histiocytic granuloma with Langhans giant cells (arrow).

Clinical features

Symptoms

Genital TB usually occurs between the age of 20 and 40 years. The common symptoms are **malaise**, **low-grade fever**, **pelvic pain** and **menstrual abnormality** (Box 14.4). Some women may be asymptomatic and the disease may be diagnosed during investigation of infertility. **Amenorrhoea** occurs due to intrauterine adhesions, destruction of the endometrium or general ill health and weight loss associated with extensive TB. **Ascites** causes abdominal distension. **Infertility** is common in women with active and treated infection. This is mainly due to tubal damage, block, peritubal adhesions and endometrial changes. Adhesions give rise to **chronic pelvic pain**, and local lesions on the cervix and vagina may cause **blood stained discharge**.

Box 14.4 Symptoms of genital tuberculosis

- Constitutional
  - Low-grade fever
  - Malaise
- Menstrual
  - Heavy menstrual bleeding
  - Amenorrhoea
  - Oligomenorrhoea
- Infertility
- Pelvic pain
- Abdominal distension
- Abdominal mass
- Blood stained vaginal discharge

Signs

General signs of TB such as weight loss and fever may be present. Lymphadenopathy involving cervical or iliac nodes may be palpable. If there is gross ascites, it is clinically obvious, but small amount of fluid is visible only on imaging. The typical 'doughy' abdomen indicates associated abdominal TB. Hydrosalpinx or tubo-ovarian mass may be palpable on abdominal/pelvic examination. Advanced stages with pelvic adhesions may result in 'frozen pelvis'.

Clinical evaluation

History

In developing countries, TB is still commonly encountered. Whenever a patient presents with low-grade and persistent fever, weight loss and malaise TB should be suspected. Detailed history is important to ascertain the presence of other symptoms such as menstrual disturbances, secondary amenorrhoea, infertility, abdominal distension and pelvic pain.

Physical examination

The clinical signs are similar to chronic PID. A systematic and thorough examination is necessary to arrive at the diagnosis (Box 14.5).

Box 14.5 Physical examination in genital tuberculosis

- General examination
  - Fever
  - Loss of weight
- Abdominal examination
  - Ascites, doughy abdomen
  - Mass-encysted ascites
- Per speculum examination
  - Ulcer on vulva/vagina/cervix
- Pelvic examination
  - Fixed uterus
  - Adnexal mass
  - Frozen pelvis

Investigations

Since the incidence of TB is on the decrease, a high index of suspicion is necessary for early diagnosis. In a young girl who is not sexually active, presence of tubo-ovarian mass or pyosalpinx should arouse suspicion of TB. In older women with ascites, ovarian cancer must be ruled out. Tubo-ovarian mass, pyosalpinx and frozen pelvis are seen in chronic PID due to other organisms as well.

Endometrial biopsy should be performed in the premenstrual phase; samples should be taken from cornual region. With onset of menstruation, the endometrium is shed and the diagnosis may be missed. Tissue should be sent in formalin for histological examination and in saline for culture (Box 14.6).

Box 14.6 Endometrial biopsy

- Histology
- Fluorescent antibody technique
- Culture
- PCR
- NAAT
- Xpert MTB/RIF assay

NAAT, nucleic acid amplification test; *PCR*, polymerase chain reaction; *MTB*, *Mycobacterium tuberculosis*; *RIF*, rifampicin.

- Confirmation of diagnosis by histology, culture or nucleic acid amplification test (NAAT) can be difficult in some cases.
- Polymerase chain reaction (PCR) has been found to be useful in rapid and improved diagnosis of TB.
- Xpert *M. tuberculosis/rifampicin* (MTB/RIF) assay is a rapid molecular assay that permits rapid diagnosis through detection of *M. tuberculosis* DNA and simultaneous identification of rifampicin drug resistance. This has been recommended for diagnosis of pulmonary and extrapulmonary TB by the WHO. This test may replace the conventional culture and histopathology in future.

Ultrasonography may be helpful in identifying the pelvic mass (Fig. 14.3) and tubal dilatation or pyosalpinx. **Chest X-ray** may show coexistent pulmonary TB, and if suspicious lesions are found, sputum should be checked at least thrice for AFB.

Hysterosalpingogram should be avoided if TB is suspected. But if it is performed during evaluation of infertility, the typical appearance, as listed in Box 14.7, is highly suggestive (Fig. 14.4).

Box 14.7 Hysterosalpingography in genital tuberculosis

- Calcification in adnexa
- Tubal block at the isthmus
- Multiple constrictions (beaded appearance)
- Rigid tube
- Extravasation of contrast

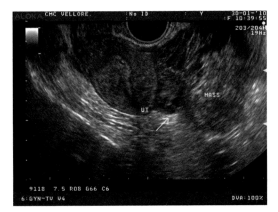

Figure 14.3 Ultrasonography in a woman with suspected pelvic TB. A complex tubo-ovarian (arrow) mass is seen adjacent to the uterus. *TB*, tuberculosis.

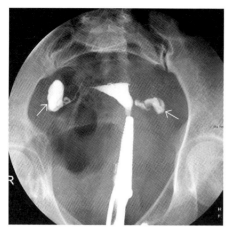

Figure 14.4 Hysterosalpingogram in a woman with infertility and past history of TB. Tubes show terminal dilatation (arrows), and there is no spill of contrast indicating bilateral tubal block. *TB*, tuberculosis.

Laparoscopy is required when diagnosis cannot be established and the index of suspicion is high (Box 14.8; Fig. 14.5). It may also be performed as part of evaluation of infertility. When suspicious lesions are found, peritoneal biopsies are taken for histopathology and AFB culture.

Management

Treatment of genital TB is with medications; surgery is indicated in very few cases.

- **Multiple drug therapy** is the mainstay of treatment. Short-term treatment for 6–9 months is effective for genital TB.

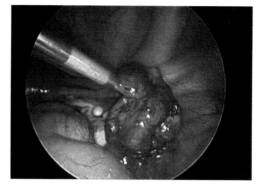

Figure 14.5 Laparoscopy in a woman with infertility revealing tubo-ovarian mass due to TB. The tubes are thickened, bunched up and dilated. There are peritubal adhesions. *TB*, tuberculosis.

Box 14.8 Laparoscopy in genital tuberculosis

- Tubercles on visceral surface and peritoneum
- Pyosalpinx
- Tubo-ovarian mass
- Caseation
- Peritoneal biopsy

- Directly observed treatment short course (DOTS) is not necessary in the developed countries and for women in higher socioeconomic class in developing countries since compliance and adherence to treatment is good. For patients from the lower socioeconomic strata in developing countries, DOTS is recommended.
- The Revised National Tuberculosis Control Program recommendations (2013) for treatment of TB are given in Table 14.2.

Table 14.2 WHO guidelines for treatment of TB (DOTS)

Category of patients	Type of patient	Regimen	
		Intensive phase	Continuation phase
I	• Sputum smear positive • Sputum smear negative • Extrapulmonary (includes genital and others)	$2H_3R_3Z_3E_3$	$4H_3R_3(E_3)$
II	• Smear-positive relapse • Smear-positive failure • Smear-positive treatment after default • Others	$2H_3R_3Z_3E_3S_3/1H_3R_3Z_3E_3$	$5H_3R_3E_3$

DOTS, directly observed treatment short course; *E*, ethambutol (1200 mg); *H*, isoniazid (600 mg); *R*, rifampicin (450 mg); *S*, streptomycin (750 mg); *TB*, tuberculosis; *Z*, pyrazinamide (1500 mg).

- **For patients with newly diagnosed TB in India, where level of isoniazid resistance is high, ethambutol should be added in the continuation phase of 4 months.**
- Since multiple drugs are used, it is important to watch for side effects.
- Isoniazid should be taken after breakfast.
- Liver function tests should be performed before starting rifampicin and should be repeated if the patient has vomiting and right upper quadrant pain. Liver enzymes are elevated more than twice the normal level; rifampicin, pyrazinamide and isoniazid (INAH) should be withdrawn till enzymes normalize and then reintroduced one after the other (rifampicin first, INAH second) so as to identify and avoid the offending drug.
- Rifampicin, a hepatic enzyme inducer, interacts with several drugs, so care must be taken while prescribing other medications. Oral contraceptives must be avoided.
- If ethambutol is added, the patient should be counselled about potential visual complications and should be advised to seek help early if new visual symptoms arise.

Monitoring response to treatment

This is mandatory so that decision regarding changeover to second-line therapy and surgical intervention can be made at the appropriate time (Box 14.9). Clinical response should be assessed monthly and endometrial biopsy should be performed every 3 months. The anti-TB drug regimen may have to be modified depending on the sensitivity report at the initial follow-up visit.

Clinical follow-up should continue even after treatment is completed since late recurrences

---

Box 14.9 Monitoring response to therapy in genital tuberculosis

- Assess constitutional symptoms
- Size of the pelvic mass and ascites
  - Clinical
  - Ultrasonogram
- ESR
- Endometrial biopsy

ESR, erythrocyte sedimentation rate.

---

and resistance are known. If there is no response to therapy, changeover to second-line drugs is indicated.

Surgical intervention

The indications for surgical intervention are listed in Box 14.10.

Box 14.10 Indications for surgical intervention in genital tuberculosis

- Persistent symptoms
  - Fever
  - Pain
  - Ascites
- Persistent pelvic mass
- Progression of disease
- Presence of fistulae
- When the diagnosis is in doubt

Type of surgery depends on the extent of disease found at laparotomy. In young women, ovarian conservation should be attempted and unilateral adnexectomy may be performed if the disease is confined to one ovary. Often hysterectomy and bilateral salpingo-oophorectomy are required. Dense adhesions increase the risk of bowel and bladder injury.

Key points

- Tuberculosis (TB) of the female genital tract is a common cause of tubal infertility and menstrual abnormality in the developing world. Incidence is variable; it is about 5–10% in infertile women.
- Genital TB is always almost secondary, caused by *Mycobacterium tuberculosis*. *Mycobacterium bovis* is the organism when the primary lesion is in the gastrointestinal tract.
- The fallopian tubes are involved in 75–100% of the cases. Endometrium is involved in 30–80% of the cases and the ovaries in 9–11%.

- Tubal pathology may be in the form of endosalpingitis, exosalpingitis or interstitial salpingitis.
- Since the endometrium is shed every month, the infection does not spread to the myometrium or progress further.
- Tuberculous peritonitis may be wet or dry.
- Women with genital TB may be asymptomatic or present with low-grade fever, pelvic pain, menstrual irregularity, infertility or secondary amenorrhoea.

Key points *(Continued)*

- Physical examination may reveal ascites, mass in the abdomen, fixed uterus or a frozen pelvis.
- Endometrial biopsy, performed in the premenstrual phase, may reveal tubercle bacilli. Histopathological examination reveals granulomatous lesion with epithelioid cells and Langhans giant cells.
- Ultrasonography may reveal pelvic mass, hydrosalpinx or pyosalpinx. Laparoscopy may be required when diagnosis cannot be established and the index of suspicion is high.
- Management is by antituberculous therapy using combination of drugs as recommended by the World Health Organization.

Self-assessment

Case-based questions

Case 1

An 18-year-old student presented with low-grade fever, weight loss, weakness and amenorrhoea of 6 months' duration. Examination revealed BMI of 19, moderate ascites and left-sided pelvic mass of 5 × 6 cm size.

1. What conditions will you consider?
2. What investigations will you order?
3. If diagnosis cannot be arrived at by investigations, how will you proceed?
4. What is the management if it is tuberculosis?

Case 2

A 48-year-old multipara presented with progressive abdominal distension of 6 months' duration. She also complained of loss of weight, loss of appetite and vague abdominal discomfort. Her menstrual cycles were infrequent and scanty. On examination, BMI was 25; ascites was present but no definite abdominal or pelvic mass.

1. What conditions will you consider?
2. What investigations will you order?
3. How will you confirm your diagnosis?
4. If the diagnosis is abdominal tuberculosis, what is the treatment?

Answers

Case 1

1. **(a)** Genital tuberculosis with tubo-ovarian mass
   (b) Ovarian malignancy
2. Ultrasound scan, ESR, complete blood count, ascitic fluid examination for lymphocytes and malignant cells, endometrial biopsy, tumour markers (CA 125 may be elevated in both conditions).

3. Laparoscopy/laparotomy and peritoneal biopsy.
4. **(a)** Isoniazid, rifampicin and pyrazinamide for 2 months followed by rifampicin and isoniazid for 4 months
   (b) Response monitored by clinical assessment, ultrasonogram and ESR

Case 2

1. **(a)** Ovarian cancer
   (b) Gastrointestinal cancer
   (c) Abdominal TB
2. **(a)** Ultrasonography (abdominal and transvaginal) for pelvic mass, nature of the mass
   (b) Doppler studies for resistance index, ESR, CA 125, carcinoembryonic antigen (CEA)
   (c) CT scan if required
3. **(a)** Ascitic tap
   (b) Cytological examination of fluid for white cells, lymphocytes and malignant cells
4. **(a)** Antituberculous therapy with isoniazid, rifampicin and pyrazinamide for 2 months followed by isoniazid and rifampicin for 4 months
   (b) Response monitored by clinical assessment, ESR and ultrasonography

Long-answer question

1. How do you diagnose endometrial tuberculosis? Discuss the treatment of endometrial tuberculosis in a 28-year-old patient.

Short-answer questions

1. Tuberculous salpingitis
2. Medical treatment of female genital tuberculosis

15 | Endometriosis

Case scenario

Mrs GK, 30, came to the clinic, looking depressed and tense. She was a mother of a 5-year-old child and wanted another one desperately. Mrs GK had developed congestive dysmenorrhoea and deep dyspareunia during the past 2 years, and this had become a constant dull ache in the pelvis for the past 1 year. She consulted a local specialist, underwent a laparoscopy and was told that she had extensive endometriosis and her tubes were severely damaged. She had come for opinion regarding further management.

Introduction

Endometriosis is a common, benign condition that affects adolescent girls and women in the reproductive age group. It can be associated with mild or severe, debilitating symptoms. The pathogenesis of this disorder is not clearly understood and optimal treatment is controversial.

Definition

Endometriosis is defined as the presence of endometrial glands and stroma outside the uterus. It is a benign condition but has several similarities to malignancy such as disease progression, local invasion and widespread dissemination. Endometriosis is different from adenomyosis where the endometrial tissue is seen in the myometrium.

Prevalence

Prevalence varies with the category of women studied and methods used for diagnosis. Overall, endometriosis occurs in about 8–10% of the population. It is seen in 12–30% of women with chronic pelvic pain and almost 50% of women with infertility.

Risk factors

Factors that are associated with an increased risk of endometriosis are given in Box 15.1.

- Menstrual cycle
  - Early menarche
  - Heavy menstrual bleeding
  - Short menstrual cycles
- Delayed childbearing
  - Voluntary/involuntary
- Nulliparity/low parity
- Higher social class
- History of endometriosis in first-degree relatives
- Lower body mass index
- Obstructive Müllerian anomalies
- Exposure to dioxins

Multiparity, prolonged lactation, high body mass index and diet rich in vegetables and fruits are protective against endometriosis.

Pathogenesis

There are several theories regarding the development of endometriosis (Box 15.2).

Box 15.2 Theories of development of endometriosis

- Implantation theory
- Coelomic metaplasia theory
- Induction theory
- Venous and lymphatic dissemination
- Immunological theory
- Genetic factors
- Molecular defects

Implantation theory

Originally proposed by Sampson, this theory postulates that endometrial fragments transported through the tubes into the peritoneal cavity by retrograde menstruation are responsible for the development of endometriosis. In support of this theory are the observations shown in Box 15.3.

Retrograde menstruation occurs in 80–90% of women and is physiological. There must be additional factors that induce the growth of these endometrial cells in the ectopic location in some women but not in others. In these susceptible women, the regurgitated endometrium develops into endometriosis on the peritoneum, ovary or deep within the cul-de-sac.

Box 15.3 Observations in support of Sampson's implantation theory

Endometriosis is common in
- Women with obstructive Müllerian anomalies
- Women with short and heavy menstrual cycles
- Dependent portions of the pelvis
  - Ovary
  - Cul-de-sac
  - Uterosacral ligaments
  - Rectovaginal septum
  - Posterior surface of the uterus

Coelomic metaplasia theory

Meyer has postulated that the cells of the original coelomic membrane undergo metaplasia into endometrial tissue. The serosal layer of all intra-abdominal organs arises from the coelomic epithelium, which is considered multipotent. What causes this metaplasia is not known.

Induction theory

This theory proposes that degenerating menstrual endometrium releases endogenous factors that induces metaplasia of the coelomic epithelium. This is an extension of the coelomic metaplasia theory.

Venous and lymphatic dissemination

Vascular and lymphatic dissemination of endometrial cells can potentially explain the occurrence of endometriosis in the cervix, vagina and vulva, gastrointestinal tract, lungs, pleural cavity, surgical scars and lymph nodes.

Immunological theory

Decreased cellular immunity to endometriotic tissue has been demonstrated in women with endometriosis. This results in reduced clearance of shed endometrial cells from the peritoneal cavity. The immunological changes may also cause an alteration in the function of macrophages that secrete cytokines and growth factors that enhance the implantation of endometrial cells and development of endometriosis.

Genetic factors and molecular defects

Genetic factors A familial predisposition to endometriosis has been documented. There is a sevenfold increase in the incidence in relatives of women who have the disease. One of 10 women with endometriosis will have a sister or mother with the disease. The disease also tends to be severe and occurs at an earlier age in women with a history of disease in a first-degree relative. The inheritance is polygenic.

Molecular defects Biologically important molecular abnormalities such as activation of oncogenic pathways and biosynthetic cascades causing increased production of cytokines, growth factors, oestrogens and prostaglandins have been identified. They contribute to the development of endometriosis.

Possible pathogenic mechanism

Research has now revealed that several biologically active substances are produced in the ectopic endometrial tissue that are responsible for the various stages in the development of endometriosis from implanted endometrium (Box 15.4).

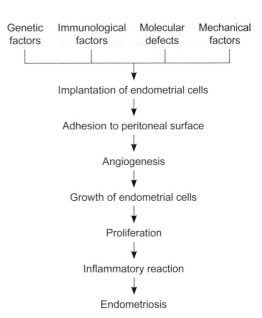

Figure 15.1 Mechanism of pathogenesis of endometriosis.

Box 15.4 Biologically active substances produced in ectopic endometrium

- Cytokines — Adhesion to peritoneal surface
- MMP — Invasion
- VEGF-A — Angiogenesis
- Growth factors — Growth
- Oestrogen — Proliferative change
- Prostaglandin — Inflammation

MMP, matrix metalloproteinase; *VEGF-A*, vascular endothelial growth factor-A.

The production of these substances could be genetically determined. Immunological and genetic factors also determine the survival of regurgitated endometrial cells, their adhesion to peritoneum and growth.

The pathogenesis of endometriosis currently proposed is shown in Fig. 15.1.

Pathology

Classification and macroscopic appearance of pelvic endometriosis

Endometriosis is classified into three types (Box 15.5).

Superficial endometriosis of pelvic endometriosis

This is otherwise called **peritoneal endometriosis**. These lesions are usually seen in the

---

Box 15.5 Classification of pelvic endometriosis

- Superficial or peritoneal endometriosis
- Ovarian endometriosis
- Deep infiltrating endometriosis

---

dependent portion of the pelvis. The most common sites are surface of ovaries, usually involving both sides. Pelvic peritoneum over the anterior and posterior surfaces of the uterus, pouch of Douglas, uterosacral ligaments and broad ligaments are the other common sites. Endometriotic deposits may be seen on cervix, vagina and, rarely, vulva. Pelvic nodes are involved in 30% of women.

Gross appearance of superficial endometriosis varies depending on whether the lesions are early and recent or old and long-standing (Box 15.6; Fig. 15.2). Early lesions are pink, red or haemorrhagic and become brown or black with time. Eventually the discolouration disappears and the lesions appear white.

Superficial endometriosis cannot be palpated on clinical examination. It is difficult to visualize on imaging, and diagnosis is by laparoscopy.

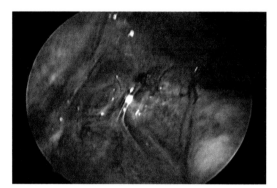

Figure 15.2 Superficial or peritoneal endometriosis. Old, long-standing disease appears dark brown.

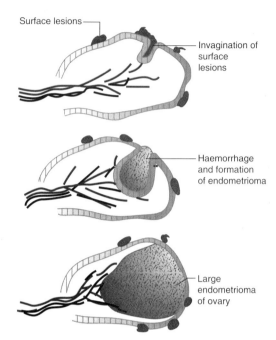

Figure 15.3 Diagrammatic representation of formation of ovarian endometrioma. Superficial lesions on the ovarian surface invaginate and form cysts, which eventually enlarge and are filled with old blood.

Ovarian endometriosis

Endometriosis of the ovary may be of two types:

- Superficial implants that occur as part of peritoneal endometriosis
- Deep ovarian endometriosis or endometrioma

Endometrioma occurs by inversion and invagination of the ovarian cortex with superficial endometriotic deposits (Fig. 15.3).

Grossly, endometriomas are located on the antimesenteric surface of the ovary and cause adhesion of the ovary to the posterior peritoneum. Cyst wall is white or yellow and the cyst is filled with thick, chocolate-coloured fluid (Fig. 15.4a and b); hence, such cysts are known as 'chocolate cysts'. Most women with ovarian endometriosis have associated deep infiltrating endometriosis.

Ovarian endometriomas, when large, can be detected on pelvic examination. They have thick, fibrotic cyst walls with adhesions to surrounding structures. In 30% of cases, both ovaries are involved. Ovarian endometrioma is usually associated with more extensive pelvic endometriosis. Typical features at laparotomy/laparoscopy are listed in Box 15.7 and shown in Fig. 15.5.

Deep infiltrating endometriosis

This is also known as posterior pelvic endometriosis. By definition, the lesions extend >5 mm

beneath the peritoneum. They are usually located in the rectovaginal space but may involve uterosacral ligaments, cervix, bowel or ureters. The lesions cause inflammatory reaction and adhesion formation and can mimic malignancy (Fig. 15.6a and b).

The lesions can be felt on pelvic and per rectal examination as tender induration and nodularity. They can be visualized on imaging, but the extent or depth cannot be assessed at laparoscopy.

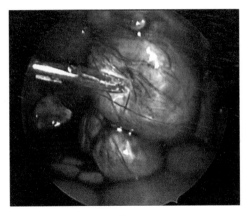

a.

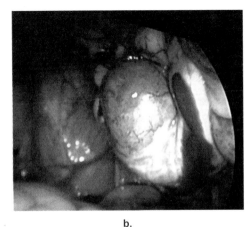

b.

Figure 15.4 Ovarian endometrioma. **a.** Large ovarian endometrioma with white cyst wall. **b.** Chocolate-coloured fluid is seen flowing from inside the cyst.

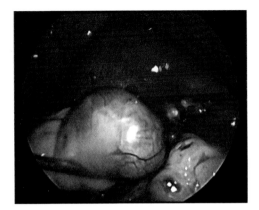

Figure 15.5 Bilateral ovarian endometrioma. Uterus is seen with adhesions on the posterior surface between the uterus, right tube and right ovary.

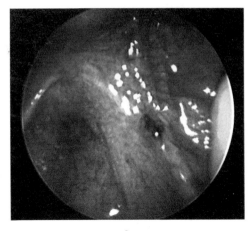

a.

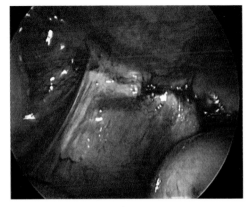

b.

Figure 15.6 Deep infiltrating endometriosis. **a.** Endometriotic deposits on the right uterosacral ligament. **b.** Endometriotic deposits in the pouch of Douglas obscuring the uterosacral ligaments and forming adhesions.

Extrapelvic endometriosis

Endometriotic implants on the ovaries, tubes, uterine surfaces, pelvic side walls and pelvic peritoneum are referred to as **pelvic endometriosis**. **Extrapelvic endometriosis** includes lesions elsewhere in the peritoneal cavity, other body cavities or surgical scars (Fig. 15.7). It can occur in any organ system but is not frequently encountered. Overall, less than 12% of all cases of endometriosis are extrapelvic. The common sites are listed in Box 15.8.

Microscopic appearance

Microscopically, endometriotic lesions consist of **endometrial glands** and **stroma**.

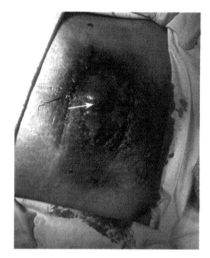

Figure 15.7 Endometriosis of the abdominal scar following caesarean section. The lesion appears as a bluish black (arrow) nodule on the scar. The area has been painted with Betadine.

Box 15.8 Common sites of extrapelvic endometriosis

- Urinary tract
  - Bladder
  - Ureters
- Gastrointestinal tract
  - Sigmoid colon
  - Rectum
  - Ileocaecal area
  - Appendix
  - Small bowel
- Surgical scars
  - Caesarean section
  - Episiotomy
- Pulmonary and thoracic
  - Lungs
  - Pleura

Hemosiderin-laden macrophages are often seen. Glands may reveal secretory or proliferative activity. Deep infiltrating lesions are surrounded by fibrous and smooth muscle tissue. In women with endometriosis of long duration, the typical endometrial glands and stroma may not be present in the cyst wall. Positive histology confirms the diagnosis, but negative histology does not exclude it.

Risk of malignancy in endometriosis

Rarely, ovarian clear cell carcinoma and endometrioid carcinoma can develop in endometriosis.

Therefore, endometriosis in the perimenopausal and postmenopausal age should be excised completely when surgery is undertaken. Since malignant transformation seems to be oestrogen dependent, oestrogen replacement therapy should be administered under supervision in postmenopausal women with known endometriosis. Endometriosis-associated ovarian cancer has a better prognosis.

Clinical features

Endometriosis is most commonly seen in the reproductive age group. It is rare before menarche and regresses after menopause. It can also occur in young girls and occasionally in the perimenopausal age as well.

Symptoms

Endometriosis is a chronic disease with several symptoms. The symptoms typically associated with endometriosis are listed in Box 15.9. Endometriosis should be suspected in women with infertility, dysmenorrhoea, dyspareunia and chronic pelvic pain. But the disease can be asymptomatic even when the disease is advanced.

Pain

Pain during menstruation, defaecation, ovulation and sexual intercourse, and chronic pelvic pain are commonly associated with endometriosis.

- Dysmenorrhoea is usually secondary, starts before the onset of bleeding, continues throughout the menstrual period and extends into postmenstrual phase. The pain worsens

Box 15.9 Symptoms of endometriosis

- Pain
  - Severe dysmenorrhoea
  - Chronic pelvic pain
  - Ovulation pain
  - Pain on defaecation
  - Deep dyspareunia
- Menstrual abnormalities
  - Heavy menstrual bleeding
  - Premenstrual spotting
- Cyclic bowel, bladder symptoms
- Infertility
- Chronic fatigue

progressively with duration of the disease, is very severe causing incapacitation and does not respond to simple analgesics.

- Chronic pelvic pain is a distressing symptom, felt as a deep-seated pain in the pelvis, radiates to the back and worsens during menses.
- Dyspareunia is usually described as pain deep in pelvis during sexual intercourse. It is due to direct pressure on the pouch of Douglas or uterosacral ligaments.
- Pain on defaecation and dysuria, bleeding per rectum and urethra may be experienced cyclically when disease involves the bowel or bladder.
- The severity of the pain bears no relationship to the severity of the disease, but endometrioma and deep infiltrating disease are almost always associated with pain.

The causes of pain are as listed in Box 15.10.

Box 15.10 Causes of pain in endometriosis

- Peritoneal inflammation
- Activation of nociceptors
- Nerve irritation with deep infiltration
- Tissue damage
- Local production of prostaglandins
- Adhesion formation
- Collection of blood in endometriotic implants

Menstrual abnormalities

Like heavy menstrual bleeding and premenstrual spotting, menstrual abnormalities are usually due to associated anovulation and abnormal follicular development.

Cyclic bowel, bladder symptoms

In endometriosis involving the bladder, cyclic haematuria can occur. Cyclic bleeding from the rectum is less common.

Infertility

Endometriosis is a common cause of infertility. The prevalence of endometriosis is 30–45% in infertile women. There are several mechanisms by which endometriosis leads to infertility. These are listed in Box 15.11. Infertility can occur with even mild endometriosis, although it is more commonly associated with moderate to severe disease.

Box 15.11 Causes of infertility in endometriosis

- Ovulatory dysfunction
  - Abnormal folliculogenesis
  - Anovulation
  - Luteal phase defect
  - Luteinized unruptured follicle syndrome
- Immunological alterations
  - Decreased sperm survival
  - Altered immunity
- Peritoneal factors
  - Intraperitoneal inflammation
  - Local production of prostaglandins/cytokines
- Interference with implantation
  - Endometrial dysfunction
- Mechanical factors
  - Anatomical distortion of tubes
  - Interference with ovum pick-up
  - Altered tubal motility
  - Peritubal adhesions
- Interference with coital function
  - Dyspareunia
- Sperm inactivation
  - Phagocytosis by macrophages
  - Inactivation by antibodies

Signs

In women with early and minimal endometriosis, symptoms may be present without any signs. When the endometriomas are large, pelvic mass may be palpable abdominally. Typically, the masses are fixed to surrounding structures due to recurrent bleeding and resultant fibrosis. Retroverted and fixed uterus, tender uterosacral ligaments and nodules in the pouch of Douglas are characteristic features of endometriosis.

Clinical evaluation

History

Since endometriosis is a disease of varied symptoms, a detailed history is important. Physical signs may be minimal, but the clinician should suspect endometriosis when the typical symptoms of congestive dysmenorrhea, dyspareunia or chronic pelvic pain are present in a young woman presenting with infertility. Other symptoms should also be asked for.

Physical examination

Physical examination may not reveal any abnormality in women with minimal superficial endometriosis. Larger and advanced lesions can be detected on examination (Box 15.12). Deep infiltrating lesions in the rectovaginal area and uterosacral ligaments are better felt when examination is performed during menstruation. Vaginal lesions may be seen as bluish nodules in the posterior fornix on speculum examination.

Box 15.12 Physical examination in endometriosis

- Abdominal examination
  - Mass arising from the pelvis
  - Located in iliac fossae
  - Tender
  - Not freely mobile
- Per speculum examination
  - Vaginal lesions
- Pelvic examination
  - Fixed retroverted uterus
  - Adnexal mass
    - Tender
    - Fixed
  - Tender uterosacral ligaments
- Per rectal/rectovaginal examination
  - Tenderness in the pouch of Douglas
  - Nodules in the pouch of Douglas

Investigations

Even with typical symptoms and signs, diagnosis of endometriosis cannot be made with certainty.

Imaging

It is of limited value except in ovarian endometrioma as shown in Box 15.13. Ovarian endometrioma >2 cm in size can be diagnosed on transvaginal ultrasonogram and appears as cystic mass with middle-level echoes with or without internal septations on ultrasonography (Fig. 15.8). Magnetic resonance imaging can identify lesions >1 cm and rectovaginal nodules and is useful in the evaluation of extensive endometriosis (Fig. 15.9).

Box 15.13 Investigations in endometriosis

- Ultrasonogram abdominal/transvaginal
  - Not useful in superficial endometriosis
  - Not accurate in deep infiltrating endometriosis
  - Useful in ovarian endometrioma
    - Ovarian mass
      - Cystic mass
      - Low-level internal echoes
      - Hyperechoic foci in the wall
    - Hydroureteronephrosis
- Magnetic resonance imaging
  - Not useful in superficial endometriosis
  - Less accurate in deep infiltrating endometriosis
  - Useful in ovarian endometriomas
    - Endometrioma larger than 1 cm
    - Rectovaginal nodules
- Doppler ultrasound
  - Not very useful
- Barium studies
  - In severe bowel endometriosis
- Intravenous urography
  - Severe endometriosis
  - Suspected ureteric involvement
- CA 125
  - Levels elevated in endometriosis
  - Not useful as diagnostic tool

CA 125

CA 125 is a marker used in epithelial ovarian cancers. Levels are elevated in endometriosis but vary widely. Sensitivity of this test for diagnosis of endometriosis is low. Therefore, it is not a diagnostic tool in endometriosis but may be used to detect recurrence.

Laparoscopy

Visual inspection of the pelvis at laparoscopy is the gold standard for the diagnosis of endometriosis. The pelvic structures should be grasped and mobilized and the location and extent of all lesions and adhesions noted (Fig. 15.10a–c). Laparoscopy is useful for diagnosis, obtaining sample for histology and therapy (Box 15.14).

Biopsy should be taken when the ovarian endometrioma is more than 3 cm in diameter and in deep infiltrating disease to confirm diagnosis and exclude the rare possibility of malignancy.

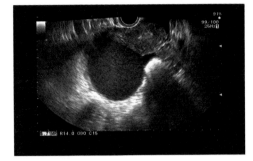

a.

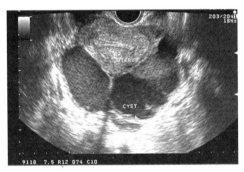

b.

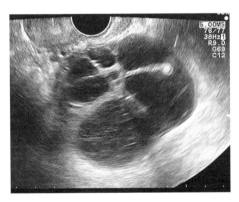

c.

Figure 15.8 Ultrasonographic pictures with ovarian endometriosis. It appears as cysts with middle-level echoes with or without septae. **a.** Unilateral ovarian endometrioma. **b.** Bilateral ovarian endometrioma. **c.** Endometrioma appearing as multiloculated cyst with middle level echoes.

Laparoscopy is very useful in visualization of superficial peritoneal endometriosis and ovarian endometriomas. However, deep infiltrating lesions are not well visualized at laparoscopy and their extent is difficult to determine. Adhesions

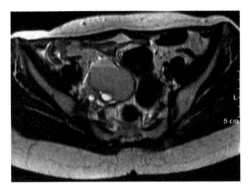

a.

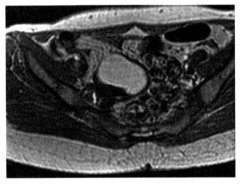

b.

Figure 15.9 Magnetic resonance imaging, endometriotic cysts in the right ovary, T2- and T1-weighted images. **a.** T2-weighted image: Right adnexa shows multiloculated cyst with one large and several small locules. **b.** T1-wieghted image: The largest locule is hyperintense and smaller ones are hypointense. This signifies haemorrhage in various stages of evolution.

may, sometimes, prevent visualization of even superficial endometriosis.

There is no specific timing during menstrual cycle for performing laparoscopy, but it should not be performed within 3 months of hormonal therapy since it may lead to underdiagnosis.

Box 15.14 Role of laparoscopy in endometriosis

- Visualization of lesions
- Staging the disease
- Biopsy for histology
- Evaluation of the extent of adhesions
- Therapeutic intervention if required

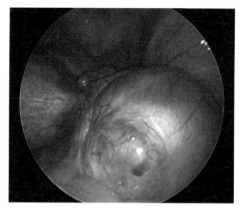

a.

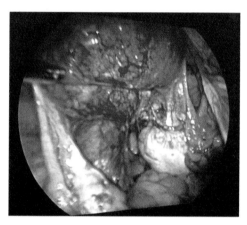

b.

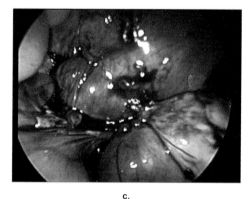

c.

Figure 15.10 Pelvic endometriosis seen at laparoscopy. a. Large endometrioma. b. Extensive adhesions obliterating the pouch of Douglas. The right tube is bunched up and adherent to the ovary. c. Extensive pelvic endometriosis with dense adhesions between uterus, tubes and ovaries.

Classification and staging of endometriosis

The revised American Fertility Society (r-AFS) classification, which is also adapted by the American Society for Reproductive Medicine (ASRM) in 1996 (Fig. 15.11), is widely used. Points are allocated for size, depth and location of endometriotic lesions, periovarian adhesions and pouch of Douglas obliteration. The total score is then used to stage the disease as in Box 15.15.

This staging system classifies deep infiltrating disease as stage 1. Interobserver variability in staging is high and does not help in predicting disease progression, rate of recurrence or severity of symptoms, but it is the best available tool to describe the extent of disease and plan management.

American Society for Reproductive Medicine: revised classification of endometriosis

Patient's name _____ Date _____
Stage I (minimal)   1–5
Stage II (mild)   6–15   Laparoscopy___ Laparotomy___ Photography ____
Stage III (moderate) 16–40   Recommended treatment _____
Stage IV (severe)   >40   _____
Total _____   Prognosis_____

	Endometriosis	<3 cm	1–3 cm	>3 cm
Peritoneum	Superficial	1	2	4
	Deep	2	4	6
Ovary	R Superficial	1	2	6
	Deep	4	10	20
	L Superficial	1	2	4
	Deep	4	16	20
	Posterior cul-de-sac obliteration	Partial		Complete
		4		40
	Adhesions	<1/3 enclosure	<1/3–2/3 enclosure	>2/3 enclosure
Ovary	R Filmy	1	2	4
	Dense	4	8	16
	L Filmy	1	2	4
	Dense	4	8	16
	Adhesions	<1/3 enclosure	<1/3–2/3 enclosure	>2/3 enclosure
Tube	R Filmy	1	2	4
	Dense	4	8'	16
	L Filmy	1	2	4
	Dense	4	8'	16

*If the fimbriated end of the fallopian tube is completely enclosed change the point assignment to 16.
Denote appearance of superficial implant types as red [(R), red, mid-pink, flamelike, vesicular blobs, clear vesicles], white [(W) specifications, peritoneal defects, yellow-brown], or black [(B) black, haemosiderin deposits, black]. Denote percent of total described as R_____% and B_____%. Total should equal 100%.

Figure 15.11 The revised American Fertility Society classification and scoring of endometriosis. Points are added together to calculate the score. According to the total score, the disease is staged.

- Stage 1 (minimal)   Score 1–5
- Stage 2 (mild)   Score 6–15
- Stage 3 (moderate)   Score 16–40
- Stage 4 (severe)   Score >40

Management

There is no known permanent cure for endometriosis, and the best available is **bilateral oophorectomy**. Since this is not acceptable in young, infertile women, other methods of treatment to relieve pain and improve fertility have to be resorted to.

- Short-term goals of the treatment are relief of pain and improvement of fertility.
- Long-term objectives are prevention of disease progression and recurrence after therapy.

Empirical treatment

In women with symptoms suggestive of endometriosis where fertility is not an issue, empirical treatment with progestogens or combined oral contraceptive pills can be tried without laparoscopic confirmation of diagnosis. Proper counselling is important and analgesics are used in addition. Treatment can be continued for up to 6 months. Gonadotropin-releasing hormone (GnRH) analogues can also be used, but they are more expensive.

Expectant management

A wait-and-watch policy or expectant management can be considered in perimenopausal women.

In women with minimal endometriosis, progression occurs in 30–60% within a year; hence, expectant management cannot be recommended. The disease does not progress after menopause; hence, perimenopausal women can be safely observed.

Medical management

This is indicated for

- Relief of pain
- Prevention of progression of disease

Ectopic endometrium responds to ovarian oestrogen and progesterone similar to uterine endometrium. Cyclic changes in response to these hormones are responsible for the symptoms of endometriosis. Therefore, suppression of ovarian steroid production should theoretically eliminate symptoms and disease progression.

- All medical therapies act by suppressing ovulation, and thereby ovarian steroidogenesis. Hence, medical treatment is undertaken only in women in whom immediate fertility is not desired. The purpose of medical management is pain relief. Symptoms recur after discontinuation of treatment in 5–15% of cases in the first year and 40–50% of cases in 5 years.
- Duration of medical therapy is usually for 6–12 months. Depot medroxyprogesterone can be continued for 2 or more years, but loss of bone mineral density should be kept in mind. Calcium supplementation is mandatory. Levonorgestrel intrauterine system (LNG-IUS) can be continued indefinitely.
- There is strong evidence that combined oral contraceptive pills, progestins, GnRH agonists and danazol are equally effective in relieving pain, but the main difference is in the cost and side effects.

Preparations used in medical treatment are listed in Table 15.1.

Nonsteroidal anti-inflammatory agents

Since inflammation plays a major role in the pathogenesis of endometriosis, anti-inflammatory agents such as nonsteroidal anti-inflammatory drugs (NSAIDs) are effective in reducing pain. They are generally used as a first-line therapy in the treatment of dysmenorrhoea and pelvic pain, and once hormonal therapy is started, they may be used as an adjunct.

Progestins

Progestins cause decidualization of endometriotic deposits and later atrophy. They are generally used orally continuously for 6–9 months and are effective in reducing pain. Medroxyprogesterone acetate in doses of 20–30 mg/day is recommended. Women are amenorrheic while they are on treatment, but breakthrough bleeding can occur. This can be managed with small doses of oestrogen. Depot medroxyprogesterone acetate (DMPA) is used when treatment is required for a longer duration and infertility is not an issue.

Table 15.1   Drugs used in medical management of endometriosis

Drug group	Preparation	Dose
NSAIDs	Mefenamic acid	500 mg thrice daily
Progestins		
Oral	MPA	30 mg daily
Oral	Lynestrenol	10 mg daily
Oral	Norethisterone	20 mg daily
IM depot	MPA	150 mg 3 monthly
LNG-IUS		
COC pills		
Oral	Ethinyl oestradiol	30 μg daily
Oral	Levonorgestrel	0.15 mg once daily
GnRH analogues		
IM depot	Leuprolide	3.75 mg monthly
SC depot	Goserelin	3.6 mg monthly
Antigonadotropin		
Oral	Danazol	600–800 mg daily
Oral	Gestrinone	1.25–2.5 mg twice weekly

COC, combined oral contraceptive; *GnRH*, gonadotropin-releasing hormone; *IM*, intramuscular; *LNG-IUS*, levonorgestrel intrauterine system; *MPA*, medroxyprogesterone acetate; *NSAID*, nonsteroidal anti-inflammatory drug; *SC*, subcutaneous.

It is, therefore, useful in young girls and older women.

Levonorgestrel intrauterine system

This is another route through which progesterone can be administered when long-term treatment is required. Suppression of menstruation and significant relief of pain, dysmenorrhoea and dyspareunia have been noticed. LNG-IUS has been found to be useful in rectovaginal endometriosis, superficial endometriosis and recurrent endometriosis after surgery. The intrauterine system can be left in the uterus for up to 5 years.

Combined oral contraceptive pills

Combination pills containing 30 μg of ethinyl oestradiol + 0.5 mg of levonorgestrel or 0.15 mg of desogestrel are the first-line drugs in symptomatic peritoneal endometriosis and endometriomas of <3 cm in size. They cause atrophy of the lesions, induce amenorrhoea and relieve symptoms. They can be used for 6–12 months continuously. Cyclic administration has not been found to be as effective. Side effects are minimal and the treatment is cost-effective.

GnRH agonists

These suppress the pituitary gonadotropins, producing a condition of pseudomenopause. The ovarian steroid production is in turn suppressed and the lesions undergo atrophy. Several preparations are available, and most are used as subcutaneous or intramuscular injection monthly. They cause symptoms of hypo-oestrogenism and reduction in bone mineral density. Hence, they are not used for more than 6 months and add-back therapy is generally included to reduce side effects (*see* Chapter 23, *Hormone therapies in gynaecology*). The drugs are expensive and are not better than other drugs in providing symptomatic relief. Hence, they are not the first-line drugs in management of endometriosis.

Antigonadotropins

They act by suppressing hypothalamic–pituitary–ovarian axis and cause increase in androgen and decrease in oestrogen levels.

Danazol was popular for the treatment of endometriosis in the past, but due to the androgenic side effects, it has now been replaced by other drugs. In doses of 600–800 mg daily, it causes amenorrhoea and significant relief of symptoms. Weight gain, fluid retention, acne, hirsutism and oily skin are side effects that are unacceptable.

Gestrinone has a complex action on oestrogen, progesterone and androgen receptors. Symptom relief is similar to that observed with danazol and side effects are also similar.

New medical approaches

Medical treatment of endometriosis has been mainly hormonal with a view to suppress oestrogen production. With better understanding of the pathogenesis at the molecular level, new therapeutic approaches are being tried. The newer drugs are listed in Box 15.16.

Surgical management

Surgical intervention is required in the following situations:

- Ineffective medical management
- Chronic pelvic pain
- Ovarian endometrioma
- Infertility

The goal of surgical treatment is to remove all the visible disease and release all adhesions.

Box 15.16 Newer drugs in endometriosis

- Selective progesterone receptor modulators
  - Mifepristone
  - Mesoprogestins
- GnRH antagonists
- Aromatase inhibitors
  - Letrozole
  - Anastrozole
- Selective oestrogen receptor modulators
  - Raloxifene
- TNF-α inhibitors
- Angiogenesis inhibitors
- Matrix metalloproteinase inhibitors
- Immunomodulators
  - Pentoxifylline
- ER-β antagonists

ER-β, oestrogen receptor beta; GnRH, gonadotropin-releasing hormone; TNF-α, tumour necrosis factor alpha.

Surgery may be conservative where the uterus and ovaries are preserved or radical where hysterectomy and bilateral salpingo-oophorectomy is performed (Box 15.17). Surgery can be laparoscopic or open.

Box 15.17 Surgery in endometriosis

- Conservative surgery
  - Cauterization of lesions
  - Laser vaporization of lesions
  - LUNA
  - Adhesiolysis
  - Cyst aspiration and irrigation
  - Cystectomy
  - Vaporization of inner cyst wall
  - Excision of rectovaginal nodules
- Radical surgery
  - Hysterectomy with
    - Bilateral salpingo-oophorectomy
    - ±Bowel resection
    - ±Ureteric resection and anastomosis/reimplantation

LUNA, laparoscopic uterosacral nerve ablation.

Type of surgery performed will depend on various factors as listed in Box 15.18.

Currently, evidence suggests that even in minimal to mild (stages 1 and 2) endometriosis, surgery relieves pain and improves fertility. In moderate to severe disease (stages 3 and 4), effect on fertility is uncertain and assisted reproductive techniques may have to be resorted to. But relief of pain does occur after surgery. In all stages of endometriosis, surgery limits progression of the disease (Box 15.19).

Box 15.18 Factors determining the type of surgery in endometriosis

- Age
- Stage of the disease
- Severity of pain
- Associated infertility
- Prior medical treatment

Box 15.19 Results of surgery in endometriosis

- Relieves pain
- Improves fertility
- Limits disease progression

Surgical management of superficial endometriosis

Laparoscopic surgery is feasible in most women. Diagnosis can be confirmed and therapeutic procedures can be performed at the same sitting. All visible diseases including those on ovarian surface should be resected or cauterized using electrocautery/laser. Adhesions should be released and resected (Box 15.20). Laparoscopic uterosacral nerve ablation (LUNA) performed along with resection of lesions relieves pain, but it is not useful when used alone.

Box 15.20 Surgical management of superficial endometriosis

- Coagulation of superficial lesions
  - Electrocautery
  - Laser
- Adhesiolysis
- LUNA

LUNA, laparoscopic uterosacral nerve ablation.

Surgery for ovarian endometrioma

Laparoscopic surgery is feasible in most women with endometrioma. Smaller endometriomas of diameter <3 cm can be aspirated, but evidence suggests that larger lesions should be excised leaving the ovarian cortex. The inner cyst wall of the remaining portion of the cyst is peeled off or cauterized (Box 15.21; Fig. 15.12a and b).

> **Box 15.21 Surgery for ovarian endometrioma**
>
> - Size <3 cm
>   - Aspiration and irrigation
>   - Vaporization/excision of inner wall
>   - Occasionally, cystectomy
> - Size >3 cm
>   - Cystectomy

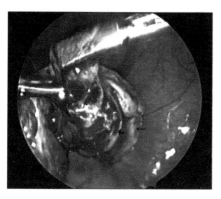

a.

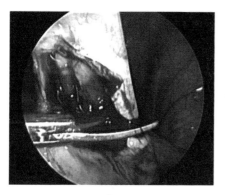

b.

Figure 15.12 Laparoscopic surgery for ovarian endometrioma. **a.** The inner lining is peeled off from the outer cyst wall and removed. **b.** The outer cyst wall is being trimmed.

Surgical management of deep infiltrating endometriosis

For deep infiltrating endometriosis and advanced-stage disease with gastrointestinal or urinary tract involvement, thorough preoperative evaluation and team approach is required. Laparoscopic or laparoscopic-assisted vaginal approaches may be feasible, but many women with deep infiltrating disease require laparotomy and radical surgery (Box 15.22). If the woman is in the premenopausal age, hormone replacement therapy is required after bilateral oophorectomy.

> **Box 15.22 Management of deep infiltrating and advanced endometriosis**
>
> - Preoperative evaluation
>   - Ultrasonography
>   - Magnetic resonance imaging
>   - Barium enema
>   - Intravenous urography
> - Preoperative preparation
>   - Bowel preparation
>   - Ureteric catheterization
> - Surgical procedure
>   - Hysterectomy with
>   - Bilateral salpingo-oophorectomy
>   ± Bowel resection
>   ± Ureteric resection and anastomosis/reimplantation

Treatment of infertility in endometriosis

Successful pregnancies occur in minimal, mild and moderate endometriosis after medical and surgical treatment. Overall spontaneous pregnancy rate is low. Ovulation induction, controlled hyperstimulation with intrauterine insemination, in vitro fertilization (IVF) or intracytoplasmic sperm injection (ICSI) may be required. This is dealt with in Chapter 22, *Infertility*.

Preoperative and postoperative medical therapy

Preoperative therapy with danazol, progestin or GnRH agonist improves disease scores. It may make surgery easier but does not alter the results of surgery. Postoperative therapy after conservative treatment does not delay the recurrence of pain or disease recurrence as per the currently available evidence.

Hormone therapy after hysterectomy and oophorectomy

Oestrogen alone can cause reactivation of symptoms, and, rarely, endometrioid carcinoma may develop in the residual endometriotic tissue. A combination of oestrogen and progestin is recommended for these women, but the risks of breast cancer should be kept in mind.

Recurrent endometriosis

Recurrence after conservative surgery is usually managed by hysterectomy and bilateral salpingo-oophorectomy. Recurrences after hysterectomy are uncommon if both ovaries are removed. Local recurrences should be resected.

Key points

- Endometriosis is the presence of endometrial gland and stroma outside the uterus.
- There are several theories regarding the development of endometriosis. These include implantation theory, coelomic metaplasia theory, induction theory and immunological theory. Genetic and molecular factors have also been implicated.
- Severe biologically active substances such as cytokines, matrix metalloproteinase (MMP), vascular endothelial growth factor-A (VEGF-A), growth factors and prostaglandins have been implicated in endometriosis.
- Pathologically, endometriosis is classified into superficial endometriosis, ovarian endometriosis and deep infiltrating endometriosis. Endometriosis can also occur at extrapelvic sites.
- Risk factors for endometriosis include early menarche, delayed childbearing, low parity, high social class, Müllerian anomalies and environmental factors.
- Symptoms of endometriosis include severe dysmenorrhoea, dyspareunia, chronic pelvic pain, menstrual abnormalities, infertility and bowel/bladder symptoms. Pain is the most predominant symptom.
- Clinical examination may reveal pelvic mass, fixed retroverted uterus, adnexal mass, tenderness and/or tender nodule in the pouch of Douglas.

- Clinical diagnosis of endometriosis cannot be made with certainty even in women with typical symptoms and signs. Imaging is of value in ovarian endometriosis.
- Visual inspection of the pelvis at laparoscopy is the gold standard for diagnosis of endometriosis.
- Staging of endometriosis is by the American Fertility Society. The disease is staged as stage 1, 2, 3 and 4.
- Management of endometriosis may be medical or surgical. Medical management is by progestogens, combined oral contraceptive pills, gonadotropin-releasing hormone (GnRH) analogues or antigonadotropins. Levonorgestrel intrauterine system (LNG-IUS) is also being used currently.
- Surgical management in endometriosis may be conservative or radical. Conservative surgery consists of cauterization, adhesiolysis, laser vaporization, cyst aspiration, cystectomy or excision of endometriotic nodule.
- Definitive treatment of endometriosis is by hysterectomy with bilateral salpingo-oophorectomy. Bowel resection and/or ureteric resection and anastomosis may be required in addition.
- Infertility in women with endometriosis may require assisted reproductive technique.

Self-assessment

Case-based questions

Case 1

An 18-year-old college student presents with severe congestive dysmenorrhoea of 2 years' duration, not responding to NSAIDs. Clinical examination is noncontributory.

1. What is the next step in evaluation?
2. If superficial endometriosis is diagnosed, what is the management?
3. How will you counsel the patient and her parents?

Case 2

A 38-year-old lady, mother of one child, presents with secondary dysmenorrhoea and dyspareunia. She has been on NSAIDs and combination oral contraceptive pills for 6 months without much relief of symptom.

1. How will you evaluate her clinically?
2. What investigation will you order?

3. If the diagnosis is rectovaginal endometriosis with ovarian endometrioma of 6 cm and stage 4 disease, what is the management?
4. What is the postoperative management?

Answers

Case 1

1. Abdominal ultrasonogram may be noncontributory. Transvaginal ultrasonogram is not possible. Therefore, laparoscopy is required.
2. (a) Cauterization of endometriotic lesions at laparoscopy
   (b) Combination oral contraceptive pills continuously for 6 months

   Alternatively, injection DMPA 150 mg IM 3 monthly can be used for 1–2 years.

3. (a) The patient will be amenorrheic while on treatment.

(b) Menstruation will resume after stopping the medication.

(c) Breakthrough bleeding can occur and doctor should be contacted.

(d) Early marriage is recommended since the disease can recur and progress.

(e) Subfertility is common and treatment may be required.

Case 2

1. (a) General examination
   (b) Abdominal examination for masses
   (c) Per speculum examination to look for bluish nodules in the posterior fornix
   (d) Pelvic examination for ovarian mass, tenderness, nodules in the pouch of Douglas, tenderness, fixity of uterus
   (e) Rectal examination for induration of uterosacral ligaments
   (f) Rectovaginal examination for deep infiltrating rectovaginal nodules
2. (a) Abdominal and transvaginal ultrasonography to look for ovarian mass, hydroureteronephrosis, size of rectovaginal nodules

(b) Barium enema

(c) Intravenous urography

3. Laparotomy, hysterectomy with bilateral salpingo-oophorectomy, excision of rectovaginal nodules, excision of all lesions.

4. Oestrogen replacement therapy.

Long-answer questions

1. Discuss the aetiology, clinical features and medical management of endometriosis.
2. Define endometriosis. Discuss the diagnosis and management of a case of endometriosis in a 35-year-old woman with one child.

Short-answer questions

1. Chocolate cyst of the ovary
2. Surgical treatment of endometriosis
3. Staging of endometriosis
4. Deep infiltrating endometriosis
5. Pathogenesis of endometriosis

16 | Chronic Pelvic Pain

Case scenario

Mrs BA, 35, a housewife, mother of three children, presented to an outpatient clinic with a history of chronic pelvic pain, which increased on physical exertion and movement. Her husband had a small shop, selling bicycle parts. She was very keen on undergoing a tubal ligation after the last delivery, but her husband refused due to religious reasons. She conceived 2 years ago and had a termination of pregnancy performed by an untrained dai in her village. She developed sepsis and was hospitalized for 2 weeks. She also complained of painful menstruation, pain starting 3–4 days prior to the onset of bleeding. She was quite incapacitated and found it difficult to carry out her day-to-day activities and take care of her small children. This had caused a lot of anxiety, tension and depression. The couple had also incurred a lot of expenditure by way of investigations and treatment elsewhere.

Introduction

Chronic pelvic pain (CPP) is a challenging problem because of its complex aetiology and poor response to treatment. Since the condition is not well understood, it is poorly managed. A multidisciplinary approach involving a gynaecologist, urologist, gastroenterologist, psychiatrist and sometimes other specialists is necessary for proper management. It is seen in primary care as frequently as asthma or backache.

Definition

Pain is defined by the International Association for the Study of Pain as an unpleasant sensory and emotional experience associated with actual or potential tissue damage. **CPP is defined as noncyclic pain of at least 6 months' duration, unrelated to menstruation, intercourse or pregnancy.** The pain should involve the pelvis, abdominal wall at or below the umbilicus, lower back and/or buttocks. It should be severe enough to cause disability or necessitate medical care (Box 16.1). In some conditions, in addition to the chronic persistent pain, there may be cyclic pain or pain related to menstruation or sexual intercourse.

CPP is most common in women in the reproductive age, especially between 26 and 30 years, but can occur from as early as age 18 to 50. It must be differentiated from dysmenorrhoea (which is related to menstrual cycle) and dyspareunia (which is related to sexual intercourse).

Box 16.1 Chronic pelvic pain

- Nature
  - Noncyclic pain
- Duration
  - 6 months or more
- Location
  - Lower abdomen, below umbilicus
  - Low back
  - Buttocks
- Prevalence
  - 15–20%
- Age group
  - Reproductive age group

Prevalence

The prevalence is variable, depending on the population studied. Severe pain necessitating treatment is found in 4% of population, but milder degrees of pain occur in 15–25%.

Risk factors

Risk factors for CPP are difficult to determine due to multiple aetiological factors. In general, the risk factors for the various gynaecological and nongynaecological conditions and history of physical and sexual abuse and past psychiatric disorders increase the risk of CPP.

Pathogenesis and aetiology

Fresh tissue damage causes acute pain. Chronic pain continues long after the tissue injury heals.

Pain perception involves peripheral and central nervous systems, and is influenced by other social, psychological and environmental factors. Various modulators such as prostaglandins, vasoactive peptides and endorphins also play a role. Pain may arise from any pelvic organ or referred to the pelvic area. Twenty-five to 30% of women with CPP have more than one aetiology. Specific conditions giving rise to CPP are listed in Box 16.2. No cause may be found even after thorough evaluation in some women, posing a challenge to the attending physician.

Box 16.2 Causes of CPP

- Gynaecological conditions
  - Endometriosis
  - Chronic pelvic inflammatory disease
  - Pelvic adhesions
  - Adenomyosis
  - Ovarian remnant/residual ovary syndromes
  - Pelvic congestion syndrome
  - Leiomyoma
- Urological conditions
  - Interstitial cystitis
  - Urethral syndrome
  - Chronic urinary tract infection
- Gastrointestinal conditions
  - Irritable bowel syndrome
  - Inflammatory bowel disease
- Musculoskeletal disorders
  - Separation of pubic symphysis
  - Sacroiliitis
  - Myofascial pelvic pain syndrome
- Neurological conditions
  - Nerve entrapment
  - Neuropathic pain
- Psychosomatic disorders
  - Anxiety
  - Depression
  - Sexual dysfunction

CPP, chronic pelvic pain.

Gynaecological conditions

Endometriosis

Characteristically, women with endometriosis present with secondary dysmenorrhoea and dyspareunia, but deep infiltrating disease can cause chronic pain (Fig. 16.1). Pain is not related to the extent or severity of endometriosis. This condition is dealt with in detail in Chapter 15, *Endometriosis*.

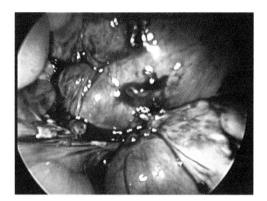

Figure 16.1 Endometriosis with extensive adhesions. Bilateral ovarian endometriomas are seen. Both ovaries are adherent to each other and to the posterior uterine surface. Bands of adhesion to other pelvic structures can also be seen. Uterine body, tubes and pouch of Douglas are covered by adhesions.

Chronic pelvic inflammatory disease

CPP is a well-known presentation of chronic pelvic inflammatory disease. This may be due to the formation of adhesions or local production of substances that modulate pain. Clinical diagnosis is difficult. Patient may give a past history of sexually transmitted disease (STD), intrauterine contraceptive device (IUCD) insertion, or puerperal or postabortal sepsis. Associated vaginal discharge, dysmenorrhoea and dyspareunia are common. Laparoscopy is required to confirm the presence of adhesions or tubo-ovarian mass (Fig. 16.2). This is discussed in detail in Chapter 13, *Infections of the upper genital tract.*

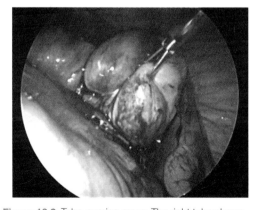

Figure 16.2 Tubo-ovarian mass. The right tube shows hydrosalpinx and is adherent to the ovary forming a mass. Band of adhesion is seen running from the pelvic wall to the mass. This is usually seen in chronic pelvic inflammatory disease.

Genital tuberculosis

Genital tuberculosis must be kept in mind while evaluating CPP in developing countries such as India. Other symptoms include general ill health, menstrual disturbances and abdominal distension due to ascites. This is dealt with in more detail in Chapter 14, *Tuberculosis of the female genital tract.*

Pelvic adhesions

Adhesions between structures in the pelvis may be caused by infection, endometriosis or prior surgery (Fig. 16.3). Dense, vascular adhesions are more likely to cause pain. Nerve fibres and sensory neurotransmitters have been identified in the adhesions. These may play a role in the causation of pain. Release of dense adhesions has been shown to relieve pain in some series, but a *Cochrane* systematic review found no significant benefit with this intervention.

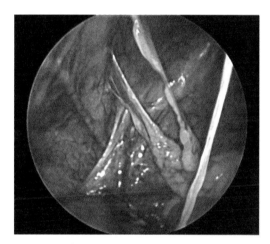

Figure 16.3 Pelvic adhesions. Strands of adhesions are seen between anterior abdominal wall and pelvic structures. This usually occurs after abdominal surgery.

Adenomyosis

Although the usual presentation in adenomyosis is dysmenorrhoea and heavy menstrual bleeding, some women present with CPP. This condition is dealt with in detail in Chapter 10, *Benign diseases of the uterus.*

Ovarian remnant and residual ovary syndromes

In severe endometriosis or pelvic inflammatory disease with extensive adhesions, a small amount of ovarian tissue that is left behind during oophorectomy may become entrapped in adhesions. This is called **ovarian remnant syndrome** and can be the cause for CPP. One or both ovaries left behind during hysterectomy can also be buried in adhesions and give rise to pelvic pain and dyspareunia. This is called the **residual ovary** or **entrapped ovary syndrome**. The ovary that is entrapped develops follicular cysts or haemorrhages and the pain is usually cyclic with a dull, additional, noncyclic component.

Pelvic congestion syndrome

This condition is associated with dilatation of veins and stasis of blood in the pelvis giving rise to CPP, pressure, heaviness, dyspareunia and exacerbation of pain after prolonged standing. The aetiology is not known. Dilated veins may be visualized at laparoscopy, but diagnosis is usually made by venography. Characteristic venographic findings are dilatation of uterine and ovarian veins with reduced venous clearance.

The gynaecological causes of CPP and their clinical features are summarized in Table 16.1.

Table 16.1 Gynaecological causes of CPP

Condition	Associated features
Endometriosis	• Dysmenorrhoea • Dyspareunia
Pelvic inflammatory disease	• History of STD, acute PID, IUCD • Dysmenorrhoea • Dyspareunia
Adhesions	• History of prior surgery, PID, endometriosis • Pain on movement
Adenomyosis	• Heavy menstrual bleeding • Dysmenorrhoea
Ovarian remnant/ trapped ovary syndrome	• History of hysterectomy • Cyclic exacerbation of pain
Pelvic congestion syndrome	• Dyspareunia • Pain on standing

CPP, chronic pelvic pain; *IUCD*, intrauterine contraceptive device; *PID*, pelvic inflammatory disease; *STD*, sexually transmitted disease.

Urological conditions

Interstitial cystitis

Interstitial cystitis is an inflammatory condition associated with pain in suprapubic, vaginal and urethral areas, dysuria, frequency and urgency.

The pain increases as the bladder distends and is relieved by voiding. Many women with interstitial cystitis have irritable bowel syndrome (IBS), allergies and dyspareunia. Diagnosis is by cystoscopy, which reveals characteristic submucosal oedema and petechiae and glomerulations. Women with this condition may not complain of bladder symptoms unless specifically questioned.

Urethral syndrome

In addition to chronic pain, women with this condition have symptoms of urethral irritation such as frequency, postvoid fullness, incontinence and dyspareunia. Postmenopausal oestrogen deficiency is the most common cause, but surgical trauma and chlamydial infection can also cause urethral syndrome.

Chronic and recurrent urinary tract infections

Chronic and recurrent urinary tract infections (UTIs) with or without partial obstruction and stasis of urine can give rise to CPP in addition to other urinary symptoms and fever.

The urological conditions giving rise to CPP and their clinical features are summarized in Table 16.2.

Table 16.2 Urological causes of CPP

Condition	Associated features
Interstitial cystitis	• Dysuria • Frequency • Pain on bladder filling • Allergies • Irritable bowel syndrome
Urethral syndrome	• Dysuria • Frequency • Incontinence • Postvoid fullness
Chronic/recurrent UTI	• Dysuria • Frequency • Systemic symptoms

CPP, chronic pelvic pain; *UTI*, urinary tract infection.

Gastrointestinal conditions

Irritable bowel syndrome

This is a functional bowel disease and a common cause of CPP. The Rome criteria used for diagnosis of IBS include intermittent or constant pain with altered stool frequency, stool form, stool passage, bloating sensation and/or passage of mucus. Women with IBS also have associated dyspareunia, chronic low backache and bladder dysfunction.

Inflammatory bowel disease

Chronic, recurrent inflammatory bowel disorders including ulcerative colitis can give rise to CPP and bloody diarrhoea.

Musculoskeletal disorders

Pain arising from bones or joints due to trauma or inflammation can present as CPP. Pain is generally associated with movement and worsens by the end of the day. Typical examples are separation of pubic symphysis and inflammation of the sacroiliac joint. Poor posture and muscle dysfunction can also give rise to pain. Spasm of levator ani or any other group of muscles in the pelvis has been found in women with no other demonstrable organic pathology. This condition is known as myofascial pelvic pain syndrome (MPPS). 'Trigger points' can be identified in these women with muscle spasm. Pressure on these points elicits intense pain similar to that experienced by the patient at other times.

Neurological conditions

Nerve entrapment

Nerves can be entrapped in scar tissue, at the edge of the rectus muscle, in abdominal incisions and as they pass through narrow foramina. Ilioinguinal nerve, genitofemoral nerve, cutaneous nerves and sacral nerve can be involved. Pain may be localized to abdominal wall, thigh, groin or back depending on the nerve involved. Associated bladder, bowel and sexual dysfunction may be present.

Neuropathic pain

Involvement of pelvic nerves in fibrotic diseases such as endometriosis, infiltration by malignancy and pain syndromes such as coccydynia or vulvodynia are also the causes of CPP.

The gastrointestinal, musculoskeletal and neurological conditions giving rise to CPP are summarized in Table 16.3.

Psychosomatic disorders

Women with anxiety, stress, personality disorders, depression and somatization disorders can

Table 16.3 Gastrointestinal, musculoskeletal and neurological causes of CPP

Condition	Associated features
Gastrointestinal conditions	
Irritable bowel syndrome	• Altered stool frequency/consistency • Altered stool passage • Bloating • Passage of mucus
Inflammatory bowel disease	Bloody diarrhoea
Musculoskeletal conditions	• Pain on movement • Worsen by end of the day • Trigger points
Neurological conditions	• Location depends on the nerve involved • Bladder, bowel, sexual dysfunction

CPP, chronic pelvic pain.

present with CPP. There is a strong correlation between childhood and adult sexual abuse, substance abuse and CPP. Therefore, women with CPP require expert and sensitive approach and a thorough evaluation of the past and present social and emotional problems.

Clinical features

Symptoms

Apart from the presenting symptom of pelvic or lower abdominal pain or backache, the other symptoms depend on the cause of pain. Women with CPP are often frustrated since they may have already consulted several specialists. Women who have psychosomatic disorders may present with multiple nonspecific symptoms.

There are some symptoms associated with CPP that are indicators of the underlying serious pathology (Box 16.3). When any of these are present, the patient should be evaluated thoroughly by the respective specialists.

Signs

Signs vary with the aetiology of the pain. Women with gynaecological causes of pain may have a mass arising from pelvis in case of large endometriotic cysts. Pelvic examination may reveal an enlarged uterus in adenomyosis, adnexal mass, tenderness and induration of uterosacral ligaments in endometriosis, tender fixed tubo-ovarian masses in chronic pelvic inflammatory disease and tuberculosis. Trigger points can be identified.

Clinical evaluation

History

Since CPP is a disorder with complex aetiology, predisposing factors and associated conditions, a thorough history to assess the physical, mental and social status is important (Box 16.4). It is important to give adequate time at the initial consultation to listen to the patients and allay their fears.

Physical examination

This should include general examination, gynaecological examination and evaluation of other systems (Box 16.5). Referral to other specialists is decided upon by the nature of symptoms.

Investigations

Investigations will depend on provisional diagnosis arrived at after history taking and physical examination (Box 16.6). Transvaginal ultrasonogram is useful for making a diagnosis of ovarian endometrioma, tubo-ovarian mass, adenomyosis (Figs 16.4–16.6) and residual/remnant ovary syndrome. Laparoscopy is considered the 'gold standard' in the evaluation of CPP and is useful for the diagnosis of endometriosis, pelvic adhesions and pelvic congestion syndrome (Figs 16.7 and 16.8). But in more than 50% of women, laparoscopy may be negative. This may help in

reassuring the patient or sometimes increases the anxiety. Therefore, appropriate preoperative counselling is mandatory.

Box 16.6 Investigations in CPP

- Full blood count
- VDRL
- Urinalysis and midstream culture
- Vaginal swab for culture/*Chlamydia*
- Abdominal and transvaginal ultrasonogram
  - Endometriosis
  - Tubo-ovarian mass
  - Adenomyosis
  - Residual/remnant ovary
- Urological and GI evaluation
- Laparoscopy
  - Endometriosis
  - Pelvic congestion syndrome
  - Adhesions
  - PID
- MRI and CT scan
  - When appropriate

CPP, chronic pelvic pain; *CT*, computed tomography; *GI*, gastrointestinal; *MRI*, magnetic resonance imaging; *PID*, pelvic inflammatory disease; *VDRL*, Venereal Disease Research Laboratory.

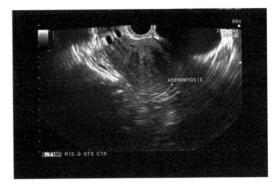

Figure 16.5 Ultrasonogram showing adenomyosis. The myometrium at the fundus is thickened and reveals areas of mixed echogenicity. There is definite demarcation from the myometrium.

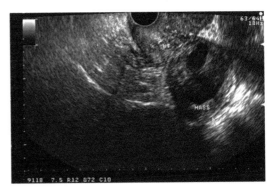

Figure 16.6 Ultrasonogram showing tubo-ovarian mass. The mass has mixed echogenicity indicating dilated tube and ovary bunched up together to form a mass.

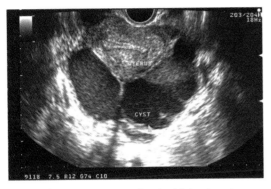

Figure 16.4 Ultrasonogram showing bilateral ovarian endometrioma. The ovaries with endometriotic cysts (endometrioma) are seen adherent to the posterior aspect of the uterus.

Magnetic resonance imaging (MRI) and computed tomography (CT) scan are rarely indicated. Other investigations such as cystoscopy, barium studies and venography are undertaken when required.

Management

Treatment consists of medical and surgical interventions. Women with definitive diagnosis of

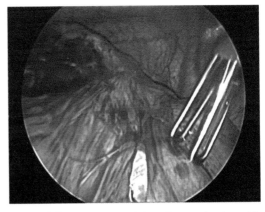

Figure 16.7 Laparoscopy; picture shows extensive pelvic adhesions, reaching up to the uterine fundus. The left ovary is seen through the adhesions. The fundus of the uterus and left tube are visible.

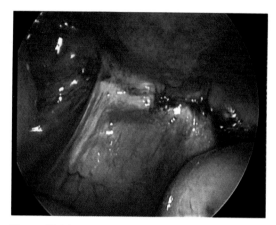

Figure 16.8 Laparoscopy; picture shows endometriosis. Note the blue and black puckered spots on the uterosacral ligaments and peritoneum of the pouch of Douglas.

gynaecological conditions should be given specific treatment. Those with established urological, gastrointestinal, neurological or psychiatric conditions should be referred for multidisciplinary management.

Medical management

The following is the first line of management for most women with CPP:

- Counselling regarding lifestyle modification, dietary adjustment and analgesics are important first-line therapies.
- Nonsteroidal anti-inflammatory drugs (NSAIDs) are effective in mild-to-moderate pain.
- Ovarian suppression with combined pill, medroxyprogesterone or gonadotropin-releasing hormone (GnRH) analogues can be tried for 3–6 months even without laparoscopic evaluation in suspected cases of endometriosis.
- Ongoing proven pelvic inflammatory disease may be treated with antibiotics. However, there is no room for empirical treatment with antibiotics.
- Women with pelvic congestion also respond to ovarian suppression.
- IBS can be managed by dietary adjustment, antidepressants and antispasmodics on the basis of clinical diagnosis.
- When depression is the predominant feature, antidepressants are helpful. They are effective

in vulvodynia and other neurological pain syndromes when used along with gabapentin. Musculofascial pain syndrome also responds to antidepressants and gabapentin.

Drugs used in treatment of CPP are listed in Box 16.7.

Box 16.7 Drugs used in medical management of CPP

- NSAIDs
- Drugs for ovarian suppression
  - Medroxyprogesterone acetate
    - Oral 50 mg daily
    - IM 150 mg 3-monthly
  - Combined oral contraceptive pills
    - Once a day for 21 days/month
  - GnRH analogues
    - 3.6 mg once in 28 days
- Antidepressants
  - Amitriptyline
    - 25–50 mg daily
  - Fluoxetine
    - 20 mg daily
  - Sertraline
    - 50–100 mg daily
- Gabapentin
  - 300 mg two or three times per day
- Levonorgestrel IUS

CPP, chronic pelvic pain; *GnRH*, gonadotropin-releasing hormone; *IM*, intramuscular; *IUS*, intrauterine system; *NSAID*, nonsteroidal anti-inflammatory drug.

Surgical management

Surgery is of limited value in the management of CPP. Stage 3 or 4 endometriosis, and remnant and residual ovarian syndromes may require surgical intervention. Adhesiolysis does not relieve pain except in severe vascular adhesions. There is no evidence to support the use of other surgical procedures such as nerve ablations and neurectomy (Box 16.8).

Other interventions

Other modalities of treatment are used with varying results in the management of CPP (Box 16.9).

A simple algorithm for the evaluation and management of CPP is given in Fig. 16.9.

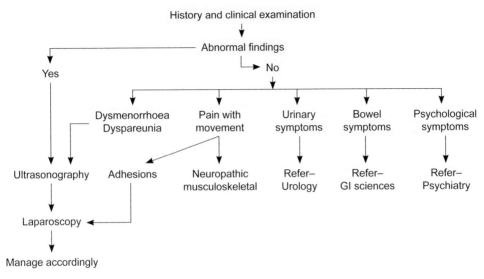

Figure 16.9 Algorithm for evaluation and management of CPP. *CPP*, chronic pelvic pain; *GI*, gastrointestinal.

Box 16.8 Surgical management of CPP

- Adhesiolysis
  - Moderate-to-severe vascular adhesions
- Oophorectomy
  - Residual/remnant ovarian syndrome
- Hysterectomy + oophorectomy
  - Stage 3 or 4 endometriosis
- Uterosacral nerve ablation
  - Endometriosis, unexplained pain
- Presacral neurectomy
  - Endometriosis, unexplained pain

CPP, chronic pelvic pain.

Box 16.9 Other interventions in the management of CPP

- Static magnetic therapy
- Ultrasound therapy
- Trigger point injections
- Acupuncture
- Transcutaneous electrical nerve stimulation
- Photographic reinforcement
- Writing therapy

CPP, chronic pelvic pain.

Key points

- Chronic pelvic pain (CPP) is defined as noncyclic pain of at least 6 months' duration, unrelated to menstruation, intercourse or pregnancy. It is a challenging problem and requires multidisciplinary approach. It is most common during the reproductive age.

- Pain may arise from any pelvic organ or may be referred to the pelvic area. There may be more than one aetiological factor. CPP may be caused by gynaecological, urological, gastrointestinal, musculoskeletal, neurological or psychosomatic conditions.

- The gynaecological conditions causing CPP are endometriosis, chronic pelvic inflammatory disease, pelvic adhesions, adenomyosis, ovarian remnant/ residual ovary syndrome and pelvic congestion syndrome. These conditions give rise to other associated symptoms such as dyspareunia, pain on exertion or movement and dysmenorrhoea.

- A detailed history is mandatory in CPP. In many patients, this helps in identifying the organ system involved. History should include location of pain, precipitating factors, type of pain, intensity and other associated symptoms such as dysmenorrhoea and dyspareunia. History of previous surgery, sepsis and sexual abuse is important.

- If CPP is associated with symptoms such as bleeding per vaginum or rectum, pelvic mass, weight loss, postcoital bleeding, alteration in bowel habits or history of suicidal tendencies, significant underlying pathology should be suspected and the patient referred for further evaluation.

- Physical examination in CPP should include general examination, a gynaecological evaluation, rectal

(Continued)

Key points *(Continued)*

examination and evaluation of the spine and sacroiliac joints.

- Ultrasonography, both transvaginal and abdominal, is useful in identifying organic pelvic pathology. Laparoscopy is the gold standard for evaluation. Computed tomography (CT) scan and magnetic resonance imaging (MRI) are rarely indicated.
- Women with definitive diagnosis of pelvic pathology should be managed accordingly.
- Counselling is an essential component of managing women with CPP.
- Medical management of CPP consists of nonsteroidal anti-inflammatory drugs (NSAIDs), gonadotropin-

releasing hormone (GnRH) analogues to suppress ovarian function, gabapentin, antidepressants and antispasmodics.

- Surgical intervention is required only in women with severe endometriosis and residual/remnant ovary. Uterosacral nerve ablation and presacral neurectomy have been tried in unexplained CPP with some success.
- Other interventions such as ultrasound therapy, trigger point injections, writing therapy and photographic reinforcement may be of value in some women with CPP.

Self-assessment

Case-based questions

Case 1

A 35-year-old lady, mother of three children with a history of one termination of pregnancy followed by sepsis, presents with a history of CPP of 1-year duration. Pain is brought about by physical exertion and increases on movement. She also has congestive dysmenorrhoea.

1. What is the next step in the evaluation?
2. What diagnosis would you consider?
3. What investigations would you ask for?
4. How will you manage?

Case 2

A 25-year-old single lady, software engineer, presents with CPP of 2 years' duration. No abnormality is detected on physical examination. The patient is not very communicative.

1. What further information would you try to obtain?
2. What is the management?

Answers

Case 1

1. General examination followed by abdominal examination to ascertain the location of pain; look for any abdominal or pelvic mass and tenderness.
2. (a) Intra-abdominal adhesions—CPP with pain on physical exertion and movement
   (b) Chronic pelvic inflammatory disease—Postabortal sepsis, dysmenorrhoea and CPP
   (c) Adenomyosis—Multipara, dysmenorrhoea and CPP

3. Abdominal and transvaginal ultrasonogram to look for uterine size, adenomyosis, tubo-ovarian mass.
4. (a) Counselling regarding the possibility of adhesions
   (b) Analgesics for CPP
   (c) Mefenamic acid 500 mg thrice daily during menstrual cycles for dysmenorrhoea

Case 2

1. History of sexual abuse, premarital sex, termination of pregnancy, stress, symptoms of depressive illness, social history, dysmenorrhoea.
2. If symptoms are suggestive of psychosomatic disorder, refer to a psychiatrist for full evaluation and treatment.

   If not, counselling, reassurance, analgesics and amitriptyline 25 mg daily.

Long-answer questions

1. A 38-year-old lady presents with a history of CPP. Discuss the evaluation and management.
2. What are the causes of CPP? Discuss the management of a 28-year-old lady with CPP, dyspareunia and congestive dysmenorrhoea.

Short-answer questions

1. Pelvic congestion syndrome
2. Role of laparoscopy in CPP
3. Uterosacral nerve ablation
4. Residual ovarian syndrome
5. Ovarian remnant syndrome

Gynaecological Endocrinology and Infertility

17 Paediatric and Adolescent Gynaecology

Case scenario

A young lady walked into a clinic one afternoon, looking distraught and carrying a 4-year-old child. She had noticed vaginal bleeding in the child an hour ago and wondered if the child had some serious illness or cancer. The mother was also worried about sexual abuse.

Introduction

Although paediatric and adolescent gynaecological problems need to be managed by specialists interested in this area, there are some common problems in this group of girls that every doctor should be aware of. Some of these problems can easily be managed by a primary care physician provided there is a basic knowledge of the pathophysiology of the conditions. Some of the conditions are physiological and require only reassurance.

Disorders in the neonatal period

Circulating maternal oestrogen crosses the placenta and acts on the internal and external genital organs and breast tissue of the neonate. These effects subside in 2 weeks. The effects of maternal oestrogen on the neonate are given in Box 17.1.

Box 17.1 Effects of oestrogen in the neonate

- Enlargement of the breast
- Discharge from the breast
- Mucoid vaginal discharge
- Blood stained vaginal discharge

Hydrocolpos

A membrane or transverse vaginal septum can occlude the vagina leading to the collection of mucoid discharge, causing distension of the vagina. The condition presents as pelvic mass in prepubertal girls but can also occur in the neonate. The membrane can be visualized on examination, and simple incision to drain the fluid can cure the condition.

Disorders in childhood

Managing gynaecological disorders in childhood requires patience, understanding and tact. The parents are usually worried and anxious. The child may be uncooperative.

- The examination room should be child friendly. One parent, preferably the mother, must be present during the examination to reassure the child and ensure cooperation.
- General examination and examination of the other systems should be performed before proceeding with examination of the genitalia. Occasionally, examination may have to be performed under anaesthesia.
- If a sample of discharge is required for examination, it can be obtained with a moistened swab or using a small feeding tube attached to a syringe.
- A colposcope can be used to visualize the vulva under magnification. A nasal speculum or fibre optic scope can be inserted through the hymenal orifice under anaesthesia for visualization of vagina.

A few disorders commonly seen in childhood are given in Box 17.2.

Box 17.2 Common disorders in childhood

- Vulvovaginitis
- Labial adhesions
- Lichen sclerosis of the vulva
- Vaginal bleeding

Vulvovaginitis

Factors predisposing to vulvovaginitis

Under the influence of maternal oestrogen, the lining squamous epithelium of vagina is many cell layered and the cells are rich in glycogen at birth. The ovaries are inactive and the effects of maternal oestrogen wear off gradually. The epithelium becomes thin, glycogen content decreases, the pH becomes alkaline and the protective effect of acid secretions no longer exists. The vaginal epithelium is, therefore, more prone to infection. Since the labial fat pads and pubic hair are absent in the child, introitus is also more exposed to infection. Poor local hygiene may also contribute to the problem (Box 17.3).

Box 17.3 Factors predisposing to vulvovaginitis

- Deficiency of oestrogen
  - Thinning of vaginal epithelium
  - Decrease in glycogen content
  - Alkaline pH
- Absence of labial fat pad
- Lack of labial hair
- Poor hygiene

Causes of vulvovaginitis

Common causes of vulvovaginitis are as in Box 17.4. Vulvovaginitis is nonspecific in 75% of children and due to specific organisms in 25%. The child presents with pruritus and soreness in the vulva with or without discharge.

Box 17.4 Aetiology of vulvovaginitis in children

- Nonspecific
  - Poor hygiene
  - Allergy
  - Foreign body
- Specific
  - Group A β-haemolytic *Streptococcus*
  - Other bacteria
    - Pinworm
    - *Candida*
    - *Trichomonas*

Nonspecific vulvovaginitis

This is more common than specific infections.

Poor vulvar hygiene is seen in many children. Back-to-front wiping brings the organisms from the perianal region forward into the vagina and is responsible for recurrent infection in some children. Allergy to chemicals in the toilet soap and detergent is a common problem. Occasionally, foreign body may be the cause, but the discharge is bloodstained and foul smelling in such cases.

Management of nonspecific vulvovaginitis consists mainly of counselling the parents (Box 17.5). Bland nonmedicated creams usually suffice.

Examination under anaesthesia is necessary if foreign body is suspected. Purulent discharge may be treated with a short course of antibiotics such as amoxicillin with clavulanate.

- Counselling
  - Improve hygiene
  - Avoid chemicals—Use mild soap and detergent
  - Encourage front-to-back wiping
- Bland nonmedicated creams
- 1–2.5% hydrocortisone ointment for allergy
- EUA, removal of foreign body
- If discharge purulent
  - Short course of antibiotics

EUA, examination under anaesthesia.

Specific vulvovaginitis

This is seen in only 20–25% of children. It is often secondary to respiratory or enteric infections. The common organism is group A β-haemolytic *Streptococcus*, although, rarely, enteric bacteria have also been isolated. Candidal infection is rare unless the child is immunosuppressed. Pinworm infection can occur from perianal region. Trichomoniasis is rare. Gonococcal infection is caused by sexual abuse. Vaginal discharge must be sent for culture to identify the organism.

Management is as outlined in Box 17.6. The dosage of drugs depends on the weight of the child.

Box 17.6 Management of specific
vulvovaginitis

- Local oestrogen cream to relieve soreness and pruritus
- 1% hydrocortisone ointment if symptoms severe
- Antibiotics as per culture report
- Mebendazole for pinworm infestation
- Clotrimazole cream for candidiasis
- Oral metronidazole for trichomoniasis

Labial adhesions

The labia minora adhere to each other giving the appearance of fusion (Fig. 17.1). It is said to be due to oestrogen deficiency and the resultant thinning of epithelium. Fusion starts posteriorly and extends anteriorly. Associated poor perineal hygiene is usually seen.

Management is simple and is by application of local oestrogen cream for 2 weeks. The adhesions may separate spontaneously or can be easily separated. Betamethasone cream 0.05% can be used in difficult cases.

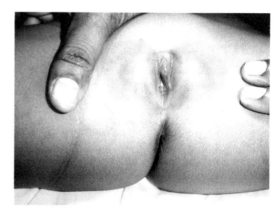

Figure 17.1 A 2-year-old child with labial adhesions. The labia minora appears fused and the introitus is not visible.

Lichen sclerosis

This has a tendency to affect the genital area especially in children. Symptoms are intense pruritus, soreness, dysuria, blood-stained discharge or bleeding and pain on defaecation. The vulval skin looks white, atrophic, parchment-like and excoriated. Diagnosis is clinical. Treatment is with local 2.5% hydrocortisone cream initially, followed by 1% hydrocortisone cream if response is observed. Alternatively, clobetasone ointment 0.05% may be used twice daily for 6–12 weeks. Attention to local hygiene is important.

Vaginal bleeding

Vaginal bleeding in the neonatal period is common due to sudden withdrawal of maternal oestrogen. No treatment is required, but the parents must be reassured. Bleeding during childhood may be due to several causes as outlined in Box 17.7.

Presence of foreign body must always be excluded in a child who presents with vaginal bleeding. Associated purulent discharge may be present. Trauma may be accidental, but sexual abuse must be ruled out by careful history taking.

Vulvar condylomas due to papillomavirus may be acquired prenatally from the mother. Lichen sclerosis has already been discussed earlier in this chapter. It can cause vaginal bleeding.

Exogenous oestrogen use must be kept in mind. These are usually administered as creams or alternative therapy. Precocious puberty is discussed

- Foreign body
- Trauma
- Sexual abuse
- Exogenous oestrogen
- Vulvar lesions
  - Condyloma
  - Lichen sclerosis
- Precocious puberty
  - Central
  - Peripheral
- Tumours
  - Sarcoma botryoides
  - Granulosa cell tumour of the ovary
- Bleeding from other sites
  - Urethra
  - Rectum

later in the chapter. Granulosa cell tumour of the ovary is one of the conditions leading to precocious puberty (*see* Chapter 31, *Malignant diseases of the ovary and fallopian tube*).

Tumours of the genital tract are rare but can occur in childhood. Sarcoma botryoides is discussed in Chapter 27, *Preinvasive and invasive diseases of the vulva and vagina* and granulosa cell tumour of the ovary is discussed in Chapter 31, *Malignant diseases of the ovary and fallopian tube*.

Bleeding due to a urethral caruncle or from the rectum must also be considered and ruled out by careful clinical examination.

Management

Careful history taking and clinical examination are mandatory. Examination under anaesthesia is required if foreign body is suspected. Vaginal tumours can also be visualized and biopsy taken under anaesthesia. Ultrasonography is useful in the diagnosis of ovarian tumours.

Disorders in adolescence

Adolescence is the time during which endocrinal changes of puberty, sexual development and growth occur. Social and psychological adaptation to the hormonal changes of puberty goes on throughout adolescence. Disorders seen during this period are the result of aberrations in hormone production and psychological maladaptation.

Physiology of puberty

Puberty is the time during which sexual maturation takes place resulting in reproductive capacity. Menarche is the onset of menstruation and is one of the many events in puberty, but is an external manifestation of hypothalamic–pituitary–ovarian function. It is an important event since it is an obvious parameter of sexual maturity. The terms used are as given in Box 17.8.

Box 17.8 Terminology used in physiology of puberty

- Puberty — Time of sexual maturation
- Gonadarche — Activation of gonads by the pituitary hormones resulting in production of ovarian hormones
- Menarche — Onset of menstruation
- Thelarche — Onset of breast development
- Adrenarche — Activation of production of androgens by the adrenal cortex
- Pubarche — Appearance of pubic hair

Puberty occurs between the ages 8 and 16 years, and includes breast development, pubic and axillary hair development, growth spurt and onset of menstruation. The age of onset and progression of puberty are influenced by genetic, socioeconomic and environmental factors. Age at menarche is also variable and seems to occur earlier now due to changing lifestyle and nutrition.

The events of puberty start with 'awakening' of the hypothalamus. What triggers the initiation of pubertal hypothalamic function is not known. There is an increase in activators and decrease in inhibitors of gonadotropin-releasing hormone (GnRH) secretion. The endocrine changes are depicted in Fig. 17.2. The hypothalamus releases GnRH in a pulsatile fashion. The pituitary gland responds by releasing gonadotropins, namely follicle-stimulating hormone (FSH) and luteinizing hormone (LH). These act on the ovary causing synthesis and release of sex steroids—Oestrogen and progesterone. They act on breast, uterus and other target organs and lead to breast development and menstruation. Under the influence of oestrogen, uterus and cervix also grow and reach the adult proportion of 2:1. The early menstrual cycles are anovulatory and irregular. The endometrium differentiates into basal functional layer and shows the characteristic changes under the influence of gonadal hormones.

Other pubertal changes

Body weight and composition

Body mass increases at puberty. There is increase in lean body mass and fat mass. The latter is more in girls. Excessive weight gain can occur, depending on individual nutritional status. Obesity in adolescence can later lead to metabolic syndrome.

Bone growth

Linear bone growth is essential for increase in height. Bone mineralization peaks a few months after peak height velocity, and this leads to increase in requirement of calcium and vitamin D. Deficiency in these can increase the risk of osteoporosis and fracture.

Clinical examination of the adolescent girl

History taking and examination of the adolescent requires tact and sensitivity. It should be least stressful for the patient and parents. History and examination should be as described in Box 17.11. History of sexual activity is important but may be asked in privacy. Pelvic examination should not be performed unless indicated. The procedure should be discussed with the patient and her parents. In girls who are not sexually active, if internal examination is indicated, it should be performed rectally. Speculum examination should be avoided, if possible.

Box 17.11 Clinical examination of adolescent girl

- History
  - Age of onset of menarche
  - Past history of childhood illness
  - Family history
  - Sexual history
- Examination
  - Height, weight, body mass index
  - Breast—Tanner stage
  - Pubic and axillary hair—Tanner stage
  - Abdominal examination—Masses
  - External genitalia
  - Hymen
  - Rectal examination where required

Common problems at puberty

Some common problems at puberty are listed in Box 17.12. These problems arise due to nutritional deficiencies, hormonal changes and blood loss during menstruation.

Box 17.12 Common problems at puberty

- Anaemia
- Acne
- Abnormal uterine bleeding
- Obesity
- Injuries to epiphyseal growth plates
- Scoliosis
- Psychological problems

Disorders of puberty

Common disorders in adolescence are disorders of growth and disorders of puberty. Growth disorders are beyond the purview of this book. Disorders of puberty may be precocious puberty or delayed puberty. This chapter will deal with precocious puberty. Delayed puberty will be discussed in Chapter 18, *Primary amenorrhoea*. Another common condition is heavy menstrual bleeding during puberty, which is dealt with in Chapter 7, *Abnormal uterine bleeding*.

Precocious puberty

By definition, puberty is said to be precocious when it occurs before the age of 8 years. Menarche before age of 9 years is also considered precocious. Classification according to aetiology is given in Box 17.13.

In some children, isolated **premature thelarche** or isolated **premature pubarche/ adrenarche** is seen. However, these are uncommon. These are usually nonprogressive variants of puberty.

Central precocious puberty

This is due to early secretion of gonadotropins (gonadotropin dependent), resulting in stimulation of ovarian function. All the changes of puberty occur in the same order.

- Idiopathic gonadotropin secretion is the most common.

- Central precocious puberty (gonadotropin-dependent)
  - Idiopathic
  - Intracranial tumours/cysts
  - Infections
  - Trauma
  - Malformations
  - Gene mutations
- Peripheral precocious puberty (gonadotropin-independent)
  - Oestrogen-secreting ovarian tumours
  - Sex hormone–secreting adrenal tumours
  - McCune–Albright syndrome
  - Exogenous oestrogen exposure
  - Primary hypothyroidism

- Tumours, cysts, trauma or inflammation affecting the hypothalamus or pituitary can give rise to central precocious puberty. Tumours must be looked for by imaging.

Peripheral precocious puberty

This is due to secretion of sex hormones by ovary or adrenal gland (gonadotropin independent).

- Exposure to exogenous oestrogen should be excluded.
- Granulosa cell tumour or granulosa–theca cell tumours of the ovary are uncommon. They present with bleeding and pelvic mass.
- McCune–Albright syndrome is a condition where gonadotropin receptors are activated early. This can affect other endocrine glands as well. The syndrome is associated with polyostotic fibrous dysplasia and café-au-lait spots. Follicular cysts of the ovary are usually present.
- Severe primary hypothyroidism can also cause precocious puberty.

Management

The aims of treatment in precocious puberty are as follows:

- To avoid psychological problems due to precocious development
- To prevent reduction in final height that results from early fusion of epiphysis under the influence of oestrogen

Evaluation

History and physical examination should be thorough (Box 17.14). Estimation of serum FSH and LH levels is useful for differentiating central from peripheral precocious puberty. Thyroid-stimulating hormone (TSH) estimation is required when thyroid dysfunction is suspected. High serum oestradiol level indicates peripheral precocity such as an oestrogen-secreting ovarian tumour. Determination of bone age is important for treatment decisions. Imaging by pelvic ultrasonography or magnetic resonance imaging of the brain, if required, will identify ovarian tumours or central nervous system lesions.

- History
  - Age
  - Meningitis
  - Encephalitis
  - Trauma
  - Symptoms of increased intracranial pressure
  - Exogenous hormones
- Examination
  - Height, weight, skin lesions, bony deformity
  - Breast—Tanner stage
  - Pubic and axillary hair—Tanner stage
  - Abdominal/pelvic mass
  - Café-au-lait spots
- Investigations
  - Bone age
  - Serum FSH, LH, TSH, oestradiol
  - Ultrasound scan to rule out ovarian/adrenal mass
  - MRI to rule out intracranial lesions
  - Other hormone levels when indicated

FSH, follicle-stimulating hormone; LH, luteinizing hormone; TSH, thyroid-stimulating hormone.

Treatment

Most girls with isolated premature thelarche or adrenarche require only reassurance. Counselling is an important aspect of management. The earlier the onset of puberty, the more likely that treatment will be needed. Girls who present with precocious puberty before age 6 usually require treatment.

Treatment of central precocity is by suppression of gonadotropin production with GnRH analogues, given 3-weekly till normal age of puberty is reached. Continuous stimulation with GnRH analogues suppresses gonadotropin production. Some tumours require surgical removal.

Tumours of the ovary or adrenal gland causing peripheral precocity should be removed surgically. Exogenous steroids should be discontinued.

McCune–Albright syndrome is treated by aromatase inhibitors that interfere with peripheral aromatization of androgen to oestrogens, thereby reducing oestrogen levels. Drugs used are letrozole, anastrozole or testolactone. Tamoxifen has also been used in peripheral precocity, with good results.

Treatment is summarized in Box 17.15.

Box 17.15 Treatment of precocious puberty

- Central precocious puberty
  - GnRH analogues 3.5 mg SC 3-weekly
  - Surgery for tumours, if required
- Peripheral precocious puberty
  - Surgical intervention for ovarian/adrenal tumours
  - Aromatase inhibitors
    - Letrozole
    - Testolactone
    - Anastrozole
  - Tamoxifen
  - Treatment of thyroid dysfunction

GnRH, gonadotropin-releasing hormone; *SC*, subcutaneously.

Key points

- Gynaecological problems are not uncommon during childhood and adolescence. Some of them can be managed by a primary care physician, but most need referral to a specialist.

- Maternal oestrogen that crosses the placenta can act on the genital organs of the neonate and cause vaginal discharge, bleeding, breast enlargement or discharge from the breast.

- During childhood, several factors such as low oestrogen levels and the resultant alkaline pH of the vagina, thin vaginal epithelium and absence of labial fat pad exposing the introitus predispose to vaginal infections.

- Labial adhesions also occur due to oestrogen deficiency and can be easily managed by local oestrogen cream and manual separation.

- Vulvovaginitis in the child is nonspecific in 75% of the cases and is due to poor hygiene, allergy or foreign body.

- Specific vulvovaginitis is secondary to respiratory or enteric infections.

- Lichen sclerosis in children affects the genital area and presents with intense pruritus, soreness, discharge and pain.

- Vaginal bleeding in children is most often due to foreign body, trauma or sexual abuse. Precocious puberty and vaginal or ovarian tumours are uncommon causes of bleeding.

- Examination under anaesthesia is required if presence of foreign body is suspected.

- Puberty is the period during which secondary sexual characteristics develop and sexual maturation occurs.

It includes gonadarche, thelarche, adrenarche and menarche. Puberty occurs between 8 and 16 years of age.

- Awakening of the hypothalamus is followed by gonadotropin-releasing hormone (GnRH) production. This acts on the pituitary and causes release of follicle-stimulating hormone (FSH), luteinizing hormone (LH), adrenocorticotrophic hormone (ACTH) and growth hormone (GH). Growth spurt is an essential component of puberty.

- Breast development is dependent on oestrogen and progesterone. Axillary and pubic hair development is dependent on adrenal androgen production.

- Disorders of puberty may be precocious puberty or delayed puberty.

- Precocious puberty can be central or peripheral. Central precocity is due to intracranial lesions, trauma, infections of central nervous system or malformations. Peripheral precocity may be due to sex hormone–secreting tumours of the ovary/adrenal gland, McCune–Albright syndrome or exogenous steroids.

- Precocious puberty can cause premature fusion of epiphyses of long bone and lead to short stature. Therefore, early diagnosis and treatment are important.

- Counselling and reassurance are essential components of treatment of precocious puberty. Central precocity is treated with GnRH analogues. Peripheral precocity is usually treated with aromatase inhibitors. Surgical intervention is required for tumours of the brain and ovary.

Self-assessment

Case-based questions

Case 1

A 5-year-old child is brought by her mother with a history of pruritus vulva. The mother also noticed vaginal discharge on the underclothes.

1. What conditions would you consider?
2. How will you proceed further with history, examination and investigations?
3. How will you manage this child?

Case 2

A 4-year-old child is brought with a history of vaginal bleeding associated with discharge.

1. How will you proceed with history taking and physical examination?
2. What diagnosis would you consider?
3. How will you manage this child?

Answers

Case 1

1. Vulvovaginitis, lichen sclerosis.
2. (a) History of dysuria, bloody discharge, pain
   (b) Use of soaps and detergents
   (c) Examination of the vulva to look for lesions of lichen planus and scratch marks
   (d) Discharge—Nature, colour, odour, purulent or not, blood-stained or not
   (e) Presence of pinworms

(f) Swab for culture if purulent
(g) Local hygiene
3. (a) Advice on hygiene, technique of washing, avoidance of chemicals, soaps and detergents
   (b) Bland nonmedicated cream
   (c) 25% hydrocortisone or 0.05% clobetasone ointment if due to allergy or lichen sclerosis
   (d) Appropriate antibiotics for bacterial/fungal infections

Case 2

1. Nature of discharge—Purulent, foul smelling, blood stained, frank blood.
     Local examination to look for discharge, bleeding.
2. Foreign body in the vagina, vaginal tumour.
3. (a) Examination under anaesthesia, removal of foreign body
   (b) Biopsy if vaginal tumour

Long-answer question

1. Discuss the physiology of puberty. What are the causes of precocious puberty? Discuss the evaluation and management of a 7-year-old girl with precocious puberty.

Short-answer questions

1. Vulvovaginitis in children
2. Causes of vaginal bleeding in childhood
3. Physiology of puberty

18 | Primary Amenorrhoea

Case scenario

Miss LM, 19 was brought to the clinic by her parents because she had not had a menstrual bleed. Parents had noticed normal growth and normal breast development that started at 10 years of age. Their elder daughter had started menstruation at age 17. Therefore, they had hoped that this girl would start menstruating sooner or later. When this had not happened till age 18, their neighbours and friends had felt that they had waited long enough. But the parents were construction workers earning daily wages and were worried about the expenses involved. But when she completed 19 years and still did not menstruate, they were worried and brought her for evaluation.

Introduction

Normal pubertal changes begin with linear growth and are followed by breast development, development of pubic and axillary hair and onset of menstruation. Delay can occur in the entire process of puberty or just the onset of menstruation. This may be a simple delay or involve a host of anatomical and physiological abnormalities. Evaluation and management of this condition is, therefore, complex and requires a multidisciplinary approach.

Definition

Primary amenorrhoea is defined as absence of menstruation by age 16 in the presence of secondary sexual characteristics and normal growth. The changes of puberty generally occur between ages 8 and 16 (*see* Chapter 17, *Paediatric and adolescent gynaecology*). Growth spurt and weight gain occur between ages 9 and 12. Breast development starts around 9 years of age followed by pubic and axillary hair growth. Menstruation starts between 12 and 13 years of age. The age at which these occur varies, but some breast development is generally seen by age 12. Absence of secondary sexual characteristics by age 14 warrants investigation or close follow-up.

Aetiology

Normal puberty depends on normal hypothalamic–pituitary–ovarian function and normally developed end organs. Causes of primary amenorrhoea are multiple and can be due to problems at different levels in this axis or other endocrinal dysfunction (Fig. 18.1; Box 18.1).

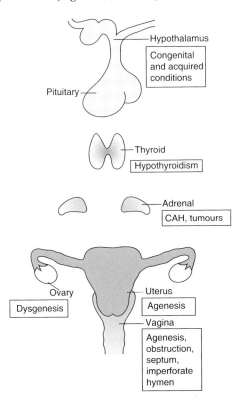

Figure 18.1 The causes of primary amenorrhoea. Abnormalities may be at any level in the hypothalamic–pituitary–ovarian axis, uterus or other endocrine function. *CAH*, congenital adrenal hyperplasia.

Clinical classification

The abnormality in primary amenorrhoea may be anatomical, endocrinological or genetic. However, a clinical classification is useful and

---

Box 18.1 Causes of primary amenorrhoea

- Hypothalamic–pituitary functioning
  - Congenital
    - Isolated GnRH deficiency
    - Multiple pituitary hormone deficiencies
  - Acquired
    - Hydrocephalus
      - Infections
      - Trauma
      - Empty sella syndrome
      - Tumours
    - Functional hypothalamic amenorrhoea
      - Anorexia nervosa
      - Exercise
      - Stress
- Ovarian dysgenesis
  - Turner syndrome and its variants
  - XX/XY gonadal agenesis
- Uterus
  - Uterovaginal agenesis
  - Menstrual outflow obstruction
- Adrenal
  - Congenital adrenal hyperplasia
    - 17α-Hydroxylase deficiency
  - Androgen-secreting tumours
- Thyroid
  - Prepubertal/juvenile hypothyroidism
- Others
  - Androgen-insensitivity syndrome
  - 5α-Reductase deficiency
  - Constitutional delay
  - Prior chemotherapy or radiotherapy

GnRH, gonadotropin-releasing hormone.

---

practical for evaluation, diagnosis and management. This is shown in Box 18.2.

Box 18.2 Clinical classification of primary amenorrhoea

Primary amenorrhoea with
- Normal secondary sexual characteristics
- Absent secondary sexual characteristics
- Heterosexual development

Primary amenorrhoea with normal secondary sexual characteristics

Presence of secondary sexual characteristics, especially breast development, is used as the criterion for categorization into this group.

- Presence of secondary sex characteristics is an evidence of normal oestrogen production indicating normal ovaries and hypothalamic–pituitary–ovarian function.
- The pathology may be in the uterus/vagina, peripheral resistance to androgens or a simple constitutional delay.
- Based on the presence or absence of uterus, the causes of amenorrhoea are listed in Box 18.3. Uterovaginal agenesis and complete androgen insensitivity are common causes of primary amenorrhoea in this category.
- When uterus is present, constitutional delay or outflow obstruction must be considered. Other conditions such as prolactinomas and polycystic ovarian syndrome (PCOS) are usually seen in older girls and more often present with secondary amenorrhoea.

Box 18.3 Primary amenorrhoea with normal secondary sexual characteristics

- Uterus absent
  - Uterovaginal agenesis
  - Complete androgen-insensitivity syndrome
- Uterus present
  - Outflow obstruction
  - Prolactinoma
  - Early-onset PCOS
  - Weight loss/anorexia
  - Constitutional delay

PCOS, polycystic ovarian syndrome.

Uterus absent

Uterovaginal agenesis

Uterovaginal agenesis, also known as Rokitansky–Mayer–Kuster–Hauser (RMKH) syndrome, is the second most common cause of primary amenorrhoea (the first being Turner syndrome). Classification of various anomalies of the Müllerian ducts has been dealt with in Chapter 2, *Development of the female genital tract: Normal and abnormal.*

- The uterus in uterovaginal agenesis is usually very rudimentary, external genitalia are those of normal female and the vagina is a dimple of about 1.5 cm. The ovaries are normal (Fig. 18.2).
- Serum follicle-stimulating hormone (FSH) is in the normal range, and clinical examination and ultrasound scan will establish the diagnosis.

- Associated renal anomalies are common and should always be looked for.

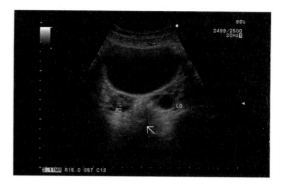

Figure 18.2 Ultrasonographic appearance in Müllerian agenesis. Both ovaries are visualized; they contain follicles. Uterus is seen as a small rudimentary structure (arrow).

Complete androgen-insensitivity syndrome

Complete androgen-insensitivity syndrome is the most important differential diagnosis when girls present with primary amenorrhoea, breast development and absent uterus.

- It is an X-linked recessive disorder and 'sisters' with the same clinical presentation are seen.
- In this condition there is an abnormality in the androgen receptors in all tissues. Due to androgen receptor insensitivity, the Wolffian structures do not develop, but Müllerian structures regress since anti-Müllerian hormone (AMH) production is normal.
- Karyotype is XY; gonad is testes. Testes may be present in the labia majora, inguinal canal or intra-abdominally. The girls have female external genitalia, but the vagina is short and blind.
- Peripheral conversion of androgen to oestrogen occurs and the oestrogen thus produced is responsible for breast development. Axillary and pubic hair are scanty or absent since the androgen receptors in the hair follicles do not respond to adrenal androgens.
- Serum testosterone levels are as in the normal male (>200 mg/mL); serum FSH is moderately elevated since the pituitary androgen receptors are not responsive to androgen.
- The chances of malignancy developing in the gonad with Y chromosome are about 20%. Therefore, surgical removal of the gonad is mandatory but can be delayed till 18 years to

permit breast development and epiphyseal closure.

Uterus present

Outflow obstruction

Obstruction to the outflow of menstrual blood leads to collection of blood in the genital tract above, a condition known as **cryptomenorrhoea**.

- This could occur due to imperforate hymen, transverse vaginal septum or absent vagina in the presence of a normal uterus (American Society of Reproductive Medicine—ASRM class I). These are discussed in Chapter 2, *Development of the female genital tract: Normal and abnormal.*
- They present with cyclic abdominal pain at puberty, which may later become persistent pain
- In girls with transverse vaginal septum and imperforate hymen, the vagina distends with blood forming a haematocolpos and pushes the uterus up into the abdomen. The collection of blood extends into the uterus and tubes forming haematometra and haematosalpinx (Fig. 18.3a and b).
- The imperforate hymen can be seen as a bluish bulging membrane at the introitus. In vaginal atresia, haematometra occurs immediately.
- Urinary retention can occur due to pressure on the urethra by the haematocolpos.
- Bilateral ovarian endometriosis can result due to prolonged retrograde menstruation. Since development of kidneys and urinary tract is closely linked to development of Müllerian ducts, anomalies of the kidneys and urinary tract are common in these girls.
- Diagnosis is by clinical examination including per rectal examination and examination under anaesthesia. Ultrasound scan can detect haematocolpos/haematometra, but MRI has been found to be an excellent tool for diagnosing the exact site and nature of anomaly. Serum FSH levels are in the normal range.

Prolactinoma

Prolactin-secreting tumours of the pituitary usually cause secondary amenorrhoea, but, occasionally, the tumour may develop prepubertally giving rise to primary amenorrhoea. This is discussed in detail in Chapter 19, *Secondary amenorrhoea and polycystic ovarian syndrome.*

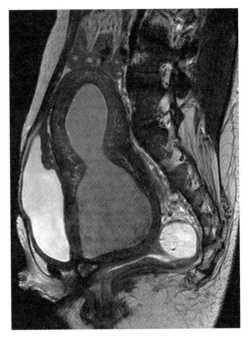

a.

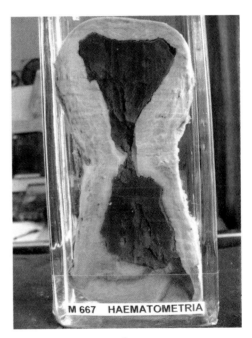

b.

Figure 18.3 Hematometra and hematocopos. a. Magnetic resonance imaging in a patient with transverse vaginal septum. Haematocolpos and haematometra are seen. b. Coronal section through a specimen of uterus and vagina. It shows haematocolpos and haematometra with brownish discolouration due to collected blood.

Early onset PCOS

Polycystic ovarian disease also usually occurs a few years after puberty and the presentation is usually with secondary amenorrhoea, but, occasionally, girls with very early onset of PCOS are seen. Management is discussed in Chapter 19, *Secondary amenorrhoea and polycystic ovarian syndrome*.

Weight loss, anorexia, stress and exercise

These can give rise to hypothalamic dysfunction. Gonadotropin-releasing hormone (GnRH) secretion is abnormal, the luteinizing hormone (LH) surges do not occur and basal level of LH may be low or normal. Follicular development and ovulation do not take place.

Constitutional delay

Normally, menarche occurs within 2 years of development of secondary sexual characteristics. In some girls, this may be delayed due to inadequate pulsatility of GnRH production. But menstruation eventually sets in. In this common disorder, maternal age at menarche is usually delayed and is a very useful clinical clue.

Primary amenorrhoea with absent secondary sexual characteristics

Primary amenorrhoea with nondevelopment of secondary sexual characteristics is usually due to endocrine or chromosomal abnormalities.

- Absence of secondary sexual characteristics indicates absence of oestrogen. This may be due to absent ovaries or unstimulated ovaries.
- Primary ovarian failure is usually due to a chromosomal defect such as Turner syndrome. Physical examination will reveal other stigmata, especially a short stature.
- Unstimulated ovaries result from defects at the hypothalamic–pituitary level.
- Hypothalamic/pituitary defects are also associated with short stature since growth hormone production and thyroid hormone axis are affected in most situations. Therefore, accurate measurement of height is important in these girls.
- Using the height percentile and standard deviation score, they are categorized into short stature and normal height (Box 18.4).

Box 18.4 Primary amenorrhoea with absent secondary sexual characteristics

- Normal height
  - Isolated GnRH deficiency
  - XX/XY gonadal dysgenesis
  - Turner mosaic
- Short stature
  - Turner syndrome
  - Hypothalamic/pituitary lesions—Congenital/acquired

GnRH, gonadotropin-releasing hormone.

Normal height

Isolated GnRH deficiency

There is no GnRH production by the hypothalamus even though the pituitary is normal. Some of these girls have associated anosmia and the condition is called **Kallman syndrome**. Growth hormone production is normal; therefore, height is normal. Serum FSH is low, but stimulation of the pituitary with GnRH yields normal FSH and LH response.

XX/XY gonadal dysgenesis

The karyotype is XX or XY, but gonads do not develop. Phenotype is female and Müllerian structures are present. They respond to exogenous oestrogen administration by withdrawal bleeding. Serum FSH is elevated, normally in the menopausal range (>40 mIU/mL). Karyotyping establishes the diagnosis.

Turner mosaic

The most common mosaicism seen in girls with primary amenorrhoea is 45X0/46XX. The physical stigmata of Turner syndrome may not be present and ovaries may contain a few follicles. Ovulation and oestrogen production are infrequent and serum FSH is elevated. Karyotyping is essential for making the diagnosis.

Short stature

Turner syndrome and its variants

This is the most common cause of primary amenorrhoea seen in clinical practice.

- The syndrome is characterized by the absence of one X chromosome (45X0). Deletions involving short or long arm of the X chromosome also occur.

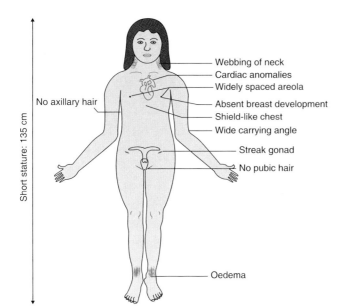

Figure 18.4 Stigmata in Turner syndrome.

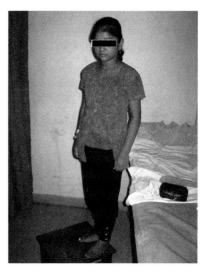

Figure 18.5 A 23-year-old girl with primary amenorrhoea due to pituitary failure. Short stature and sexual infantilism are evident.

- In Turner syndrome, the Müllerian structures are developed; although external genitalia are of a female, ovaries are represented by a band of fibrous tissue called **streak gonads**.
- Other stigmata generally seen are webbed neck, short stature, wide carrying angle, widely spaced nipples, shield chest, and disorders of the heart and kidneys.
- Secondary sexual characteristics do not develop (Fig. 18.4). Height may be normal in mosaics and other stigmata may not be present.
- Serum FSH is elevated and is normally in the menopausal range. Karyotyping is essential to exclude the presence of Y chromosome that necessitates removal of the gonad.

Hypothalamic/pituitary lesions

The lesions can be congenital or acquired.

Congenital lesions Various syndromes involving deficiency of multiple pituitary hormones are known to occur. They involve gonadotropins, growth hormones, thyroid-stimulating hormone and adrenocorticotropic hormone. Hence, the individuals are short statured, gonads are unstimulated and serum FSH levels are low (<5 mIU/mL).

Acquired lesions Neonatal and early childhood infections can lead to the hydrocephalus

and destroy the hormone-producing cells of the hypothalamus. Tumours such as craniopharyngioma, trauma to the base of skull and empty sella syndrome can present with primary amenorrhoea, sexual infantilism and short stature (Fig. 18.5).

Primary amenorrhoea with heterosexual development

A small number of girls may develop signs of virilization at the time of puberty. This could be due to

- Late-onset congenital adrenal hyperplasia
- Partial androgen insensitivity
- 5α-Reductase deficiency

Congenital adrenal hyperplasia is usually diagnosed in the neonatal period. These children have to take adequate steroid replacement for normal pubertal development to occur. The late-onset congenital adrenal hyperplasia is commonly due to 21-hydroxylase deficiency. This usually presents with secondary amenorrhoea and is discussed in Chapter 19, *Secondary amenorrhoea and polycystic ovarian syndrome*. However, the less common types with 17- and 11-hydroxylase deficiencies present with primary amenorrhoea and hypertension. Girls with

11-hydroxylase deficiency also have heterosexual development.

The other two conditions are uncommon.

Clinical evaluation

History

A detailed history and physical examination are the key to diagnosis and management. Although the list of causes is extensive, the most common conditions should be thought of first, namely constitutional delay, Turner syndrome and Müllerian anomaly, in that order. Androgen insensitivity can occur in siblings. They may also give a history of surgery for inguinal hernia in childhood. History should include all the details given in Box 18.5.

Physical examination

Physical examination should be systematic, as sequenced in Box 18.6. Pelvic examination may be inappropriate, but external genitalia can be examined and the bulging bluish membrane of imperforate hymen should be looked for. Vaginal depth can be assessed using the little finger or a metal catheter. Per rectal examination can be performed when required. This will reveal the distended vagina in cases of haematocolpos or a bulky uterus in haematometra. Examination under anaesthesia may be required in some girls with outflow obstruction. Associated renal anomalies should always be excluded in girls with Müllerian anomalies.

Box 18.5 History in primary amenorrhoea

- Age
- Growth chart, if available
- Age at onset of thelarche
- Abdominal pain
- Any disorder of smell perception
- Family history
- Siblings
- Maternal age at menarche
- Neonatal/childhood encephalitis
- Inguinal/abdominal surgery
- Prior radiotherapy/chemotherapy

Box 18.6 Physical examination in primary amenorrhoea

- Height
- Weight
- Blood pressure
- Breast development—Tanner staging
- Pubic hair and axillary hair—Tanner staging
- Arm span/upper segment and lower segment ratio
- Features of Turner syndrome
- Abdominal mass
- External genitalia
- Inguinal hernia, gonad in labia/inguinal region
- Clitoromegaly/signs of virilization
- Depth of vagina/bulging bluish membrane
- Per rectal examination

Investigations

After history and physical examination, most patients can be categorized into two groups:

- **Group 1:** Girls with normal secondary sexual characteristics
- **Group 2:** Girls without normal secondary sexual characteristics

Girls with normal secondary sexual characteristics

Girls in Group 1 need an ultrasonogram to determine the presence of uterus and rule out renal anomalies.

- If uterus is absent and ovaries are not visualized on imaging, karyotyping should be performed to exclude androgen-insensitivity syndrome.
- Ovaries with follicles may be visualized in uterovaginal agenesis. Karyotyping clinches the diagnosis.
- If uterus is present, signs of outflow obstruction should be looked for. Magnetic resonance imaging is useful in determining the exact level of obstruction.
- If there is no obstruction, estimation of serum FSH, LH and prolactin levels will help differentiate between the various conditions described in Fig. 18.6.

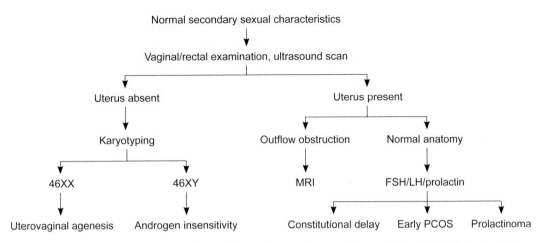

Figure 18.6 Evaluation of primary amenorrhoea with normal secondary sexual characteristics. *FSH*, follicle-stimulating hormone; *LH*, luteinizing hormone; *MRI*, magnetic resonance imaging; *PCOS*, polycystic ovarian syndrome.

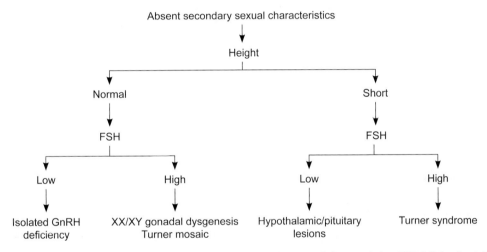

Figure 18.7 Evaluation of primary amenorrhoea with absent secondary sexual characteristics. *FSH*, follicle-stimulating hormone; *GnRH*, gonadotropin-releasing hormone.

Girls without normal secondary sexual characteristics

Height (linear growth) is an important criteria used to differentiate between various conditions in Group 2.

- Normal height indicates normal growth hormones and absence of chromosomal abnormalities causing short stature.

- Girls in Group 2 need estimation of serum FSH. If the value is >40 mIU/mL, it is indicative of ovarian failure and karyotyping is required (Fig. 18.7).

Management

Management consists of counselling, surgical intervention when required and hormone therapy. It is important to discuss the prognosis for menstrual function, sexual function and reproductive function.

Girls with no uterus should be counselled carefully since menstruation and reproduction are not possible, although sexual function can be achieved through vaginoplasty. **Those with Y chromosomes** (androgen insensitivity and XY gonadal dysgenesis) should have gonadectomy around 18 years of age allowing for breast development and epiphyseal closure.

Outflow obstruction needs surgical intervention depending on the site and nature of anomaly, as outlined in Chapter 2, *Development of the female genital tract: Normal and abnormal.*

Patients with **ovarian** and **hypothalamic/pituitary failure** should have hormone therapy to induce breast development and menstruation. It is important to start with low-dose oestrogen (20 µg ethinyl oestradiol) alone at 10–11 years and add progesterone 2 years later or after the first breakthrough bleed, whichever is earlier. The patients should be placed on long-term hormone therapy with conjugated equine oestrogen 0.625 mg and medroxyprogesterone 2.5 mg daily to prevent complications. Management is outlined in Table 18.1.

Table 18.1 Management of primary amenorrhoea

Condition	Management
Normal secondary sexual characteristics	
Outflow obstruction	Surgical treatment
Androgen insensitivity	• Gonadectomy • Hormone therapy
Prolactinoma	Medical/surgical management
PCOS	Medical management
Constitutional delay	Observation
Functional hypothalamic amenorrhoea	Lifestyle modification
Amenorrhoea	• Hormone therapy • Ovulation induction with gonadotropins
Absent secondary sexual characteristics	
Hypothalamic/pituitary lesions	• Hormone therapy • Surgery for tumours • Ovulation induction
XY gonadal dysgenesis	• Gonadectomy • Hormone therapy • ART with donor oocyte
XX gonadal dysgenesis	• Hormone therapy • ART with donor oocyte
Turner syndrome and variants	• Hormone therapy • ART with donor oocyte

ART, assisted reproductive technique; *PCOS*, polycystic ovarian syndrome.

Key points

- Primary amenorrhoea is defined as absence of menstruation by age 16. Absence of secondary sexual characteristics by age 14 warrants investigations.
- Causes of primary amenorrhoea are multiple and can be due to problems at any level in the hypothalamic–pituitary–ovarian axis or due to other endocrinal dysfunction.
- For purposes of evaluation and diagnosis, primary amenorrhoea is classified into primary amenorrhoea with (a) normal secondary sexual characteristics, (b) absent secondary sexual characteristics and (c) heterosexual development.
- Girls with secondary sexual characteristics are further classified into those with uterus and those without it. Uterovaginal agenesis and androgen-insensitivity syndrome are common disorders and have a similar clinical presentation. They are differentiated by karyotyping.
- When uterus is present, outflow obstruction or delayed puberty must be considered. Other conditions such as prolactinomas and polycystic ovarian

syndrome usually occur in older girls but can rarely present as primary amenorrhoea.
- Absence of secondary sexual characteristics indicates absent or unstimulated ovaries. Linear growth is also affected when the condition involves growth hormone production or when a chromosomal defect causing short stature is present.
- Ovaries are absent (streak gonads) in primary ovarian failure. The most common condition is Turner syndrome. Girls with this syndrome are short and have other stigmata as well.
- Thorough and detailed history and physical examination are important in arriving at a diagnosis of primary amenorrhoea and classifying it into clinical categories. Investigations can be thus minimized.
- Vaginal examination may be difficult to perform and not warranted in most girls. But rectal examination may be required.
- Investigations in primary amenorrhoea depend on the clinical categorization. Karyotyping is essential when chromosomal anomalies are suspected. Outflow

(Continued)

Key points *(Continued)*

obstruction and uterovaginal agenesis are confirmed by ultrasonography and/or MRI. Serum follicle-stimulating hormone (FSH) is elevated in ovarian failure but low in hypothalamic–pituitary failure.

- Counselling regarding menstrual, sexual and reproductive functions and possible outcome of

treatment is mandatory. Surgical intervention is required for outflow obstruction. Gonadectomy is mandatory in all patients with a Y chromosome. Girls with hypothalamic–pituitary failure, primary ovarian failure and androgen insensitivity require hormone replacement therapy.

Self-assessment

Case-based questions

Case 1

A 17-year-old girl presents with a history of primary amenorrhoea. She has no other significant history. On examination, her height is 155 cm and weight 50 kg. Her breast development is Tanner stage 4, and pubic hair and axillary hair are absent. Bilateral inguinal masses are noted.

1. What is the next step in clinical evaluation?
2. What investigations will you order?
3. If karyotype is 46XY, what is your diagnosis?
4. How will you manage?

Case 2

A 16-year-old girl is brought with a history of absent breast development and primary amenorrhoea. On examination, her height is 135 cm and there is a cardiac murmur.

1. What investigations will you order?
2. If karyotype is 45X0, what is the diagnosis and management?
3. If she wants to conceive, what advise will you give her?

Answers

Case 1

1. Examination of external genitalia and per rectal examination to ascertain the presence of uterus. Ultrasonogram to confirm it.
2. If uterus is absent, karyotyping.
3. Androgen-insensitivity syndrome.
4. (a) Gonadectomy at age 18.
   (b) Hormone therapy—Start with combined pill till axillary and pubic hair growth is achieved and later

change to Premarin 0.625 mg daily; continue till age 50.
   (c) Counselling—Need for long-term hormone therapy:
       (i) Possibility of normal sexual function
       (ii) Inability to menstruate and bear a child

Case 2

1. Serum FSH and karyotyping.
2. Diagnosis: Turner syndrome. Management:
   (a) Hormone therapy:
       (i) Starting with oestrogen and adding progesterone later
       (ii) Long-term continuous hormone therapy required
   (b) Counselling:
       (i) Need for long-term hormone treatment
       (ii) Possibility of normal sexual function
3. Assisted reproduction with donor oocyte.

Long-answer question

1. What are the causes of primary amenorrhoea? How will you evaluate a 17-year-old girl with primary amenorrhoea?

Short-answer questions

1. Cryptomenorrhoea
2. Turner syndrome
3. Aetiology of primary amenorrhoea
4. Uterovaginal agenesis
5. Androgen-insensitivity syndrome

19 | Secondary Amenorrhoea and Polycystic Ovarian Syndrome

Case scenario

Miss HA, 18, a student in a local engineering college, came to the clinic with a history of amenorrhoea for 8 months. Her menstrual cycles had become irregular in the past 2 years. She had also gained about 9 kg weight in the past 2 years and had noticed excessive hair growth on her face, arms and thighs. She was busy preparing for her examinations and attending various coaching classes during the past 2 years and had no exercise. During her spare time, she watched television and played computer games.

Introduction

Amenorrhoea or the absence of menstruation can occur after regular menstrual cycles for a few months or years. This can occur due to disorders of the hypothalamus, pituitary, ovary or the genital tract. Evaluation and management requires a clear understanding of the physiology and endocrinology of menstruation, and therefore should be by a team of endocrinologist, gynaecologist and infertility specialist.

Definition

Secondary amenorrhoea is defined as the absence of menstruation for 6 months or more in a woman with previous spontaneous regular cycles or a period equal to the duration of three cycles if previous cycles are irregular.

Consequences of secondary amenorrhoea

Although the absence of menstruation may not lead to any harm in the short term, the associated or causative problems can have undesirable consequences (Box 19.1).

Causes of secondary amenorrhoea

Physiological conditions

Secondary amenorrhoea can be physiological in the following situations:

- Pregnancy
- Lactation
- Menopause

Pregnancy must be ruled out in all women of reproductive age with secondary amenorrhoea before considering pathological causes.

> **Box 19.1 Consequences of secondary amenorrhoea**
>
> - Psychological
>   - Anxiety
>   - Altered self-image
>   - Loss of self-esteem
> - Possible decrease in fertility
> - Hypo-oestrogenism
>   - Short term
>   - Hot flashes
>   - Night sweats
>   - Vaginal dryness
>   - Dyspareunia
>   - Urinary symptoms
>   - Long term
>   - Osteoporosis
>   - Coronary heart disease
> - Hyperoestrogenism
>   - Endometrial hyperplasia
>   - Increased risk of endometrial carcinoma
> - Hyperinsulinaemia/insulin resistance
>   - Metabolic syndrome
> - Hirsutism

Pathological conditions

Normal menstrual cycle indicates normal functioning of the complex hypothalamic–pituitary–ovarian axis and normal uterus. Abnormality at any level in this axis or uterus can cause amenorrhoea. Systemic diseases such as liver disease and chronic debilitating illnesses, obesity and acute weight loss and some drugs can also cause amenorrhoea. Causes of secondary amenorrhoea are listed in Box 19.2 and diagrammatically represented in Fig. 19.1.

Hypothalamic causes

Hypothalamic conditions account for nearly 30% of all causes of secondary amenorrhoea. These are listed in Box 19.3.

Functional hypothalamic amenorrhoea

In this disorder, there is a decrease in gonadotropin-releasing hormone (GnRH) secretion, leading to decreased pulsatile secretion of luteinizing hormone (LH), absence of midcycle surge and

> **Box 19.2 Pathological causes of secondary amenorrhoea**
>
> - Hypothalamic
> - Pituitary
> - Ovarian
> - Uterine
> - Other endocrinopathies
>   - NCCAH
>   - Hypothyroidism
>   - Cushing syndrome

NCCAH, nonclassic congenital adrenal hyperplasia.

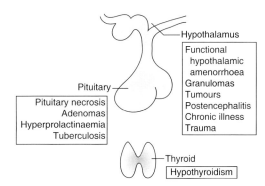
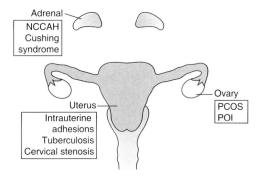

Figure 19.1 Diagrammatic representation of the causes of secondary amenorrhoea at various levels. *NCCAH*, nonclassic congenital adrenal hyperplasia; *PCOS*, polycystic ovarian syndrome; *POI*, primary ovarian insufficiency.

anovulation. Serum follicle-stimulating hormone (FSH) levels are low or normal.

- This can be caused by emotional stress, weight loss and vigorous exercise. Chronic illnesses that are associated with weight loss and renal or liver dysfunction also lead to a hypogonadotropic state acting through the hypothalamus.

- Functional hypothalamic amenorrhoea
  - Stress
  - Weight loss
  - Weight gain
  - Athletic amenorrhoea
  - Genetic
- Granulomas
  - Tuberculosis
  - Sarcoidosis
- Tumours
- Postencephalitis
- Chronic illness
- Trauma

- **Vigorous exercise** causes release of catechol oestrogens and endogenous opioids, which act on the hypothalamus to suppress GnRH production.
- **Weight loss** of more than 10–15% of ideal body weight is associated with amenorrhoea. There is a pathological condition called **anorexia nervosa**, which is usually seen in teenage girls. It is an extreme form of eating disorder and leads to severe weight loss and amenorrhoea.
- **Obesity** is a common cause of secondary amenorrhoea. Obese women convert the androgens to oestrone, and this causes a chronic hyperoestrogenic state. Leptins produced by the fat cells also inhibit GnRH secretion by the hypothalamus. This leads to a situation of chronic anovulation and amenorrhoea. The condition can be mistaken for polycystic ovarian syndrome (PCOS). Features of hypothalamic amenorrhoea are summarized in Box 19.4.

Other hypothalamic causes

Granulomatous lesions such as tuberculosis and sarcoidosis, tumours of the hypothalamus, chronic illnesses, sequelae of encephalitis and trauma lead to hypothalamic dysfunction and low levels of GnRH and gonadotropins. Circulating oestrogen level is also low; therefore, there is no bleeding with progesterone administration.

Pituitary causes

Disorders of the pituitary contribute to about 15–20% cases of secondary amenorrhoea (Box 19.5).

- Most often due to change in weight or stress
- Lack of LH pulsatility and midcycle surge
- No ovulation
- Low oestrogen levels
- No withdrawal bleeding with progesterone

LH, luteinizing hormone.

- Pituitary necrosis
  - Sheehan syndrome
- Tuberculosis
- Tumours
  - Pituitary adenomas
- Hyperprolactinaemia
  - Microadenoma
  - Macroadenoma

Pituitary necrosis—Sheehan syndrome

Pituitary necrosis occurs most often following postpartum haemorrhage (PPH) and the resulting hypotension. This condition is known as **Sheehan syndrome**.

- These patients can have panhypopituitarism involving thyroid and adrenal glands as well.
- Most often, patients present several years after PPH with recurrent episodes of vomiting and hypotension requiring hospitalization and intravenous (IV) fluids and unless specifically questioned may not even mention the PPH that occurred years ago.
- There is a history of failure to lactate, weight loss, breast atrophy, depigmentation of the areolae, hypotension and symptoms of hypothyroidism.
- Levels of thyroid-stimulating hormone (TSH), plasma cortisol, prolactin, FSH and LH are low, and there is no response to progesterone challenge.

Infiltrative lesions of the pituitary and **tuberculosis** are also causes of gonadotropin deficiency.

Pituitary adenomas are not always associated with hyperprolactinaemia but can cause gonadotropin deficiency and amenorrhoea. Other features of excess growth hormone or Cushing disease are generally associated.

Hyperprolactinaemia

Hyperprolactinaemia usually presents with amenorrhoea and galactorrhoea, although galactorrhoea may be absent in some. Prolactin secretion is under the inhibitory control by the hypothalamus through dopamine. Serotonin and thyrotropin-releasing hormone are the stimulators of prolactin. Hyperprolactinaemia is associated with reduction in GnRH and gonadotropin production through direct effect on the hypothalamus and pituitary. Secondary to gonadotropin deficiency, oestrogen levels are low and patients generally do not have withdrawal bleeding with progesterone. It should be remembered that values up to 25 ng/mL are normal in women of reproductive age.

- Hyperprolactinaemia can be caused by physiological, pharmacological and pathological conditions (Box 19.6).
- History of drugs that cause hyperprolactinaemia and serum TSH to exclude hypothyroidism are the first steps in evaluation of hyperprolactinaemia.
- If TSH is elevated and primary hypothyroidism is diagnosed, no further tests are necessary and thyroxine therapy can be instituted.
- If hypothyroidism has been excluded, a serum prolactin level of >200 ng/mL is indicative of prolactinomas. Prolactin levels between 25 and 75 ng/mL indicate functional hyperprolactinaemia or drug-induced hyperprolactinaemia. Levels between 75 and 200 ng/mL may be due to microprolactinoma, stalk compression by nonfunctional pituitary tumours or drugs.
- If visual fields are normal, a patient with prolactin >200 ng/mL can be started on treatment with dopamine agonists without any further tests. If visual field defects are present on perimetry, imaging of the pituitary with CT scan/MRI is required to determine the size and extent of the tumour (Fig. 19.2).
- If prolactin levels are between 75 and 200 ng/mL and the patient is on drugs that cause the increase, the patient may be reassured. If pituitary microprolactinoma or other tumours are suspected, further imaging and treatment are warranted.

The characteristic features of pituitary amenorrhoea are listed in Box 19.7.

Ovarian causes

Disorders of the ovary or ovarian failure result in insufficient oestrogen and/or progesterone

---

Box 19.6 Causes of hyperprolactinaemia

- Physiological conditions
  - Stress
  - Pregnancy
  - Lactation
  - Irritative lesions of the chest wall
- Drugs
  - Antihypertensives
    - α-Methyldopa
    - Verapamil
    - Reserpine
  - Antipsychotics
    - Phenothiazines
    - Haloperidol, risperidone
    - Tricyclic antidepressants
  - Dopamine receptor antagonists
    - Metoclopramide
  - Antiemetics
- Pathological conditions
  - Hypothyroidism
  - Prolactinomas
    - Microadenoma
    - Macroadenoma
  - Hypothalamic pituitary tumours

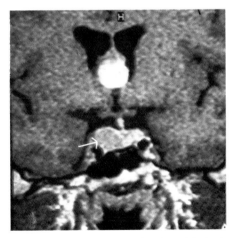

Figure 19.2 Magnetic resonance imaging of the brain showing prolactinomas (arrow). The pituitary stalk is seen deviated to the left and the tumour is on the right side of the gland.

production to cause cyclic changes in the endometrium. This can lead to secondary amenorrhoea (Box 19.8). Ovarian disorders are the most common causes of secondary amenorrhoea.

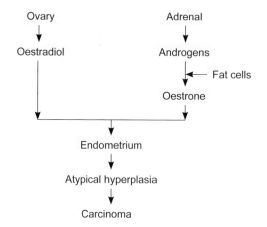

Figure 19.6 Endometrial changes in polycystic ovarian syndrome.

should be evaluated for this and advised preventive and therapeutic measures.

Diagnostic criteria for PCOS

Several professional groups have proposed different diagnostic criteria for PCOS. However, the American Society for Reproductive Medicine/European Society of Human Reproduction and Embryology (ASRM/ESHRE) consensus group opinion (Rotterdam, 2003) criteria for diagnosis of PCOS have been accepted now. These criteria are shown in Box 19.12.

Box 19.12 Rotterdam criteria for diagnosis of PCOS

Any two out of the following three:
- Oligo-ovulation and/or anovulation
- Hyperandrogenism (clinical and/or biochemical)
- Polycystic ovaries (by ultrasonography)

PCOS, polycystic ovarian syndrome.

The criteria for ultrasound diagnosis of polycystic ovaries are as in Box 19.13 and Fig. 19.7. The ovaries appear enlarged and pearly white with multiple follicles at laparoscopy (Fig. 19.8).

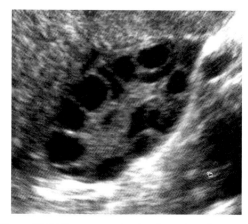

Figure 19.7 Ultrasonography showing polycystic ovary. Multiple follicles arranged along the ovarian cortex, 'the necklace sign'.

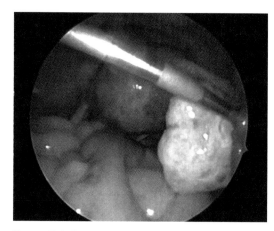

Figure 19.8 Polycystic ovary visualized through laparoscope. The right ovary is enlarged and pearly white, and has multiple follicles.

Box 19.13 Ovarian morphology on ultrasound

- Twelve or more follicles
- Each follicle 2–9 mm in diameter
- Ovarian volume >10 cm³

Diagnosis of PCOS

Initial evaluation is by history and physical examination.

A clinical diagnosis of PCOS can be made with reasonable certainty in women with obesity, menstrual irregularity (fewer than eight menstrual cycles per year or cycle length >35 days), oligo-ovulation and clinical signs of androgen excess with or without infertility. Ultrasonography and further investigations are not necessary.

There is no consensus regarding investigations for diagnosis of PCOS.

• Although the Rotterdam diagnostic criteria have been agreed upon, the ultrasonographic diagnosis requires experienced sonologist and the diagnostic criteria must be strictly adhered to. Moreover, these ultrasonographic features are found in 20% of normal adults.
• Serum LH:FSH ratio is not useful since only 50% of women with PCOS have elevated LH.
• In women with hirsutism, serum free testosterone can help to differentiate between PCOS and other conditions such as androgen-producing tumours. However, it is not a diagnostic test for PCOS.
• Insulin resistance, abnormal plasma glucose levels and dyslipidaemia are metabolic effects and not diagnostic tests.
• Serum prolactin and TSH levels should be measured in obese women.

Primary ovarian insufficiency

This condition was formerly known as premature ovarian failure and premature menopause. **Primary ovarian insufficiency (POI) is defined as ovarian failure with high FSH levels, occurring before 40 years of age.**

In this condition, the patient presents with secondary amenorrhoea and the ovaries have no oocytes; there is no folliculogenesis or ovarian hormone production. Serum FSH levels rise due to lack of negative feedback by oestrogens. Some women may have intermittent LH surges and ovulation.

There are two major categories of POI:

• POI associated with follicle depletion
• POI with no follicle depletion

POI with follicle depletion

Causes of POI with follicle depletion are given as follows:

• Chromosomal disorders such as fragile X syndrome or partial deletion of X chromosome or other somatic chromosomal defects.

• Autoimmune ovarian destruction associated with lymphocytic infiltration of ovaries. Autoimmune failure can also be part of polyglandular failure, involving the pancreatic islets, thyroid, parathyroid and adrenal glands.
• Following chemotherapy with ovariotoxic drugs, especially alkylating agents such as cyclophosphamide, or following radiotherapy to the abdomen and pelvis.

Women with POI present with symptoms of hypo-oestrogenism and are prone to all the long-term problems of menopause such as osteoporosis and coronary heart disease. The endometrium is atrophic and does not bleed with administration of progesterone.

Diagnosis is by elevated levels of serum FSH (>40 mIU/L) in a woman with secondary amenorrhoea or infrequent menstruation. Evaluation should include tests for other endocrine deficiencies and karyotyping.

Occasional ovulation can occur; pregnancies have been reported. This must be borne in mind while counselling these women.

POI without follicular depletion

Formerly known as resistant ovary, this condition is characterized by amenorrhoea and ovaries with follicles that do not develop under FSH stimulation. The defect may be in FSH receptors, oestradiol precursor production or aromatase function. Clinical presentation is similar to POI with follicular depletion; FSH levels are high. Ovarian biopsy is diagnostic but is not recommended as a routine since it does not contribute to the management.

The salient features of amenorrhoea due to ovarian causes are summarized in Box 19.14.

Box 19.14 Features of amenorrhoea due to ovarian causes

• PCOS is the most common
  – Diagnosis is clinical
  – Withdrawal bleeding with progesterone positive
• POI is most often autoimmune
  – Elevated FSH
  – No withdrawal bleeding with progesterone

FSH, follicle-stimulating hormone; *PCOS*, polycystic ovarian syndrome; *POI*, primary ovarian insufficiency.

Uterine causes

Secondary amenorrhoea can be due to damage to the endometrium (Box 19.15).

- Intrauterine adhesions
- Tuberculosis
- Cervical stenosis

Intrauterine adhesion (Asherman syndrome) is caused by vigorous curettage postpartum or after an abortion. The **basal layer** of the endometrium is scraped off, and adhesions form in the uterine cavity.

Genital tuberculosis can also cause amenorrhoea. This is dealt with in Chapter 14, *Tuberculosis of the female genital tract*.

Cervical stenosis that occurs following operations such as cone biopsy, cervical amputation and Fothergill surgery can cause obstruction to the menstrual flow and amenorrhoea associated with abdominal pain. The hormone levels are normal, but there is no withdrawal bleeding with progesterone.

Salient features of amenorrhoea due to uterine causes are listed in Box 19.16.

Box 19.16 Salient features of uterine causes of secondary amenorrhoea

- Intrauterine adhesions—The most common
- Normal FSH/LH
- No withdrawal bleeding with progesterone

FSH, follicle-stimulating hormone; *LH*, luteinizing hormone.

Thyroid and adrenal endocrinopathies

Endocrinopathies involving thyroid, adrenal and other glands can cause amenorrhoea (Box 19.17).

Box 19.17 Thyroid and adrenal
           endocrinopathies causing
           secondary amenorrhoea

- Hypothyroidism
- Cushing disease
- NCCAH

NCCAH, nonclassic congenital adrenal hyperplasia.

Hypothyroidism with elevated TSH causes hyperprolactinaemia and amenorrhoea. Dry skin, puffiness of face, pedal oedema, pallor and slow-relaxing ankle jerks are important clues to the diagnosis.

Cushing disease can be secondary to overproduction of adrenocorticotropic hormone (ACTH) by the pituitary or primary abnormality in the adrenal gland. In pituitary ACTH-dependent Cushing disease, the elevated ACTH causes hyperpigmentation of skin and stimulates adrenal androgen production as well and causes hirsutism. The excess cortisol production from the adrenal causes suppression of GnRH and gonadotropins causing secondary amenorrhoea. Other clinical features of Cushing disease such as truncal obesity, nuchal fat pads, purple abdominal striae, hypertension, proximal muscle weakness and osteoporosis are usually seen (Fig. 19.9). In early stages, Cushing disease can closely resemble PCOS and is, therefore, an important differential diagnosis for PCOS.

Congenital adrenal hyperplasia (CAH) due to 21-hydroxylase deficiency occurs in the classic form in the neonate and nonclassic or milder form in the adult. The classic form presents with ambiguous genitalia and electrolyte imbalance. The nonclassic congenital adrenal hyperplasia (NCCAH) manifests at puberty. Clinical spectrum is varied and hyperandrogenism can cause hirsutism alone or mild virilization in addition. Serum levels of 17α-hydroxyprogesterone and dehydroepiandrosterone (DHEA) are elevated. This is discussed further in Chapter 20, *Hirsutism and virilization.*

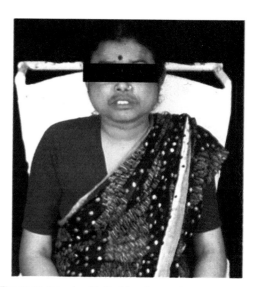

Figure 19.9 Lady with Cushing disease. Note the moon facies and obesity.

Clinical evaluation

History

Thorough history and clinical examination are mandatory before ordering investigations. Important details in history are listed in Box 19.18.

Box 19.18 History taking in secondary amenorrhoea

- Age
- Parity
- Menstrual history
  - Duration of amenorrhoea
  - Prior irregular/regular cycles
- History of recent loss/gain in weight
- Tuberculosis
- Obstetric history
  - Postpartum haemorrhage
  - Curettage
  - Lactation
- Galactorrhoea
- Symptoms of menopause
  - Hot flushes
  - Mood changes
  - Sleep disturbances
  - Vaginal dryness
- Endocrinopathies
  - Symptoms of thyroid, adrenal disease
- Family history
  - Autoimmune diseases
  - Obesity
  - Diabetes mellitus
- History of medications
- History of radiotherapy
- History of chemotherapy

Physical examination

History should be followed by physical examination (Box 19.19).

Further evaluation

Further evaluation should be performed in a stepwise manner.

- The possibility of pregnancy must be kept in mind in all women presenting with secondary amenorrhoea. This has to be ruled out by a urine pregnancy test or serum β-human chorionic gonadotropin (hCG) test.

Box 19.19 Physical examination in secondary amenorrhoea

- Height, weight, body mass index
- Blood pressure
- Signs of hyperandrogenism
  - Acne
  - Hirsutism
  - Virilization
  - Alopecia
- Signs of insulin resistance
  - Acanthosis nigricans
- Breast examination
  - Galactorrhoea
  - Atrophy
- Thyroid enlargement
- Features of thyroid/adrenal disease
- Pelvic examination
  - Signs of oestrogen deficiency
  - Cervical stenosis
  - Size of uterus

- If the pregnancy test is negative, the next step is measurement of serum FSH, LH, prolactin and TSH.
- Assessment of oestrogen status may be by estimation of serum oestradiol levels or progesterone challenge test.
- **Progesterone challenge test** is performed using any of the preparations given in Box 19.20. This helps to detect endogenous oestrogen production, which primes the endometrium and makes it respond to progesterone by withdrawal bleeding. Withdrawal bleeding can occur 2–10 days after completing the dose. The test is especially useful in low-resource settings where hormonal evaluation is expensive and/or unavailable. Positive test indicates the presence of oestrogen.

Box 19.20 Progesterone challenge test

- Medroxyprogesterone acetate 10 mg for 7–10 days
- Norethisterone 5 mg for 7–10 days
- Micronized progesterone 400 mg oral for 7–10 days

- Normal FSH, TSH and prolactin levels and positive progesterone challenge test are indicative of PCOS, or late-onset 21-OH deficiency. LH may be moderately elevated in PCOS.
- Normal TSH, prolactin and normal or low-normal FSH and LH and negative progesterone challenge test indicate hypothalamic

disorder. They should be evaluated further by magnetic resonance imaging and other tests.

- Low FSH, LH, prolactin and TSH and negative response to progesterone challenge indicate pituitary failure, most often due to necrosis.
- High serum FSH indicates POI. Progesterone challenge test is usually negative. Karyotyping and tests to exclude polyglandular failure should be performed.
- High serum prolactin indicates hyperprolactinaemia. If levels are >200 ng/mL (tumour range), MRI of the pituitary is the next step. If levels are lower, other causes such as drugs, thyroid dysfunction and microprolactinomas must be excluded.
- Elevated TSH occurs in hypothyroidism.
- If all hormonal levels are normal, progesterone challenge test is negative and there is a history of uterine curettage, tuberculosis or surgery, uterine causes must be suspected. Oestrogen–progesterone challenge test can be performed in these women.

Oestrogen–progesterone challenge test The endometrium is primed with oestrogen (ethinyl oestradiol 10 μg daily or conjugated equine oestrogen 1.25 mg daily) for 2 weeks and progesterone added during the third week. Bleeding is expected to occur within a week after stopping the hormones. Failure to bleed indicates endometrial pathology such as Asherman syndrome or tuberculosis.

Endocrine workup is required to make a diagnosis at this stage (Fig. 19.10).

Management

Management consists of

- Counselling
- Treatment of the underlying cause
- Achieving fertility
- Prevention of long-term complications
- Counselling is the first and most important step in the management. Some of the pathological conditions cannot be cured and resumption of spontaneous menstruation or achieving fertility is not possible. Some conditions such as PCOS and hypo-oestrogenic amenorrhoea are associated with long-term complications and require long-term preventive therapy. These should be discussed in detail with the patient.
- Treatment is mostly medical, although surgical intervention is occasionally required. Medical

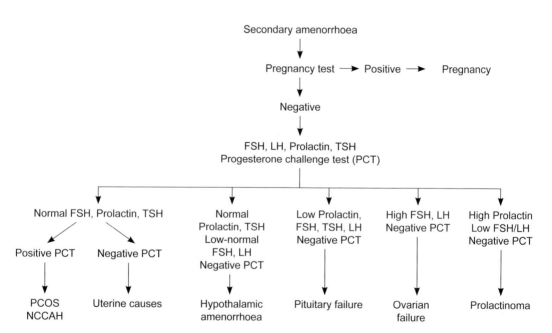

Figure 19.10 Evaluation of secondary amenorrhoea. *FSH*, follicle-stimulating hormone; *LH*, luteinizing hormone; *LOCAH*, late-onset congenital adrenal hyperplasia; *PCOS*, polycystic ovarian syndrome; *POI*, primary ovarian insufficiency; *TSH*, thyroid-stimulating hormone.

treatment of hirsutism and infertility associated with PCOS is dealt with in Chapter 20, *Hirsutism and virilization*, and Chapter 22, *Infertility*.

- Women with hypothalamic amenorrhoea need psychotherapy, weight optimization and lifestyle modification. Oral contraceptive (OC) pills can be tried for re-establishing menstrual cycles but may not be effective. These women are prone to osteoporosis: therefore, calcium and vitamin D supplementation is required.
- Pituitary necrosis results in deficiency of gonadotropins, TSH and ACTH. The patients require thyroxin and steroid replacement in addition to OC pills. Calcium and vitamin D supplementation is mandatory.
- The first step in management of hyperprolactinaemia is to discontinue drugs that increase prolactin levels and treat hypothyroidism, if present. Both macroprolactinoma and microadenoma are treated initially with dopamine agonists—Bromocriptine or cabergoline. Bromocriptine is used in doses of 1.25–2.5 mg daily and is less effective in decreasing prolactin levels. Dose of cabergoline is 0.25–0.5 mg once a week. Transsphenoidal surgery is indicated only when there is no response to treatment or in giant macroadenomas.
- Management of PCOS is complex. Treatment depends on the patient's age, clinical features and desire for pregnancy. Lifestyle modification and weight optimization are mandatory for all women with PCOS to prevent long-term complications.
  - Adolescents with menstrual irregularity are treated with OC pills or progestin alone, given for 7–10 days every month. Management of hirsutism is discussed in Chapter 20, *Hirsutism and virilization*. Insulin resistance and abnormal glucose tolerance are indications for metformin.
  - Women in the reproductive years may, in addition, require treatment for infertility. Ovulation induction by clomiphene with or without metformin is required. This is discussed further in Chapter 22, *Infertility*. Even after completion of family, progestins for 7–10 days once a month or alternate months is advisable to prevent endometrial hyperplasia and carcinoma.
- Treatment of POI is with OC pills that should be continued till age 50. Polyglandular failure requires replacement of other hormones as well. Calcium and vitamin D supplementation is essential.

- Intrauterine adhesions (Asherman syndrome) are diagnosed by hysteroscopy or hysterosalpingography. The adhesions can be broken down by hysteroscopic resection. An intrauterine device can be inserted following this and OC pills administered for three to six cycles to prevent reformation of adhesions.
- Cervical stenosis should be managed by dilatation of cervix.

Management of secondary amenorrhoea is summarized in Table 19.2.

Table 19.2 Management of secondary amenorrhoea

Diagnosis	Management
Hypothalamic amenorrhoea	• Lifestyle modification • Weight optimization • OC pills • Calcium/vitamin D supplementation • Gonadotropin therapy for infertility • Surgery for tumours
Pituitary causes	
Pituitary necrosis	• OC pills, other hormones as required • Calcium/vitamin D supplementation
Tumours	Surgery/radiation
Hyperprolactinaemia	• Cabergoline/bromocriptine • Rarely surgery
Tuberculosis	• Anti-TB treatment • OC pills/other hormones
Ovarian causes	
PCOS	• Lifestyle modification • OC pills for menstrual irregularity • Metformin for glucose intolerance • Ovulation induction • Antiandrogens for hirsutism
POI	• OC pills • Calcium/vitamin D supplementation
Uterine causes	
Intrauterine adhesions	• Hysteroscopic adhesiolysis • OC pills
Tuberculosis	Anti-TB treatment
Cervical stenosis	Surgical intervention
Other causes	
NCCAH	• Dexamethasone • OC pills/antiandrogens
Hypothyroidism	Eltroxin

NCCAH, nonclassic congenital adrenal hyperplasia; *OC*, oral contraceptive; *PCOS*, polycystic ovarian syndrome; *POI*, primary ovarian insufficiency; *TB*, tuberculosis.

Key points

- Secondary amenorrhoea is defined as the absence of menstruation for 6 months or more in a woman with previous regular cycles or a period equal to the duration of three cycles if previous cycles were irregular.
- Secondary amenorrhoea is associated with psychological consequences, decrease in fertility, short- and long-term effects of hypo-oestrogenism and long-term effects of hyperoestrogenism.
- Secondary amenorrhoea may be due to abnormalities at the level of the hypothalamus, pituitary, ovary, uterus or other endocrinopathies.
- Hypothalamic amenorrhoea is most often functional, due to change in weight or stress. Gonadotropin and oestrogen levels are low and there is no withdrawal bleeding with progesterone.
- Pituitary necrosis, pituitary adenomas, tuberculosis (TB) and hyperprolactinaemia are the common pituitary causes of secondary amenorrhoea.
- Hyperprolactinaemia usually presents with amenorrhoea and galactorrhoea. It may be due to usage of medications, hypothyroidism or prolactinomas.
- Pituitary amenorrhoea is associated with low gonadotropin and oestrogen levels and there is no withdrawal bleeding with progesterone.
- Ovarian causes of secondary amenorrhoea are polycystic ovarian syndrome (PCOS) and primary ovarian insufficiency (POI). PCOS is the most common condition.
- As per the American Society for Reproductive Medicine (ASRM) criteria, PCOS is diagnosed when any two of the following three criteria are present: (a) oligo-ovulation and/or anovulation; (b) hyperandrogenism; (c) polycystic ovaries.
- Definite criteria for diagnosis of polycystic ovaries on ultrasonography have been laid down.
- Clinical features of PCOS include menstrual irregularities, infertility, obesity, signs of hyperandrogenism and acanthosis nigricans. Several endocrinological abnormalities may be present.
- Metabolic syndrome, endometrial cancer and breast cancer are the known consequences of PCOS.
- Amenorrhoea due to ovarian causes is associated with elevated follicle-stimulating hormone (FSH) or luteinizing hormone (LH)/FSH ratio. Withdrawal bleeding with progesterone is present in PCOS but absent in POI.
- Uterine causes of secondary amenorrhoea include intrauterine adhesions (Asherman syndrome), TB and cervical stenosis. Serum gonadotropin levels are normal and there is no withdrawal bleeding with progesterones.
- Detailed history and physical examination are mandatory in the evaluation of women with secondary amenorrhoea.
- Subsequent evaluation is by serum FSH, LH, prolactin and thyroid-stimulating hormone (TSH) levels. Oestrogen status may be assessed by progesterone challenge test.
- Based on the levels of these tests, a diagnosis can be arrived at, further targeted investigations performed and treatment planned.
- Treatment is mostly medical. All women with obesity, PCOS and anorexia require lifestyle changes and weight optimization.
- Women with hypo-oestrogenism must receive combination oral contraceptive (OC) pills till age 50 and calcium and vitamin D supplementation to prevent long-term complications.

Self-assessment

Case-based questions

Case 1

A 35-year-old lady, mother of three children, presents with a history of secondary amenorrhoea since last delivery, lethargy and generalized weakness.

1. What specific details will you ask for in history?
2. What will you look for on clinical examination?
3. What is the next step in evaluation?
4. If progesterone challenge test is negative, what investigations will you order?

5. If FSH and LH are <5 mIU/mL, what is your diagnosis? How will you manage?

Case 2

An 18-year-old college student with a history of irregular cycles since menarche presents with amenorrhoea of 8 months' duration. Her height is 162 cm; weight is 75 kg.

1. What will you look for on clinical examination?
2. If she has withdrawal bleeding with progesterone, what is the probable diagnosis?
3. What investigations will you order?

4. What do you expect the results of investigations to be?
5. What is the management?

Answers

Case 1

1. Postpartum haemorrhage, lactation, symptoms of hypothyroidism and adrenal deficiency.
2. Body mass index, blood pressure, breast atrophy.
3. Progesterone challenge test.
4. Serum FSH, LH, thyroid function test, TSH, plasma cortisol.
5. Diagnosis: Sheehan syndrome—Amenorrhoea since delivery, symptoms of deficiency of other pituitary hormones, low FSH and LH.
   Management:
   (a) Hormone replacement therapy
   (b) Thyroxine, if required
   (c) Hydrocortisone, if required
   (d) Calcium supplements

Case 2

1. Blood pressure, hirsutism, acanthosis nigricans, galactorrhoea, signs of virilization such as clitoromegaly.
2. PCOS.
3. Serum FSH, LH, prolactin, TSH, pelvic ultrasonography.
4. (a) Elevated LH/FSH ratio
   (b) Mildly elevated prolactin
   (c) Normal TSH
   (d) Polycystic ovaries
5. (a) Weight reduction
   (b) Combination pill to regularize cycles
   (c) Spironolactone or cyproterone for hirsutism
   (d) Long-term follow-up for metabolic syndrome

Long-answer question

1. What are the causes of secondary amenorrhoea? How will you evaluate a 17-year-old girl with secondary amenorrhoea?

Short-answer questions

1. Sheehan syndrome
2. Clinical features and diagnosis of PCOS
3. Primary ovarian insufficiency
4. Progesterone challenge test

20 | Hirsutism and Virilization

Case scenario

Miss BL, 18, an engineering student, was brought by her mother with a history of increased hair growth on the face, arms and thighs. She had gained about 12 kg of weight after moving to the hostel 2 years earlier. Her menstrual cycles had become more and more delayed and her last menstrual period was 4 months ago. The increase in facial hair had become an embarrassment and she had to shave once every 5 or 6 days. Her friends had been passing comments about her weight and facial hair due to which Miss BL had become withdrawn, depressed and homebound. Her parents were concerned about her menstrual irregularity and its effects on her reproductive function.

Introduction

Hirsutism and virilization are signs of hyperandrogenism. The pathophysiology of hyperandrogenism is complex. In addition to hirsutism and virilization, there may be other subtle manifestations such as acne, alopecia and oily skin. Clinically obvious features of hyperandrogenism have a marked psychological impact on the patient and need a team approach by the gynaecologist, endocrinologist, dermatologist and cosmetologist.

Definitions

Hirsutism is defined as excessive growth of terminal hair in a male distribution in women. It specifically refers to growth of midline hair over the upper lip, chin, hair on the chest, abdomen, back, linea alba, inner thighs and upper limbs (Fig. 20.1a–c). In women, these areas normally do not have terminal hair.

Isolated hirsutism is usually gradual in onset and is due to mild increase in circulating androgen or increased sensitivity of pilosebaceous units to androgen. Menstrual irregularity and amenorrhoea are common in women with hirsutism, but they may have regular menstrual cycles (Box 20.1). Serum total testosterone levels are normal or only mildly elevated, usually <1.5 ng/mL. If there is no associated virilization, underlying ovarian or adrenal neoplasm is unlikely.

Box 20.1 Hirsutism

- Excessive growth of terminal hair
- Male pattern
- Mild hyperandrogenism
- Normal/mild-to-moderate elevation of testosterone (<1.5 ng/mL)
- Gradual onset
- Associated menstrual irregularity may or may not be present
- Not caused by neoplasm

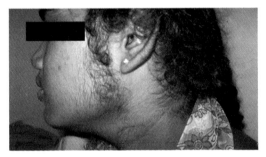

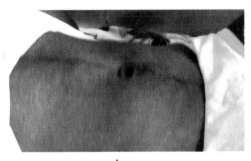

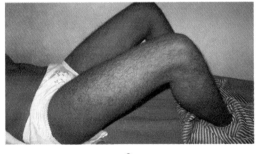

Figure 20.1 Hirsutism. a. Increased facial hair. b. Increased abdominal hair. c. Increased hair on thighs and legs.

Virilization is defined as the presence of signs of masculinization in women. These include, in addition to hirsutism, breast atrophy,

deepening of voice, temporal balding, clitoromegaly, increased libido and increased muscle mass (Box 20.2; Fig. 20.2a–c). Virilization results from a more severe form of hyperandrogenism,

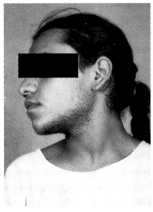

a.

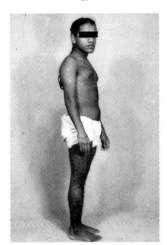

b.

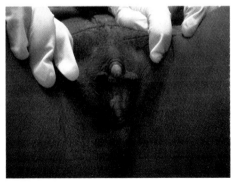

c.

Figure 20.2 An 18-year-old girl with virilization shows (a) increased facial hair with frontal balding; (b) breast atrophy and increased muscle mass; (c) clitoromegaly.

and it usually develops rapidly. Women with virilization are usually amenorrhoeic, serum testosterone levels are elevated to >2 ng/mL and underlying ovarian/adrenal neoplasm should always be suspected.

Box 20.2 Virilization

- Signs of masculinization
- Uncommon
- Rapid development
- Marked hyperandrogenism
- Elevated testosterone levels (>2 ng/mL)
- Associated with amenorrhoea
- Always rule out neoplasma

Hypertrichosis refers to increase in androgen-independent terminal hair over trunk and limbs. The condition may be familial or due to some drugs such as phenytoin sodium.

Other clinical signs of hyperandrogenism The pilosebaceous unit is sensitive to androgens. Increase in androgen level can give rise to other clinical manifestations, as shown in Box 20.3.

Box 20.3 Other clinical signs of hyperandrogenism

- Acne
- Oily skin
- Alopecia involving scalp hair

Pathophysiology of hair growth

Adult body hair are of three types:

1. *Vellus hair:* Fine hair that covers most of the body
2. *Terminal hair:* Dark, thick hair that grows in certain parts of the body
3. *Sexual hair:* Terminal hair that is sensitive to androgens, located in the midline of the body such as lip, chin, back, chest, pubic area, thighs, arms and also axilla
- Normal levels of androgens stimulate the growth and pigmentation of sexual hair.
- Higher levels of androgens convert vellus hair into terminal sexual hair, causing hirsutism.
- High androgen levels can cause conversion of the terminal scalp hair into vellus hair, leading to alopecia and frontal balding.

Hair growth cycle

This consists of three phases as in Box 20.4. The duration of each phase is variable depending on the site, age, and genetic and hormonal factors. It may extend from few weeks to few months.

Box 20.4 Hair growth cycle

- Anagen phase: Active growing phase
- Catagen phase: Rapid involution phase
- Telogen phase: Resting phase

Physiology of androgens

Androgens are produced by ovaries, adrenal glands and peripheral tissues. Adrenal and ovarian androgen biosynthesis is shown in Fig. 20.3. In peripheral tissues (predominantly skin), androstenedione and dehydroepiandrosterone (DHEA) are converted to testosterone.

The circulating androgens are listed in Box 20.5.

Box 20.5 Circulating androgens

- Testosterone
- Androstenedione
- DHEA
- DHEAS

DHEA, dehydroepiandrosterone; *DHEAS*, dehydroepiandrosterone sulphate.

- In normal women, both ovary and adrenal glands contribute equally to the production of testosterone and androstenedione. However, 80% of DHEA is produced by adrenal glands and only 20% by ovary.
- Major portion (80%) of the testosterone is bound to sex hormone–binding globulin (SHBG); only the free fraction is biologically active.
- DHEA and androstenedione are bound to albumin.
- Testosterone is converted to active form, dihydrotestosterone (DHT), by the enzyme 5α-reductase in the target tissue.
- DHT and testosterone are the most potent androgens, whereas androstenedione and DHEA are weak androgens.
- In hirsute women, major proportion of testosterone is from the ovary.

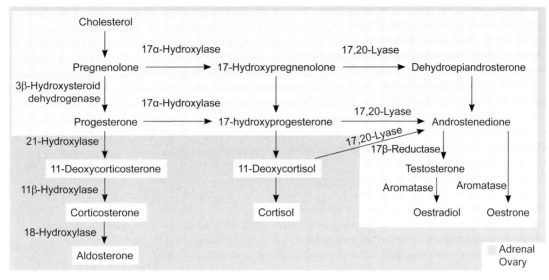

Figure 20.3 Steroid biosynthesis in adrenal gland and ovary.

Pathogenesis of hyperandrogenism

Hirsutism can result from hyperandrogenism due to abnormality at any of the several sites listed in Box 20.6.

Box 20.6 Pathogenesis of hyperandrogenism

- Increased production of androgens
  - Ovary
  - Adrenal
- Exogenous administration of androgens
  - Medications
- Increased proportion of unbound androgens
  - Decrease in SHBG levels
- Peripheral disorders of androgen metabolism
  - Increase in 5α-reductase
- Abnormalities of androgen receptors
  - Increase in androgen receptors in hair follicles
  - Increased sensitivity of hair follicles to androgens

SHBG, sex hormone–binding globulin.

Causes of hyperandrogenism

Increased production of androgens

Conditions that give rise to increased androgen production are listed in Box 20.7. Virilization is caused by marked increase in testosterone levels and is, therefore, not seen in polycystic ovarian syndrome (PCOS).

Box 20.7 Increased production of androgens

- Ovarian androgens
  - PCOS
  - Stromal hyperthecosis
  - Luteomas of pregnancy
  - Tumours
    - Sertoli–Leydig cell tumours
    - Gynandroblastomas
    - Steroid (lipoid) cell tumours
- Adrenal androgens
  - Congenital adrenal hyperplasia
  - Tumours
    - Adenomas
    - Carcinomas
    - Cushing syndrome

PCOS, polycystic ovarian syndrome.

Ovarian hyperandrogenism

Polycystic ovarian syndrome

This is the most common cause of hyperandrogenism. Definition and clinical features of PCOS have been discussed in detail in Chapter 19, *Secondary amenorrhoea and polycystic ovarian syndrome*. Characteristic presentation is that of a young girl with obesity, menstrual irregularity, hyperandrogenism, infertility and hirsutism. Insulin resistance and dyslipidaemia are common.

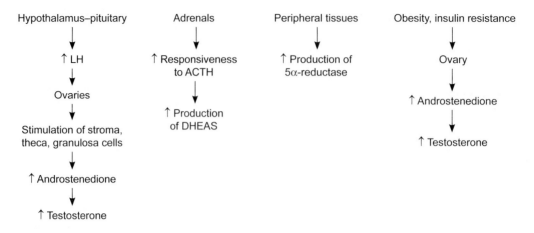

Figure 20.4 Abnormalities causing hyperandrogenism in PCOS. *ACTH*, adrenocorticotropic hormone; *DHEAS*, dehydroepiandrosterone sulphate; *LH*, luteinizing hormone; *PCOS*, polycystic ovarian syndrome.

Hyperandrogenism in PCOS is the result of several abnormalities (Fig. 20.4), namely:

- Increase in luteinizing hormone (LH) secretion by the pituitary results in stimulation of the ovarian stroma, theca and granulosa cells to produce more testosterone and androstenedione.
- Adrenal glands secrete more dehydroepiandrosterone sulphate (DHEAS) due to hyperresponsiveness to circulating adrenocorticotropic hormone (ACTH).
- An increase in 5α-reductase production has been demonstrated in the peripheral tissue.
- In addition, obesity and the associated insulin resistance lead to hyperinsulinaemia. This stimulates ovarian androgen production.
- The serum total testosterone usually does not exceed 2 ng/mL. Therefore, although hirsutism is common, virilization is seldom seen in PCOS.

Ovarian hyperthecosis

Ovarian hyperthecosis refers to the presence of luteinized theca cells in the ovarian stroma, which secrete increasing amounts of testosterone.

- Ovaries are enlarged with increase in ovarian stroma, to about 6–7 cm, but not polycystic.
- Women with this disorder initially present with hirsutism, acne and virilization, insulin resistance and hyperinsulinaemia. Obesity may or may not be present. The disorder is more common in postmenopausal women. In

premenopausal women, it may be difficult to differentiate it from PCOS.

- The androgens are converted to oestrogens in the peripheral tissues, increasing the risk of endometrial hyperplasia and cancer, especially in postmenopausal women.
- Diagnosis is by elevated testosterone level (>1.5 ng/mL), normal or low LH and follicle-stimulating hormone (FSH), normal DHEA and 17-hydroxyprogesterone (17-(OH)P) levels associated with ovarian enlargement.

Luteoma of pregnancy

This is a benign hyperplasia of the ovary that causes virilization in the foetus and mother. The condition regresses spontaneously after delivery.

Androgen-producing tumours

Androgen-producing tumours of the ovary are mostly sex cord stromal tumours (SCSTs) and are uncommon.

- Sertoli–Leydig cell tumours are low-grade malignant tumours and are usually diagnosed at an early stage. They occur in the reproductive age.
- Steroid cell tumours are rare SCSTs, composed of cells that resemble steroid hormone–secreting cells.
- Leydig cell tumours, stromal luteomas and other unspecified steroid cell tumours come under this category. Leydig cell tumours (hilus cell tumours) and stromal luteomas occur in the postmenopausal age and are benign.

- Other unspecified steroid cell tumours, also known as lipoid cell tumours, occur in younger women, and secrete androgen, oestrogen or ACTH and can cause hirsutism and virilization. Although of low-grade malignant behaviour, they can metastasize and recur.
- Gynandroblastomas are rare tumours containing ovarian and testicular elements. They are also generally seen in young women with a mean age of 30 years.

Salient clinical and diagnostic features of ovarian conditions causing hyperandrogenism are summarized in Table 20.1.

Table 20.1 Ovarian hyperandrogenism

Disease	Clinical features	Diagnostic tests
PCOS	• Obesity • Menstrual irregularity • Hirsutism • Virilization	• Mild elevation of T • Typical picture on U/S
Stromal hyperthecosis	• Hirsutism • Virilization • Obesity +/− • Menstrual irregularity • Gradual progression	• Elevated T >1.5 ng/mL • No elevation of LH, FSH, DHEA • Ovaries enlarged, but not polycystic
Luteoma of pregnancy	• Hirsutism • Virilization • Occurs in pregnancy	• Elevated T • Regresses after delivery
Tumours	• Hirsutism • Virilization • Rapid progression • Reproductive or older age • Pelvic mass	• Marked elevation of T >2 ng/mL • Ovarian mass on U/S

DHEA, dehydroepiandrosterone; FSH, follicle-stimulating hormone; LH, luteinizing hormone; PCOS, polycystic ovarian syndrome; T, testosterone; U/S, ultrasound.

Adrenal hyperandrogenism

Congenital adrenal hyperplasia/late-onset 21-hydroxylase deficiency

- Congenital adrenal hyperplasia (CAH) is an **autosomal recessive disorder** that results from an enzymatic defect in the cortisol synthesis pathway.
- Deficiency of 21-hydroxylase is the most common, but 11β-hydroxylase defects can also occur.

- The classic form is congenital and manifests as sexual ambiguity and electrolyte disturbances in the newborn.
- The nonclassic or milder form of congenital adrenal hyperplasia (NCCAH) presents at or after puberty and accounts for 1.5–2% of cases of hirsutism. They also have menstrual irregularity, acne, obesity and virilization. **Hirsutism is more marked than in PCOS.**
- Linear growth is affected due to early epiphyseal closure as a result of early hypothalamic–pituitary–gonadal axis activation (Fig. 20.5).

Pathophysiology
Androgen biosynthesis and the enzymes involved at each step are given in Fig. 20.3.

When 21-hydroxylase is deficient, the substrates, namely DHEA and 17α-hydroxyprogesterone, accumulate in the system. They are converted to testosterone in the peripheral tissues. The lack of cortisol leads to compensatory increase in ACTH production and the androgen production increases further.

Elevation of 17α-hydroxyprogesterone to >6 ng/mL is diagnostic of 21-hydroxylase deficiency. When the levels of 17-(OH)P are between 2.5 and 6 ng/mL, further evaluation by ACTH stimulation test is required to confirm the diagnosis.

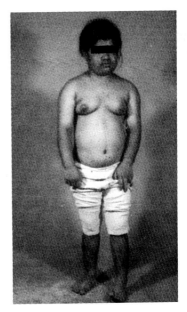

Figure 20.5 A 17-year-old girl with late-onset 21-hydroxylase deficiency—Short stature, hirsutism and increased muscle mass.

Deficiency of 11β-hydroxylase is associated with hypertension and hypokalaemia due to accumulation of 11-deoxycortisol and deoxycorticosterone, which are weak mineralocorticoids.

Pathophysiology of NCCAH is summarized in Box 20.8.

Box 20.8 Pathophysiology of congenital adrenal hyperplasia

- Deficiency of enzyme 21-hydroxylase
- Accumulation of androgenic substrates/precursors [17-(OH)P and DHEA]
- Conversion of 17-(OH)P and DHEA to testosterone in peripheral tissues
- Increase in ACTH due to lack of negative feedback
- Further increase in androgens

ACTH, adrenocorticotropic hormone; *DHEA*, dehydroepiandrosterone; *17-(OH)P*, 17-hydroxyprogesterone.

Adrenal tumours

They are **adenomas** and **carcinomas** and secrete DHEAS and androstenedione, which get converted into testosterone peripherally. Markedly elevated levels of DHEAS usually indicate adrenal tumour. They can be visualized on CT scan or MRI. These tumours of the adrenal glands are rare.

Cushing syndrome It refers to the effects of excess of circulating glucocorticoids as a result of exogenous administration or endogenous production. The most common cause of excessive endogenous production is Cushing disease, which is excessive production of glucocorticoids by the adrenal gland secondary to increase in ACTH levels. This can cause hirsutism and menstrual irregularity. This is because ACTH stimulates adrenal androgen production as well.

These women have other clinical features of Cushing disease such as obesity, purple abdominal striae, nuchal fat pad, proximal weakness, bone pains, menstrual irregularity, secondary diabetes mellitus and hypertension (Fig. 20.6a and b). In these patients, hirsutism and virilization, if present, tend to be mild and the other clinical features of Cushing disease dominate the clinical picture. The condition can be mistaken for PCOS, and further evaluation by dexamethasone suppression tests is required to establish the diagnosis.

Salient clinical and diagnostic features of various disorders of the adrenal glands causing hyperandrogenism are summarized in Table 20.2.

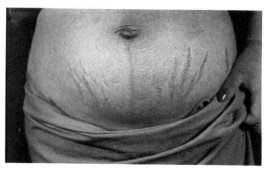

a.

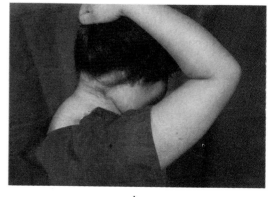

b.

Figure 20.6 Cushing syndrome. a. Purplish striae on the abdominal wall. b. Nuchal fat pad.

Table 20.2 Adrenal hyperandrogenism

Condition	Clinical features	Diagnostic tests
NCCAH	• Obesity • Hirsutism • Virilization • Hyperpigmentation • Menstrual irregularity +/−	• Elevated 17α-hydroxyprogesterone (>6 ng/mL) • Elevated DHEA
Cushing syndrome	• Obesity • Hirsutism • Hypertension • Other features of Cushing syndrome	• Elevated cortisol • Positive dexamethasone suppression test
Tumours	• Rapid progression • Hirsutism • Virilization • Menstrual irregularity	• Markedly elevated DHEA • Markedly elevated T (>2 ng/mL)

DHEA, dehydroepiandrosterone; *NCCAH*, nonclassic congenital adrenal hyperplasia; *T*, testosterone.

Drug-induced hirsutism

Drugs that can cause hirsutism are listed in Box 20.9.

Box 20.9 Drugs causing hirsutism

- Oral contraceptives
- Danazol
- Diazoxide
- Phenytoin sodium
- Anabolic steroids
- Testosterone
- Thyroxin
- Cyclosporin
- Glucocorticoids

Increased proportion of unbound androgens

This is generally due to reduction in SHBG. Oestrogens increase SHBG level, but androgens decrease it. Therefore, conditions that cause hyperandrogenism (Box 20.10) also reduce the SHBG levels and cause further increase in serum levels of the bioavailable androgens.

Box 20.10 Causes of decrease in SHBG

- Exogenous androgens
- PCOS
- Classic and nonclassic congenital adrenal hyperplasia
- Cushing syndrome
- Obesity
- Hyperinsulinaemia
- Hyperprolactinaemia
- Excess growth hormone
- Hypothyroidism

PCOS, polycystic ovarian syndrome; *SHBG*, sex hormone–binding globulin.

Peripheral disorder of androgen metabolism and abnormalities in androgen receptors

This is otherwise known as **idiopathic hirsutism**.
- The condition is familial and is the second most common cause of hirsutism.
- **The androgen levels are not elevated.**
- There is no associated ovulatory dysfunction, menstrual irregularity, virilization, obesity or metabolic syndrome.

- Increase in 5α-reductase activity in the hair follicles has been demonstrated in some women.
- An increase in the androgen receptors or increased sensitivity of the receptors to androgens may also contribute to idiopathic hirsutism.

Clinical evaluation

History

Various details pertaining to age of onset, rapidity of progression, associated menstrual irregularity and other associated symptoms must be obtained (Box 20.11).

Box 20.11 History

- Age
- Age of onset
- Rapidity of progression
- Severity
  - Frequency of hair removal
- Associated menstrual irregularity
  - Oligomenorrhoea
  - Amenorrhoea
- Voice changes
- Virilization
- Weight gain
- Family history of hirsutism
- Medications

Onset at puberty indicates PCOS or NCCAH, but onset at older age may be due to tumours of the ovary. Rapid progression indicates tumours. Frequency of hair removal is an indirect indicator of severity or of the psychological impact on the patient. A positive family history is usually present in PCOS, nonclassic congenital adrenal hyperplasia (NCAH) and idiopathic hirsutism. Hirsutism with virilization is indicative of excess testosterone production and, therefore, tumours of the ovary or adrenal. Associated amenorrhoea indicates moderate to severe elevation of androgen levels.

Physical examination

Documentation of the severity of hirsutism is mandatory. Ferriman–Gallwey scoring system is generally used. This scoring system quantitates the hair growth in nine androgen-sensitive areas;

each area gives scores from 0 to 4, adding up to a total score of 36. A score of 8 or more is considered as hirsutism (Fig. 20.7). Scoring also helps in the assessment of response to therapy. Clinical signs of virilization must be looked for since subsequent evaluation depends on the presence or absence of virilization. Clitoromegaly is a definite indication of virilization. It is defined as a clitoral index (length × width) of 35 mm^2 or length >10 mm. General examination, abdominal and pelvic examination, and examination of the breast to look for signs of Cushing syndrome, virilization, pelvic tumour and galactorrhoea are mandatory (Box 20.12).

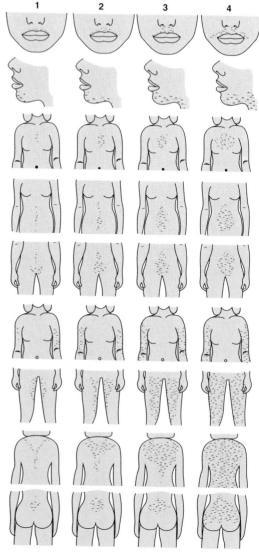

Figure 20.7 Pictorial representation of Ferriman–Gallwey scoring system. Hair on nine areas are given scores from 1 to 4, giving a maximum score of 36.

Box 20.12 Clinical evaluation in hirsutism

- General examination
  - Obesity (BMI)
  - Acanthosis nigricans
  - Signs of Cushing syndrome
  - Blood pressure
  - Oily skin
  - Frontal balding
- Hirsutism score
- Breast examination—Galactorrhoea
- Abdominal examination
  - Striae
  - Pelvic mass
- External genitalia
  - Clitoromegaly
- Pelvic examination
  - Adnexal mass

BMI, body mass index.

Investigations

Investigations depend on clinical diagnosis. A simple algorithm for clinical diagnosis is shown in Fig. 20.8.

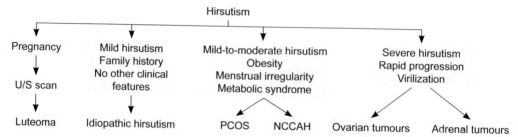

Figure 20.8 Clinical diagnosis of aetiology of hirsutism. *NCCAH*, nonclassic congenital adrenal hyperplasia; *PCOS*, polycystic ovarian syndrome; *U/S*, ultrasound.

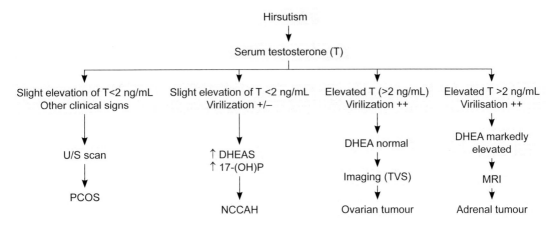

Figure 20.9 Investigation of hirsutism. *DHEA*, dehydroepiandrosterone; *DHEAS*, dehydroepiandrosterone sulphate; *NCCAH*, nonclassic congenital adrenal hyperplasia; *PCOS*, polycystic ovarian syndrome; *T*, testosterone; *TVS*, transvaginal ultrasound scan; *U/S*, ultrasound.

- With history and clinical examination, iatrogenic and pregnancy-related hirsutism can be ruled out.
- If hirsutism is familial and mild (score 8–12), and there is no associated menstrual abnormality, virilization, metabolic syndrome or obesity, a diagnosis of idiopathic hirsutism can be made and treatment started.
- If hirsutism is moderate (score 12–15), associated with obesity, menstrual irregularity and insulin resistance, PCOS and NCCAH are possibilities. Serum testosterone, DHEA and 17-(OH)P levels should be asked for.
- In women with marked hirsutism (score >15) or virilization, estimation of serum testosterone and DHEAS will help in identifying the source of androgen as ovary or adrenal. Very high levels of DHEA are indicative of adrenal tumours. Imaging of ovary and adrenal is necessary to confirm diagnosis.
- If signs of Cushing syndrome are present, plasma cortisol estimation and dexamethasone suppression tests are required.

An algorithm for evaluation is given in Fig. 20.9.

A serum testosterone is required in all except idiopathic hirsutism. Additional tests are required depending on clinical diagnosis or suspicion.

Management

Management depends on the severity of hirsutism, underlying pathology and fertility concerns.

The modalities of management are listed in Box 20.13.

Box 20.13 Management of hirsutism and virilization

- Cosmetic and physical measures
- Medical treatment
- Surgical treatment

Cosmetic and physical measures

These are useful for women with mild hirsutism, especially idiopathic, and as an adjunct to medical treatment in moderate and severe hirsutism. They are also useful while awaiting response to medical therapies. Cosmetic therapies are listed in Box 20.14.

Medical treatment

Most women who use cosmetic measures will experience regrowth of hair and require medical therapy. All women with hyperandrogenism require medical treatment as well.

Response to medical treatment becomes clinically evident only after 6 months of therapy. It has to be continued for 9 months to 1 year before significant effect is observed because of the long duration of hair growth cycle.

Eflornithine hydrochloride cream has been found to be useful in facial hirsutism. It is a cell cycle inhibitor that inhibits ornithine decarboxylase, which is required for hair growth. It is expensive, but effective. It can be combined with laser therapy.

Combined OC pills

- Combined oral contraceptive (OC) pills are the treatment of choice in majority of women with hirsutism, especially when there is associated menstrual irregularity.
- They act by inhibiting LH secretion and ovarian and adrenal androgen production, and increasing SHBG. In addition, they regularize the menstrual cycles.
- OC pills containing 30 μg of ethinyl oestradiol are more effective. There is very little difference between the androgenic and the nonandrogenic progestin-containing OCs. Drospirenone has definite antiandrogenic effects, but there is a higher risk of venous thromboembolism.
- OC pills are the first line of treatment in PCOS and NCCAH.

Glucocorticoids

Glucocorticoids are not very effective in treatment of hirsutism, although they suppress ACTH production and serum androgen levels. They are not recommended for treatment of hirsutism, according to 2008 Endocrine Society guidelines.

GnRH agonists

They reduce androgen levels by suppressing pituitary gonadotropins and thereby ovarian androgens. However, they are not used as primary treatment of hirsutism because they cause hypo-oestrogenism and are expensive. Therefore, they are recommended only in women with severe ovarian hyperandrogenism (PCOS/hyperthecosis) who do not respond to OC pills or antiandrogen therapy.

Antiandrogens

Antiandrogens are effective in reducing hirsutism and act at the androgen receptor level or on the enzyme 5α-reductase. The drugs are listed in Table 20.3. They can be used alone or in combination with OC pills. Flutamide is hepatotoxic.

Table 20.3 Medical treatment of hirsutism

Drug	Mechanism of action	Indication	Dose
Eflornithine hydrochloride	Inhibits ornithine decarboxylase	PCOS, hyperthecosis	
Combined OC pills	• Suppresses pituitary LH • Suppresses ovarian T • Increases SHBG	PCOS	1 tablet daily, cyclic
GnRH agonist (Leuprolide)	Suppresses pituitary LH	PCOS, hyperthecosis	3.6 mg IM monthly
Spironolactone	Inhibits androgen binding to receptors	Idiopathic, moderate to severe	50–100 mg twice daily
Cyproterone acetate	Inhibits androgen binding to receptors	Idiopathic hirsutism	50–100 mg during days 5–15 with ethinyl oestradiol
Flutamide	Inhibits androgen binding to receptors	Severe hirsutism	250 mg twice daily
Finasteride	5α-reductase inhibitor	Idiopathic, moderate to severe	5 mg daily

GnRH, gonadotropin-releasing hormone; LH, luteinizing hormone; OC, oral contraceptive; PCOS, polycystic ovarian syndrome; SHBG, sex hormone–binding globulin; T, testosterone.

Surgical treatment

Surgery is required in women with significant clitoromegaly (Box 20.15). Androgen-secreting ovarian tumours and postmenopausal hyperthecosis are managed by oophorectomy. If the tumour is large or malignant, hysterectomy with bilateral oophorectomy may be required. Adrenalectomy is the treatment of choice for adrenal tumours (Box 20.15).

Box 20.15 Surgical treatment

- Clitoromegaly — Clitoridal reduction
- Sertoli–Leydig cell tumour ⎫
- Lipoid cell tumour   ⎬ Oophorectomy
- Hilus cell tumour   ⎪
- Stromal hyperthecosis ⎭
- Adrenal adenoma ⎫ Adrenalectomy
- Adrenal carcinoma ⎭

Key points

- Hirsutism and virilization are the result of excessive androgen production by the adrenals or ovaries.
- Hirsutism is the excessive growth of terminal hair in a male distribution. The androgen levels are mildly elevated. Menstrual irregularity may be associated.
- Virilization is the presence of signs of masculinization in women. The androgen levels are markedly elevated and are associated with amenorrhoea.
- There are three types of adult body hair: Vellus hair, terminal hair and sexual hair.
- The hair growth cycle takes 3–6 months to complete and consists of anagen phase, catagen phase and telogen phase.
- The circulating androgens are testosterone, androstenedione, dehydroepiandrosterone (DHEA) and DHEA sulphate. About 80% of testosterone is bound to globulin and only the free fraction is biologically active.
- Hirsutism can result from increased androgen production, exogenous androgen administration, increase in the proportion of unbound androgen or peripheral disorders of androgen metabolism.
- Increase in ovarian androgen production can be due to polycystic ovarian syndrome (PCOS), hyperthecosis or androgen-producing tumours of the ovary.
- Adrenal androgen production increases in congenital adrenal hyperplasia and adrenal tumours.
- PCOS is the most common cause of hyperandrogenism and hirsutism.
- Several drugs can cause hirsutism.
- Clinical evaluation of hirsutism should include a detailed history and thorough physical examination. Special attention must be paid to blood pressure, obesity, frontal balding, Ferriman–Gallwey score, galactorrhoea, clitoromegaly and adnexal mass.
- Serum testosterone and DHEA levels must be measured as the initial step in the diagnostic workup of hirsutism. Markedly elevated testosterone levels in a woman with virilization indicate the presence of ovarian or adrenal tumour.
- Management of hirsutism is by cosmetic and physical measures and medications. Virilization may require surgical intervention.
  - Medical treatment must be continued for 9 months to 1 year before significant improvement is noticed. Drugs that suppress androgen production or antiandrogens may be used.
  - Surgical intervention may be clitoridectomy, oophorectomy or adrenalectomy.

Self-assessment

Case-based questions

Case 1

An 18-year-old medical student presents with a 2-year history of weight gain and irregular cycles and increased hair growth on the face and arms. She is forced to shave once in 2 weeks. There is no family history of similar problems.

1. What clinical features will you look for?
2. What is your provisional diagnosis?
3. What investigations will you order?

4. How will you manage?

Case 2

A 20-year-old girl presents with a history of increased hair growth of 4 years' duration. There is no menstrual irregularity. BMI is 21. Mother and sister have similar history. She uses depilatory cream every 2–3 weeks.

1. What clinical features will you look for?
2. What is your provisional diagnosis?
3. What investigations will you order?
4. How will you manage?

Answers

Case 1

1. BMI, blood pressure, extent of hirsutism, Ferriman–Gallwey score, signs of virilization—Clitoromegaly, frontal balding, breast examination, abdominal examination for striae.
2. PCOS, rule out NCCAH.
3. **(a)** If there is no virilization and hirsutism is mild to moderate, it is PCOS.
   (i) Blood tests—Sugar level, lipid profile
   (b) If clitoromegaly is present and hirsutism is moderate to severe, consider
   (i) NCCAH
   (ii) Serum DHEA and 17α-hydroxyprogesterone
4. Both are managed by
   (a) Weight reduction
   (b) Combination OC pills for hirsutism and menstrual irregularity
   (c) Surgery for clitoromegaly if required

Case 2

1. Severity of hirsutism, FG score, breast examination, signs of virilization.
2. Idiopathic hirsutism.
3. If no other clinical abnormality detected, no investigations are required.
4. Since hirsutism is moderate and needs hair removal, give spironolactone 100 mg daily, eflornithine cream for facial application daily or laser therapy.

Long-answer question

1. An 18-year-old girl presents with hirsutism. How will you evaluate? Discuss the management.

Short-answer questions

1. Virilization
2. Androgen-secreting tumours of the ovary
3. Nonclassic congenital adrenal hyperplasia
4. Medical management of hirsutism

21 | Menopause

Case scenario

Mrs AP, 50, walked into the menopause clinic looking distraught. She was a housewife, mother of two children who had spent her entire lifetime looking after the family. Her menstruation had stopped 1 year ago and she was miserable, depressed and irritable, had several hot flushes through the day and night, and could hardly sleep for 3–4 hours. Her husband was a busy executive and travelled a lot; her children had grown up and left home. She was lonely and felt unwanted.

Introduction

Menopause is a crucial period in a woman's life. Quality of life declines during this period due to the various problems associated with oestrogen deficiency and ageing. With increasing life expectancy of women all over the world, 25–30% of a woman's life is in the postmenopausal period. Coping with the pressures of modern life and the mood swings of menopause together can be overwhelming. Attention to the health and emotional needs of these women is important for the individual, family and community.

Definition

Menopause is defined as cessation of menses for a period of 12 months or more in a woman aged 40 or above. It is a retrospective diagnosis that can be made with certainty only after 12 months of amenorrhoea in the **appropriate age group**. It is an indication of ovarian follicular depletion and resultant oestrogen deficiency.

Cessation of menstrual periods in younger women aged 40 or younger was called premature menopause earlier, but this term is not used anymore. It is included under primary ovarian insufficiency.

Age at menopause

The mean age of menopause varies with the ethnic group. It is 51 years in the West, but occurs earlier in certain other populations. Exact figure for India is not available, but small population studies have identified 45 years as the mean age.

The age at menopause is primarily determined genetically. Other factors affecting age at menopause are listed in Box 21.1. High socioeconomic status, low parity, smoking and factors that affect ovarian follicular function are associated with an earlier age at menopause.

Box 21.1   Factors affecting age at menopause

- Genetic factors
- Ethnicity
- Socioeconomic status
- Parity
- Smoking
- Prior ovarian surgery
- Prior chemotherapy
- Prior radiotherapy

Menopause can be surgically induced by bilateral oophorectomy and ovariotoxic chemotherapy or radiation. Symptoms after surgical menopause have an abrupt onset.

Stages of reproductive ageing

A woman's menstrual cycles go through the following stages:

- Reproductive years
- Menopausal transition (perimenopause)
- Menopause
- Postmenopause

Reproductive years

This is divided into early and late. The late reproductive years precede onset of menopausal transition and are of variable duration. The cycles are ovulatory but may be short and progesterone levels are low. The fertility potential is decreased.

Menopausal transition or perimenopause

This is the period preceding the menopause characterized by irregular menses and missed periods associated with increase in follicle-stimulating hormone (FSH) levels (>20 IU/mL). Heavy and prolonged menstrual bleeding can occur. The duration of menopausal transition varies from 2 to 8 years. Rapid oocyte depletion and decline in ovarian function occurs.

Menopause

Following a few years of perimenopause, there is the cessation of menses. This is known as the final menstrual period (FMP). When this amenorrhea persists for 12 months, it is termed menopause.

Postmenopause

This is the period following menopause or final menstrual period. The first years are considered early postmenopause, and the later years are referred to as late postmenopause.

Menopausal transition, menopause and postmenopause are depicted in Fig. 21.1. This has been further modified in 2011 as Stages of Reproductive Aging Workshop +10 (STRAW+10) staging system for reproductive aging in women.

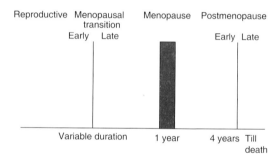

Figure 21.1 Menopausal transition, menopause and postmenopause.

Physiology of menopause

As mentioned earlier, depletion of ovarian follicles is the cause of cessation of menstruation. The hypothalamic–pituitary–ovarian axis is intact and functional.

- The ovary of the newborn girl child has nearly 1 million oocytes. The number of oocytes decreases gradually with age and more rapidly from about 37 years. This oocyte depletion is attributed to apoptosis.
- With reduction in the number of oocytes, the hormones produced by the granulosa cells, namely oestrogen and inhibin, also decrease. This removes the negative feedback inhibition of gonadotropin production and leads to increase in FSH levels (>40 IU/mL).
- Luteinizing hormone (LH) level also increases but to a lesser extent (>20 IU/mL; Fig. 21.2).

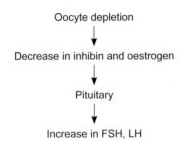

Figure 21.2 Physiology of menopause. *FSH*, follicle-stimulating hormone; *LH*, luteinizing hormone.

- Ovarian reserve and level of anti-Müllerian hormone decrease.
- The cycles become anovulatory and there is no progesterone production. The ovarian stroma, however, continues to produce some oestrogen and androgens.
- The adrenal androgen production also continues, though at a lower level. The androgens are converted in peripheral fat tissue into oestrone, which is a weak oestrogen.
- Unopposed action of oestrone on the endometrium leads to proliferative changes,

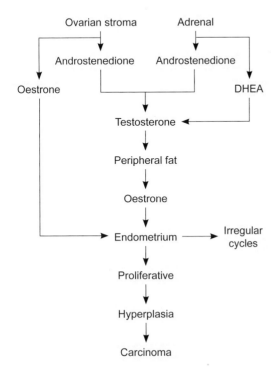

Figure 21.3 Oestrogen production in postmenopausal period and its effect on the endometrium. *DHEA*, dehydroepiandrosterone.

hyperplasia and, sometimes, carcinoma (Fig. 21.3). This risk is more in obese women in whom peripheral oestrone production is higher due to the increased fat mass.

Effects of menopause

These are mainly due to hypo-oestrogenic state, which influences the functioning of various organ systems of the body. The effects can be classified depending on their time of onset (Box 21.2).

Box 21.2 Effects of menopause

- Immediate
- Intermediate
- Long term

Immediate effects

The immediate effects of hypo-oestrogenism are mainly vasomotor symptoms, mood swings and sexual dysfunction (Box 21.3). Hot flushes and mood swings are experienced by some women even during menopausal transition. Some of the immediate effects of menopause can be distressing but are self-limiting.

Box 21.3 Immediate effects of menopause

- Vasomotor symptoms
  - Hot flushes
  - Sweating
  - Palpitations
- Urinary symptoms
  - Dysuria
  - Increased frequency
  - Recurrent lower UTI
- Mood disturbances
  - Depression
  - Anxiety
  - Irritability
- Insomnia
- Cognitive dysfunction
  - Memory loss
  - Poor concentration
  - Tiredness
  - Lack of motivation
- Sexual dysfunction
  - Dyspareunia
  - Decreased libido

UTI, urinary tract infection.

Vasomotor symptoms

Vasomotor symptoms or hot flushes are experienced by 75% of women and are severe in 10–15%. They usually reduce in number and severity by 2–3 years but can continue up to 10 years. Hot flush is an acute sensation of heat and skin changes, including sweating. It is mediated by noradrenaline and serotonin at the hypothalamus. There is an increase in core body temperature during the flushes and peripheral vasodilatation. The causation is not well understood and is thought to be due to increased FSH levels or reduction in oestrogen levels. Hot flushes can cause sleep deprivation and irritability. They respond dramatically to oestrogen.

Urinary symptoms

Increased frequency, urgency and dysuria are common troublesome symptoms in postmenopausal women. The lining epithelium of the lower urinary tract is also dependent on oestrogen for its integrity; oestrogen deprivation at menopause induces changes in urothelium. These changes predispose to frequent lower urinary tract infections.

Mood disturbances

Fluctuating oestrogen levels can lead to reduction in central neurotransmitters such as serotonin and cause mood changes such as depression and anxiety. Oestrogen replacement can ameliorate these symptoms, but some progestogens can increase it.

Vaginal dryness

Vaginal dryness due to lack of oestrogen is a distressing symptom, but women may not complain about this unless specifically asked. Vaginal dryness causes dyspareunia.

Sexual dysfunction

Reduction in androgen level leads to decreased libido. This, combined with dyspareunia, causes sexual dysfunction early in menopause.

Insomnia and cognitive dysfunction

Insomnia can be due to hot flushes or depression. Cognitive dysfunction is caused by effects of hypo-oestrogenic state on oestrogen receptors of the central nervous system.

Intermediate effects

These begin a few years after menopause and continue to worsen (Box 21.4). Similar to the immediate effects, they can also affect quality of life.

Box 21.4 Intermediate effects

- Genital atrophy
- Effects on collagen
  - Skin changes
  - Urodynamic effects
  - Pelvic organ prolapse

Genital atrophy

Oestrogen deficiency leads to thinning of vaginal mucosa, loss of superficial keratinized layer, reduced secretion by the vaginal glands and increase in vaginal pH. These changes give rise to dryness, dyspareunia and bleeding. The increase in vaginal pH may lead to local infections. Local and systemic oestrogens are effective in alleviating these symptoms.

Effects on collagen

Collagen is the main component of supports of the uterus, bladder and urethra. Lack of oestrogen leads to reduction in collagen support and atrophy of the ligaments and mucosa of vagina and urethra. This causes urodynamic changes and pelvic organ prolapse, stress incontinence, urgency and increased frequency of urination.

Skin changes Postmenopausal skin changes are thinning due to loss of collagen, easy bruising, vulnerability to trauma and infection.

Urodynamic effects Atrophy of the ligaments that support the bladder, bladder neck and vagina can lead to pelvic organ prolapse and urodynamic changes. Urge incontinence and stress incontinence are common problems.

Pelvic organ prolapse Oestrogen deficiency causes atrophy of the pelvic ligaments and other tissues leading to pelvic organ prolapse. Women who have early stage prolapse may experience worsening.

Long-term effects

The long-term effects clinically manifest later and increase morbidity and mortality (Box 21.5).

Box 21.5 Long-term effects

- Osteoporosis
- Cardiovascular effects
- Dementia

Osteoporosis

Osteoporosis is one of the well-known long-term effects of oestrogen deficiency.

- Postmenopausal osteoporosis is due to oestrogen deficiency and affects trabecular bone (Box 21.6).
- Oestrogen receptors are present in osteoblasts and osteoclasts. Oestrogens increase osteoblastic activity and decrease osteoclastic activity.
- In the oestrogen-deficient state, bone resorption is increased, especially in the vertebrae, femoral neck and distal radius. The phase of bone formation is shortened, the net result being osteoporosis.
- The loss of bone mineral density is the highest in the first 5 years, but the effects manifest much later.

Box 21.6 Postmenopausal osteoporosis

- Due to oestrogen deficiency
- Affects trabecular bone
- Reduction in BMD
  - 2.5% per year/5 years
  - 1% per year thereafter
- Increased fracture risk

BMD, bone mineral density.

- Risk of postmenopausal osteoporosis (bone mineral density) is affected by several other factors that can further increase the severity (Box 21.7).
- The predominant symptom of osteoporosis is backache. Women can present with vertebral fractures giving rise to severe pain (Fig. 21.4).
- Some women present only with progressive kyphosis without a history of symptomatic vertebral fracture.
- There is increased susceptibility to other pathological fractures at other sites as well.
- Bone mass can be assessed by several methods, but dual-energy X-ray absorptiometry (DEXA) is the gold standard.

Box 21.7 Risk factors for osteoporosis

- Low body mass index
- Genetic—Family history of osteoporosis
- Peak bone mass at puberty
- Poor dietary calcium intake
- Poor vitamin D status
- Multiparity
- Exposure to sunlight
- Alcohol and smoking
- Drugs
  - Corticosteroids
  - Long-term anticonvulsants (e.g. phenytoin)
- Other endocrine disorders
  - Cushing syndrome
  - Hyperparathyroidism
  - Hyperthyroidism

Cardiovascular disease

Coronary heart disease (CHD) is the leading cause of death in postmenopausal women. Incidence of CHD is three times lower in premenopausal women compared to that in men. However, the incidence rapidly increases after menopause to equal that in men. The lower incidence in premenopausal women is due to the protective effect of oestrogen. Oestrogen acts in several ways to decrease the risk of CHD (Box 21.8).

Box 21.8 Protective effect of oestrogen on cardiovascular disease

- Decrease in low-density lipoproteins
- Increase in high-density lipoproteins
- Decrease in total cholesterol
- Nitric oxide–mediated coronary vasodilatation
- Direct effect on endothelium
- Direct effects on reduction of atheroma

The risk is increased by several factors such as diabetes, hypertension, obesity and dyslipidaemia. But oestrogen status increases the risk independent of other factors. Primary ovarian insufficiency and oophorectomy increase the risk severalfold.

Dementia

Oestrogens have a direct effect on neuronal growth, neurotransmitter production and vasculature of the central nervous system. Oestrogen deficiency can cause cognitive decline.

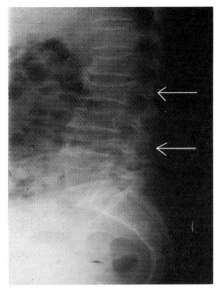

a.

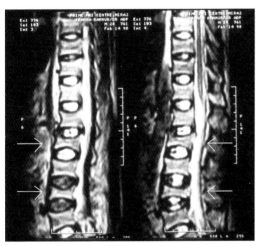

b.

Figure 21.4 Postmenopausal osteoporosis with vertebral fracture. a. X-ray lumbar spine showing fracture of L2 and L4 vertebrae (arrows). The vertebral body is collapsed while the intervertebral discs appear broader. b. Magnetic resonance imaging of vertebral column showing fracture and collapse of lumbar vertebrae (arrows).

Dementia, especially Alzheimer disease, is seen usually in older women. The effect of oestrogen therapy in improving dementia is controversial.

In addition, **osteoarthritis**, **impaired balance** and **increase in body fat** that occur postmeno-pausally are also related to and worsened by oes-trogen deficiency.

Clinical evaluation

History

History should focus on a woman's lifestyle, assessing symptoms and their severity and risk factors for long-term effects (Box 21.9).

Box 21.9 History in menopausal women

- Age
- Age at menopause
- Irregular menstrual cycles
- Type of menopause
  - Spontaneous/iatrogenic
- Symptoms
  - Vasomotor
  - Mood swings
  - Dyspareunia/vaginal dryness
  - Urge/stress incontinence/frequency
  - Back pain
- Family history
  - Osteoporosis
  - Coronary heart disease
  - Breast cancer
- Lifestyle
  - Dietary calcium/vitamin D
  - Exposure to sunlight
  - Exercise
  - Smoking, alcohol
- Medical problems
  - Diabetes/hypertension
  - Dyslipidaemia
- Drugs
  - Corticosteroids
  - Thyroxine

Physical examination

General and systemic examination to rule out or assess the severity of medical problems and evidence of oestrogen deficiency will help in decision regarding hormone therapy (HT) or other modalities of treatment (Box 21.10). The woman may be in menopausal transition or postmenopausal.

Investigations

In a woman in the menopausal age with amen-orrhoea of more than 1 year or irregular men-strual cycles and typical symptoms, serum FSH for confirmation of menopause is not required.

When in doubt regarding menopausal status, serum FSH estimation is useful (Box 21.11).

Since women in the menopausal age may have underlying medical problems, some basic investigations are necessary (Box 21.12). Further investigations will depend on the woman's age, duration of menopause, lifestyle and pre-existing medical problems.

Serum calcium, phosphorus and 25-hydroxyvitamin D levels should be estimated in women with nutritional calcium deficiency and poor sunlight exposure.

DEXA should be performed in the following situations:

- All women who are more than 5 years postmenopausal
- Women above the age of 55 years (especially in Indian women in whom menopause is known to occur early)
- Postmenopausal women with a history of one or more risk factors for osteoporosis
- Women with a history of fractures

Lumbar spine, hip and forearm are usually studied. The results are reported as T-scores. A T-score of +2.5 to –1 is considered normal, –1 to –2.5 indicates osteopenia and lower than –2.5 indicates osteoporosis (Fig. 21.5).

Mammography is mandatory in women with high-risk factors for breast cancer. It is advisable to perform mammography before starting HT in women who are not on annual mammographic screening.

Management

All perimenopausal and postmenopausal women need counselling regarding lifestyle modification and supplements to prevent long-term effects of menopause.

Lifestyle modification

This consists of measures to reduce the risk of osteoporosis and improve the quality of life (Box 21.13).

Calcium and vitamin D supplementation

All perimenopausal and postmenopausal women should receive 1–1.5 g of elemental calcium and 400–800 IU of vitamin D daily.

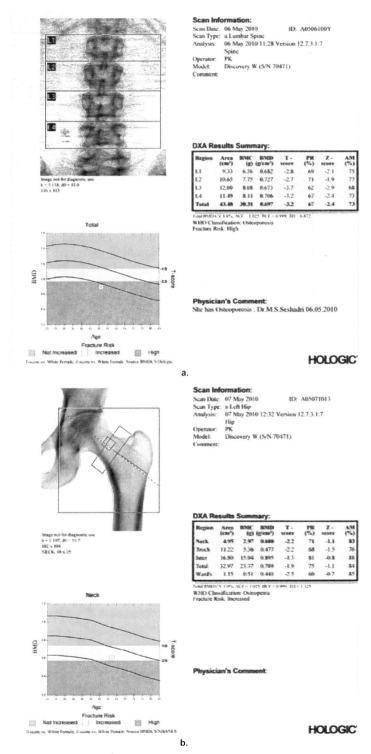

Figure 21.5 DEXA. a. DEXA of lumbar spine. T-score is –3.2, indicating osteoporosis. b. DEXA of hip. T-score is –1.9, indicating osteopenia. *DEXA*, dual-energy X-ray absorptiometry.

Treatment options

These are directed at specific symptoms.

Women in menopausal transition

Women in menopausal transition usually present with irregular menstrual cycles with or without menopausal symptoms such as hot flushes and mood swings. They can be treated with low-dose combination pills containing 20 μg of ethinyl oestradiol. This can be continued till menopause (Fig. 21.6). This regularizes the menstrual cycles and is effective against hot flushes and other symptoms. This can be continued till menopause. However, to know if menopause has occurred, the pill should be stopped for 2–4 weeks once a year and serum FSH measured. If it is in the menopausal range (>40 IU/mL), a switch to menopausal HT may be considered after discussion with the woman.

Postmenopausal women

Postmenopausal women with various symptoms require specific treatment. Younger women should be given medications to prevent long-term effects on the cardiovascular system and bones.

Menopausal hormone therapy (MHT)

This was earlier referred to as **hormone replacement therapy**. Replacement of oestrogen to alleviate the symptoms of oestrogen deficiency is the basis of HT. In women with intact uterus, unopposed oestrogen use can lead to endometrial hyperplasia and cancer. Therefore, progesterone should be added either continuously or cyclically.

Beneficial effects of MHT

- MHT is effective against
  - Vasomotor symptoms
  - Mood swings
  - Vaginal dryness
  - Urogenital atrophy
- MHT (both combined and oestrogen alone) prevents postmenopausal osteoporosis. The risk reductions are similar with oestrogen alone and oestrogen–progestin combinations. Risk of fracture at hip, vertebrae and wrist is reduced significantly.
- MHT has a beneficial effect on CHD in young women with premature ovarian insufficiency and postmenopausal women aged 50–59 years, <10 years postmenopausal.
- MHT reduces all-cause mortality in the same group of women.
- Combined HT reduces risk of type 2 diabetes and insulin resistance.

Adverse effects of MHT
HT has adverse effects that can be minor or major.

Minor adverse effects The minor adverse effects (Box 21.14) can be managed by counselling prior to starting HT and adjustment of dosage.

> **Box 21.14 Minor adverse effects**
>
> - Nausea
> - Bloating
> - Weight gain (1–2 kg)
> - Fluid retention
> - Breakthrough bleeding
> - Breast tenderness

Major adverse effects The main concerns regarding use of HT are the major adverse effects (Box 21.15).

Cardiovascular effects

- Observational studies performed three decades ago have shown that HT is the best treatment for postmenopausal symptoms, alters lipid profile favourably and protects against cardiovascular disease and osteoporosis.

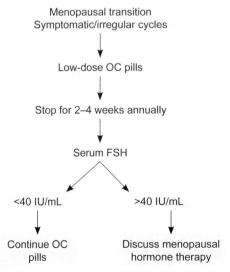

Figure 21.6 Management of menopausal transition. *FSH*, follicle-stimulating hormone; *OC*, oral contraceptive.

Box 21.15 Major adverse effects

- Cardiovascular effects
  - Venous thromboembolism
  - Pulmonary embolism
  - Thrombogenic stroke
  - Coronary heart disease
- Malignancies
  - Breast cancer
  - Endometrial cancer

- In 2002, results of a large multicentric trial known as Women's Health Initiative Trial, which included 16,608 women with a mean age of 63 years, were published. The study showed that there was an increase in breast cancer, CHD, venous thromboembolism (VTE) and stroke in hormone users, although there was a reduction in hip fracture.
- However, subsequent analysis of the data of the same trial and other prospective trials has established that the major adverse effects are related to
  - Age
  - Years since menopause
- Cardiovascular effects are much higher in older women (>60 years) who are more than 10 years postmenopausal, women with high-risk factors such as diabetes, hypertension and dyslipidaemia, and smokers.
- The major adverse effects are also more with combination of oestrogen and progesterone. Use of oestrogen alone is much safer.
- The progestin component of MHT is responsible for increase in CHD and breast cancer.
- In younger women (50–59 years) and in women who are <10 years postmenopausal, even with combined HT, there is a
  - Lower risk of CHD
  - Lower mortality rate
- Both combined HT and oestrogen alone increase the risk of thrombotic stroke and VTE (including deep vein thrombosis and pulmonary embolism). However, the absolute risk is insignificant.

Malignancies

The two malignancies that are of concern with MHT are endometrial and breast cancers.

Endometrial cancer Risk of endometrial cancer increases when oestrogen is used alone. But when progestin is added in the recommended dose, there is no increase in risk of hyperplasia or cancer. Progestin can be used as continuous or cyclic regimen.

Ovarian cancer There is a small increase in risk of ovarian cancer in oestrogen-only and combined HT users. The absolute risk is very low.

Breast cancer Several studies have shown a small increase [relative risk (RR) 1.4] in breast cancer after 5 years of use of combined HT. The risk is related to dose and duration of HT. However, oestrogen taken alone does not increase the risk. Combined HT should be used with caution in women with a family history of breast cancer and is probably best avoided in those who had previous breast cancer.

Summary, conclusions and current recommendations

- Oestrogen replacement is the best known treatment for vasomotor symptoms, mood changes, vaginal symptoms and urinary symptoms. It should be used for the relief of these symptoms unless there are contraindications.
- It is the best known therapy for prevention of osteoporosis, when compared with all other medications available. However, it should not be used solely for this purpose in postmenopausal women.
- Oestrogens have a cardioprotective effect when used immediately after menopause, but, currently, they are not recommended for primary prevention of cardiovascular disease.
- The lowest effective dose of oestrogen should be used. Vaginal oestrogen is recommended for urogenital symptoms.
- It should be combined with a minimum dose of progestin in women with intact uterus.
- It should be used for the lowest duration. Duration of therapy should be preferably 3 years but can be extended to 7 years.
- Younger women with premature ovarian insufficiency or early surgical menopause can use it till 50 years of age.

Summary and conclusions are given in Box 21.16.

Decision making regarding HT

- Counselling regarding risks and benefits of HT should be thorough.
- Risk assessment should be performed and women with high or moderate risk should not be prescribed MHT.
- The decision to use MHT must be individualized.

Box 21.16 Summary and conclusions of studies on HT

- Hormone therapy is useful in immediate postmenopausal symptomatic women.
- In older women, risk of CHD, stroke and VTE is increased.
- This increase is more in
  - Women with pre-existing cardiovascular risk factors
  - Age >60 years
  - Duration of menopause >10 years
- The same risk does not exist in younger menopausal women with POI.
- Risk of breast cancer increases after 5 years of use of combined HT.
- Risk of CHD and breast cancer is associated with addition of progestin.
- Vaginal oestrogens should be used for urogenital atrophy and vaginal dryness.
- The minimum required dose should be used.
- Duration should be 3 years, can be extended if required
- Hormone therapy should not be used purely for prevention of CHD or osteoporosis.

CHD, coronary heart disease; *HT*, hormone therapy; *POI*, premature ovarian insufficiency; *VTE*, venous thromboembolism.

- The final decision regarding HT rests with the patient.

Preparations and dosage
- Oral oestrogens have a more favourable effect on the lipid profile. The most common formulation used is conjugated equine oestrogen (Premarin) 0.625 mg daily. 17-β oestradiol 1mg/day can also be used.
- Transdermal oestrogens and implants do not have the hepatic effects. Transdermal preparations are also associated with less risk of VTE.
- Vaginal oestrogens are absorbed minimally and are very effective in women with vaginal dryness, dyspareunia and urinary symptoms. They can be used in older women as well.
- Progestins should be used in addition to oestrogen in women with intact uterus. Combination of conjugated oestrogen 0.625 mg daily with medroxyprogesterone acetate (MPA) 2.5 mg daily or MPA 5 mg for 12 days in a month is recommended. This is the minimum effective dose of progesterone to prevent endometrial hyperplasia.
- Currently, micronized progesterone (200 mg/day for 12 days or 100 mg/day continuously) is

also being used. This is considered to have less cardiovascular effects and less increase in risk of breast cancer.

HT can be prescribed as systemic or local formulations (Box 21.17).

Box 21.17 Formulations of oestrogen and progesterone

- Oral
  - Oestrogens
    - CEE — 0.625 mg daily
    - 17β-Oestradiol — 1 mg daily
  - Progestins
    - MPA — 2.5 mg daily (or) 5 mg daily for 10 days/month
    - Micronized progesterone — 100 mg daily/200 mg for 12 days/month
- Transdermal patches and gels
  - Oestradiol patches — 25–50 µg once/twice weekly
  - Oestradiol gel — 1.25 g daily
- Implants
  - Oestradiol — 25–50 mg once in 3 months
- Local preparations
  - Creams
    - Conjugated oestrogen — 0.05–2 g daily
    - Oestradiol cream (0.01%) — 0.05–2 g daily
  - Oestradiol vaginal tablets — 1 tablet/day
  - Oestradiol vaginal rings — 1 ring once in 3 months

CEE, conjugated equine oestrogen; *MPA*, medroxyprogesterone acetate.

Other treatment options

Several other options are available as alternatives to MHT for management of the menopausal woman (Box 21.18). They have variable effects on the menopausal symptoms, endometrium, breast, bone and cardiovascular system.

- Selective oestrogen receptor modulators (SERMs) such as raloxifene prevent osteoporosis but have no beneficial effects on genitourinary symptoms and may actually worsen vasomotor symptoms.

- Tibolone is a selective tissue oestrogen activity regulator (STEAR), effective against all the symptoms, and protects the bone, but its cardiovascular effects are a matter of controversy. It may worsen hypertension and may increase the risk of stroke.
- Combination of bazedoxifene and oestrogen combines the advantages of oestrogen and SERM, without the side effects of either. This is not in routine use.
- In women with moderate to severe vasomotor symptoms in whom HT is contraindicated, other drugs such as clonidine, gabapentin and serotonin reuptake inhibitors (SSRIs; e.g. paroxetine, citalopram and venlafaxine) can be used. Of these, desvenlafaxine has been found to be the most effective.
- Osteoporosis can be treated by bisphosphonates administered weekly (alendronate), monthly (ibandronate) or yearly (IV zoledronic acid). Bisphosphonates are now the drug of choice for treatment of established osteoporosis.
- Calcitonin nasal spray is useful in patients with painful vertebral crush fractures.

- Daily subcutaneous synthetic human parathormone 1–34 has been shown to increase bone density and decrease fracture risk and is used in osteoporosis refractory to other medications.
- Both calcitonin and parathormone are quite expensive at present.

Alternative therapies

Alternative therapies are required for symptomatic women in whom there are contraindications for the use of HT (Box 21.19) and in women who do not wish to take HT due to personal preferences.

The options are several, but they are poorly studied. Phytoestrogens are the most widely used. These are present in soy preparations. Reduction in hot flushes, vaginal symptoms and improvement in bone mineral density have been reported with phytoestrogens. Other alternative therapies are listed in Box 21.20.

Key points

- Menopause is defined as cessation of menstruation for 12 months or more in a woman aged 40 years and above. The mean age at menopause varies with the ethnic groups; it is 51 years in Western countries.
- The period preceding the menopause is called the period of menopausal transition. During this period, the menstrual cycles become irregular and follicle-stimulating hormone (FSH) levels are moderately elevated.
- Menopause is the result of oocyte depletion in the ovary with the associated fall in oestrogen and inhibin levels. The cycles are anovulatory and there is no progesterone production.
- Androgens produced from the ovarian stroma and adrenal glands are converted into oestrone. Unopposed action of this on the endometrium can cause irregular bleeding, endometrial hyperplasia and carcinoma. This risk is markedly increased in obese women.
- Hypo-oestrogenic state of menopause gives rise to several symptoms such as hot flushes, mood disturbances, insomnia and urinary symptoms.
- Intermediate effects that set in a few years later include genital atrophy, urodynamic changes and pelvic organ prolapse.
- Late effects are mainly osteoporosis and cardiovascular changes. Osteoporosis predominantly affects trabecular bones such as spine, femoral neck and radius. This results in increased risk of fractures. Several risk factors increase the risk of osteoporosis.
- Cardiovascular effects are due to changes in the high- and low-density lipoproteins, effects on the vascular endothelium and other factors.
- Clinical evaluation of postmenopausal women should include a history of symptoms, family history and details of lifestyle. General examination and examination of the breasts, spine and pelvis are mandatory.
- Basic investigations should be performed in all women. Dual-energy X-ray absorptiometry (DEXA), assessment of vitamin D levels and mammography should be performed where indicated.
- Lifestyle modification including adequate dietary intake of calcium, exposure to sunlight and weight-bearing exercises should be advised. Supplementation of 1–1.5 g of calcium and 1000–1500 units of vitamin D is essential.
- Hormone therapy (HT) is the best known treatment for vasomotor symptoms, mood changes, vaginal symptoms and prevention of osteoporosis. Decision regarding HT should be made after discussing the indications, contraindications and adverse effects with the patient.
- Other treatment options such as raloxifene, tibolone and selective serotonin reuptake inhibitors (SSRIs) should be considered when HT is contraindicated. Bisphosphonates and other drugs are available for the treatment of osteoporosis.
- Several alternative therapies are available, but are poorly studied.

Self-assessment

Case-based questions

Case 1

A 45-year-old lady presents with irregular menstrual cycles every 45–60 days with slight increase in flow lasting for 7–8 days. She has occasional hot flushes for the past 6 months.

1. What details would you like in history?
2. What examination will you do?
3. If her history and examination are unremarkable, how will you manage?

Case 2

A 50-year-old lady presents with a history of hot flushes 10 per day and 4 per night, irritability and insomnia. She attained menopause 1 year ago. BMI is 26 and there are no other risk factors.

1. What points will you focus on in history?
2. How will you evaluate?
3. How will you manage?

Case 3

A 48-year-old lady presents with a history of menopause 1 year ago with no symptoms. Her BMI is 30.

1. What details will you ask for in history?
2. How will you evaluate?
3. How will you manage?

Answers

Case 1

1. (a) Severity of hot flushes, mood changes
   (b) Family history of breast and endometrial cancer
   (c) History of diabetes, hypertension, dyslipidaemia
   (d) Dietary calcium intake and sunlight exposure
2. (a) General examination, blood pressure, BMI
   (b) Pelvic examination, cervical smear

3. (a) Prescribe low-dose combination pills cyclically.
   (b) Perform annual check-up.
   (c) Estimate serum FSH annually.
   (d) Continue till FSH levels indicate menopause.
   (e) Evaluate need for HT at menopause.

Case 2

1. History same as in Case 1.
2. (a) General, breast and pelvic examination and cervical smear
   (b) Haemoglobin, blood sugar, lipid profile
3. (a) Lifestyle modification—Walking, sunlight exposure 30 minutes daily; dietary advice—Calcium 1000 mg daily and vitamin D 800 IU/day.
   (b) Counsel regarding HT—Benefits outweigh risks. If willing, HT—tab CEE (Premarin) 0.625 mg + tab MPA 2.5 mg daily.
       Evaluate 3 months later; continue for 5 years if no side effects are observed.
   (c) Perform annual check-up, mammogram 3-yearly.

Case 3

1. (a) Details of menopausal symptoms—Vasomotor, genital, urinary
   (b) Family history of breast cancer, CHD, diabetes, hypertension
   (c) Diet, exercise, sunlight exposure
2. (a) General, breast and pelvic examination
   (b) Cervical smear
   (c) Haemoglobin, blood sugar, lipid profile
3. (a) Lifestyle modification
   (b) Counselling regarding weight reduction—(i) walking 5 km/day (1 hour) for 5 days/week, (ii) 1400-cal diet with 500 mL of milk daily, (iii) calcium 1 g/day with vitamin D 800 IU/day
   (c) No HT since she is asymptomatic and obese

Long-answer question

1. Discuss the merits and demerits of postmenopausal hormone therapy.

Short-answer questions

1. Pathophysiology of menopause
2. Postmenopausal osteoporosis

22 | Infertility

Case scenario

Mrs and Mr VR came to the OPD one Tuesday morning. They had been married and sexually active for 5 years, but Mrs VR had not conceived. Her periods were irregular and she was also overweight. Her parents and in-laws were beginning to worry, and the pressure was taking its toll on their relationship. All in all, it was a bit too much to bear, and the couple was confused and anxious.

Introduction

Couples presenting with an inability to conceive need special attention and care by a gynaecologist, reproductive endocrinologist and sometimes psychiatrist since the problem is complex and may involve one or both the partners. Infertility causes a lot of distress and emotional problems and must be handled with sensitivity and understanding. With the availability of assisted reproductive techniques (ARTs), the prognosis has improved considerably in recent years.

Definitions

Infertility is defined as the failure of a couple to conceive after 1 year of unprotected sexual intercourse in women <35 years of age, and after 6 months of unprotected sexual intercourse in women >35 years of age.

Primary infertility is the inability to conceive in a couple who has had no prior pregnancies.

Secondary infertility is the inability to conceive in a couple who has had at least one prior conception, which may have ended in a live birth, stillbirth, miscarriage, induced abortion or ectopic pregnancy.

Fecundability is the probability of achieving pregnancy within one menstrual cycle.

Prevalence

Prevalence of infertility is about 10–15% in couples of reproductive age. Prevalence increases with age. About 80% of women conceive within 1 year of marriage and 90% within 2 years.

Aetiology

For pregnancy to occur, ovulation, ovum transport by the tubes, presence of normal sperms, fertilization and implantation in the uterine cavity are all essential. Infertility can be due to problems in the male, female or both partners. In some couples, aetiology is unknown, often referred to as unexplained infertility (Box 22.1).

Box 22.1　Aetiology of infertility

- Male factors: 30%
- Female factors: 40–55%
- Both male and female factors: 10–20%
- Unexplained: 10–15%

Female factors causing infertility

The female factors may be problems at the level of ovary, uterus, fallopian tubes, cervix or peritoneum (Box 22.2; Fig. 22.1).

Box 22.2　Female factors causing infertility

- Ovulatory dysfunction: 40%
- Tubal factors: 40%
- Uterine factors: 10%
- Cervical factors: 5%
- Peritoneal factors: 5%

Ovulatory dysfunction

Ovulation is critical to conception. In ovulatory dysfunction, there is oligo-ovulation or anovulation with associated abnormalities of production of ovarian hormones. This can interfere with the preparation of endometrium for implantation and luteal support thereafter. Ovulatory dysfunction can be classified into decreased or absent ovarian reserve and oligo-ovulation or anovulation.

Decreased ovarian reserve

The number of resting or nongrowing primordial follicles is referred to as the ovarian reserve. Fertility decreases with decreasing ovarian reserve. The main reasons for reduced or absent

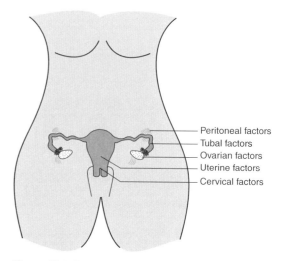

Peritoneal factors
Tubal factors
Ovarian factors
Uterine factors
Cervical factors

Figure 22.1 Female factors causing infertility—Ovarian, tubal, uterine, cervical and peritoneal.

ovarian reserve are advancing maternal age, primary ovarian insufficiency (POI) and resistant ovary (Box 22.3).

Box 22.3　Reasons for reduced or absent ovarian reserve

- Advanced maternal age
- Primary ovarian insufficiency
- Resistant ovary

With advancing maternal age, the quality and number of oocytes decrease and this in a normal woman becomes critical after the age of 35 years. This can occur early in women with POI. POI and resistant ovary are dealt with in Chapter 19, *Secondary amenorrhoea and polycystic ovarian syndrome*. Several tests are used to determine the ovarian reserve, but none have a high sensitivity or specificity (Box 22.4). Estimation of serum follicle-stimulating hormone (FSH), serum anti-Müllerian hormone and transvaginal ultrasonogram is generally used. Low antral follicle count and small ovaries indicate poor ovarian reserve.

Anovulation

Absence of ovulation and infrequent ovulation (oligo-ovulation) are common causes of infertility. The World Health Organization (WHO) classifies disorders of ovulation into three types (Box 22.5).

- Serum FSH day 3
  - >15 mIU/mL
- Serum AMH
  - <8.1 pmol/L
- Transvaginal ultrasound
  - Antral follicle count
    - >10 follicles of 2–10 mm diameter
  - Mean ovarian volume
    - >3 mL
- Serum inhibin
  - <400 pg/mL
- Clomiphene citrate challenge test
  - 100 mg clomiphene from day 5 to 9
  - FSH on days 3 and 10 (<10 mIU/mL)
  - Oestradiol on day 3 (<80 pg/mL)

AMH, anti-Müllerian hormone; *FSH*, follicle-stimulating hormone.

Box 22.5 **WHO classification of disorders of ovulation**

- Type I: Hypogonadotropic hypogonadism
  - Low FSH, LH
  - Low oestradiol
- Type II: Normogonadotropic hypogonadism
  - Normal FSH
  - Normal oestradiol
- Type III: Hypergonadotropic hypogonadism
  - High FSH, LH
  - Low oestradiol

FSH, follicle-stimulating hormone; *LH*, luteinizing hormone; *WHO*, World Health Organization.

Type I: Hypogonadotropic hypogonadism

Women in this group are amenorrheic and anovulatory. Disorder may be in the hypothalamus or pituitary, congenital or acquired. Low gonadotropin-releasing hormone (GnRH) production by the hypothalamus leads to low levels of FSH and luteinizing hormone (LH), lack of ovarian stimulation and low oestradiol levels. There is no ovulation. Pituitary disorders such as Sheehan syndrome or weight loss–related disorders such as anorexia nervosa are associated with low FSH and LH production. Treatment of infertility in this group is by ovulation induction with gonadotropins with or without ARTs.

Hyperprolactinaemia causes decrease in GnRH secretion, leading to anovulation, amenorrhoea and galactorrhoea. Elevated prolactin may be due to tumours, drugs or hypothyroidism. The condition is discussed in detail in Chapter 19, *Secondary amenorrhoea and polycystic ovarian syndrome*.

Type II: Normogonadotropic hypogonadism

The most common condition under this group is polycystic ovarian syndrome (PCOS), which is also the most common cause of anovulation. Clinical features, diagnosis and sequelae of PCOS are discussed in Chapter 19, *Secondary amenorrhoea and polycystic ovarian syndrome*. Women with late-onset congenital adrenal hyperplasia, and adrenal and ovarian tumours are also included in this group, but these conditions are uncommon.

Type III: Hypergonadotropic hypogonadism

In this group of women, the primary problem is ovarian failure with failure of folliculogenesis and resultant low oestradiol. This stimulates FSH production by the pituitary. Primary ovarian failure due to Turner syndrome or Turner mosaic, ovarian radiation or chemotherapy and POI comes under this group. Treatment of infertility in this group is by ART with donor oocyte.

Tubal factors

The ovum that is released is usually picked up by the fimbriae of the tubes and transported into the tubal lumen, where it is fertilized by the sperm. Patent tubes with normal motility and normal ciliary action of the inner lining are essential for conception. Tubal damage is usually the result of pelvic infection (*see* Chapter 13, *Infections of the upper genital tract*). Scarring and adhesion formation lead to tubal occlusion, formation of hydrosalpinx, destruction of cilia and interference with tubal motility. Endometriosis causes anatomical distortion of the tubes, although they may be patent. They cause peritubal adhesions, kinking or tubal occlusion. Causes of tubal damage are as listed in Box 22.6. Tubal factors are common causes of secondary infertility.

Uterine factors

Implantation of the fertilized ovum and further growth of the embryo takes place in the uterus. Congenital and acquired abnormalities of the uterus can interfere with this process (Box 22.7).

Congenital abnormalities

Several congenital abnormalities of the uterus and vagina give rise to primary amenorrhoea (*see*

Box 22.6 Causes of tubal damage

- Pelvic infection
  - Chlamydial infection
  - Gonococcal infection
  - Postabortal infection
  - Puerperal infection
  - Genital tuberculosis
- Tubal pregnancy
- Endometriosis
- Pelvic surgery

Box 22.7 Uterine factors

- Congenital abnormalities
- Acquired abnormalities
  - Endometrial polyps
  - Intrauterine adhesions
  - Submucous leiomyomas
  - Tuberculosis

Chapter 18, *Primary amenorrhoea*). Following surgical correction of congenital anomalies, infection and endometriosis may ensue and result in tubo-ovarian damage leading to infertility. Other anomalies such as bicornuate and septate uterus cause recurrent miscarriage.

Acquired abnormalities

Leiomyomas that are subserous, however large, do not interfere with conception. Submucous leiomyomas and cornually located myomas that occlude the tubes can cause infertility. Anovulation and endometrial hyperplasia that are often associated with myomas also contribute. **Endometrial polyps** can interfere with implantation and must be removed. **Intrauterine adhesions** occur following repeated curettage and can be dense and fibrous in some cases (Asherman syndrome). These women are amenorrheic and infertile. **Tuberculous endometritis** is associated with amenorrhoea and infertility.

Cervical factors

Cervical factors account for 5% of cases of infertility and are caused by cervical stenosis, scarring or abnormalities of cervical mucus–sperm interaction. Scarring and stenosis can also cause changes in the cervical mucus. These usually occur following surgical procedures outlined in Box 22.8. Occasionally, pin hole os or cervical stenosis may be congenital.

Box 22.8 Causes of cervical stenosis and scarring

- Congenital
- Postsurgical
  - Dilatation of cervix
  - LEEP
  - Conization
  - Amputation
  - Fothergill operation

LEEP, loop electroexcision procedure.

The cervical mucus undergoes changes during menstrual cycle under the influence of hormones. During ovulation, the mucus becomes thin, its sodium content and elasticity increases, and microchannels are formed to facilitate sperm passage. When these changes do not occur due to hormonal abnormality or antioestrogenic effect of drugs, sperm movement through the cervix can be affected. In addition, agglutinating antisperm antibodies have been demonstrated in the cervical mucus of infertile couples. These cause agglutination of the sperms and impair their motility.

Peritoneal factors

The uterus, tubes and ovaries are located in the peritoneal cavity. Diseases of the peritoneal cavity can cause infertility by several mechanisms as outlined in Box 22.9. The main causes of peritoneal damage are endometriosis and pelvic inflammatory disease (PID) including genital tuberculosis.

Box 22.9 Infertility due to peritoneal factors

- Adhesions
  - Peritubal
  - Periovarian
- Tubal obstruction
- Kinking
- Formation of rigid tubes
- Tubo-ovarian mass
- Interference with peritoneal fluid production

Endometriosis

Endometriosis is an important aetiological factor for infertility. It is discussed in detail in Chapter 15, *Endometriosis*. Several possible mechanisms have been identified for causation of infertility in endometriosis (*see* Chapter 15, *Endometriosis*): Moderate and severe endometriosis causes tubal damage, adhesions and kinking, but minimal endometriosis is also associated with a high incidence of infertility probably due to immunological alterations and coital dysfunction. Inflammatory mediators such as cytokines and tumour necrosis factor cause changes in peritoneal and tubal environment. Luteal phase disorders, oligo-ovulation and luteinized unruptured follicle (LUF) syndrome are also common. The stage of the disease does not correlate with the risk of infertility.

Pelvic inflammatory disease

Infection by *Chlamydia trachomatis* and *Neisseria gonorrhoeae,* and genital tuberculosis are known to be associated with a high risk of tubal damage, adhesions and infertility. *Mycoplasma hominis* and *Ureaplasma urealyticum* are other organisms that have been implicated. Postabortal or puerperal sepsis can lead to tubal damage and peritubal adhesions and cause secondary infertility.

Genital tuberculosis

Genital tuberculosis is an important cause of infertility in developing countries. Failure to conceive is due to tubal damage, peritoneal involvement with adhesions and endometritis.

Immunological factors

Antisperm antibodies

These are present in the semen, cervical mucus, serum and ovarian follicular fluid. They may be immunoglobulin G (IgG), immunoglobulin M (IgM) or immunoglobulin A (IgA). They are found in about 10–12% of infertile couples, but also in some normal fertile men and women. They affect the semen quality and interfere with sperm capacitation and motility, and fertilization.

Male factors in infertility

Male factors alone or in combination with female factors contribute to about 40% of cases of infertility. Structurally and functionally normal sperms in sufficient numbers must be deposited in the vagina for fertilization of the ovum.

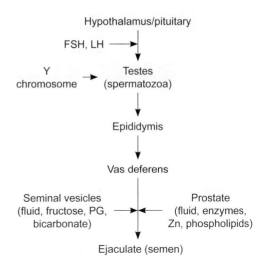

Figure 22.2 Spermatogenesis. *FSH*, follicle-stimulating hormone; *LH*, luteinizing hormone; *PG*, prostaglandin.

Any defect in the production, maturation and/or transport of sperms can lead to infertility.

The testis has two types of cells: Sertoli cells that are responsible for spermatogenesis and production of inhibin and Leydig cells that produce testosterone. Spermatogenesis is directed by genes on the Y chromosome. FSH and LH secreted by the pituitary gland stimulate spermatogenesis and production of testosterone. The spermatozoa then mature in the epididymis (Fig. 22.2), and are transported through the vas deferens. The seminal fluid from the seminal vesicles contributes to the semen volume and contains fructose for nutrition, prostaglandins and bicarbonate. The prostatic gland secretions provide additional seminal fluid volume, enzymes and proteases. The sperms undergo capacitation when they come in contact with cervical mucus. This process is essential for fertilization. Male factor is classified into pretesticular, testicular or post-testicular factors.

Pretesticular causes

These are disorders at the level of hypothalamus/pituitary or other peripheral organs (Box 22.10).

Testicular causes

These affect **testicular spermatogenesis** or **testosterone production**. The conditions are listed in Box 22.11. Most men with these disorders have oligospermia or azoospermia.

Box 22.10 Pretesticular causes of infertility

- Hypothalamic disorders
  - Hypogonadotropic hypogonadism
  - Tumours
  - Infiltrative diseases
    - Tuberculosis
    - Sarcoidosis
    - Histiocytosis
  - Drugs
- Pituitary disorders
  - Congenital
  - Tumours
  - Radiation
  - Granuloma
- Peripheral organs
  - Adrenal disorders
  - Liver failure

Box 22.11 Testicular causes of infertility

- Chromosomal abnormalities
  - Klinefelter syndrome
  - Mixed gonadal dysgenesis
  - Partial androgen insensitivity
  - Genetic disorders of spermatogenesis
- Local conditions
  - Varicocele
  - Cryptorchidism
  - Trauma
  - Orchitis
  - Radiation
  - Chemotherapy
  - Tight underclothing
- Substance abuse
  - Alcohol, smoking, caffeine
  - Occupational exposure to heat and toxins

Varicocele is the most common correctable cause of male infertility and should always be excluded. Those with grade 2 or 3 varicocele need surgical intervention.

Post-testicular causes

The problem may be in sperm motility, transport or ejaculation. The post-testicular causes are given in Box 22.12. In these cases, spermatogenesis is normal.

Unexplained infertility

Unexplained infertility accounts for 10% of cases of infertility. A diagnosis of unexplained

Box 22.12 Post-testicular causes of infertility

- Abnormalities of epididymis
- Congenital block in the ducts
- Congenital bilateral absence of vas deferens
- Acquired blocks in the ejaculatory ducts
  - Infection
  - Trauma
- Antisperm antibodies
- Erectile dysfunction
- Idiopathic male infertility

infertility is made when all investigations are normal. More detailed evaluation may uncover some subtle causes, but some remain unexplained. Some contributory factors to unexplained infertility are listed in Box 22.13.

Box 22.13 Contributing factors to unexplained infertility

- Luteal phase defect
- Luteinized unruptured follicle syndrome
- Minimal endometriosis
- Small endometrial polyps
- Hyperprolactinaemia
- Subtle cervical factors
- Implantation failure
- Immunological causes
- Psychological factors

Luteal phase defect

This condition is also known as luteal phase deficiency or luteal phase dysfunction (LPD). Deficient progesterone production during postovulatory or luteal phase leads to inadequate secretory changes in the endometrium. This makes it unsuitable for implantation and can cause infertility and early pregnancy loss. Diagnosis of luteal phase defect is made when two endometrial biopsies taken in two consecutive cycles during the luteal phase show a delay of more than 2 days beyond the actual cycle day in the histological development of the endometrium. Alternatively, midluteal progesterone levels have also been used but a definite cut-off level is difficult to determine. *The clinical relevance of this condition has been questioned and diagnostic methods are not reliable. The causative role of luteal phase defect in infertility is not proven.*

Luteinized unruptured follicle syndrome

When the dominant follicle undergoes luteinization without rupture and release of the ovum, it is referred to as LUF syndrome. Pregnancy cannot occur, but progesterone production occurs along with all other changes associated with ovulation. The condition is rare and is seen in some women with endometriosis.

Clinical evaluation

Both female and male partners should be evaluated. The male partner should be present at the first visit and subsequently when treatment is planned so that the couple has a full grasp of the diagnosis and management. These should be discussed elaborately before evaluation is begun (Box 22.14).

Box 22.14 Points to be discussed with the couple

- Clinical evaluation of both the partners
- Diagnostic tests
  - Male
  - Female
- Sequence of tests
- Timing of tests
- Total duration
- Cost
- Probability of unexplained infertility in 10%
- Prognosis

History

Female partner

A detailed history regarding duration of infertility, sexual history, past and family history, menstrual history and details of prior treatment should be obtained (Box 22.15).

- It is important to differentiate between primary and secondary infertility since the approach to investigation is different in both cases.
- If the woman has regular cycles with spasmodic dysmenorrhoea and midcycle pain, she is probably ovulating.
- Congestive dysmenorrhoea and dyspareunia indicate endometriosis.

Box 22.15 History—Female partner

- Age
- Number of years married
- Contraception used
- Sexual history
  - Frequency per week
  - Dyspareunia
- Menstrual history
  - Menstrual cycles
  - Dysmenorrhoea
  - Midcycle bleeding/pain
- Obstetric history
  - Previous pregnancy
  - Postabortal/puerperal sepsis
  - Curettage
- Medical illnesses
  - Polycystic ovarian syndrome
  - Diabetes/hypertension
  - Tuberculosis/sexually transmitted diseases
- Family history
  - Genetic mutations
  - Family history of infertility
- Personal history
  - Medications
  - Galactorrhoea
  - Previous surgery
- Pelvic surgery
  - Tubal/ovarian
  - Bowel/bladder
- Smoking/alcohol/substance abuse

- History of previous pelvic surgery or previous abortion/delivery followed by sepsis suggests pelvic adhesions and tubal block.
- Obese woman with irregular cycles, hirsutism and acanthosis nigricans may have PCOS.

Male partner

A similar detailed history from the male partner is mandatory (Box 22.16).

Physical examination

The couple must undergo a thorough physical examination (Boxes 22.17 and 22.18).

The male partner should be evaluated along with the female.

Investigations

Investigations to identify the cause of infertility are required in most cases. Couples who are young, married for a short duration and unaware

- Age
- Occupation
- Smoking/alcohol/substance abuse
- Sexual history
  - Erectile dysfunction
  - Premature ejaculation
- Anosmia, hyposmia
- Past history
  - Surgery
    - Herniorrhaphy/hydrocelectomy
    - Surgery for undescended testes
- Injury
- Infections
  - Mumps
  - Orchitis
  - Epididymitis
  - Sexually transmitted diseases
- Medications

Box 22.17 Examination of the female

- General examination
  - Body mass index
  - Blood pressure
  - Signs of hyperandrogenism
    - Acne
    - Hirsutism
    - Acanthosis nigricans
- Breast examination
  - Galactorrhoea
- Signs of thyroid dysfunction
- Abdominal examination
  - Mass arising from the pelvis
  - Scars of surgery
- Speculum examination
  - Cervical stenosis
  - Scarring of the cervix
- Pelvic and rectal examination
  - Uterine size
  - Adnexal mass/tenderness
  - Nodules in POD
  - Induration of uterosacrals

POD, pouch of Douglas.

Box 22.18 Examination of the male

- General examination
  - Body proportions
  - Body mass index
  - Blood pressure
  - Hair growth
  - Gynaecomastia
- Examination of the genitalia
  - Testicular volume, consistency
  - Epididymal fullness/tenderness/thickening
  - Varicocele
  - Vas deferens

Box 22.19 Investigations of the female partner

- Tests for ovulation
- Tests for tubal patency
- Tests to exclude peritoneal factors
- Tests for uterine pathology
- Tests for cervical factors

Female partner

Investigations of the female are classified as in Box 22.19.

Tests for ovulation

Documentation of ovulation is an important component of evaluation of infertility.

Tests used for detection of ovulation are as follows:

- Midluteal serum progesterone
- Basal body temperature (BBT) chart
- Urinary/serum LH
- Transvaginal sonography
- Endometrial biopsy
- Regular menstrual cycles indicate ovulation. Midcycle pain or **mittelschmerz** and spotting also indicate ovulation. Confirmation by midluteal progesterone is adequate when history indicates ovulatory cycles.
- However, women with irregular cycles require more tests to confirm ovulation and ascertain the cause of anovulation.
- Kits for detection of LH surge by urinary LH measurement are easy to use. This and the day 21 progesterone measurement are the tests commonly used now.

Midluteal serum progesterone Serum progesterone level >3 ng/mL on day 21 of a 28-day cycle is indicative of ovulation in women with

of fertile period can be counselled and investigations can be undertaken after 6 months or 1 year. Secondary infertility is most often due to tubal factor, and if history suggests ovulatory cycles, tubal patency tests or laparoscopy should be performed first.

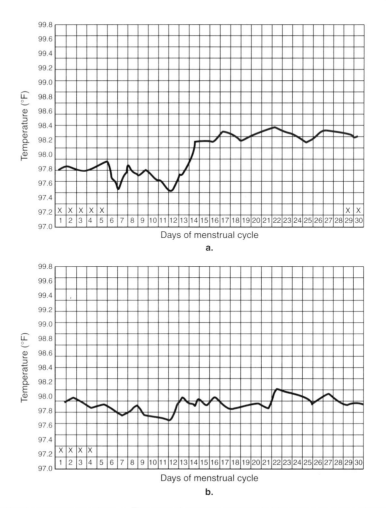

Figure 22.3 Basal body temperature chart. **a.** The normal ovulatory pattern is biphasic with a rise of temperature to about 0.4°F after ovulation. **b.** The anovulatory temperature pattern shows no rise of temperature.

regular cycles. But since progesterone is secreted in pulses, single measurement lacks sensitivity. Value of 10 ng/mL indicates adequate luteal support and is associated with higher pregnancy rates. This is the test performed in most centres now to confirm ovulation.

Basal body temperature chart Progesterone has a thermogenic effect and the body temperature rises by 0.2°C or 0.4°F immediately after ovulation. The temperature should be checked daily from day 1 of the cycle, on awakening, before any activity and recorded on a graph. Ovulatory cycles have a biphasic temperature pattern (Fig. 22.3). Although it is the cheapest way of confirming ovulation, it is not useful for predicting the exact time of ovulation. Ovulation can be identified only retrospectively; therefore, it cannot be used for timing of intercourse. Although correlation with transvaginal ultrasound is poor, in centres where progesterone estimation is not available and as preliminary evaluation of ovulatory function, BBT is useful.

Urinary/serum LH Ovulation occurs about 36 hours after LH surge. Serial measurement of urinary LH starting 3–4 days prior to the predicted LH surge is used to predict ovulation. Commercial kits are available for home use and LH level of >40 mIU/mL is considered to indicate a surge. Correlation with transvaginal ultrasound is good. Serum LH levels are not useful for home monitoring.

Transvaginal sonography Serial sonographic examination of the ovaries is used to visualize the

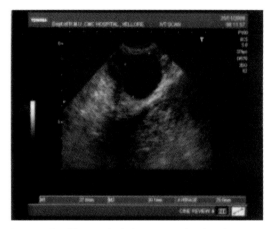

Figure 22.4 Transvaginal ultrasonography showing preovulatory dominant follicle of 20 mm in size.

- Midluteal serum progesterone
  - Currently used as routine by most
  - Done on day 21
  - >3 ng/mL confirms ovulation
- BBT chart
  - Inexpensive, used in peripheral centres
  - Biphasic pattern in ovulatory cycles
- Urinary LH
  - Commercial kits
  - Indicates LH surge
  - Occurrence of ovulation 34–36 hours later
  - Surge suggested by a level >40 mIU/mL
- Transvaginal ultrasonogram
  - Serial scans from day 10
  - Monitors development of follicle and rupture
  - Dominant follicle 18–20 mm preovulation
  - Follicle collapses postovulation
  - Expensive, cumbersome
  - Used in ART cycles
- Endometrial biopsy
  - Routinely used in some centres
  - Secretory change indicates ovulation
  - Performed on days 24–26
  - Can diagnose LPD and TB

ART, assisted reproductive technique; *BBT*, basal body temperature; *LH*, luteinizing hormone; *LPD*, luteal phase defect; *TB*, tuberculosis.

development of the dominant follicle and its subsequent collapse after ovulation. Scans must be performed from day 10 and the follicular growth monitored. Ovulation occurs when the follicle enlarges to 18–20 mm (Fig. 22.4). Measurement of endometrial thickness is also used to assess the adequacy of endometrial preparation for implantation. Trilaminar endometrium with a thickness of >8 mm is considered favourable. This test is too cumbersome and expensive for routine evaluation of ovulatory dysfunction. It is extensively used to monitor ovulation during ovulation induction.

Endometrial biopsy Progesterone secreted after ovulation by the ovary causes secretory changes in the endometrium and prepares it for implantation. Biopsy of the endometrium has been used to document these endometrial changes as indirect evidence of ovulation. Biopsy should be performed between days 24 and 26 of the cycle. Secretory changes confirm ovulation, and dating of endometrial changes is used to diagnose luteal phase defect. Tuberculous endometritis can also be diagnosed by histological examination of endometrial biopsy and culture for tubercle bacilli.

The salient features of the tests for ovulation are listed in Box 22.20.

Assessment of ovarian reserve

This should be performed in women of age >35 years and when history is suggestive of POI. The tests are described earlier in this chapter.

Tests for tubal and peritoneal factors

These factors can be assessed together by laparoscopy. Other tests are specifically used to detect tubal block (Box 22.21). When only tubal factor is suspected, hysterosalpingography (HSG) is usually the first-line test.

Hysterosalpingography

This is used as the primary test for tubal evaluation in most women unless there is a history of prior pelvic surgery, PID or endometriosis.

- HSG is performed by injecting radio-opaque water- or oil-soluble dye through the cervix and taking X-ray films under fluoroscopy.
- As dye is injected, it flows through the uterus and tubes and spills into the peritoneal cavity, and can be visualized (Fig. 22.5).
- The procedure is performed during the follicular phase (between days 6 and 10), after menstrual bleeding stops, to avoid exposure of a fertilized ovum to radiation in case the woman has conceived during the cycle.

- Uterine abnormalities, polyps, rigidity of the tube, beading, hydrosalpinx and site of tubal block can be diagnosed by HSG. The test has a high negative predictive value, sensitivity of 65% and specificity of 83%. It is not reliable for detection of peritubal adhesions or tubal function.
- HSG also has a therapeutic effect since it flushes the tubes and may dislodge mucus and cellular debris blocking the tubes.
- If performed during menstruation, venous intravasation of dye can occur. In the presence of active infection, peritonitis can occur. Occasionally, reactivation of old infection can occur.
- Women at a high risk for infection or those found to have dilated tubes should be given oral doxycycline 100 mg twice daily for 5 days after the procedure. An antispasmodic administered before the procedure reduces pain and relieves tubal spasm.
- Complications of HSG include uterine perforation, infection and allergy to the dye. Women may experience mild to moderate postprocedural pain, which responds to analgesics.

Hysterosalpingo-contrast sonography (HyCoSy)

After injection of echogenic contrast medium into the uterus, ultrasonography is used to visualize the uterus and tubes. It is quick and easy and has a high accuracy.

Saline infusion sonography

Infusion of saline into the uterine cavity through the cervix and visualization by transvaginal sonography is known as saline infusion sonography or sonohysterosalpingography. Endometrial polyps, septae and spill of saline into the peritoneal cavity through patent tubes can be visualized. It is easy to perform and can be combined with ultrasound evaluation of ovaries and/or uterus.

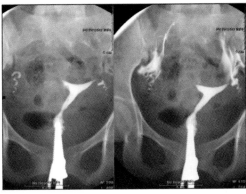

a.

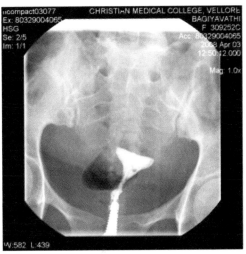

b.

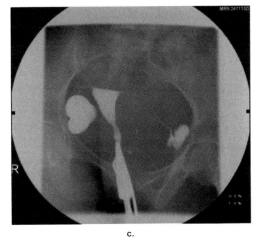

c.

Figure 22.5 Hysterosalpingography. **a.** Bilateral spill of contrast. Both tubes are visible and there is contrast seen in peritoneal cavity. **b.** Bilateral cornual block. The tubes are not visible. **c.** Bilateral hydrosalpinx with no spill of contrast. The tubes are visible and end in dilated bulbous terminal hydrosalpinx on both sides.

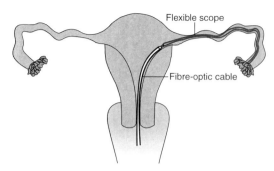

Figure 22.6 Diagrammatic representation of falloposcopy. The fibre-optic cable is seen in the uterine cavity with flexible microendoscope attached to it.

Falloposcopy

Falloposcope is a flexible microendoscope used for visualization of the tubal lumen during hysteroscopy (Fig. 22.6). Information regarding the tubal lining and tubal block can be obtained. Tube can be cannulated under falloposcopic guidance. This is not available or used as a routine.

The details of tests for tubal factor are summarized in Box 22.22.

Laparoscopy

- Peritubal, ovarian and peritoneal factors can be evaluated by laparoscopy (Box 22.23).
- The procedure needs anaesthesia and hospitalization and is more invasive and expensive than HSG.
- Therefore, it is not included as a part of the initial evaluation. It is performed in women with a history suggestive of PID, endometriosis and prior surgery, and in those who fail to conceive after initial therapy.
- Methylene blue is injected during laparoscopy, and spill of dye through the fimbrial end confirms tubal patency (Fig. 22.7). Peritubal adhesions (Fig. 22.8a), endometriosis (Fig. 22.8b), tubo-ovarian mass and small myomas can be identified by laparoscopy.
- Adhesiolysis and excision or ablation of endometriosis and excision of endometriomas can be performed during laparoscopy. Ovarian drilling can also be performed in women with PCOS, if indicated.

Tests for uterine factors

- Abnormalities of uterine cavity, intrauterine adhesions and polyps can be diagnosed by various tests listed in Box 22.24.

Box 22.22 Tests for tubal patency

- Hysterosalpingography
  - Injection of radio-opaque dye into the uterus
  - X-rays and fluoroscopy
  - Performed in follicular phase
  - Can visualize uterine septae, polyps, hydrosalpinx, site of tubal block
  - Contraindicated if active infection, bleeding
  - High sensitivity for diagnosing tubal block
- Hysterosalpingo-contrast sonography
  - Injection of echogenic contrast medium into uterus
  - Ultrasonography to view the uterus, tubes, ovary
  - As sensitive as hysterosalpingography
  - Quick and easy
- Saline infusion sonography
  - Injection of saline into the uterine cavity
  - Transvaginal ultrasonogram
  - Can diagnose polyps, septae
  - Tubal block
  - Can be combined with ultrasonography for other evaluation
- Falloposcopy
  - Flexible microendoscopy of the tube
  - Performed along with hysteroscopy
  - Visualization of tubal lumen
  - Tubal cannulation under guidance
  - Not used as routine

Box 22.23 Laparoscopic evaluation

- Tubes
  - Peritubal adhesions
  - Tubal block
  - Tubal motility
  - Condition of fimbriae
  - Hydrosalpinx
- Ovaries
  - Endometrioma
  - Adhesions
  - Polycystic ovaries
  - Tubo-ovarian mass (TB/PID)
- Uterus
  - Myomas
  - Uterine anomalies
- Peritoneal factors
  - Endometriosis
  - Postinflammatory adhesions
  - Tuberculosis

PID, pelvic inflammatory disease; *TB*, tuberculosis.

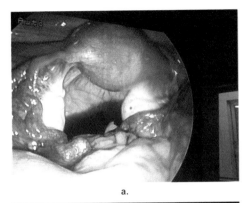

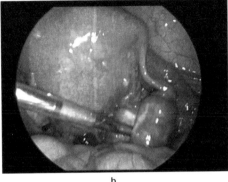

Figure 22.7 Laparoscopy in women with infertility. **a.** Uterus, both tubes and ovaries are seen. Bilateral free spill of dye is seen and there is methylene blue dye collected in the pouch of Douglas. **b.** Right tube with hydrosalpinx. The distal dilated end is filled with dye, but there is no spill indicating that the tube is blocked.

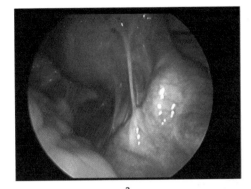

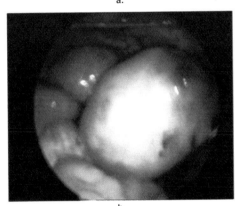

Figure 22.8 Laparoscopy. **a.** Peritubal adhesions. Strands of adhesions are seen between the tube and the uterine surface. **b.** Large ovarian endometrioma of the right ovary.

Box 22.24 Tests for uterine factors

- Hysterosalpingography
- Transvaginal ultrasonography
- Saline infusion sonography
- Hysteroscopy

- Uterine anomalies do not always interfere with conception but more often cause recurrent pregnancy loss.
- Ultrasonography helps in determining the size, number and location of myomas (Fig. 22.9).
- Saline infusion sonography is superior to HSG for detection of uterine anomalies. It also delineates polyps better than transvaginal ultrasonography.
- Hysteroscopy is the best tool for visualizing the uterine cavity. Resection of septum (Fig. 22.10) and polypectomy can also be performed in the same sitting.

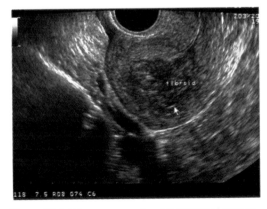

Figure 22.9 Ultrasonogram showing intramural myoma close to the uterine cavity but not distorting it.

Tests for cervical factors

Postcoital test

This test is performed to look for local antisperm antibodies and assess the quality of cervical

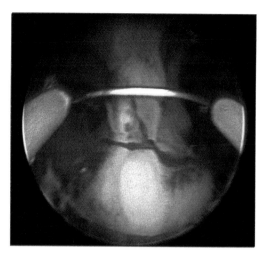

Figure 22.10 Hysteroscopic resection of uterine septum in a woman with septate uterus. The septum has been partially resected. The two halves of the uterine cavity are seen on either side.

Box 22.25 Postcoital test

- To assess
  - Cervical mucus
    - Spinnbarkeit
    - Ferning
  - Sperm–mucus interaction
- Performed 1–2 days prior to the ovulation
- Within few hours of intercourse
- Five motile sperms/HPF considered normal
- Poor reproducibility and sensitivity
- Does not alter the management
- Not used now

HPF, high-power field.

Box 22.26 Other investigations in the female partner

- Anovulatory women
  - Hirsutism, virilization: Testosterone, DHEA, 17(OH)P
  - Galactorrhoea: Prolactin, TSH
  - Obesity: Blood sugar, lipid profile
- History suggestive of infection
  - Cervical swab for *C. trachomatis*

DHEA, dehydroepiandrosterone; *17(OH)P*, 17-OH progesterone; *TSH*, thyroid-stimulating hormone.

mucus (Box 22.25). Couple should be asked to have intercourse 1–2 days prior to the predicted time of ovulation and present to the clinic within a few hours. Cervical mucus is removed with sponge forceps or aspirated and placed on a slide. Spinnbarkeit or stretchability of the mucus is tested by placing a coverslip on the mucus and stretching the mucus. Due to the effect of oestrogen, the mucus stretches to 8–10 cm. A drop of mucus is allowed to dry on the slide and examined under the microscope to look for ferning. This, when present, indicates preovulatory oestrogen effect.

The mucus is examined for presence of sperms. The presence of about five motile sperms per high-power field indicates normal sperm–mucus interaction. Absence of sperms or clumping of sperms can be due to incorrect timing, infection, medications with antioestrogenic action on the cervical mucus [clomiphene citrate (CC)] or abnormal mucus–sperm interaction. The tests lack reproducibility, sensitivity, uniform methodology and criteria for assessment. An abnormal test does not alter the management of unexplained infertility. The test has no place now in the evaluation of infertility.

Other investigations Apart from the tests discussed so far, additional tests may be required in some women (Box 22.26). In women with anovulation and signs of hyperandrogenism or galactorrhoea, further endocrine evaluation is required. Chlamydial infection must be ruled out by cervical swab in women with a history suggestive of infection.

Male partner

Nearly 70% of the conditions that cause male infertility can be diagnosed with history, physical examination and semen analysis.

Semen analysis

Semen analysis is the single most important test in the evaluation of male fertility. The sample is collected after 2–3 days of abstinence. Normal semen parameters according to the WHO (2010) are listed in Box 22.27.

White blood cells in the semen may indicate epididymitis or prostatitis. Round cells are either lymphocytes or immature germ cells. Presence of round cells suggests a defect in spermatogenesis. When semen analysis is abnormal, the male partner should be referred for further investigations to a urologist/reproductive medicine specialist.

Box 22.27   Normal semen analysis (WHO criteria)

• Volume	1.5 mL or more
• pH	>7.2
• Sperm concentration	15 million/mL or more
• Total sperm number	39 million/ejaculate
• Progressive motility	32% or more
• Total motility (progressive + nonprogressive)	40% or more
• Morphology	Normal morphology 4% or more
• Viability	58% or more alive

WHO, World Health Organization.

Further evaluation of the male

Further investigations are listed in Box 22.28.

Box 22.28   Further investigations in the male partner

- Endocrine evaluation
  - Follicle-stimulating hormone
  - Luteinizing hormone
  - Prolactin
  - Serum testosterone
- Karyotyping
  - Klinefelter syndrome
  - Y microdeletions
- Genetic testing
- Transrectal ultrasonography
  - Ejaculatory duct obstruction
- Scrotal ultrasonography
  - Evaluation of testes, epididymis
- Vasography
  - Patency of vas deferens
- Testicular biopsy
  - Spermatogenesis, atrophy

Hormonal evaluation is required to assess hypothalamic–pituitary function. Genetic abnormalities are common in men with abnormal semen characteristics. In men with azoospermia, normal serum FSH and normal spermatogenesis on testicular biopsy indicate obstruction. The site of obstruction is identified by ultrasonography and vasography. Testicular atrophy due to orchitis and other causes can also be diagnosed by biopsy. But since other methods of sperm retrieval are available, testicular biopsy is seldom undertaken now.

Management of infertile couple

All couples should be advised regarding lifestyle modification, weight reduction to ideal body weight and cessation of smoking/alcohol. Management depends on several factors as listed in Box 22.29.

Box 22.29   Factors for management decision

- Age, both male and female
- Duration of infertility
- Cause of infertility
- Prior treatment failure

Counselling regarding fertile period

- In young couples with duration of infertility <1 year, if no abnormality is found on history, physical examination and semen analysis, advise may be given regarding
  - Lifestyle modification
    - Cessation of smoking, alcohol consumption
    - Weight optimization
    - Avoidance of stress
  - Timing of intercourse
- The **fertile period** extends from 5 days prior to ovulation to the day of ovulation (6 days). Urinary LH kits, if available, can be used for timing of ovulation. BBT charts are not very precise for this purpose.
- Randomized trials have shown that weight reduction of 5–10% of body weight can restore ovulation and result in pregnancy in obese women.
- Further investigations can be delayed for 6 months to 1 year.

Treatment of ovulatory dysfunction

Ovulation induction

This is the treatment of choice for women with ovulatory dysfunction. Drugs used for this are listed in Box 22.30.

Box 22.30 Drugs used for ovulation induction

- Ovulation-inducing agents
  - Clomiphene citrate
  - Gonadotropins
    - Human menopausal gonadotropin
    - Recombinant FSH
  - Aromatase inhibitors
    - Letrozole
    - Anastrozole
- Drugs used to facilitate ovulation induction
  - Insulin sensitizers
    - Metformin
    - Pioglitazone

FSH, follicle-stimulating hormone.

Drugs used for ovulation induction

Clomiphene citrate It has a predominantly antioestrogenic and some oestrogenic action (Box 22.31). It combines with oestrogen receptors and competitively inhibits the negative feedback of oestrogen on the hypothalamus, thus increasing GnRH production. This stimulates pituitary gonadotropin secretion and ovulation.

Box 22.31 Clomiphene citrate

- Binds to oestrogen receptors
- Increases secretion of gonadotropin-releasing hormone
- Dose 50 mg once daily from day 2 to 6
- Increased by 50 mg every cycle to 150 mg daily
- Follicular response monitored
- Total duration—Six cycles

Clomiphene is used for ovulation induction in oligo-ovulation or anovulation as seen in PCOS (WHO type II). It is not useful in hypo-oestrogenic states (WHO types I and III).

- The initial dose is 50 mg daily taken on days 2–6 of the cycle. Ovulation is expected on day 14.
- Ovulation may be confirmed by LH surge using urinary LH kits, BBT chart or midluteal progesterone. However, follicular monitoring by transvaginal ultrasound is used currently in most women.
- Follicular monitoring is performed from day 12. Dominant follicular size of 18–20 mm on days 13–14 indicates good ovarian response (Fig. 22.11).
- If there is no response, dose is increased to 100 mg and then to 150 mg in the subsequent

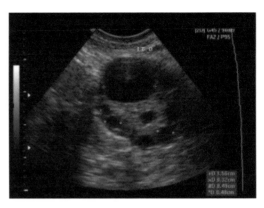

Figure 22.11 Follicular monitoring in a woman with polycystic ovarian syndrome on ovulation induction with clomiphene citrate. Ultrasonography shows polycystic ovaries with one dominant follicle.

cycles. If there is response, the drug is continued for 3–6 months.
- Women who do not conceive after 6 months of therapy are considered clomiphene failures and alternative treatments should be considered.
- About 80% of women ovulate in the first three cycles. The pregnancy rate is lower probably due to antioestrogenic action on the endometrium and cervical mucus.
- Multifoetal pregnancy is a complication of CC therapy.

Aromatase inhibitors
This class of compounds inhibits aromatase, an enzyme involved in conversion of androgens to oestrogens. Ovarian oestradiol production is suppressed, negative feedback inhibition of the hypothalamus is reduced and GnRH production is increased. These drugs have the added advantage that they promote monofollicular development; therefore, multiple pregnancy is not a concern.

Letrozole is the most widely used aromatase inhibitor. The dosage is 2.5–5 mg for 5 days from day 3 to 7. Randomized trials have shown that live birth rate and ovulation rates are higher with letrozole compared to those with clomiphene, especially in women with body mass index (BMI) >30 kg/m^2.

There have been concerns regarding the teratogenic effects of letrozole. However, studies have shown that congenital anomalies are not increased.

Letrozole is currently recommended by many as first-line drug in women with higher BMI and second-line drug after clomiphene in women with lower BMI. *However, aromatase inhibitors are currently not approved by the Food and Drug Administration (FDA) for ovulation induction.*

Another drug in this group is **anastrozole**, which is less effective in ovulation induction than letrozole and is not recommended for this purpose.

Gonadotropins

In women who do not ovulate with CC ± metformin, the next step is ovulation induction with gonadotropins. They are used as first-line drugs in hypogonadotropic anovulation (WHO type I). Human menopausal gonadotropin (hMG) contains FSH and LH. Human chorionic gonadotropin (hCG) has only LH activity. The recombinant FSH has specific FSH activity.

Gonadotropins are used alone or in combination with CC. Treatment begins with 50–75 mIU/mL of FSH on day 5 of the cycle given intramuscularly (IM) and the dose is stepped up using transvaginal ultrasound monitoring of follicular size. When follicular size is optimal, hCG 5000 IU is administered IM to trigger ovulation.

Gonadotropins are used in PCOS when there is no response to clomiphene and in women with hypopituitarism.

Complications of gonadotropin therapy are multifoetal pregnancy and ovarian hyperstimulation syndrome (OHSS). Gonadotropins are also expensive.

Drugs used to facilitate ovulation induction

Insulin sensitizers The most common cause of anovulation is PCOS. Insulin resistance plays a major role in the pathophysiology of PCOS; reducing insulin levels has been shown to restore normal ovarian function.

- *Metformin:* Metformin, which is a biguanide, is the drug that has been studied extensively. In addition to reducing insulin resistance, metformin also helps in weight reduction (Box 22.32). It is used along with CC in women with PCOS and glucose intolerance who do not respond to CC. Addition of metformin has been shown to improve pregnancy rates. The dose of metformin is 500 mg thrice daily or 850 mg thrice daily.
- *Pioglitazone:* An insulin sensitizer, pioglitazone has been used in place of metformin. Large trials are not available. Weight gain due to water retention is a problem.

Glucocorticoids Women with clinical features of PCOS and elevated dehydroepiandrosterone sulphate (DHEAS) may respond to a combination of CC and dexamethasone.

Dopamine agonists In women with hyperprolactinaemia associated with anovulation, bromocriptine or cabergoline is used for ovulation induction. Treatment should be stopped once pregnancy is diagnosed.

Other drugs used for ovulation induction are listed in Box 22.32.

> **Box 22.32 Other drugs used in ovulation induction**
>
> - Aromatase inhibitors
>   - Inhibit aromatization of androgen to oestrogen
>   - Letrozole is the drug of choice
>   - Dosage is 2.5–5 mg daily for 5 days from day 3 to 7
>   - Live birth rates higher in obese women
>   - Used as second line in PCOS, first line in obese PCOS
>   - Teratogenic effects not increased
>   - Not approved by the FDA
> - Gonadotropins
>   - hMG has FSH and LH activity
>   - hCG has LH activity
>   - hCG triggers ovulation
>   - Can be used alone or with CC
>   - Monitor with serum oestradiol
>   - Start with 50–75 IU IM daily
>   - Adverse effects
>   - OHSS
>   - Multifoetal pregnancy
> - Insulin sensitizers
>   - Metformin
>   - Reduces insulin resistance
>   - Used along with CC in PCOS
>   - 850 mg two to three times daily
>   - Pioglitazone
>   - Can be used to reduce insulin resistance
>   - Causes water retention and weight gain
> - Glucocorticoids
>   - Used in women with elevated DHEAS
> - Dopamine agonists
>   - Used in hyperprolactinaemia with anovulation
>   - Bromocriptine or cabergoline may be used
>
> CC, clomiphene citrate; DHEAS, dehydroepiandrosterone sulphate; FDA, Food and Drug Administration; FSH, follicle-stimulating hormone; hCG, human chorionic gonadotropin; hMG, human menopausal gonadotropin; IM, intramuscular; LH, luteinizing hormone; PCOS, polycystic ovarian syndrome.

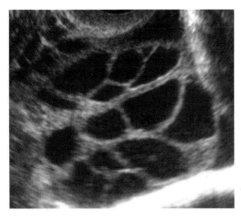

Figure 22.12 Ultrasonogram showing ovarian hyperstimulation in a patient on ovulation induction after administration of hCG. *hCG*, human chorionic gonadotropin.

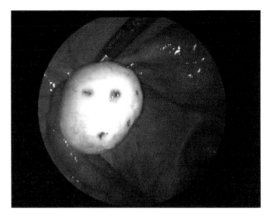

Figure 22.13 Laparoscopic view of ovary after ovarian drilling in a woman with PCOS. *PCOS*, polycystic ovarian syndrome.

Complications of ovulation induction

Ovarian hyperstimulation syndrome This syndrome is characterized by ovarian enlargement (Fig. 22.12) with abdominal distension, ascites, hypotension, oliguria, haemoconcentration, and gastrointestinal and respiratory problems (Box 22.33). They usually develop after administration of hCG to trigger ovulation or, occasionally, in early pregnancy due to endogenous hCG secretion. According to severity, OHSS is classified into grades 1–5. Treatment is by fluid replacement and supportive therapy. This can be prevented by close monitoring of serum oestradiol and follicular development, and withholding hCG if there are too many follicles or if oestradiol levels are too high.

Box 22.33 Complications of ovulation induction

- Ovarian hyperstimulation syndrome
  - Ovarian enlargement
  - Ascites, haemoconcentration, oliguria
  - Occurs with gonadotropin therapy
  - Managed conservatively
  - Replacement of fluids/albumin
- Multifoetal pregnancy
  - Twins with clomiphene citrate
  - Higher-order pregnancies with gonadotropins

Multifoetal gestation Twins and higher-order multiple pregnancies occur with ovulation-inducing agents. Higher-order multifoetal pregnancies are usually seen when gonadotropins are used, whereas twin pregnancies are a complication of clomiphene therapy.

Laparoscopic ovarian drilling

In women with PCOS who do not respond to ovulation induction by CC, ovarian drilling has been found to be as effective as gonadotropin therapy. The risk of OHSS and multiple pregnancies is also less. Ovarian drilling is performed laparoscopically by electrocautery, laser or harmonic scalpel (Fig. 22.13). The fall in androgen levels due to destruction of androgen-producing theca cells in the ovarian stroma restores normal hormonal function and ovulation. Postoperative adhesions occur in 20% of patients.

Treatment of tubal factors

- Tubal factors may be adhesions or tubal block. Tubal occlusion can be in the proximal or distal part of the tube.
- Proximal occlusion includes block at the intramural portion, isthmus or ampulla of the tube. Distal occlusion involves the fimbria.
- The success of treatment with tubes that are badly damaged is low, the risk of ectopic pregnancy is high, and in vitro fertilization (IVF) is recommended in women with sever tubal disease and in older women.
- Methods used to treat tubal occlusion are listed in Box 22.34.
- The optimal treatment should be chosen carefully (Box 22.35). Tubal microsurgery can be performed by laparotomy or laparoscopy.

Treatment of proximal tubal occlusion

Selective salpingography can be performed when proximal block is detected during HSG. Catheter is placed under fluoroscopic guidance at the tubal ostium and contrast injected under pressure. This displaces mucus or debris that is blocking the tube.

Radiologically guided cannulation is performed if the tube does not open up with selective salpingography. A guidewire is introduced into the tube under radiological guidance. High rate of success is reported with this procedure in women with proximal occlusion.

Hysteroscopic cannulation is easier to perform and used more often than radiologically guided cannulation. Pregnancy rates are the same as for tubal microsurgery. This procedure is less invasive.

Microsurgical procedures are resorted to if attempts to cannulate the tube fail. If the block is in the isthmus or ampulla, resection of the blocked portion of the tube and reanastomosis is the procedure of choice. Women who have undergone sterilization procedures and request reversal are also candidates for resection and

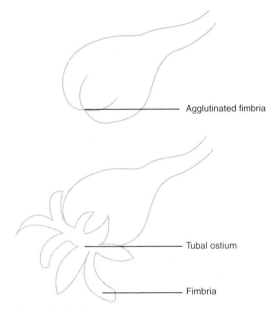

Figure 22.14 Diagrammatic representation of neosalpingostomy. The fimbriae that are agglutinated are separated and the ostium is opened.

anastomosis. If the intramural portion of the tube is blocked, tubocornual anastomosis is done.

Treatment of distal tubal occlusion

Distal tubal occlusion can be due to peritubal adhesions, occluded fimbriae or hydrosalpinx.

Fimbrioplasty is the release of peritubal adhesions and fimbrial phimosis.

Neosalpingostomy is creating a new tubal opening when the distal tube is blocked (Fig. 22.14).

Salpingectomy Women with hydrosalpinx have a poor prognosis for fertility, especially when the hydrosalpinx is >3 cm in size. The endosalpinx is usually destroyed and the fluid in the hydrosalpinx may be embryotoxic. Therefore, resection of the hydrosalpinx followed by IVF is recommended.

Treatment of peritoneal factors

Treatment of endometriosis is outlined in Chapter 15, *Endometriosis*. Pregnancy rates in minimal endometriosis increase with ovulation induction with CC followed by intrauterine insemination (IUI). Adhesions caused by PID or endometriosis can be released by laparoscopic

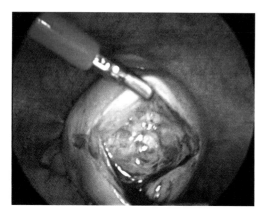

Figure 22.15 Laparoscopic myomectomy in an infertile woman with myoma. Capsule has been incised and the myoma is visible.

adhesiolysis, but adhesions can recur. IVF may be the best option in many of these women.

Treatment of uterine factors

Myomectomy is not indicated in women with infertility, except in selected circumstances. Submucous myomas and myomas that contribute to tubal occlusion and/or distort the cavity must be removed (Fig. 22.15). In women with unexplained infertility and myoma, myomectomy has been shown to improve fertility rate. Treatment of uterine factors is listed in Box 22.36.

Endometrial polyps must be removed by hysteroscopic polypectomy and the pregnancy rate improves by 30%. Intrauterine adhesions should be broken by hysteroscopic adhesiolysis. Congenital anomalies of the uterus and vagina that interfere with conception may be corrected surgically.

Treatment of cervical factors

Postcoital test (PCT) is not recommended as a routine in the workup of women with infertility. Active infection of the cervix should be treated. In women with abnormal PCT or unexplained infertility thought to be due to cervical factors, IUI is the treatment of choice.

Box 22.36 Treatment of uterine factors

- Endometrial polyp: Hysteroscopic polypectomy
- Myoma: Myomectomy, if indicated
- Intrauterine adhesions: Hysteroscopic adhesiolysis
- Congenital anomalies: Surgical correction

Treatment of male infertility

Management of male infertility is challenging. Treatment is not available or has poor results in azoospermia and conditions such as Klinefelter syndrome and other chromosomal abnormalities.

Counselling regarding cessation of smoking, alcohol, lifestyle modification, avoiding tight underclothing and regular exercise is the first step in the management.

Varicocele may or may not be associated with abnormal semen count. The benefits of surgical intervention are controversial. It is recommended that if clinically evident, varicocele must be corrected surgically.

Abnormal semen analysis may be abnormalities in the sperm, seminal fluid or both. Terminology used to describe semen abnormalities is given in Box 22.37.

Box 22.37 Abnormal semen analysis: Terminology

• Aspermia	Absence of semen (no ejaculate)
• Azoospermia	Absence of sperm in semen
• Oligozoospermia	<15 million sperms/mL of semen
• Asthenospermia	Decreased sperm motility (<32% progressive motility, <40% progressive + nonprogressive motility)
• Teratozoospermia	Abnormal sperm morphology
• Hypospermia	Low semen volume

Aspermia can be due to erectile dysfunction (ED), psychogenic factors or retrograde ejaculation. Treatment is outlined in Box 22.38. Supportive therapy is essential in the management of ED. Underlying conditions such as

---

Box 22.38 Management of aspermia

- Erectile dysfunction
  - Supportive psychotherapy
  - Treatment of underlying conditions
  - Drugs
    - Papaverine
    - Sildenafil citrate
  - IUI
- Retrograde ejaculation
  - IUI/IVF with washed sperm

IUI, intrauterine insemination; *IVF*, in vitro fertilization.

uncontrolled diabetes must be treated. Several drugs including antihypertensives can cause ED. These should be looked into. Sildenafil is now used in the treatment of ED.

Retrograde ejaculation occurs in neuropathic disorders. Sperms can be collected from the urine, washed and used for IUI or IVF.

Treatment of azoospermia depends on the cause, whether it is pretesticular, testicular or post-testicular (Box 22.39). Hypogonadotropic hypogonadism due to hypothalamic or pituitary disease may be treated with GnRH analogues or gonadotropins, respectively. Obstructive azo-ospermia can be corrected surgically by end-to-end anastomosis of epididymis or vasoepididy-mostomy depending on the site of obstruction. Aspiration of sperm from testis or epididymis followed by IVF is more successful in many cases of testicular or post-testicular azoospermia.

Box 22.39 Treatment of azoospermia

- Pretesticular azoospermia
  - GnRH therapy
  - hCG followed by hMG
  - Donor insemination
- Testicular azoospermia
  - TESE
  - (or) TESA
  - Donor insemination
- Post-testicular azoospermia
  - End-to-end anastomosis of epididymis
  - Vasoepididymostomy
  - MESA
  - (or) PESA

GnRH, gonadotropin-releasing hormone; *hCG*, human chorionic gonadotropins; *hMG*, human menopausal gonadotropin; *MESA*, microsurgical epididymal sperm aspiration; *PESA*, percutaneous epididymal sperm aspiration; *TESA*, testicular sperm fine needle aspiration; *TESE*, testicular sperm extraction.

Management of unexplained infertility

Chances of spontaneous pregnancy are high in unexplained infertility. Hence, lifestyle changes, advice regarding fertile period and wait and watch policy should be adopted for at least 6 months. If conception does not occur, further treatment is warranted (Box 22.40). Empirical use of CC for ovulation induction usually has poor pregnancy rates. IUI with superovulation using CC, gonadotropins or a combination is more effective. Long-standing unexplained infertility should be treated by IVF.

Box 22.40 Management of unexplained infertility

- Expectant management
  - Lifestyle changes
  - Fertile period
- Intrauterine insemination
  - Without superovulation
  - With superovulation
    - Clomiphene citrate
    - Gonadotropins
- In vitro fertilization

Artificial insemination

Artificial insemination refers to the procedure by which the sperm suspension is injected into the uterine cavity or cervical canal of the woman.

- This may be performed with partner's semen or donor semen.
- The procedure may be intracervical (ICI) or IUI. IUI has a better success rate and is more widely used (Box 22.41).
- It is used in couples with unexplained infertility, male factor infertility, cervical factor and minimal or mild endometriosis.
- IUI can be performed with or without supero-vulation. Clomiphene or gonadotropins are used for inducing superovulation. IUI with superovulation has a higher success rate.
- The semen is processed prior to IUI to remove prostaglandins and semen proteins and con-centrate the sperms. Sperm migration or den-sity gradient techniques may be used to select the motile sperms.

Box 22.41 Intrauterine insemination

- Indications
  - Unexplained infertility
  - Male factor
  - Cervical factor
  - Minimal or mild endometriosis
- Semen processing
- Superovulation with CC or gonadotropins
- Timing of ovulation
  - Follicular monitoring
  - hCG to trigger ovulation

CC, clomiphene citrate; *hCG*, human chorionic gonadotropin.

- If the total number of motile sperms in the processed sample is 5–10 million, pregnancy rate of 10% can be obtained.
- The procedure should be performed around the time of ovulation, when follicle reaches the appropriate size. Ovulation may be triggered by administration of hCG and insemination performed 36 hours later.

Assisted reproductive techniques

When traditional treatment of infertility is unsuccessful or when effective treatment is not available, ART is the option. ART includes procedures in which an oocyte is retrieved and fertilized by a sperm. The procedures are listed in Box 22.42.

- **IVF:** This consists of steps listed in Box 22.43.

  Controlled ovarian hyperstimulation is by downregulation with GnRH analogues and ovulation induction with gonadotropins. GnRH antagonists are also being used for downregulation. The oocyte is aspirated on the day when the follicle is 17–18 mm in size. Fertilization is performed in vitro. The embryo is transferred on day 2/3. Blastocyst transfer is performed in some cases on day 5. Luteal support is provided with vaginal progesterone.

- **Assisted fertilization techniques:** Intracytoplasmic sperm injection (ICSI) is used in couples with male factor infertility. Cumulus cells surrounding the ovum are removed and single sperm is injected through the zona pellucida into the cytoplasm (Fig. 22.16). Sperms retrieved by testicular sperm fine needle aspiration (TESA), percutaneous epididymal sperm aspiration (PESA), testicular sperm extraction (TESE) or microsurgical epididymal sperm aspiration (MESA) can be used. When the zona of the embryo is thick, assisted hatching (AH) is performed prior to embryo transfer to facilitate implantation.

- **Gamete intrafallopian transfer:** The ovum retrieved after hyperstimulation along with the prepared sperms is placed into the fallopian tube. The fertilization takes place in the tube. This procedure is not suitable for tubal factor infertility but can be used in unexplained and mild male factor infertility.

- **Zygote intrafallopian transfer:** The egg is fertilized as for IVF but transferred into the tube

---

Box 22.42　Assisted reproductive techniques

- IVF
- Assisted fertilization techniques
  - ICSI
  - AH
- GIFT
- ZIFT
- Embryo cryopreservation
- IVM
- Alternatives
  - Donor oocyte
  - Donor sperm
  - Donor embryo
  - Gestational surrogacy

AH, assisted hatching; *GIFT*, gamete intrafallopian transfer; *ICSI*, intracytoplasmic sperm injection; *IVF*, in vitro fertilization; *IVM*, in vitro maturation of oocyte; *ZIFT*, zygote intrafallopian transfer.

Box 22.43　In vitro fertilization

- Pituitary downregulation with GnRH analogue
- Controlled ovarian hyperstimulation
- Ultrasound-guided oocyte aspiration
- Processing of sperm
- Laboratory fertilization
- ICSI if the sperm count is low/sample obtained by TESE, MESA, PESA
- Embryo culture
- Transcervical transfer of embryo into the uterus

GnRH, gonadotropin-releasing hormone; *ICSI*, intracytoplasmic sperm injection; *MESA*, microsurgical epididymal sperm aspiration; *PESA*, percutaneous epididymal sperm aspiration; *TESE*, testicular sperm extraction.

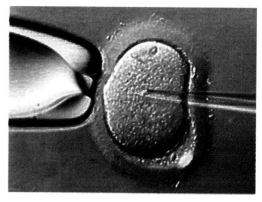

Figure 22.16 Intracytoplasmic sperm injection. The ovum is held in place by suction applied through the micropipette and sperm is injected into the cytoplasm.

laparoscopically on day 1. This procedure is rarely used.

- **Embryo cryopreservation:** Several eggs can be retrieved in a single cycle and fertilized, but only two or three are usually transferred to the uterus. The remaining embryos can be cryopreserved and used in subsequent cycles.

- **Preimplantation genetic diagnosis:** This is performed by removing a single cell from the embryo at six- to eight-cell stage for the diagnosis of single-gene defects, aneuploidy and translocations. This is usually performed when there is a family history of inherited disorders.

Key points

- Infertility may be primary (which is the inability to conceive in a couple when no prior pregnancy has occurred) or secondary (which is the inability to conceive after at least one conception has occurred).
- Infertility may be due to male factor, female factor or combined male and female factors.
- Female factors of infertility may be anovulation, tubal, uterine, peritoneal or cervical factors.
- Polycystic ovarian syndrome (PCOS) is the most common cause of anovulation.
- Tubal factors are common causes of secondary infertility. Pelvic infections, endometriosis and pelvic surgery are the important causes of tubal occlusion.
- Uterine and cervical factors of infertility may be congenital or acquired.
- Male factors of infertility are classified into pretesticular, testicular and post-testicular factors.
- Unexplained infertility accounts for 10% of all cases. It is usually due to luteal phase defect, luteinized unruptured follicle, minimal endometriosis or immunological causes.
- Basic investigations required in infertility are documentation of ovulation, hysterosalpingography (HSG) and semen analysis.
- Midluteal serum progesterone measurement is used for documentation of ovulation. Basal body temperature (BBT) can be used when progesterone assay is not available.
- HSG or laparoscopy can be used to evaluate tubal factor in infertility. Chronic pelvic inflammatory disease

- (PID) and endometriosis are the most common causes of tubal block.
- Tubal and peritoneal factors of infertility can be assessed together by laparoscopy.
- Treatment of anovulation is by lifestyle modification and ovulation induction by clomiphene citrate or gonadotropin with follicular monitoring by ultrasonography.
- Tubal microsurgery or cannulation may be attempted, but chances of ectopic pregnancy are high. Therefore, most women with tubal block require in vitro fertilization (IVF).
- Intrauterine insemination (IUI) is the treatment of choice for cervical factor of infertility.
- Male infertility can be due to pretesticular, testicular or post-testicular factors.
- If semen analysis is abnormal, further evaluation by hormonal assay, karyotyping and ultrasonography is required.
- Ejaculatory dysfunction can be treated by drugs or IUI.
- Azoospermia is treated by testicular or epididymal aspiration followed by intracytoplasmic sperm injection (ICSI) or donor insemination.
- Management of unexplained infertility is by expectant management, IUI with superovulation or assisted reproductive techniques (ARTs).
- When traditional treatment is unsuccessful or unavailable, ART is the option.

Self-assessment

Case-based questions

Case 1

A 27-year-old lady presents with a history of primary infertility for 5 years. Her menstrual cycles are irregular, for 7 days every 50–60 days, and BMI is 28.

1. What details will you concentrate on in history?
2. What will you look for on physical examination?

3. What investigations will you order?
4. If there is no male factor, how will you manage?

Case 2

A 30-year-old lady presents with a history of two miscarriages 4 years ago and failure to conceive after that. Her menstrual cycles are regular; BMI is 23.

1. What details will you concentrate on in history?

2. What will you look for on physical examination?
3. What investigations will you order?
4. If there is no male factor, how will you manage?

Answers

Case 1

1. Duration of symptoms, especially irregular cycles; excessive hair growth; prior hormonal or medical treatment; diabetes, hypertension, galactorrhoea; sexual history; history suggestive of PID, endometriosis.
2. Acne, hirsutism, galactorrhoea, acanthosis nigricans, virilization. Pelvic examination—Uterine size, ovarian enlargement.
3. (a) If hirsutism is not severe and no virilization, no galactorrhoea; she has PCOS—No endocrine workup is required. Transvaginal sonography to confirm polycystic ovaries, antral follicle.
   (b) Blood sugar, lipid profile to rule out metabolic syndrome.
   (c) Since she has primary infertility, no history of PID/endometriosis and no prior treatment, tests for tubal patency not required now.
   (d) Husband must be examined and semen analysis ordered.
4. (a) Weight reduction, exercises, lifestyle changes.
   (b) Ovulation induction with CC. Add metformin if there is no response.

Case 2

1. Details of miscarriages—Gestational age, curettage performed or not, postabortal sepsis. Prior treatment. Sexual history, dyspareunia.
2. (a) General examination
   (b) Pelvic examination: Uterine size, mobility, adnexae—Palpable/tender, mass
   (c) Tenderness in the pouch of Douglas
   (d) Induration of uterosacrals
3. Since cycles are regular, tests for ovulation are not required. TVS for uterine size, adnexal mass. HSG for tubal patency and uterine anomalies.

4. (a) If proximal tubal block is found on HSG, selective salpingography can be tried.
   (b) If distal block is found or if cannulation failed, laparoscopy, chromoperfusion and assessment for surgery are needed.
   (c) If tube is severely damaged and hydrosalpinx present, treatment is IVF after salpingectomy.
   (d) If unexplained infertility, IUI with CC can be tried.
   (e) If not successful, do IVF.

Long-answer questions

1. A 25-year-old lady, married for 5 years, presents with failure to conceive. How will you evaluate? Discuss the management of anovulation.
2. Discuss the evaluation and management of male infertility.
3. A 30-year-old lady presents with a history of two miscarriages and inability to conceive after the last miscarriage 3 years ago. Discuss the possible causes and their evaluation. How will you manage tubal block?
4. Enumerate the causes of secondary infertility. How do you manage a case of secondary infertility?

Short-answer questions

1. Basal body temperature chart
2. Tests for ovulation
3. Ovulation induction
4. Hysterosalpingogram
5. Tubal factors in infertility and their management
6. Tubal patency tests
7. Semen analysis
8. In vitro fertilization and embryo transfer
9. Intracytoplasmic sperm injection
10. Intrauterine insemination
11. Clomiphene citrate
12. Ovarian hyperstimulation syndrome
13. Male factors in infertility

23 | Hormone Therapies in Gynaecology

Case scenario

Mrs VB, 58, came to the clinic with postmenopausal bleeding for 2 weeks. She looked angry, upset and depressed. Her menopause was at age 51. She had experienced severe hot flushes and mood swing at that time and had consulted a local doctor who had prescribed oestrogen tablets. No progestogen was given. She was not counselled regarding the duration of treatment, the need for follow-up and the risks or benefits of the treatment. Since Mrs VB found the medication very effective, she continued to take it. When she noticed vaginal bleeding 2 weeks ago, she consulted a gynaecologist and was evaluated and diagnosed to have endometrial cancer due to unopposed oestrogen therapy.

Introduction

Hormones are used to treat several gynaecological conditions. The normal functioning of the reproductive system is dependent on normal hypothalamic–pituitary–ovarian function. Regulation of this is primarily through hormones. Several common disorders in gynaecology are therefore caused by abnormality in hormone production and can be treated by exogenous administration of hormones, their analogues or antagonists. Some malignancies of the genital tract can also be treated by hormones. Oral contraception and postmenopausal hormone therapy are important uses of hormones in gynaecology. Hormone therapy is associated with side effects and contraindications. It is the responsibility of the gynaecologist to evaluate the patients prior to therapy and counsel them appropriately regarding precautions, side effects and follow-up.

Gonadotropin-releasing hormone analogues

Gonadotropin-releasing hormone (GnRH) is a decapeptide, released in a pulsatile fashion by the hypothalamus. This pulsatile release is crucial for the synthesis and release of pituitary gonadotropins.

330 Essentials of Gynaecology

- Continuous administration of GnRH leads to initial transient gonadotropin stimulation followed by prolonged 'downregulation' or desensitization of the GnRH receptors in the pituitary and marked reduction in gonadotropin secretion. This is the basis of clinical use of GnRH analogues. The half-life on GnRH is only about 2–4 minutes.
- Therefore, analogues with enhanced potency and duration of action have been synthesized for clinical use. These drugs, because of their prolonged and sustained action, tend to suppress gonadotropins.
- They cannot be administered orally since they are inactivated rapidly in the gut.

Preparations and dosages

The preparations, dosages and routes of administration are given in Table 23.1.

Recombinant human GnRH (Rh GnRH) is not available for therapeutic use anymore due to the complexity of administration. GnRH agonists are used instead.

Other drugs available in this group are deslorelin and triptorelin. Triptorelin is used mainly in prostate cancer.

Clinical uses

GnRH analogues have diagnostic and therapeutic uses.

Diagnostic tests

Stimulation of the pituitary gland with Rh GnRH (gonadorelin) results in increase in serum gonadotropin levels in women with hypothalamic

Table 23.1 Preparations, dosage and route of administration of GnRH analogues

Preparation	Dosage	Route of administration
Buserelin	300 µg IN or SC daily	SC, IN
Nafarelin	400 µg IN daily	IN
Goserelin	3.6 mg implant 3-monthly	SC implant
	3.6 mg monthly	IM, depot
Leuprolide	3.75 mg IM monthly	IM, SC, depot
Histrelin	50 mg once in 12 months	SC implant

GnRH, gonadotropin-releasing hormone; IM, intramuscular; IN, intranasal; SC, subcutaneous.

failure but not pituitary failure. This stimulation test is used to differentiate between pituitary and hypothalamic amenorrhoea. In hypothalamic amenorrhoea, there is a 2.5- to 3-fold increase in follicle-stimulating hormone (FSH) and luteinizing hormone (LH) levels after GnRH stimulation, but in pituitary amenorrhoea, there is no such response. In central precocious puberty, basal FSH and LH levels are in the postpubertal range and GnRH stimulation causes a 2.5- to 3-fold increase in serum levels. In contrast, in peripheral isosexual precocity, the basal levels of FSH and LH are low or normal and there is no increase after GnRH administration.

Therapeutic uses

Therapeutic uses of GnRH are listed in Box 23.1.

Box 23.1 Therapeutic uses of GnRH analogues

- Pulsatile administration
  - Hypothalamic amenorrhoea
  - Infertility
  - Downregulation prior to ovulation induction
  - Ovulation induction in hypothalamic dysfunction
- Daily or monthly administration
  - Central precocious puberty
  - Endometriosis
  - Uterine myomas to reduce size preoperatively
  - Abnormal uterine bleeding
  - Preparation of the endometrium for transcervical resection
  - Hormone-responsive breast cancer
  - Cryptorchidism and prostatic cancer in males

GnRH, gonadotropin-releasing hormone.

Side effects

Since the analogues suppress pituitary gonadotropins, the ovarian steroidogenesis is also suppressed and a hypo-oestrogenic state similar to menopause is created. The side effects are listed in Box 23.2.

Box 23.2 Side effects of GnRH analogues

- Hot flushes
- Vaginal dryness
- Insomnia
- Dyslipidaemia
- Decrease in bone mineral density

GnRH, gonadotropin-releasing hormone.

Add-back therapy

Due to the side effects, GnRH therapy is usually limited to 6 months. If treatment is required for a longer duration, add-back therapy with oestrogens or combined oral contraceptive (OC) pills is used. When oestrogens are contraindicated, tibolone may be considered.

Gonadotropin-releasing hormone antagonists

GnRH antagonists are synthetic peptides developed to overcome the disadvantages of agonists.

- GnRH antagonists are also used for downregulation. They act on the GnRH receptors and are faster.
- They do not cause the initial increase in gonadotropins that occurs with GnRH analogues. They have been used for rapid downregulation prior to ovulation induction.
- Due to the hypersensitivity reactions, they are not recommended for routine use yet. GnRH antagonists currently available are listed in Box 23.3.

Box 23.3 GnRH antagonists

- Cetrorelix: SC
- Ganirelix: SC
- Abarelix: SC, depot
- Degarelix: SC

GnRH, gonadotropin-releasing hormone; SC, subcutaneous.

Gonadotropins

- FSH stimulates follicular growth and production of oestrogen.
- LH triggers ovulation, stimulates progesterone production, sustains the corpus luteum and supports implantation.

Commercially available FSH and LH are used mainly for these functions.

Preparations and dosages

FSH is extracted from the urine of postmenopausal women (menotropins). Menotropins contain equal amount of FSH and LH. Urofollitropin

Table 23.2 Preparations and dosages of gonadotropins

Hormone	Brand name	Dose (IU)	Route of administration
Menotropins (FSH)	Pergonal	75	IM
	Repronex	75	IM
Urofollitropin (uFSH)	Bravelle	75	SC
Recombinant (rFSH)	Gonal-f	50	SC
	Puregon	50	SC
	Follistin	50	SC
Chorionic gonadotropin (LH)	Pregnyl	1000–5000	IM
	Profasi	5000	IM
	Novarel	5000	IM

FSH, follicle-stimulating hormone; IM, intramuscular; LH, luteinizing hormone; SC, subcutaneous.

is the highly purified form. FSH is also synthesized using recombinant DNA technology.

Human chorionic gonadotropin (hCG), which mimics LH, is extracted from the urine of pregnant women (chorionic gonadotropin). Recombinant forms of LH are under trial. The preparations and dosage are listed in Table 23.2. Recombinant FSH and LH are expensive and not used as a routine.

Clinical uses

Gonadotropins are also used for diagnostic and therapeutic purposes.

Diagnostic tests

hCG stimulation is used to stimulate testosterone production and thus detect Leydig cell function. In gynaecological practice, this test is used in children with ambiguous genitalia to see if testes are present or if testicular components are present in the gonad.

Therapeutic uses

The therapeutic uses of gonadotropins are listed in Box 23.4. Their main use is in the management of infertility.

Side effects

The well-known side effects of the use of gonadotropins in ovulation induction are multifoetal pregnancy and ovarian hyperstimulation

Box 23.4 Therapeutic uses of gonadotropins

- FSH and LH (hCG)
  - Infertility
    - Induction of ovulation
    - Hyperstimulation in ART
  - Hypogonadotropic hypogonadism and cryptorchidism in males
- hCG alone
  - Recurrent pregnancy loss
  - Luteal support in IVF

ART, assisted reproductive technique; *FSH*, follicle-stimulating hormone; *hCG*, human chorionic gonadotropin; *IVF*, in vitro fertilization; *LH*, luteinizing hormone.

syndrome (OHSS). For details refer to Chapter 22, *Infertility*.

Prolactin inhibitors

Prolactin is produced by the pituitary gland and plays a major role in the preparation of breasts for lactation. It is not used for therapeutic purposes.

- Hyperprolactinaemia is a condition of prolactin excess (*see* Chapter 19, *Secondary amenorrhoea and polycystic ovarian syndrome*). Drugs that inhibit prolactin production are used in the treatment of hyperprolactinaemia, suppression of lactation and treatment of mastalgia.
- They also decrease the size of prolactinomas (benign tumour of the pituitary gland).

Preparations and dosages

The preparations available are listed in Table 23.3.

All the drugs are dopamine receptor agonists. Bromocriptine is the first drug found to have prolactin-lowering effects but is seldom used now. All except quinagolide are ergot derivatives.

Table 23.3 Drugs used to inhibit prolactin production

Preparation	Dosage (mg)	Route of administration
Bromocriptine	2.5–7.5	Oral/vaginal daily
Cabergoline	0.25–0.5	Oral twice weekly
Quinagolide	0.1–0.5	Oral daily
Pergolide	0.025–0.5	Oral daily

Cabergoline has a longer half-life, has more selective receptor activity, is more effective and has fewer side effects. Because of the twice-weekly dosage, adherence to therapy is also better. This is the drug of choice in the treatment of hyperprolactinaemia. A small dose of 0.25 mg twice weekly is used initially and increased gradually to 1.5–2 mg, if required. For suppression of lactation, a single dose of 1 mg is used.

Clinical uses

Prolactin inhibitors are used mainly for therapeutic purposes. Clinical uses of prolactin inhibitors are listed in Box 23.5.

Box 23.5 Therapeutic uses of prolactin inhibitors

- Hyperprolactinaemia
- Prolactinoma
- Suppression of lactation
- Mastalgia
- Infertility due to hyperprolactinaemia

Side effects

Bromocriptine and other dopaminergic agonists have several side effects, but they can be overcome by starting with a small dose and increasing gradually. The side effects also diminish with time. The side effects are listed in Box 23.6.

Box 23.6 Side effects of prolactin inhibitors

- Nausea and vomiting
- Headache
- Postural hypotension
- Nasal congestion
- CNS effects
  - Hallucinations, psychosis and insomnia

CNS, central nervous system.

Oestrogens

Oestrogens are steroid hormones produced mainly by the ovary and to a lesser extent by adipose tissue (*see* Chapter 3, *Female reproductive physiology*).

There are three main forms: oestradiol, oestrone and oestriol. Apart from their role in reproduction, they also have physiological actions on several organ systems and metabolism (Box 23.7). The pharmacological actions of synthetic oestrogenic steroids are an extension of these and are used to achieve the same effects.

Two types of oestrogen receptors are present in human tissues: α and β. The hormone acts by binding to these receptors.

Oestrogens play a major role in pubertal development of the genital tract and breast. They suppress FSH production by the pituitary. They have several metabolic actions (*see* Chapter 3, *Female reproductive physiology*). They increase the levels of high-density lipoproteins (HDLs) and reduce the levels of low-density lipoproteins (LDLs). This may have a cardioprotective effect. Increase in binding globulins with oestrogen administration reduces the levels of bioavailability of various hormones.

Oestrogens increase fasting plasma glucose. Due to the increase in coagulation factors, oestrogens can be thrombogenic. They have a major role in the prevention of osteoporosis.

Preparations and dosages

Oestrogens are absorbed from the gastrointestinal tract, skin and vagina. They can also be administered intramuscularly. On oral administration, they are metabolized in the liver to oestrone and oestradiol glucuronide, which are weak oestrogens. In the liver, they induce production of coagulation factors, triglycerides, binding proteins and lipoproteins. This is called the 'first-pass' effect. This is eliminated by transdermal administration. The first-pass metabolism is much less with ethinyl oestradiol (EE$_2$). Preparations and dosages are given in Table 23.4.

Natural oestrogens are conjugated equine oestrogen and oestradiol valerate. Others are synthetic oestrogens.

EE$_2$ is used for the treatment of hypogonadism to induce development of secondary sex characteristics. It is also a component of combined OC pills. Conjugated equine oestrogen

Box 23.7 Physiological and pharmacological actions of oestrogens

- Pubertal development of the female genital tract
- Development of the breast
- Pubertal growth spurt
- Development of secondary sexual characteristics
- Suppression of pituitary gonadotropin production
- Stimulation of LH surge
- Proliferative changes in the endometrium
- Increase in bone mineral density
- Effects on carbohydrate and protein and lipid metabolism
  - Increase in fasting glucose
  - Increase in hormone-binding proteins
  - Increase in HDL and decrease in LDL
- Increase in coagulation factors and fibrinolysis

HDL, high-density lipoprotein; *LDL*, low-density lipoprotein; *LH*, luteinizing hormone.

Table 23.4 Preparations and dosages of oestrogens

Preparation	Available dosages
Oral	
Ethinyl oestradiol (Lynoral)	0.01, 0.03, 0.05, 0.1 mg daily
Conjugated equine oestrogen (Premarin)	0.3, 0.625, 1.25 mg daily
Synthetic conjugated oestrogens (Enjuvia)	0.3, 0.45, 0.625, 1.25 mg daily
Esterified oestrogens (Estratab)	0.3, 0.625 mg daily
Micronized oestrogen (Estrace)	1–2 mg daily
17β-Oestradiol (several generics)	0.5, 1.2 mg daily
Transdermal	
Oestradiol patches (Estraderm)	0.025, 0.05 mg twice weekly
Oestradiol gel (EstroGel)	1.25 g daily
Intramuscular	
Oestradiol valerate (Delestrogen)	10, 20 mg once in 4 weeks
Oestradiol cypionate (Depo-Oestradiol)	1.5–2 mg once in 4 weeks
Intravenous	
Conjugated equine oestrogen (Premarin)	25 mg 6-hourly
Vaginal	
Oestradiol creams (Estrace, 0.01%)	Once daily
Conjugated oestrogen creams (Premarin)	0.05–2 mg daily
Oestradiol vaginal ring (Estring)	1 ring once in 3 months
Oestradiol vaginal tablet (Vagifem)	10 mcg once daily
Implants	
Oestradiol implant	25, 50, 100 mg once in 3 months

and 17β-oestradiol are used for postmenopausal hormone therapy. Micronized oestrogen and esterified oestrogens are not in common use.

Intravenous preparation or conjugated oestrogen, if available, is useful in arresting haemorrhage in women with anovulatory bleeding. The intramuscular injections and implants are used for postmenopausal hormone therapy with or without progesterone. Transdermal preparations are used for the same. Vaginal preparations are useful in postmenopausal women with urogenital symptoms.

Clinical uses

Oestrogens are used in combination with progestogens as combined OC pills for several indications apart from contraception. Uses of oestrogen are listed in Table 23.5.

Side effects

The side effects of oestrogens are listed in Box 23.8.

Contraindications

Due to the side effects, oestrogens are contraindicated in women with a history of thromboembolism, liver/gallbladder disease, breast/endometrial cancer and migraine.

Box 23.8 Side effects of oestrogens

- Nausea and vomiting
- Breast tenderness
- Migraine
- Thromboembolism
- Endometrial cancer and breast cancer with prolonged, unopposed use
- Gallbladder disease
- Stroke (in particular vertebrobasilar)
- Hepatic adenoma

Selective oestrogen receptor modulators

There are two types of oestrogen receptor (ER): ERα and ERβ. Drugs that selectively bind to or modify a particular type of receptor have a broad spectrum of actions—from antioestrogenic to oestrogenic—on different tissues. Selective oestrogen receptor modulators (SERMs) are nonsteroidal drugs that belong to this category and have oestrogenic action on bone, brain and liver, but antioestrogenic action on breast and endometrium. Therefore, all SERMs have a beneficial action on bone. SERMs also reduce the levels of LDL and triglycerides. The SERMs currently available are listed in Table 23.6.

Tamoxifen

This drug has been shown to prevent the recurrence of breast cancer in the affected breast and new cancer in the contralateral breast by 50%. It increases disease-free and overall survival. The therapy is usually given for 5 years.

Tamoxifen inhibits osteoclasts and prevents osteoporosis. It has an oestrogenic action on the endometrium, leading to increased risk of endometrial polyps, atypical hyperplasia, carcinoma and mixed Müllerian tumour. The risk of endometrial cancer is 3–5/1000 patient-years of use. When women taking tamoxifen present with abnormal uterine bleeding, endometrial assessment by transvaginal ultrasonography and endometrial biopsy are recommended.

Raloxifene

This drug is used primarily for the prevention of osteoporosis in postmenopausal women. It has also been found to be useful in women with ER-positive breast cancer.

Table 23.5 Uses of oestrogens

Indication	Preparations
In combined OC pills	Ethinyl oestradiol, mestranol
Postmenopausal hormone therapy	• Ethinyl oestrodiol oral • 17β-Oestradiol oral • Oestrodiol patch/gel/implant
For development of secondary sexual characteristics • Turner syndrome • Hypogonadotropic hypogonadism • Partial androgen insensitivity	Ethinyl oestradiol oral
Abnormal uterine bleeding	• IV conjugated oestrogen • Ethinyl oestradiol oral
Vulvovaginitis in children	• Vaginal cream • Conjugated oestrogen oral
Postmenopausal urogenital atrophy	• Vaginal cream/gel/ring/tablet • Conjugated oestrogen cream • 17β-Oestradiol cream/vaginal tablet

IV, intravenous; OC, oral contraceptive.

Table 23.6 Currently available SERMs

Drug	Usual dose (mg)	Indication
Tamoxifen	10–20	• Breast cancer • Gynaecomastia
Raloxifene	60	• Postmenopausal osteoporosis • Breast cancer
Ormeloxifene	30	• Contraception • Abnormal uterine bleeding
Arzoxifene	20	Breast cancer
Bazedoxifene	20–40	• Along with oestrogen • For prevention of osteoporosis
Lasofoxifene	0.25–5	Postmenopausal osteoporosis
Toremifene	60	Breast cancer
Ospemifene	60	Dyspareunia

SERMs, selective oestrogen receptor modulators.

Bazedoxifene

This has been used along with conjugated oestrogen in management of postmenopausal women. Vaginal dryness and dyspareunia, the usual side effects of SERMs, are countered by oestrogen and there is no increase in breast cancer risk. The two drugs act synergistically and prevent osteoporosis.

Ospemifene

This is specific for postmenopausal dyspareunia and is administered orally.

Ormeloxifene

This is also known as 'centchroman' or 'Saheli'. It is a once-a-week contraceptive that acts by causing asynchrony between ovulation and endometrial changes, thereby preventing implantation. Initial dose is 30 mg twice a week for 3 months followed by once a week thereafter. Ormeloxifene is also used in the treatment of heavy menstrual bleeding, at a dosage of 60 mg twice a week. The drug is currently also used for management of bleeding associated with uterine myoma.

Clinical uses

Tamoxifen is used extensively in women with breast cancer to prevent recurrence and tumour in contralateral breast. Raloxifene and Bazedoxifene are used for prevention of osteoporosis in postmenopausal women. Ormeloxifene has been found to be effective in reducing menstrual flow in women with heavy menstrual bleeding.

Side effects

The side effects of SERMs are listed in Box 23.9.

Box 23.9 Side effects of SERMs

- Nausea
- Hot flushes and vaginal dryness
- Endometrial polyps and hyperplasia/carcinoma—Tamoxifen
- Venous thromboembolism

SERM, selective oestrogen receptor modulator.

Antioestrogens

Unlike SERMs that have oestrogenic and antioestrogenic action, this class of drugs has antioestrogenic activity on all tissues. There are two well-known drugs in this category: Clomiphene citrate and fulvestrant.

Clomiphene citrate

Clomiphene citrate inhibits negative feedback inhibition of GnRH at the hypothalamus by oestrogen and induces ovulation. It is usually administered from day 2 to 6 of the menstrual cycle when the oestrogen levels are rising. Clomiphene citrate binds to oestrogen receptors on the hypothalamus and prevents oestrogen action. Pulsatile GnRH secretion ensues with resultant increase in FSH, follicular development and ovulation.

Dosage

The initial dose of clomiphene citrate (Clomid and Siphene) is 50 mg daily for 5 days from day 2 to 6 of the menstrual cycle. The response is monitored by serum oestradiol levels and/or follicular monitoring with ultrasonography. The dose is increased by 50 mg every cycle to a maximum dose of 150 mg/day if follicular response is not satisfactory. This can be given for six cycles.

Clinical uses

Clomiphene citrate is used for ovulation induction in women with anovulatory infertility, particularly in polycystic ovarian syndrome. A normal hypothalamic–pituitary–ovarian function and adequate oestrogen levels are mandatory for the action of clomiphene citrate. Indications are listed in Box 23.10.

Box 23.10 Clinical use of clomiphene citrate

- Anovulation
- Polycystic ovarian disease
- Unexplained infertility
- Stimulation of spermatogenesis

Side effects

Side effects are listed in Box 23.11. The antioestrogenic effect on the endometrium and cervical mucus can interfere with sperm motility. Luteal phase defect is another cause of clomiphene citrate failure. Prolonged use for more than a year has been shown to increase the risk of epithelial ovarian cancer. Hence, usage is restricted to 6 months.

Box 23.11 Side effects of clomiphene citrate

- Hot flushes
- Blurring of vision and scotoma
- Abdominal discomfort
- Nausea and vomiting
- Multifoetal pregnancy
- Luteal phase defect
- Antioestrogenic action
  - Cervical mucus
  - Endometrium
- Ovarian cancer (>1 year of use)
- Alopecia
- Ovarian hyperstimulation (rare)

Fulvestrant

Fulvestrant is similar to tamoxifen in its action and is used in women with breast cancer. It is administered monthly as intramuscular depot injections.

Oestrogen synthesis inhibitors—Aromatase inhibitors

Conversion of androgens to oestrogens requires the enzyme aromatase. The enzyme is present predominantly in granulosa cells, subcutaneous fat, liver, breast and placenta. Inhibiting this enzyme blocks oestrogen biosynthesis. Three generations of aromatase inhibitors (AIs) have been developed.

They are of two categories:

- **Type I:** These are steroidal agents (formestane and exemestane). They bind irreversibly to aromatase, thus inactivating the enzyme permanently.
- **Type II:** These are nonsteroidal agents (anastrozole and letrozole). These agents bind reversibly to aromatase and cause reversible inhibition.

Clinical uses

- Conversion of androgens to oestrogen by aromatization is the main source of oestrogen in postmenopausal women and this can be effectively blocked by AIs. Therefore, it is being used extensively in ER-positive postmenopausal breast cancer. AIs have been found to be superior to tamoxifen in randomized trials and do not stimulate the endometrium.
- In premenopausal women, the ovarian production of oestrogen is reduced with resultant increase in gonadotropins leading to follicular growth. AIs are, therefore, used for ovulation induction.
- Oestrogens cause fusion of epiphysis and arrest linear growth. Blocking oestrogen production with AIs results in increase in height in children and adolescents with short stature in congenital adrenal hyperplasia and in peripheral precocious puberty. Same antioestrogenic effect is used in the treatment of oestrogen-dependent conditions such as endometriosis and leiomyoma. It is also used in the treatment of gynaecomastia.

Current clinical uses of AIs are listed in Box 23.12. Letrozole, anastrozole and exemestane are used in breast cancer. Letrozole is used for ovulation induction and other indications are listed below.

Preparations and dosages

The currently available AIs and their dosages are listed in Table 23.7.

Vorozole and fadrozole are other drugs in this category. They are used as antineoplastic drugs in the management of breast cancer.

Box 23.12 Clinical uses of AIs

- Postmenopausal breast cancer
  - Second-line therapy: In recurrent disease
  - Adjuvant (first-line) therapy: To prevent recurrence
  - Neoadjuvant therapy: Preoperative
- Ovulation induction
- Endometriosis
- Leiomyoma and benign metastasizing myoma
- Endometrial stromal sarcoma
- Peripheral precocious puberty
- Congenital adrenal hyperplasia
- Short stature
- Gynaecomastia

AIs, aromatase inhibitors.

Table 23.7 Preparations and dosage of AIs

Preparation	Dosages (mg/day)
Letrozole	2.5
Anastrozole	1
Exemestane	25
Testolactone	50
Formestane	250–500

AIs, aromatase inhibitors.

Side effects

These are listed in Box 23.13.

Box 23.13 Side effects of AIs

- Arthralgia and arthritis
- Dyslipidaemia
- Vaginal dryness
- Coronary heart disease
- Osteoporosis
- Osteonecrosis of jaw

AIs, aromatase inhibitors.

Progesterone

There are three types of progestational agents:

- **Progesterone** is the naturally occurring hormone, secreted by the corpus luteum and placenta. It is metabolized rapidly in the liver and excreted as pregnanediol glucuronide. This first-pass effect reduces the efficacy of oral progesterone; therefore, a higher dose is needed and is usually used parenterally.

- **Progestogens** are compounds with progesterone-like action obtained from plants or animals.
- **Progestins** include the various synthetic pregestational agents. They have biological activity similar to that of progesterone.

Classification

Progestins have been classified according to structure as given in Box 23.14, and also according to the time sequence in which they were introduced as first-, second-, third-and fourth-generation progestins.

Box 23.14 Classification of progestins

- Progesterone
  - Micronized progesterone, 17-hydroxyprogesterone caproate
- C_{21} steroids
  - Megestrol acetate
- Stereoisomer of progesterone
  - Dydrogesterone
- Pregnanes
  - 17-Acetoxyprogesterone caproate
  - Medroxyprogesterone acetate
  - Chlormadinone acetate
- Estranes (19-nortestosterone derivatives)
  - Norethisterone, norethynodrel, norethindrone, lynestrenol, ethynodiol diacetate
- Gonanes
  - Norgestrel, levonorgestrel
  - Newer progestins
    - Desogestrel, gestodene, norgestimate
- Spironolactone derivative
  - Drospirenone
- Other progestins
  - Dienogest, nomegestrol, Nestorone, trimegestone, gestrinone

Pharmacological actions of progestins

Like the oestrogens, progestins have specific actions on the reproductive tract and other organs. The pharmacological effects are an extension of these physiological actions. Depending on their affinities for progesterone, androgen, oestrogen or mineralocorticoid receptors, the progestins have additional androgenic, progestogenic and other properties. Progesterone and pregnanes have only progestogenic actions, the 19-nortestosterone derivatives (estranes) have varying degrees of androgenic activity, and the spironolactone derivative, drospirenone, has mineralocorticoid activity.

Their action on the reproductive tract is dependent on prior priming by oestrogens. The pharmacological actions of progestins are listed in Box 23.15.

Box 23.15   Physiological and pharmacological actions of progestins

- Development of the glandular tissue of breast
  - Increase in mitotic activity
- Secretory changes in the endometrium
- Decidualization of the endometrium
- Maintenance of pregnancy
- Changes in cervical mucus
- Suppression of GnRH pulse
- Glucose intolerance
- Increase in LDL; decrease in HDL

GnRH, gonadotropin-releasing hormone; HDL, high-density lipoprotein; LDL, low-density lipoprotein.

Preparations and dosages

Progesterone, estranes, pregnanes and gonanes are available for use individually. The newer gonanes and drospirenone are available in combination with EE$_2$ as combined OC pills. These are listed in Table 23.8.

Clinical uses

Clinical uses of progesterone may be diagnostic or therapeutic.

Diagnostic tests

Progesterone challenge test (PCI) is used as the first step in evaluation of women with secondary amenorrhoea (see Chapter 19, *Secondary amenorrhoea and polycystic ovarian syndrome*). Bleeding following administration of progestin indicates the presence of oestrogen.

Therapeutic uses

Progestins are used extensively in gynaecology. As combined OC pills, they are used for contraception and several other indications (see the section 'Hormonal contraception'; Box 23.27). They are also used with oestrogens for postmenopausal hormone therapy. The newer progestins were developed specifically for use as

Table 23.8   Preparations and dosages of progestins

Preparation	Dosage	Route of administration
Micronized progesterone	100, 200 mg	Oral/vaginal
17-Hydroxyprogesterone caproate	250 mg	Intramuscular
MPA	2.5, 10 mg	Oral
	150 mg	Intramuscular, depot
Megestrol acetate	10 mg	Oral
Norethisterone	5 mg	Oral
Norgestrel	5 mg	Oral
Levonorgestrel	5 mg	Oral
Desogestrel	10 mg	Oral
Gestodene	75 µg (with EE$_2$)	Oral
Drospirenone	3 mg (with EE$_2$)	Oral
Norplant I and II	36, 70 mg	Subdermal
Implanon	Etonogestrel 67 mg	Subdermal
Vaginal ring	Releases 20 µg/day	Transvaginal
Progesterone (Progestasert)	38 mg	Intrauterine
Levonorgestrel (Mirena)	52 mg	Intrauterine

EE$_2$, ethinyl oestradiol; MPA, medroxyprogesterone acetate.

contraceptives along with EE$_2$. They have very few side effects. Nomegestrol is used as contraceptive implant; trimegestone is used for hormone therapy and contraception; Nestorone is used with EE$_2$ as a contraceptive. These have selective action on progesterone receptors. Progestins are used alone in other conditions (Box 23.16).

Side effects

These are listed in Box 23.17.

The newer progestins, desogestrel- and gestodene-containing OC pills, have been found to increase the risk of venous thrombosis with a large meta-analysis showing a relative risk of 1.7. The risk of myocardial infarction is, however, reduced due to their favourable effect on lipids. The non-pregnane progesterones used in hormone therapy at menopause also contribute to increased risk of venous thromboembolism.

• With oestrogens	Combined OC pills Postmenopausal hormone therapy
• Progestin-only contraception	Minipill: Norgestrel, desogestrel Depot: MPA Implants Intrauterine systems: Progesterone, levonorgestrel
• Emergency contraception	Levonorgestrel
• Abnormal uterine bleeding	Norethisterone, norgestrel
• Recurrent pregnancy loss	Micronized progesterone
• Secondary amenorrhoea with normal/increased oestrogen	Norethisterone
• Preterm labour	Micronized progesterone
• Luteal phase support in ART	Micronized progesterone
• Endometriosis	Norethisterone, MPA
• Endometrial hyperplasia	MPA, megestrol acetate
• Advanced endometrial cancer	MPA, megestrol acetate
• Postponement of menstruation	Norethisterone

ART, assisted reproductive technique; *MPA*, medroxyprogesterone acetate; *OC*, oral contraceptive.

Box 23.17 Side effects of progestins

- Nausea, vomiting
- Fatigue, somnolence
- Mastalgia
- Sodium water retention; weight gain
- Worsening of hypertension
- Depression, irritability
- Dyslipidaemia
- Thromboembolism
- Breast cancer (prolonged use)
- Osteoporosis (prolonged use)

Antiprogestins

Antiprogestins act by binding to progesterone receptors and blocking progesterone action on the target cells. The antiprogestin in common use is mifepristone, which is a derivative of norethindrone.

When administered in the luteal phase, antiprogestins cause luteolysis. This results in menses, similar to progesterone withdrawal bleeding. In early pregnancy, decidual breakdown and luteolysis occur. This releases prostaglandins, leading to myometrial contractions. If used in the late follicular phase, antiprogestins suppress LH surge.

These drugs also have antiglucocorticoid and antiandrogenic properties and cause increase in corticotropin levels. These drugs are metabolized in the liver.

Preparations

There are very few preparations available in this group (Box 23.18).

Box 23.18 Antiprogestins

- Mifepristone
- Onapristone
- Epostane

Clinical uses

Mifepristone is used mainly for termination of pregnancy before 7 weeks. It is administered orally in a dose of 600 mg followed 48 hours later by 400 µg of misoprostol orally or vaginally. Doses as low as 200 mg are also equally effective. Expulsion of products takes place within 5 days and the success rate is 90%. This is currently the recommended method of medical termination in early pregnancy. It is equally effective up to 13 weeks of pregnancy, but need for curettage is higher and bleeding is more. Mifepristone also has other uses (Box 23.19). For emergency contraception, 10 mg of mifepristone is administered after intercourse, but before ovulation. A dose of 200 mg prevents implantation.

Side effects

Side effects are listed in Box 23.20.

Selective progesterone receptor modulators

Selective progesterone receptor modulators (SPRMs) act on progesterone receptors, but

Box 23.19 Clinical uses of mifepristone

- Termination of early pregnancy
- Cervical ripening
- Endometriosis
- Uterine myoma
- Emergency contraception
- Breakthrough bleeding with depot MPA
- Leiomyoma
- Breast cancer
- Ovarian cancer
- Meningioma
- Cushing syndrome
- Psychotic depression

MPA, medroxyprogesterone acetate.

Box 23.20 Side effects of mifepristone

- Nausea, vomiting
- Uterine cramps
- Adrenal insufficiency
- Cardiac failure

unlike antiprogestins, these drugs have progestogenic and antiprogestogenic actions on different tissues.

The drugs available are ulipristal, asoprisnil and telapristone.

SPRMs are under trial in endometriosis, leiomyoma, emergency contraception and breast cancer.

Androgens

The principal androgen is testosterone. It is produced by the Leydig cells of the testes in the male and by the corpus luteum and adrenal glands in the female. The precursors, dehydroepiandrosterone and androstenedione, are weak androgens and are converted to testosterone in peripheral tissues.

Testosterone acts in three ways. In tissues where 5α-reductase is present, it is converted into dihydrotestosterone, a more potent androgen that acts on the androgen receptor. In tissues without 5α-reductase, testosterone directly acts on the androgen receptor. Testosterone is converted to oestradiol by aromatization in the peripheral tissues and this acts through oestrogen receptors. Therefore, actions of testosterone are androgenic and oestrogenic. Androgens are metabolized in the liver.

In males, androgens are responsible for the pubertal development and reproductive functions, pubertal growth spurt, muscle mass, hair distribution, body contour, fat distribution and libido. In the females, androgens are necessary for the development of axillary and pubic hair, libido, development of muscle mass and bone mineral density.

Preparations

Two main groups of androgens available are testosterone esters and 17α-alkylated androgens (Box 23.21). Due to the rapid metabolism by liver, most esters are ineffective when taken orally. Hence, intramuscular route is used for administration. Testosterone enanthate and cypionate are long-acting preparations and are administered weekly. Testosterone undecanoate is extra–long acting and is used once in 2 weeks.

Transdermal preparations, buccal tablets, subcutaneous pellets and nasal gel are also available.

The 17α-alkylated androgens are oral preparations. They are less androgenic and are hepatotoxic.

Box 23.21 Androgen preparations

- Testosterone esters
  - Testosterone enanthate
  - Testosterone cypionate
  - Testosterone undecanoate
- 17α-Alkylated androgens
  - Methyltestosterone
  - Oxandrolone
  - Fluoxymesterone
  - Danazol
- 19-Nortestosterone derivative
  - Gestrinone

Clinical uses

Testosterone and its esters are not used in women due to their androgenic effects. They are used in men with hypogonadism and other conditions of testosterone deficiency.

Gestrinone

Danazol, a weaker androgen, is used in the management of endometriosis. It acts by decreasing ovarian steroidogenesis. Therapeutic efficacy of danazol in endometriosis is comparable to other drugs, but due to the androgenic side effects its use is limited. To reduce side effects, vaginal route of administration is under trial. Clinical uses are listed in Box 23.22.

- Oral
  - Endometriosis: 600–800 mg/day
  - Fibrocystic disease of the breast: 100–200 mg/day
  - Heavy menstrual bleeding: 200 mg/day
  - Mastalgia: 50–100 mg/day
  - Immune thrombocytic purpura: 200 mg/day
  - Angioedema: 200 mg/day
  - Emergency contraception: 200 mg
- Vaginal
  - Endometriosis: 250 mg/day

Side effects

Two main concerns with danazol are the androgenic effects and hepatotoxicity (Box 23.23).

Box 23.23   Side effects of danazol

- Amenorrhoea
- Androgenic effects
  - Hirsutism
  - Acne
  - Oily skin
  - Deepening of voice
- Weight gain, fluid retention, oedema
- Altered liver enzymes
- Dyslipidaemia
- Hepatic tumours

Gestrinone

This is a 19-nortestosterone derivative with androgenic, antiprogestogenic, antioestrogenic and antigonadotropic actions. It suppresses LH surge and basal LH production by the pituitary and increases free testosterone levels. It has been used in the treatment of endometriosis and found to be as effective as GnRH for relief of symptoms. The recommended dose is 2.5 mg twice a week since it has a long half-life. About 80% of women become amenorrhoeic.

Side effects

Side effects are less severe than with danazol (Box 23.24).

Box 23.24   Side effects of gestrinone

- Nausea
- Muscle cramps
- Weight gain
- Acne
- Oily skin

Antiandrogens

Antiandrogens are used to inhibit androgens when their levels are elevated or when the androgenic effects are undesirable. In women, their principal use is in the treatment of hyperandrogenism, which manifests as acne, hirsutism, menstrual disturbances and infertility. Antiandrogens are of two categories: Drugs that decrease androgen production and drugs that inhibit androgen action (Box 23.25).

Box 23.25   Antiandrogens

- Inhibitors of testosterone secretion
  - GnRH analogues
  - Imidazoles
    - Ketoconazole
- Inhibitors of testosterone action
  - Androgen receptor antagonists
    - Cyproterone acetate
    - Spironolactone
    - Flutamide
    - Bicalutamide
    - Nilutamide
    - Enzalutamide
    - Cimetidine
  - 5α-Reductase inhibitors
    - Finasteride
    - Dutasteride

GnRH, gonadotropin-releasing hormone.

Inhibitors of testosterone secretion

GnRH analogues and imidazoles

GnRH analogues cause downregulation of the pituitary and suppress gonadotropins causing amenorrhoea.

Ketoconazole, an imidazole, is hepatotoxic and can also decrease cortisol synthesis and induce adrenal insufficiency. Therefore, it is not used for treatment of hirsutism.

Inhibitors of testosterone action

Androgen receptor antagonists

Cyproterone acetate It is a synthetic progestin with antiandrogenic and mild glucocorticoid activity. It reduces levels of testosterone and dehydroepiandrosterone sulphate (DHEAS). It also increases sex hormone–binding globulin (SHBG) levels, which results in decrease in free testosterone. It is used in a reverse sequential regimen— Cyproterone acetate 100 mg/day from day 5 to 15 and EE_2 30 µg/day from day 5 to 26 to provide contraception, to control cycle and to reduce hirsutism. This reverse sequential regimen is recommended since the drug is teratogenic and since contraception is essential during its use.

Spironolactone This is an aldosterone antagonist that also binds to androgen receptors. It suppresses testosterone synthesis and inhibits 5α-reductase activity; therefore, it is used for the treatment of hirsutism. The recommended dose is 50–200 mg daily. The drug can be used for long term and is well tolerated. Since spironolactone can cause feminization of male foetus, contraception is recommended. Menstrual irregularity is the most common side effect. This can be managed by concomitant use of progestins. It is essential to ensure that the patient has a normal serum creatinine before long-term use as the drug has a propensity to cause hyperkalaemia in patients with impaired renal function.

Flutamide This is a potent nonsteroidal antiandrogen and a weak inhibitor of testosterone biosynthesis. It is usually used with combined OC pills for better antiandrogenic efficacy and contraceptive effect in markedly hirsute hyperandrogenic women. The drug is hepatotoxic and liver functions should be checked prior to commencement and once in 3 months during treatment. Bicalutamide is less hepatotoxic and requires only once-daily administration. Nilutamide is more toxic. This group of drugs is used along with GnRH analogues for the treatment of metastatic prostatic cancer in men.

The indications, dosage and side effects of androgen receptor antagonists in routine use are listed in Table 23.9.

5α-Reductase inhibitors

Finasteride Finasteride is a specific inhibitor of 5α-reductase that converts testosterone to the more potent androgen, dihydrotestosterone. The principal use of this group of drugs is in the management of benign prostatic hyperplasia. For the treatment of hirsutism, it is used along with combined OC pills for better efficacy and for contraception to avoid feminization of a male foetus. The drug is also useful in managing male-pattern baldness in women.

Indications, dosage and side effects are listed in Box 23.26.

Hormonal contraception

Hormonal contraception is a well-accepted method of temporary contraception. It contains oestrogen–progestin combination or progestin

Table 23.9 Indications, dosage and side effects of androgen receptor antagonists

	Cyproterone	Spironolactone	Flutamide
Chemical nature	Synthetic progestin	Aldosterone antagonist	Substituted anilide
Mechanism of action	• Decreased plasma T, A-dione • Increase in SHBG • Antiglucocorticoid	• Suppression of T biosynthesis • Inhibition of 5α-reductase	• Antiandrogen • Weak inhibitor of testosterone biosynthesis
Indications	• Hirsutism • Acne	Hirsutism	Hirsutism
Dosage	100 mg/day during days 5–15 with EE_2 30 µg days 5–26	50–200 mg daily	250 mg 2–3 times/day
Side effects	• Nausea • Weight gain • Headache • Fatigue • Irregular bleeding • Teratogenic	• Menstrual irregularity • Mastalgia • Urticaria, hair loss • Hyperkalaemia • Feminization of the female foetus • Teratogenic	• Dry skin • Blue-green discolouration of urine • Hepatotoxicity • Teratogenic

EE_2, ethinyl oestradiol, SHBG, sex hormone–binding globulin

alone. This method of contraception has low failure rate, 0.1/100 women-years. The various forms of hormonal contraception are listed in Box 23.27.

Oestrogen–progestin combinations

Combination oral contraceptives (COCs), also known as combined OC pills, are popular and the most frequently used method of contraception. They are also used often for other indications in gynaecology. They consist of a combination of oestrogen, usually EE_2, occasionally mestranol, and a progestin. All the progestins used are 19-nortestosterone derivatives, except drospirenone.

Dosage

The side effects of oestrogen and progestin in the COCs are dose related. Although the earlier COCs had 50 µg of EE_2, it has now been reduced to 30–35 µg. Low-dose COCs have 20 µg of EE_2, but breakthrough bleeding can be a problem with this dose. The dose of progestin may be constant through the cycle as in monophasic pills or vary with each half or each week as in biphasic and triphasic pills. The dose of progestin is low in the first week and is increased later, thus reducing the total dose of progestins. COCs are usually administered for 21 days with a 7-day pill-free period for bleeding.

Mode of action

Combined OC pills act by inhibiting pituitary gonadotropin production. Since both oestrogens and progestins act synergistically, the combined OC pills are effective at a much lower dose. Follicular maturation and ovulation do not occur. Transdermal patches, vaginal rings and intramuscular injections bypass the 'first-pass' effect.

Preparations and dosages

There are several combinations available with different doses of EE_2 and different progestins (Table 23.10).

Extended-use preparations are available now. These can be used for 3 months continuously. They are useful in endometriosis and contraception in women who do not prefer monthly bleeding and in girls with neurodevelopmental delay where menstrual hygiene is a problem.

Noncontraceptive benefits

Although the COCs are primarily used for contraception, several other beneficial effects have emerged. COCs are therefore now used for several indications in gynaecology (Box 23.28).

Clinical uses

COCs are used for their contraceptive and noncontraceptive benefits as shown in Box 23.29.

Adverse effects

Adverse effects may be minor side effects (Box 23.30), cardiovascular and metabolic effects or related to development of neoplasia.

COCs may interfere with establishment of lactation. Therefore, they should be started only 6 weeks after delivery or after the lactation is well established. They increase the level of SHBG, thereby increasing the levels of total hormones

Table 23.10 Preparations of COCs and dosage

Preparation	Oestrogen		Progestin	
	Formulation	Dosage in µg	Formulation	Dosage in mg
Monophasic				
	EE₂	20	Levonorgestrel	0.1
	EE₂	20	Norethindrone acetate	1.0
	EE₂	25	Norethindrone	0.8
	EE₂	30	Levonorgestrel	0.2
	EE₂	30	Norgestrel	0.3
	EE₂	30	Desogestrel	0.2
	EE₂	35	Norethindrone	0.4
	EE₂	35	Norgestimte	0.3
	EE₂	35	Ethynodiol diacetate	1.0
	EE₂	50	Norgestrel	0.5
	EE₂	50	Ethynodiol diacetate	1.0
	Mestranol	50	Norethindrone	1.0
Biphasic				
	EE₂	20/10	Desogestrel	0.15
	EE₂	35	Norethindrone	0.5/1
Triphasic				
	EE₂	25	Desogestrel	0.1/0.125/0.15
	EE₂	25	Norgestimate	0.18/0.215/0.25
	EE₂	35	Norethindrone	0.5/0.75/1.0
	EE₂	35	Norethindrone	0.5/1.0/0.5
	EE₂	35	Norgestimate	0.18/0.215/0.25
Variable				
	EE₂	20/0/10	Desogestrel	0.2
	EE₂	30/40/30	Levonorgestrel	0.05/0.075/0.125
	EE₂	20/30/35	Norethindrone	1.0

COCs, combination oral contraceptives; *EE₂*, esthinyl oestrodiol.

Box 23.28 Noncontraceptive benefits of COCs

- Menstrual cycle
  - Regularity
  - Reduction in blood loss and anaemia
  - Reduction in dysmenorrhoea
- Ovary
  - Reduction in functional cysts
- Other benefits
  - Reduction in ectopic pregnancy
  - Reduction in benign breast disease
  - Prevention of endometrial, ovarian and colorectal cancer
  - Prevention of progression of endometriosis
  - Reduction in severity of rheumatoid arthritis
  - Increase in bone mineral density
  - Reduction in acne
  - Prevention of atherogenesis
  - Reduction in acute PID

COCs, combination oral contraceptives; *PID*, pelvic inflammatory disease.

by reducing the bioavailability of free hormones such as testosterone, thyroxin and cortisol.

Box 23.29 Clinical uses of COCs

- Contraception
  - Regular
  - Emergency
- Management of
  - AUB
  - Endometriosis
  - Primary and secondary amenorrhoea
  - PCOS
  - Hirsutism
- Add-back therapy
- Prevention of ovarian cancer

AUB, abnormal uterine bleeding; *COCs*, combination oral contraceptives; *PCOS*, polycystic ovarian syndrome.

Box 23.30 Minor side effects

- Nausea, vomiting
- Increase in cervical discharge
- Candidal vaginitis
- Hyperpigmentation of face
- Weight gain

Box 23.31 Cardiovascular and metabolic adverse effects of COCs

- Cardiovascular effect
  - Venous thrombosis
    - Increased risk (3/10,000)
    - More in thrombophilias
    - More in COCs with newer progestins
  - Ischaemic heart disease
    - No increase in nonsmokers
  - Stroke
    - Increased if smoker, diabetic, hypertensive
    - Increased in migraine with aura
  - Blood pressure
    - Minimal effect—Monitoring recommended
- Metabolic effects
  - Lipids and lipoproteins
    - Minimal effects
    - Effects of newer progestins favourable
  - Carbohydrate metabolism
    - No effects
  - Protein metabolism
    - Increase in SHBG
    - Increase in angiotensinogen
    - Increase in clotting factors
  - Liver
    - Cholestasis—Uncommon

COCs, combination oral contraceptives; *SHBG*, sex hormone–binding globulin.

Box 23.32 Effects of COCs on neoplasia

- Breast cancer
  - Controversial
  - Small or no increase in risk
- Cervical cancer
  - Minor increase in risk
  - Increase in HPV infection
- Endometrial cancer
  - 40% reduction with 2 years of use
  - 60% reduction with 4 or more years of use
- Ovarian cancer
  - Reduction in risk
- Liver tumours
  - Increase in benign adenomas
  - Slight increase in hepatocellular carcinoma

COCs, combination oral contraceptives; *HPV*, human papillomavirus.

Box 23.33 Contraindications to COCs

- History of venous thrombosis, embolism, thrombophilia
- Known ischaemic heart disease
- Diabetes with vasculopathy
- Severe hypertension
- History of breast, endometrial cancer
- Cholestasis, hepatic adenomas, abnormal liver function
- Undiagnosed vaginal bleeding
- Major surgery requiring immobilization
- Smokers >35 years

COCs, combination oral contraceptives.

Box 23.34 Some drugs that are interfered with by COCs

- Aspirin, acetaminophen
- Dicumarol, warfarin
- Imipramine
- Diazepam, alprazolam, temazepam
- Corticosteroids
- Aminophylline, theophylline
- Metoprolol
- Cyclosporine
- Antiretrovirals

COCs, combination oral contraceptives.

Most adverse effects are dose related. The risk is low with the currently available low-dose preparations. The cardiovascular and metabolic effects of low-dose preparations are listed in Box 23.31.

COCs increase the risk of some gynaecological cancers while protecting against others (Box 23.32).

Contraindications

Due to the known adverse effects in women with certain risk factors, use of COCs is best avoided in some women (Box 23.33).

Drug interactions

OC pills interact with a wide variety of drugs. COCs interfere with the actions of some drugs and dose of these drugs must be adjusted in COC users (Box 23.34). Some drugs, mainly hepatic enzyme inducers, reduce the effectiveness of COCs; therefore, other methods of contraception must be recommended (Box 23.35).

Return to fertility

Normal menstruation occurs on stopping the COCs in most women. Some have a period of amenorrhoea known as 'postpill amenorrhoea', which usually lasts less than 6 months. Resumption of ovulatory cycles and return to fertility occur in 2–3 months.

Other forms of oestrogen–progestin combinations

Transdermal patch and transvaginal ring The mechanism of action and adverse effects are same as those of low-dose pills. Patches (Ortho Evra) are well tolerated and convenient to use. Vaginal ring (NuvaRing) is kept for 3 weeks and new ring is inserted after a break of 1 week (Table 23.11). This is also convenient to use and has good patient acceptance.

Once-a-month injections Once-a-month intramuscular injections of oestrogen–progestin combination are available in some countries. Compliance is good. Contraceptive efficacy is excellent. Menstruation resumes within 30 days of stopping the injection. Preparations available are listed in Box 23.36.

Table 23.11 Transdermal and transvaginal oestrogen-progestin combination

Transdermal patch	Transvaginal ring
• Releases EE_2 20 µg + norelgestromin 150 µg daily	• Releases EE_2 15 µg + etonogestrel 120 µg daily
• Used for 3 weeks with 1-week break before the next cycle	• Kept in place for 3 weeks, with 1-week break before the next cycle
• More breakthrough bleeding and spotting	• Less breakthrough bleeding and spotting
• Breast tenderness	• May interfere with coitus
• Skin irritation at the application site	

EE_2, ethinyl oestradiol.

New developments

The goal of new developments is to improve compliance and reduce side effects. The following are some of the new developments:

- Extended dosing with a short pill-free interval of 2–4 days
- *Lower dose of EE_2*: 10 µg of EE_2 with norethindrone 28-day regimen, 4-day progestin-free interval and 2-day EE_2-free interval
- EE_2 with drospirenone for antimineralocorticoid and an androgenic action (the risk of venous thromboembolism is higher)

Progestational contraceptives

Progestins can be used alone as contraception. They can be administered through several routes.

Oral progestins

They are also known as 'minipills'. They do not inhibit ovulation in all women. If LH surge alone is suppressed, follicular maturation may occur, but no ovulation. If basal FSH is also suppressed, follicles do not develop. In women who ovulate, luteal phase defect, cervical mucus changes and endometrial changes are not conducive to fertilization or implantation.

Minipills can be started 21 days after the delivery. They must be taken at the same time each day or at least within 3 hours of the scheduled time. Failure rate is much higher if they are delayed. Indications, benefits and disadvantages are listed in Box 23.37.

Preparations and dosage

These are listed in Box 23.38.

Injectable progestins

Intramuscular injections

Depot medroxyprogesterone acetate (DMPA) and norethindrone enanthate (NET-EN) are

Box 23.37 Benefits, indications and disadvantages of minipills

- Benefits
  - No increase in
    - Coagulability
    - Glucose intolerance
    - Blood pressure
    - Cardiovascular complications
  - Do not interfere with lactation
- Indications
  - Lactating mothers
  - History of thrombosis, hypertension
  - Smokers >35 years
- Disadvantages
  - High failure rate (2–3/100 women-years)
  - Irregular bleeding
  - Functional ovarian cysts
  - Drug interactions
  - Weight gain, depression

Box 23.38 Preparations and dosages— Progestin-only pills

- Norethindrone (Micronor): 0.35 mg
- Norgestrel (Ovrette): 0.75 mg
- Levonorgestrel (Microval): 0.30 mg
- Desogestrel (Cerazette): 0.75 mg

available for intramuscular use (Box 23.39). DMPA acts for 14 weeks and is administered once in 90 days. Failure rate is 0.4/100 women-years. Intramuscular injections inhibit ovulation and cause changes in the cervical mucus and endometrium that interfere with sperm motility and implantation.

Box 23.39 Intramuscular injections

- Benefits
  - Long-acting, good compliance
  - No interference with lactation
  - No increase in coagulability
  - Cause amenorrhoea—Reduction in anaemia
  - Reduction in PID, ectopic pregnancy
  - Reduction in endometrial cancer
- Indications
  - Lactating mothers
  - Any woman in reproductive age
  - Girls with neurodevelopmental delay
  - Endometriosis

PID, pelvic inflammatory disease.

Side effects These are listed in Box 23.40.

Box 23.40 Side effects of depot progestins

- Irregular bleeding
- Weight gain
- Depression
- Reduction in bone mineral density
- Increase in LDL; reduction in HDL
- Delay in return to fertility

HDL, high-density lipoprotein; LDL, low-density lipoprotein.

Reduction in bone mineral density has been observed with DMPA, but it recovers after the drug is stopped. The Food and Drug Administration (FDA) does not recommend the use of DMPA for more than 2 years. Irregular bleeding can be managed by small doses of oestrogen or 50 mg of mifepristone once in 2 weeks. An increase in breast cancer has been reported in the first 2 years of use, but there is no overall increase.

Preparations and dosages These are listed in Table 23.12.

Table 23.12 Preparations and dosages— Intramuscular progestins

Preparation	Dose (mg)	Frequency
DMPA	150	Once in 90 days
	300	Once in 6 months
NET-EN	200	Once in 2 months

DMPA, depot medroxyprogesterone acetate; NET-EN, norethisterone enanthate.

Subcutaneous injections

When administered subcutaneously, adequate blood levels can be achieved with a smaller dose. Contraceptive efficacy is very high and duration of action is same as that of intramuscular DMPA.

Subdermal implants

Subdermal implants were developed for prolonged duration of action. The progestin-containing devices deliver a small dose of progestin daily and are effective for 3–5 years.

Norplant

Norplant is of two types: I and II. The dosage and duration of action are given in Table 23.13.

The implants are placed on the medial aspect of the arm and removed when required. The contraceptive efficacy and patient acceptance are good. Irregular bleeding is the main side effect as with other progestin-only contraceptives.

Table 23.13 Subdermal progestin implants

Norplant I	Norplant II	Implanon
6 silastic rods	2 silastic rods	Single polymer rod
Levonorgestrel	Levonorgestrel	Etonogestrel
36 mg each	70 mg each	67 mg each
Releases 85 µg/day for 3 months, 50 µg/day for 15 months, 30 µg/day thereafter	Releases 50 µg/day	Releases 30 µg/day
Effective for 5 years	Effective for 3–5 years	Effective for 3 years

Depression occurs in a few women. Insertion and removal are easy procedures.

Progestin vaginal ring

Similar to vaginal ring with oestrogen–progestin combination, progestin-only rings are being tried. They release 20 µg of levonorgestrel daily. They are removed every 3 weeks to allow bleeding to occur. Long-acting rings that can be changed every 3 months are also under trial.

Intrauterine system

Intrauterine system (IUS) is meant for intrauterine devices that are impregnated with progestins. Progestasert, which contains 38 mg of progesterone, releases 65 µg of the hormone daily. This has been largely replaced by levonorgestrel-containing device [levonorgestrel intrauterine system (LNG-IUS), Mirena]. Mirena has 52 mg of levonorgestrel and releases 20 µg daily. It is a device with very few side effects, high efficacy and high acceptance rates, and is used for several other indications as well (Box 23.41).

Clinical uses

These are listed in Box 23.42.

Emergency contraception

Emergency contraception is used following unprotected intercourse, rape or slipping, or rupture of condom. It is also referred to as 'postcoital contraception' or 'morning after pill'.

Mechanism of action

The high dose of hormones acts by reducing tubal motility, inhibiting ovulation, making the

Box 23.41 LNG-IUS

- Contains 52 mg of levonorgestrel
- Releases 20 µg daily
- Effective for 5 years
- Mechanism of action
  - Endometrial atrophy
  - Changes in cervical mucus
  - May inhibit ovulation
- Causes amenorrhoea
- Reduces ectopic pregnancy, PID
- Failure rate 0.1%
- Side effects
  - Irregular bleeding
  - Uterine cramping

LNG-IUS, levonorgestrel intrauterine system; *PID*, pelvic inflammatory disease.

Box 23.42 Clinical uses of LNG-IUS

- Contraception
- Abnormal uterine bleeding
- Endometriosis
- Endometrial hyperplasia

LNG-IUS, levonorgestrel intrauterine system.

endometrium unsuitable for implantation or interfering with luteal function.

The methods of emergency contraception are listed in Box 23.43. The first dose is taken within 72 hours of intercourse and second dose 12 hours later.

Box 23.43 Methods of emergency contraception

- COCs (Yuzpe regime)
  - With 50 µg EE_2: 2 tablets/dose
  - With 30 µg EE_2: 4 tablets/dose
  - With 20 µg EE_2: 5 tablets/dose
- Progestin-only (plan B)
  - 0.75 mg levonorgestrel: 1 tablet/dose (or)
  - 1.5 mg levonorgestrel: Single dose
- Others
  - Mifepristone: 10 mg single dose
  - Centchroman: 60 mg/dose
  - LNG-IUS
  - Copper-bearing IUCD

COCs, combination oral contraceptives; *EE_2*, ethinyl oestradiol; *IUCD*, intrauterine contraceptive device; *LNG-IUS*, levonorgestrel intrauterine system.

Emergency contraception has good success rates. Pregnancy rate with Yuzpe method is about 3.2%, levonorgestrel is 1.1%, mifepristone is 1% and copper-bearing intrauterine contraceptive device (IUCD) is 1%. Efficacy decreases with increasing delay after intercourse. Mifepristone can be used up to 120 hours after contact and copper-bearing IUCDs must be inserted within 5 days of sexual contact. If pregnancy occurs, the drugs used do not have any adverse effect on the foetus.

Key points

- Several gynaecological disorders are treated with hormones.
- Continuous administration of gonadotropin-releasing hormone (GnRH) analogues leads to marked reduction in gonadotropin secretion. Several preparations are available. They are used mainly in assisted reproduction and treatment of amenorrhoea, endometriosis and precocious puberty.
- Gonadotropins [follicle-stimulating hormone (FSH); luteinizing hormone (LH)] are mainly used to stimulate follicular growth, trigger ovulation, stimulate progesterone production and sustain corpus luteum.
- Prolactin has no therapeutic uses. But drugs that inhibit prolactin secretion are used to treat hyperprolactinaemia and mastalgia, and suppress lactation.
- Pharmacological actions of synthetic oestrogens are an extension of their physiological action on various tissues. They play a major role in the development of genital tract and secondary sexual characteristics. They suppress pituitary gonadotropins. They have major effects on carbohydrate, protein and lipid metabolism. Oestrogens increase bone mineral density.
- Preparations of oestrogens are available for oral, transdermal, intramuscular, intravenous and vaginal administration.
- The most important use of oestrogens is as part of combination oral contraceptive (COC) pills. They are also used for postmenopausal hormone therapy, for treatment of abnormal uterine bleeding and to stimulate development of secondary sexual characteristics.
- Side effects of oestrogens must be kept in mind.
- Selective oestrogen receptor modulators are used in the prevention of breast cancer and postmenopausal osteoporosis. Ormeloxifene is also used as a contraceptive.
- The most well-known antioestrogen is clomiphene, used for induction of ovulation.
- Aromatase inhibitors have recently been introduced. They are used in the treatment of several gynaecological disorders including oestrogen receptor–positive breast cancer, precocious puberty and ovulation induction.
- Progestins include the naturally occurring progesterone and other synthetic progestational agents. Pharmacological actions of progestins are similar to their physiological actions. They cause decidualization of the endometrium and play a major role in the maintenance of pregnancy.
- Preparations of progestins are available for oral, subdermal, transvaginal and intrauterine administration.
- Progestins are used along with oestrogens or alone for contraception. Other important uses include treatment of endometriosis, abnormal uterine bleeding and advanced endometrial cancer, and for luteal phase support.
- Mifepristone is an antiprogestin used in the treatment of several gynaecological conditions.

Self-assessment

Case-based questions

Case 1

A 30-year-old lady, mother of two children, presented congestive dysmenorrhea and dyspareunia. She underwent a laparoscopy and was diagnosed to have moderate endometriosis.

1. What are the hormones that can be used in this situation?

2. What side effects would you expect with GnRH analogues?
3. What is add back therapy?

Case 2

A 23-year-old woman, delivered 5 weeks ago, breastfeeding, came for contraceptive advice.

1. What contraceptive choices will you give her?
2. What is minipill? What are the uses on minipill?
3. What are the uses of LNG-IUS?

Answers

Case 1

1. Combine OC pills, oral progestins. Depo medroxy-progesterone injections, GnRH analogues, danazol, gestrinone. Others less often used are aromatase inhibitor and mifepristone
2. Hot flushes, vaginal dryness, insomnia, decrease in bone mineral density
3. Use of combine OC pills to reduce side effects of GnRH analogues is known as add back therapy

Case 2

1. Progestin only pills, injectable progestins, implants or LNG-IUS
2. Oral progestins used for contraception is referred to as 'minipills'. They are used in breastfeeding mothers, women with history of thrombosis and hypertensives.
3. Contraception, treatment of AUB-O and AUB-E, endo-metriosis, endometrial hyperplasia

Long-answer question

1. Discuss the pharmacological actions, uses, benefits and side effects of hormonal contraception.

Short-answer questions

1. Subdermal implant, Norplant
2. Levonorgestrel intrauterine system
3. Oral contraceptive pill
4. Contraindications for combined oral pill
5. Emergency contraception
6. Minipill
7. Noncontraceptive benefits of hormonal contraceptives
8. Danazol
9. Selective oestrogen receptor modulators
10. Aromatase inhibitors
11. Mifepristone
12. Cyproterone acetate
13. Uses of GnRH analogues

Disorders of the Pelvic Floor and Urogynaecology

24 Pelvic Organ Prolapse

Case scenario

Mrs GT, a widow and mother of two sons, was brought to the gynaecology clinic with urinary retention. She hailed from a village 30 miles away and her sons were farmers. She had noticed a mass protruding through her vagina 10 years ago but was too embarrassed to talk about it. The mass had increased in size considerably in the past 1 year and she had developed urinary incontinence, difficulty in defecation and vaginal discharge. Her neighbours had told her that she may require surgery and she felt she could not afford the expense. Meanwhile, she developed acute urinary retention and had to be rushed to the hospital.

Introduction

Prolapse of the pelvic organs is a common problem. Though not life-threatening, it is a condition that affects quality of life. The condition can occur after hysterectomy as well. The prevalence is likely to increase with increasing life expectancy of women. Women, especially the poor and disadvantaged, do not seek treatment for several years. Management depends on the severity of prolapse and patient's symptoms. Evaluation by a urologist may also be required in some women.

Definition and terminology

Pelvic organ prolapse (POP) is defined as the protrusion or herniation of pelvic organs into or out of the vagina that occurs due to failure of the anatomical supports. The protrusion may involve cervix and uterus (Fig. 24.1), the vaginal vault, anterior or posterior vaginal walls, and the adjacent structures such as bladder, urethra, rectum or contents of the pouch of Douglas (Fig. 24.2a–d). Depending on the organ(s) that herniate, various terms are used (Box 24.1).

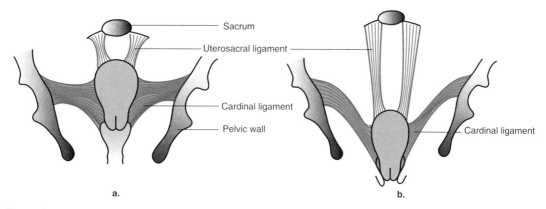

Figure 24.1 Diagrammatic representation of uterine prolapse. **a.** Normal position. **b.** Prolapse of the uterus and cervix. Note that the uterosacral and cardinal ligaments are stretched.

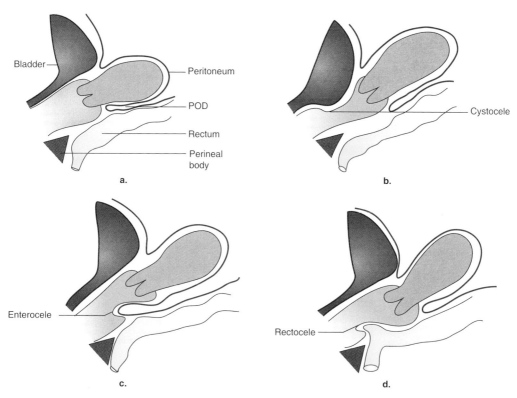

Figure 24.2 Anterior and posterior vaginal wall prolapses. **a.** Normal anatomy. **b.** Prolapse of the upper two-third of the anterior vaginal wall with the adjacent bladder (cystocele). **c.** Prolapse of the upper one-third of the posterior vaginal wall, drawing the POD with it (enterocele). **d.** Prolapse of the middle one-third of the posterior vaginal wall with the adjacent rectum (rectocele). *POD*, pouch of Douglas.

Prevalence

About 30–50% of parous women develop POP. Many are asymptomatic and have only a minor degree of prolapse and many do not report the symptoms. Globally the prevalence is 2–20%. In India, the reported overall prevalence varies from 1% to 20%. It is higher in perimenopausal and postmenopausal, multiparous women.

Surgical anatomy

To understand the pathophysiology of prolapse and to perform appropriate corrective surgery, it is important to know the surgical anatomy.

Supports of the uterus

Pelvic floor support is by a complex interaction between the muscles and the endopelvic fascia.

- The levator ani and coccygeus muscles along with their fascia form the main floor of the pelvis on which the pelvic viscera are supported (Fig. 24.3; *see* Chapter 1, *Anatomy of the female reproductive tract*).
- Condensations of the endopelvic fascia form ligaments that attach the cervix and vagina to the pelvic wall to stabilize them.
- The body of the uterus does not have strong ligamentous supports, but the cervix is held in place by the cardinal and uterosacral ligaments.
- The uterus and the upper vagina lie horizontally on the pelvic floor. The levator ani muscles have a resting tone, which keeps the pelvic floor closed and prevents any herniation.
- Normally, the ligaments are not under tension.

Supports of the vagina

Vaginal supports are important in holding the vagina, bladder, urethra and rectum in their position. They can be arbitrarily divided into levels I, II and III (DeLancey) as given in Box 24.2. They merge with each other above and below (Fig. 24.4).

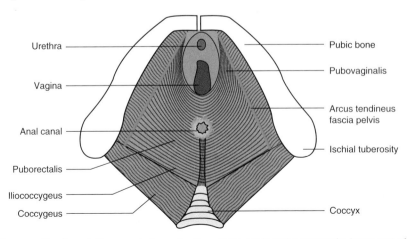

Figure 24.3 Diagram of levator ani. The muscle forms the floor of the pelvis and supports the lower part of the vagina.

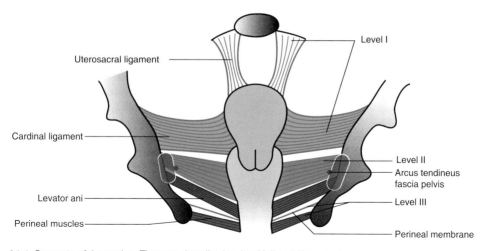

Figure 24.4 Supports of the vagina. They are described as level I, II and III supports.

Box 24.2 Supports of the vagina (DeLancey)

- Level I   Apex of   Uterosacral ligaments
             vagina/cervix   Cardinal ligaments
- Level II   Middle third of Paravaginal
             the vagina   attachment to:
                              – Arcus tendineus
                                fascia pelvis
                              – Arcus tendineus
                                rectovaginalis
- Level III Lower third of   Perineal membrane
             the vagina   Perineal body
                              Perineal muscles

Box 24.3 Defects at various levels of support of vagina

- Level I (suspension defects)
  - Descent of the cervix
  - Enterocele
  - Apical/vault prolapse
- Level II (attachment defects)
  - Cystocele
  - Rectocele
- Level III (fusion defects)
  - Gaping introitus
  - Deficient perineum
  - Urethrocele

Pathophysiology

Damage to the levator ani may be a direct damage to muscle fibres or, more often, damage to the innervation. When the muscles are damaged, the pelvic floor opens and the uterus and vagina are pushed downwards by the intra-abdominal pressure. The axis of the vagina changes and the cervix and apex of the vagina protrude into the upper vagina. The ligaments and fascia hold the organs in place initially, but stretch and yield with time.

Damage to the vaginal supports at various levels gives rise to prolapse of structures at the respective levels (Box 24.3). Supports at more than one level may be affected.

Risk factors

The aetiology of POP is multifactorial. The risk factors are broadly classified as given in Box 24.4.

Box 24.4 Risk factors in POP

- Weakening of pelvic supports
  - Pregnancy and delivery
  - Multiparity
  - Age
  - Menopause
  - Congenital defect
  - Acquired tissue abnormalities
  - Hysterectomy
  - Previous surgery for POP
- Chronic increase in intra-abdominal pressure
  - Smoking
  - Constipation
  - Chronic lung disease
  - Obesity
  - Occupational

POP, pelvic organ prolapse.

Weakening of supports

This can be due to damage to the levator ani or to the endopelvic fascia and ligaments.

Pregnancy and delivery Some weakening of ligaments and fascia occurs due to hormonal changes of pregnancy. When the foetal head passes through the vagina, there may be direct injury to the levator ani muscle, damage to nerve fibres and stretching of the fascia. The risk increases with certain obstetric factors (Box 24.5). Instrumental delivery causes tearing or stretching of ligaments when instrument is applied before full cervical dilatation.

Box 24.5 Obstetric factors that increase risk of pelvic organ prolapse

- Vaginal delivery
- Large foetus
- Injudicious instrumentation
- Prolonged second stage
- Premature bearing down
- Multiparity

Menopause Oestrogen deficiency associated with menopause causes weakening and atrophy of the ligaments and fascia of the pelvis causing POP and urinary incontinence. Pre-existing asymptomatic POP can worsen and become obvious and symptomatic after menopause. **Age** is an important independent risk factor. Postmenopausal women are also older and the changes in tissues with age may be an additional factor causing prolapse in older women.

Congenital and acquired weakness of the muscles and fascia This is associated with hypermobile joints. Neuropathies and myopathies can lead to POP. Congenital weakness of the tissues leads to POP in young, nulliparous women. These women are thin, have easy labours and have hypermobile joints due to inherited disorders of collagen, such as Marfan syndrome. Since they present at a young age, conservative surgery is required. Chances of recurrence are high since the collagen tissue is weak. Therefore, additional support with mesh is usually necessary.

Surgical procedures Surgical procedures for stress incontinence that alter the vaginal angle, prior surgery for POP and hysterectomy that may damage pelvic supports can lead to POP.

Chronic increase in intra-abdominal pressure

When the intra-abdominal pressure increases, the levator ani contracts and the uterus and vagina are compressed anteroposteriorly against the pelvic floor. When the increase in intra-abdominal pressure is frequent and chronic, pelvic floor, normal or minimally damaged, may not offer adequate support. The hiatus widens and the uterus and vagina begin to sag through it. The ligaments stretch or tear and POP occurs.

Obesity, chronic cough, smoking, constipation and occupations that involve lifting of heavy weights increase intra-abdominal pressure and can predispose to POP.

Description and quantification

There are several systems of quantification in use. Description and quantification are essential for assessment of severity of the defects, standardization of documentation, reproducibility, planning treatment and assessment of results of the therapy.

Anatomical classification

The traditional method, which is the anatomical classification, is given in Box 24.6. The introitus is the reference point in anatomical classification of POP (Fig. 24.5). **This classification is not recommended now.**

Box 24.6 Anatomical classification of POP

• Normal	Cervix at the level of ischial spines
• First degree	Cervix below the spines but above the introitus
• Second degree	Cervix at the level of introitus
• Third degree	Cervix outside the introitus
• Procidentia	Uterine fundus outside the introitus

POP, pelvic organ prolapse.

The examining fingers can be approximated above the uterine fundus lying outside the introitus in procidentia.

The anterior and posterior vaginal wall prolapses are described as in Box 24.7.

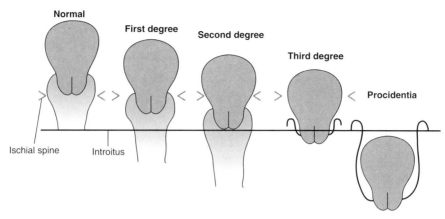

Figure 24.5 Diagram depicting anatomical classification of prolapse into first-, second- and third-degree prolapse and procidentia.

Box 24.7 Anterior and posterior vaginal wall prolapses

- Cystocele — Bulge in the upper two-third of the anterior vaginal wall
- Urethrocele — Bulge in the lower one-third of the anterior vaginal wall
- Enterocele — Bulge in the upper one-third of the posterior vaginal wall
- Rectocele — Bulge in the middle one-third of the posterior vaginal wall
- Deficient perineum — Distance between the introitus and the anal verge decreased

POP-Q system

The International Continence Society (ICS) has developed and recommended a system of quantification known as the POP-Q system, which is currently recognized as an objective, site-specific and standard system for describing POP. It is the accepted classification by the American Urogynecologic Society and the Society of Gynecologic Surgeons.

The hymen is the fixed reference point. Six reference points are identified (Table 24.1; Fig. 24.6), and the location of these points with reference to the plane of the hymen is measured and tabulated in a grid. The points above the hymen are expressed as '–' and those below as '+'; hymenal ring is '0'.

Other measurements required are as follows:

Table 24.1 Reference points in the POP-Q system

Point	Description	Range
Aa	Anterior vaginal wall, midline 3 cm proximal to external urethral meatus	–3 to +3 cm
Ba	Anterior vaginal wall, most dependent portion. Between Aa and anterior fornix	–3 cm to +tvl
C	Cervix or vaginal cuff	±tvl
D	Posterior fornix or vaginal apex, corresponds to utero-sacrals	±tvl
Ap	Posterior vaginal wall, midline 3 cm proximal to hymen	–3 to +3 cm
Bp	Posterior vaginal wall, most dependent portion. Between Ap and posterior fornix	–3 cm to +tvl

POP-Q, pelvic organ prolapse quantification; tvl, total vaginal length.

- **Genital hiatus (gh):** External urethral orifice to posterior hymenal remnant
- **Total vaginal length (tvl):** Hymenal ring to point D
- **Perineal body (pb):** Posterior hymen to middle of anal opening

Measurements are taken using a marked spatula or scale and are expressed in centimetres. The patient is examined in dorsal position while

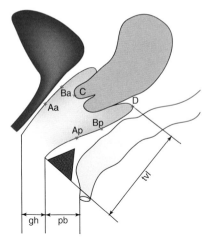

Figure 24.6 POP-Q classification. The diagram shows the reference points and measurements. *Aa* and *Ba*, points A and B on anterior vaginal wall; *Ap* and *Bp*, points A and B on posterior vaginal wall; *C*, cervix; *D*, posterior fornix; *gh*, genital hiatus; *pb*, perineal body; *tvl*, total vaginal length.

performing Valsalva manoeuvre. Total vaginal length is measured after reducing the prolapse. Once the measurements are taken, they are tabulated in a 3/3 grid shown as follows:

Aa Anterior wall	Ba Anterior wall	C Cervix or vaginal vault
gh Genital hiatus	pb Perineal body	tvl Total vaginal length
Ap Posterior wall	Bp Posterior wall	D Posterior fornix

Staging of POP

The degree of prolapse is quantified as in Box 24.8.

Modification of POP-Q system known as simplified POP-Q (S-POP-Q) has been developed. It is simpler but not in routine use.

Classification of anterior wall prolapse

The anterior vaginal wall prolapse has been further classified as in Box 24.9.

Distension of the vagina by foetal head or atrophy due to oestrogen deficiency causes an attenuation of connective tissue of the anterior vaginal wall leading to a central defect. The vaginal rugae are absent, but the lateral attachment to arcus tendineus is preserved; therefore, the lateral vaginal sulci are preserved. When anterolateral attachment of vagina to arcus tendineus

---

Box 24.8 Staging of POP

- Stage 0
  - No demonstrable prolapse
- Stage 1
  - All points ≤1 cm above the hymenal ring
- Stage 2
  - Lowest point within 1 cm of the hymenal ring (between −1 and +1)
- Stage 3
  - Lowest point >1 cm below the hymenal ring, but 2 cm less than tvl (tvl−2)
- Stage 4
  - Complete prolapse with lowest point ≥tvl−2

POP, pelvic organ prolapse; tvl, total vaginal length.

Box 24.9 Anterior vaginal wall prolapse

- Central defector distension cystocele
  - Rugae absent
  - Lateral vaginal sulci present
- Lateral (paravaginal) defector displacement cystocele
  - Rugae present
  - Lateral vaginal sulci absent

---

fascia pelvis is detached or stretched, paravaginal (lateral) defects occur. The rugae are preserved, but the bulge or prolapse is more to the side and the lateral vaginal sulci are absent on one or both sides.

Classification of posterior vaginal wall defects

The posterior vaginal wall is supported mainly by the rectovaginal septum, which is attached superiorly to the uterosacral ligaments, inferiorly to the perineal body and laterally to the arcus tendineus fasciae rectovaginalis. Lower third of the posterior vagina is supported by the perineal body. Detachment of rectovaginal septum from its upper or lower attachments and disruption of its central fibres give rise to central defects. Detachment of rectovaginal septum from the arcus tendineus fascia rectovaginalis leads to paravaginal defects.

Symptoms

Many women with POP are asymptomatic. The descent may be of a minor degree and the woman maybe unaware of the problem. But when the prolapse increases, a sensation of fullness in the vagina is usually felt. The other symptoms are listed in Box 24.10.

Fullness in the vagina

This is the most common symptom. A sensation of fullness may be felt with anterior or posterior wall prolapse or with descent of the cervix.

Mass descending per vaginum

When the prolapse descends to the introitus or below, the women can feel or see the protrusion. Initially, the prolapsed organ protrudes while straining during defaecation or lifting heavy weights, but later it protrudes all the time. The patient may also experience a feeling of pelvic pressure.

Low backache

As the cervix descends, the uterosacral ligaments are stretched and the woman experiences low backache. The ache is worse by the end of the day and is relieved by rest.

Urinary symptoms

Urinary symptoms are usually present when there is anterior vaginal wall prolapse. Urine collects in the cystocele, which is at a lower level than the bladder neck, and is not emptied during micturition. This causes a sensation of incomplete evacuation. Dysuria, frequency and urgency are due to recurrent cystitis, which is caused by stasis of urine. Stress incontinence occurs due to urethral hypermobility. Retention of urine can occur when the urethra is kinked and totally occluded as in procidentia and long-standing POP.

Bowel symptoms

When the rectocele is large, defaecation difficulties may arise. Splinting the rectum and straining during defaecation or digital evacuation are typical symptoms of rectocele. Faecal matter collecting in the rectocele may occasionally cause sensation of incomplete evacuation. Rectal symptoms are not as common as urinary symptoms.

Sexual symptoms

Damage to the levator ani causes relaxation of the pubovaginalis fibres. Damage to perineal body causes the introitus to gape. These can lead to sexual dissatisfaction and incontinence of flatus and stools. Mass protruding into or through the vagina can also interfere with normal sexual act.

Vaginal discharge/bleeding

A decubitus ulcer forms on the cervix when the cervix lies outside the introitus due to venous stasis, congestion and oedema (Fig. 24.7). This can cause discharge, which is mucoid and occasionally bloodstained. If the ulcer is traumatized, bleeding can also occur.

Clinical evaluation

History

A detailed history helps in diagnosis and decision regarding management (Box 24.11).

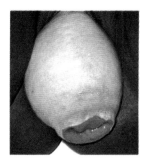

Figure 24.7 Decubitus ulcer in the most dependent part of the prolapse.

Box 24.11 History in POP

- Age
- Parity
- Symptoms
  - Fullness in the vagina
  - Mass descending per vaginum
    - On straining
    - At rest
  - Urinary symptoms
  - Bowel symptoms
  - Sexual dissatisfaction
  - Backache
  - Discharge/bleeding
- Past history
  - Connective tissue disorders
  - Myopathy/neuropathy
- Obstetric history
  - Number of pregnancies/vaginal deliveries
  - Duration of second stage
  - Size of the baby
  - Instrumental delivery
- Menopausal status
- Occupation
- Chronic cough/constipation
- Smoking
- Previous surgery
  - Surgery for prolapse
  - Hysterectomy

POP, pelvic organ prolapse.

Physical examination

Physical examination will confirm the diagnosis, and ascertain the degree/stage of prolapse and structures involved. The need for surgical correction and type of correction can also be decided upon in most women after history and physical examination (Box 24.12; Fig. 24.8a–e).

Box 24.12 Physical examination in POP

- General examination
  - Body mass index
  - Joint hypermobility
  - Other signs of myopathy/neuropathy
- Respiratory system
  - Features of COPD
- Abdominal examination
  - Abdominal mass
- Local examination
  - Vulval atrophy
  - Perineal body
  - Introitus—Gaping
  - Vaginal rugae
- Prolapse
  - POP-Q classification staging
- Tone of levator ani muscle
- Lateral vaginal sulcus
- Enterocele
- Stress incontinence
- Decubitus ulcer
- Pelvic examination
  - Uterine size, mobility, position
  - Adnexal mass
- Rectal examination
  - Rectocele
  - Tone of anal sphincter
  - Deficient perineum

COPD, chronic obstructive pulmonary disease; *POP*, pelvic organ prolapse.

- The patient should be examined in dorsal position. Sims speculum and a ruler or sponge forceps with 1-cm marks should be available.
- Postmenopausal atrophic changes can be seen in the vulva in older women. Absence of vaginal rugae indicates oestrogen deficiency or central defect.
- The patient should be asked to strain or perform Valsalva manoeuvre for taking measurements. Prolapse is then reduced to measure the total vaginal length.
- Lateral vaginal sulcus runs obliquely from the posterior aspect of the pubic bone to the ischial spine. Its absence indicates a paravaginal defect.
- Enterocele may be demonstrated in the dorsal or left lateral position. After reducing the prolapse, the posterior vaginal wall is retracted by a Sims speculum. The cervix should be pulled anteriorly by a tenaculum to expose the posterior fornix. The patient is asked to strain and

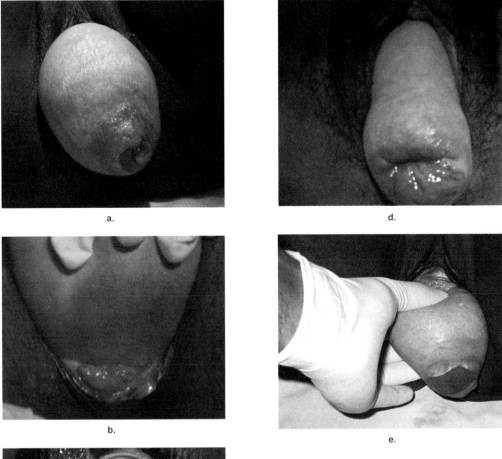

a.

b.

d.

e.

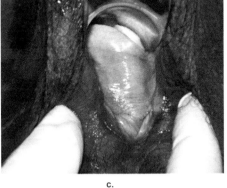

c.

Figure 24.8 Uterine, anterior wall and posterior wall prolapse. **a.** Cystocele—Bulge in the upper two-third of the anterior vaginal wall. **b.** Rectocele—Bulge in the middle third of the posterior vaginal wall. **c.** Deficient perineum. Rectocele can also be seen. **d.** Third-degree prolapse—Cervix lying outside the introitus. **e.** Procidentia—The body of the uterus lies outside the introitus; the fingers can be approximated above the uterine fundus.

the speculum is gradually withdrawn (Fig. 24.9). Enterocele appears as a bulge in the upper one-third of the vagina.

- Elongation of cervix must be looked for above (supravaginal portion) and below (portiovaginalis) the level of bladder sulcus.
- Tone of the levator muscles can be assessed by palpating the pubovaginalis fibres in the lateral wall of the lower one-third of the vagina when the patient contracts the muscle.
- Bimanual pelvic examination should be performed to assess uterine size and exclude adnexal masses.
- A rectovaginal examination is mandatory to differentiate between a high rectocele and an enterocele; look for deficient perineum. The

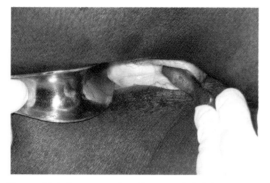

Figure 24.9 Demonstration of enterocele in left lateral position. Sims speculum is used to retract the posterior vaginal wall and the cervix is pulled towards the pubic symphysis by a tenaculum. As the speculum is withdrawn, the enterocele appears as a bulge in the upper third of the posterior vaginal wall.

anterior rectal wall can be felt to protrude into a rectocele.

- In some women, the prolapse may not be obvious in the dorsal position. These women have to be examined in a squatting or standing position.

Vaginal wall sulci

There are three sulci on the anterior vaginal wall and a lateral vaginal sulcus on each side (Box 24.13; Fig. 24.10a and b).

Box 24.13   Sulci on anterior and lateral vaginal walls

- Submeatal sulcus
  - Just above the external urethral meatus
- Transverse vaginal sulcus
  - At the bladder neck
- Bladder sulcus
  - At the level of the bladder
- Lateral vaginal sulcus
  - Along the arcus tendineus fascia pelvis

The transverse vaginal sulcus is at the level of the bladder neck. The bladder sulcus is at the level of attachment of the anterior vaginal wall to the cervix. The distance between the bladder sulcus and the cervix is normally the length of the vaginal portion of the cervix (about 1–1.5 cm), and is increased when the vaginal portion of the cervix is elongated.

The lateral vaginal sulcus is absent in paravaginal defects and helps to differentiate between

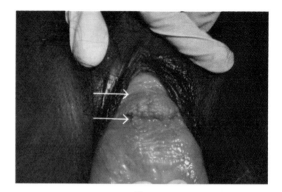

a.

b.

Figure 24.10 Sulci on the anterior vaginal wall. a. Submeatal (arrow) and transverse vaginal sulcus (double arrow). b. Bladder sulcus (arrow).

the anterior vaginal wall prolapse due to distension and displacement.

Investigations

Investigations to assess fitness for surgery, to rule out urinary tract infection and other pelvic pathology, are performed as a routine (Box 24.14).

Test for occult stress incontinence

Some women with a major degree of prolapse have no demonstrable stress incontinence due to urethral kinking. But when the prolapse is reduced and supported by sponge forceps, fingers, cotton swab or pessary, stress incontinence becomes obvious (occult stress incontinence). These women with occult stress incontinence present with incontinence after surgery for prolapse if anti-incontinence procedure is not performed simultaneously.

Other tests

Other investigations are ordered only if necessary (Box 24.15). If history is suggestive of urodynamic abnormality, urodynamic studies are indicated. They are not recommended as a routine in POP. In women with severe bowel symptoms, proctography may be performed. Magnetic resonance imaging (MRI) helps in the evaluation of the muscles and fascia and the fascial defects. But it is not recommended as a routine.

Differential diagnosis

POP must be differentiated from other conditions that present with mass descending per vaginum (Box 24.16).

A rim of cervix with pedicle going through the internal os can be felt in **endocervical/**
endometrial polyps. In **chronic inversion** of the uterus, a cervical rim is felt and traction on the protruding uterine fundus causes the cervix to move upwards. In **hypertrophic elongation of cervix**, the portiovaginalis is elongated as is obvious from the increase in distance between the external os and the bladder sulcus, and the fornices are deep (Fig. 24.11). **Gartner cyst** is a cyst on the anterolateral vaginal wall.

Management

POP is not a condition that requires immediate surgical correction. Many women continue for several years with a mild degree of prolapse and minimal symptoms. Surgical correction has a 30% chance of recurrence. Surgery can also interfere with fertility. Therefore, all factors must

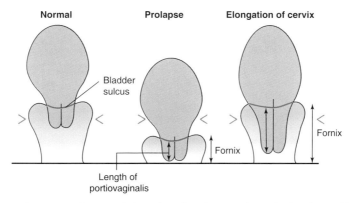

Figure 24.11 Differences between prolapse and elongation of cervix; normal state is also shown. The vaginal fornix is deep and the distance between the bladder sulcus and the external os is increased in vaginal elongation of the cervix.

be taken into consideration before management decisions are made.

Management of decubitus ulcer

Rarely, decubitus ulcer can become malignant. Ulcers should be evaluated by cytology, and if the smear is abnormal, colposcopy and directed biopsy are warranted. The prolapse should be reduced and retained in position by rest, packing or pessary. Oestrogen vaginal cream can be used in postmenopausal women to aid in healing (Box 24.17).

Box 24.17 Management of decubitus ulcer

- Smear for cytology
- Colposcopy and directed biopsy
  - Nonhealing ulcer
  - Abnormal Pap smear
- Reduction of prolapse
- Oestrogen cream if postmenopausal

Management of POP

Treatment is required in women with symptomatic or severe degrees of prolapse. Management may be conservative or surgical. Choice of treatment should take into consideration patient's age, parity, desire for future pregnancies, symptoms, degree of prolapse and associated comorbidities.

Conservative management

Nonsurgical management is chosen for several indications (Box 24.18).

Box 24.18 Indications for conservative management of pelvic organ prolapse

- Mild or moderate degree of prolapse
- Asymptomatic women
- Unfit for surgery
- Old women
- Prolapse in pregnancy
- While awaiting surgery

Conservative management is given in Box 24.19.

Vaginal pessary

Vaginal pessaries are of two types:

- Support pessaries
- Space-filling pessaries

Box 24.19 Conservative management in pelvic organ prolapse

- Weight reduction
- Lifestyle modification
- Pelvic floor exercises
- Vaginal pessary

Ring pessary, which is a support pessary, is commonly used. Inflatable space-filling pessaries preclude coital function (Fig. 24.12). Pessaries are available in different sizes and the correct size must be chosen. Pessary is commonly used for prolapse in pregnancy, for women awaiting surgery, for decubitus ulcer to heal and in frail, old women who are unfit for surgery. Long-term use can cause vaginal discharge and occasionally ulceration. The pessary has to be cleaned every 3–4 days and reinserted. The patient should be followed up after 2 and 6 weeks, and 6-monthly thereafter. Additional use of vaginal oestrogen cream reduces the chances of ulceration.

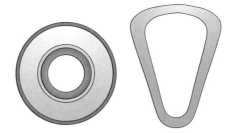

Figure 24.12 Pessaries used for conservative management of prolapse.

Surgical management

Surgery is the treatment of choice for POP. It is aimed at restoration of normal anatomy and function. Connective tissue tears are corrected, and vaginal walls and vault are supported by the strengthened ligaments. Vaginal or abdominal hysterectomy is performed along with corrective surgery whenever indicated. Surgical procedures may be

- Reconstructive procedures
- Obliterative procedures

Routes of surgery

Surgery for prolapse can be performed by

- Vaginal route
- Abdominal route

- Laparoscopically
- Combined approach

Vaginal route is most commonly used since the defects are easily corrected by this approach.

Reconstructive procedures

In women with symptomatic prolapse who are fit for surgery, reconstructive procedures are recommended. Usually uterine or vault prolapse is associated with anterior and/or posterior vaginal wall prolapse. Therefore, combination of various procedures is required.

Surgery for anterior and posterior vaginal wall prolapses

The reconstructive surgical procedures performed for anterior and posterior vaginal wall prolapses are listed in Box 24.20. The steps of various surgical procedures are given in Chapter 34, *Gynaecological surgery.*

- Most anterior vaginal wall defects are central defects and are corrected by anterior colporrhaphy. The procedure consists of plication of the fascia between the bladder and the vaginal wall (vaginal muscularis, pubocervical fascia). Site-specific repair was performed in the past for paravaginal defects. This is not performed now for anterior vaginal wall defects. Paravaginal defect repairs are not performed now.
- Enterocele repair involves reducing the contents (bowel loops) of the enterocele, obliteration of the sac and closure of the defect below it by approximation of uterosacral ligaments. This can be done by McCall culdoplasty vaginally or Moskowitz procedure abdominally.
- Rectocele repair is by posterior colporrhaphy. Other posterior wall defects can be managed by site-specific repairs. A deficient perineum or defective perineal body is repaired by perineorrhaphy. This is combined with posterior

colporrhaphy in most women with mid and low posterior wall prolapse.

Hysterectomy in the management of POP

Hysterectomy is often performed along with anterior and posterior vaginal wall repairs. This is based on the following reasons:

- The cardinal and uterosacral ligaments are damaged and the cervix along with the vaginal apex descends (uterine/apical prolapse) in most women with anterior and posterior vaginal wall prolapses.
- Hysterectomy makes it easier to perform vault suspension procedures to elevate the apex.
- If hysterectomy is not performed, uterine prolapse can recur.

Therefore, a vaginal hysterectomy is usually performed in older women (arbitrarily 35 or 40 years) who have completed family. But it must be remembered that hysterectomy is not the treatment for prolapse; corrective surgery for defects at all levels should be performed after completion of hysterectomy.

Preservation of prolapsed uterus

This is indicated in a young woman who wants to preserve uterus for reproductive or menstrual function. The prolapse in these young women is usually due to congenital defects in the supporting tissue or acquired defects. In women with strong but stretched uterosacral and cardinal ligaments, these may be shortened and used to support the cervix. Uterus-preserving surgeries are listed in Box 24.21.

- ***Fothergill or Manchester procedure:*** When the cervix is hypertrophied and there is supravaginal elongation, this is the treatment of choice. In this, the cervix is amputated to normal length; cardinal ligaments are clamped,

---

Box 24.20 Surgical procedures for anterior and posterior vaginal wall prolapse

- Anterior vaginal wall
    - Anterior colporrhaphy   Plication of pubovesicocervical fascia

- Posterior vaginal wall
    - Posterior colporrhaphy   Plication of rectovaginal fascia
    - Site-specific repair   Perirectal fascial repair at the site of defect
    - Perineorrhaphy   Approximation of pubovaginalis; repair of perineal body
    - McCall culdoplasty   Plication of uterosacrals; attaching uterosacrals to vaginal vault
    - Moskowitz procedure (abdominal)   Purse-string plication of peritoneum of POD

POD, pouch of Douglas.

cut and fixed anteriorly to the cervix to shorten the ligaments and support the cervix. Anterior colporrhaphy is usually required. If there is associated posterior vaginal wall prolapse, posterior repair is performed as well. Although the uterus may be preserved for reproductive function, amputation of the cervix reduces fertility. Cervical incompetence, cervical stenosis and recurrence of prolapse are other complications.

- *Suspension/sling procedure:* In women with weak ligaments and pelvic floor due to congenital defects, some kind of suspension procedure must be performed. These women are generally young and nulliparous or have one child. Since the cardinal and uterosacral ligaments are weak and stretched, fascia or Mersilene tape is used.

Reconstructive surgery for vaginal vault prolapse

After hysterectomy for uterovaginal prolapse, the vaginal vault has to be supported by vault suspension. When a woman presents with vault prolapse following hysterectomy, abdominal, vaginal or laparoscopic corrective surgery is required (Box 24.22).

Obliterative procedures

Obliterative procedures are performed in elderly, frail women who are unfit for major surgery. Vaginal intercourse is not possible following obliterative procedures and patients must be counselled regarding this. Procedures performed are as follows:

- Partial colpocleisis
- Total colpocleisis

Partial colpocleisis or LeFort colpocleisis is the procedure commonly performed. The epithelium of a large area of anterior and posterior vaginal walls is removed, and the anterior and posterior vaginal walls are sutured together to occlude the vagina. Tunnels are created laterally for the discharge to escape.

Total colpocleisis or colpectomy/vaginectomy refers to removal of entire vaginal epithelium and closure of vagina. This is performed rarely, in women with vault prolapse.

Concomitant surgery for stress incontinence

Many women with POP have stress incontinence and some women with major degree of prolapse, who do not have incontinence preoperatively, may develop this after surgery for POP (occult stress incontinence).

- In women with stress incontinence and POP, surgery for stress incontinence should be performed along with pelvic reconstruction. The choice of surgery depends on route of POP repair:
  - Vaginal surgery for POP should be combined with midurethral sling.
  - Abdominal surgery should be combined with Burch procedure (refer Chapter 25, *Urogynaecology*).
- Women who have occult stress incontinence may be managed by one of the following approaches:

– Concomitant stress incontinence surgery
– Surgery for POP initially and later, if required, surgery for stress incontinence

Choice of surgery

Several factors determine the choice of surgery. It is important to decide on the type of surgery that each patient requires after taking into consideration all factors. Decision must be individualized (Box 24.23).

Choice of surgery: General guidelines

The general guidelines for determining the choice of surgery in the management of POP are enumerated in Box 24.24.

Use of synthetic and biological meshes in the management of POP

Synthetic and biological 'meshes' have been used as adjuncts in the surgical management of POP. They augment the supportive tissues and provide scaffolding for fibroblast proliferation and collagen formation.

- Synthetic grafts may be absorbable or nonabsorbable.
- Biological grafts are allografts, autografts or xenografts.
- Synthetic, nonabsorbable, macroporous, monofilament meshes (Prolene mesh) are used in the management of POP (Fig. 24.13).
- They are used in women with recurrent prolapse or occasionally in primary repair of large anterior or posterior wall defects.

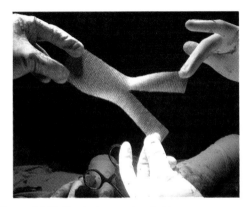

Figure 24.13 Synthetic, nonabsorbable, macroporous, monofilament mesh, used in the surgical treatment of prolapse.

Box 24.23 Factors determining the choice of surgical treatment in pelvic organ prolapse

- Age
- Parity
- Degree/stage of prolapse
- Prior surgery for prolapse
- Intra-abdominal adhesions
  - Endometriosis
  - PID
- Type of prolapse
  - Anterior vaginal wall
  - Posterior vaginal wall
  - Apical/vault
- Associated stress incontinence

PID, pelvic inflammatory disease.

Box 24.24 Choice of surgery in POP

- Older women, completed family, uterine, anterior and posterior compartment prolapses
  - Vaginal hysterectomy
  - Anterior colporrhaphy
  - Posterior colporrhaphy/site-specific repair
  - Perineorrhaphy
  - McCall culdoplasty
- Young women, not completed family, strong ligaments, uterine, anterior and posterior compartment prolapses
  - Fothergill/Manchester operation
- Nulliparous prolapse (congenital weakness of tissues)
  - Abdominal sacrocolpopexy
  - Purandare/Shirodkar/Khanna sling procedure
- Only anterior vaginal wall prolapse
  - Anterior colporrhaphy
- Only posterior vaginal wall prolapse
  - Posterior colporrhaphy
  - Perineorrhaphy
- Posthysterectomy vault prolapse
  - Sacrospinous colpopexy
  - McCall culdoplasty
  - Bilateral high uterosacral suspension
  - Abdominal/laparoscopic colpopexies
- Any POP with stress incontinence
  - Combine with anti-incontinence surgery
    - If vaginal surgery—TVT or TOT
    - If abdominal surgery—Burch procedure

POP, pelvic organ prolapse; *TOT*, transobturator tape; *TVT*, tension-free vaginal tape.

- Complications include infection, mesh erosion, chronic vaginal discharge and dyspareunia.
- They are not recommended for routine use in surgical correction of POP.

Key points

- Pelvic organ prolapse (POP) is the protrusion of the pelvic organs into or through the vagina due to failure of anatomical supports. Cervix, uterus, vaginal vault and anterior and/or posterior walls may protrude.

- Along with anterior and posterior vaginal prolapses, adjacent organs such as bladder, rectum or contents of the pouch of Douglas also herniate.

- POP is caused by damage to the levator ani muscle and the vaginal supports at various levels. There are several risk factors, but pregnancy, delivery and post-menopausal oestrogen deficiency are most common.

- Traditionally, POP is classified as first-, second- and third-degree prolapse and procidentia. Anterior and posterior wall prolapses are further divided into cystocele, urethrocele, enterocele, rectocele and deficient perineum, depending on the level of prolapse.

- The International Continence Society (ICS) has developed and recommended a quantification system known as POP-Q system. The hymen is the fixed point. Six reference points are identified and the location of these points with reference to the plane of the hymen is measured. Genital hiatus, total vaginal length and perineal body are also measured. The measurements are tabulated in a grid.

- Symptoms of prolapse include mass descending per vaginum, low backache and urinary, bowel and sexual symptoms.

- The chest and abdomen should be examined to rule out conditions causing an increase in intra-abdominal pressure. Tone of the levator ani muscle must be checked, and presence of stress incontinence and decubitus ulcer must be looked for. The prolapse should be graded according to POP-Q system.

- In addition to routine investigations, pessary test should be performed to rule out occult stress incontinence in POP.

- Conservative management in POP consists of lifestyle modification, pelvic floor exercises and vaginal pessaries.

- Surgery is the treatment of choice unless it is contraindicated or the POP is minimal. Specific reconstructive surgery should be performed for anterior and posterior vaginal wall prolapses. Site-specific repair is recommended.

- Preservation of uterus and type of surgery in POP depend on the age, parity, aetiology and type of prolapse and associated pathology. Corrective surgery for vaginal vault prolapse may be performed vaginally, abdominally or laparoscopically.

- Synthetic and biological meshes have been used as adjuncts in surgical management of POP. They are not recommended for routine use.

Self-assessment

Case-based questions

Case 1

A 52-year-old lady presents with mass descending per vaginum, minimal since 7 years but increasing progressively since 3 years. She is a mother of four children and is postmenopausal 4 years.

1. What specific details in history would you ask for?
2. The findings on local examination are given in figure below. Draw a 3/3 grid. At what stage is the prolapse?
3. There is a decubitus ulcer of 2 × 2 cm. What is the management?
4. What surgery would you recommend for this lady?

Case 2

A 28-year-old lady, mother of two children, presents with mass descending per vaginum with stress incontinence. On examination, she is found to have a stage 3 prolapse with cystocele, and no posterior wall prolapse.

1. How will you evaluate this lady?
2. What surgery would you recommend?
3. How will you counsel before surgery?

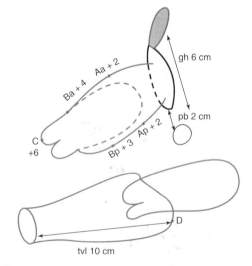

Figure Diagram depicting findings on examination of Case 1. *Aa* and *Ba*, points A and B on anterior vaginal wall; *Ap* and *Bp*, points A and B on posterior vaginal wall; *C*, cervix; *D*, posterior fornix; *gh*, genital hiatus; *pb*, perineal body; *tvl*, total vaginal length.

Answers

Case 1

1. **(a)** Symptoms:
    - **(i)** Urinary symptoms—Frequency, urgency, dysuria, stress incontinence, sensation of incomplete evacuation
    - **(ii)** Bowel symptoms—Sensation of incomplete evacuation, constipation
    - **(iii)** Sexual problems—Discharge/bleeding, back pain
   (b) Obstetric history—Vaginal deliveries, duration of second stage, instrumentation, weight of babies
   (c) Past history of any surgery
2.

Aa +2 cm	Ba +4 cm	C +6 cm
gh 6 cm	pb 2 cm	tvl 10 cm
Ap +2 cm	Bp +3 cm	D 4 cm

   Stage 3.
3. **(a)** Do a Pap smear.
   (b) Reduce the prolapse.
   (c) Apply oestrogen cream daily.
4. Vaginal hysterectomy, pelvic reconstruction that includes anterior colporrhaphy, posterior colporrhaphy, perineorrhaphy and McCall culdoplasty.

Case 2

1. Examine the prolapse; do a POP-Q classification and staging.
   (a) Routine investigations
   (b) Clinical demonstration of stress leak

2. Fothergill/Manchester repair with tension-free vaginal tape or transobturator tape.
     Or cystocele repair, Purandare or Khanna sling procedure and transobturator/tension-free vaginal tape procedure.
3. Counsel regarding chances of recurrence of prolapse and difficulty in conceiving, if she wants another child. Chances of cervical stenosis/incompetence.

Long-answer questions

1. A 32-year-old woman reports to you with a uterine prolapse. Discuss in detail the evaluation and management of this case.
2. Describe pelvic floor and discuss the aetiology of prolapse. How will you manage a lady of 55 years with third-degree uterine prolapse? Mention the steps of surgery.

Short-answer questions

1. Pessary treatment of prolapse
2. Nulliparous prolapse
3. POP-Q classification of prolapse
4. Causes of prolapse
5. Supports of the uterus
6. Enterocele
7. Fothergill surgery

25 | Urogynaecology

Case scenario

Mrs GK, 38, a bank officer and mother of three children, had gained about 8 kg weight recently and her BMI was 29. She noticed leakage of urine on sneezing or coughing since 2 years, which had gradually become worse. Now the urine leakage occurred when she lifted something heavy or even when she laughed. Such episodes at work became a source of embarrassment. She was very upset, did not sleep well and wanted treatment.

Introduction

Anatomically and developmentally, genital tract and urinary tract are closely related. Urinary tract can be affected in several gynaecological conditions, during pregnancy and childbirth. Dissection of the urinary tract is often required in pelvic surgeries. Many women with urological problems seek treatment from the gynaecologist. Knowledge of the anatomy, physiology and common urogynaecological disorders is, therefore, essential for the practice of gynaecology.

Anatomy of the bladder and urethra

The urinary bladder is a hollow structure, with capacity to increase in volume as the urine accumulates. The wall has three layers (Box 25.1). The urethra is approximately 4 cm long, located behind the pubic symphysis anterior to the vagina. The urethral wall has two layers, inner mucosa and outer muscular layer.

The intrinsic sphincter is continuous with detrusor muscle. The extrinsic sphincter has two components—The sphincter urethrae and levator ani. The sphincter urethra, which consists of striated muscle and surrounds the upper two-third of the urethra, is known as the rhabdosphincter and is responsible for urethral closure. The fibres of the distal one-third of urethra are made up of the pubourethralis fibres of the levator ani (Fig. 25.1). Under physical effort, this provides additional closure force. The pubourethral ligaments attach the urethra to pubic symphysis.

- Urinary bladder
  - Mucosa
    - Transitional epithelium
  - Detrusor muscle
    - Three layers of smooth muscles
    - Contract as one unit
  - Serosa
    - Covers anterior and superior surface
- Urethra
  - Mucosa
    - Proximal
      - Transitional epithelium
    - Distal
      - Stratified squamous epithelium
  - Muscle layer
    - Inner smooth muscle
      - Intrinsic sphincter
    - Outer circular striated muscle
      - Extrinsic sphincter
    - Upper one-third
      - Sphincter urethrae
    - Lower one-third
      - Levator ani

Innervation of urinary tract

The sympathetic supply is from T11 to L2 and parasympathetic from S2 to S4. Somatic nerve supply to the urethral sphincter and levator ani is through pudendal nerves from S2 to S4 (Box 25.2; Fig. 25.2). The sympathetic system relaxes the detrusor, closes the urethra and controls the bladder storage, whereas the parasympathetic system promotes bladder emptying. The somatic nerves from S2 to S4 reach the extrinsic sphincter and promote contraction under effort.

Box 25.2 Innervation of lower urinary tract

• Parasympathetic S2–S4	Detrusor	Contraction
	Intrinsic sphincter	Relaxation
• Sympathetic T11–L2	Detrusor	Relaxation
	Intrinsic sphincter	Contraction
• Motor fibres S2–S4 (pudendal nerve)	Levator ani and sphincter urethrae	Contraction

Physiology of micturition

As the urine fills the bladder, the bladder relaxes and stretches to accommodate the urine. At 150–200 mL, the first sensation of bladder filling is experienced. The afferent impulses pass to S2–S4 and thence to higher centres in the brainstem and cortex, which inhibit voiding until suitable time. Levator ani muscles aid the process by voluntary contraction, if required.

The inhibition is released at the appropriate time; the efferent parasympathetic impulses cause detrusor contraction and urethral sphincter relaxation. This leads to voiding of urine.

Common urological problems

The common urological problems in women are listed in Box 25.3.

Box 25.3 Common urological problems

- Urinary tract infections
- Urethral syndrome
- Urinary incontinence
- Painful bladder syndrome

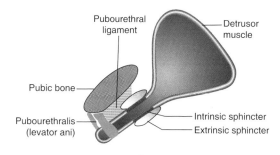

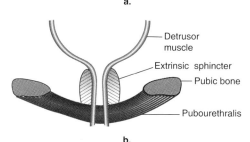

Figure 25.1 Diagrammatic representation of sphincter urethrae. a. The intrinsic sphincter is continuous with the detrusor. b. The extrinsic sphincter consists of striated muscle that surrounds the urethra in the upper one-third and the fibres of the levator ani (pubourethralis) that encircle the urethra in the lower one-third.

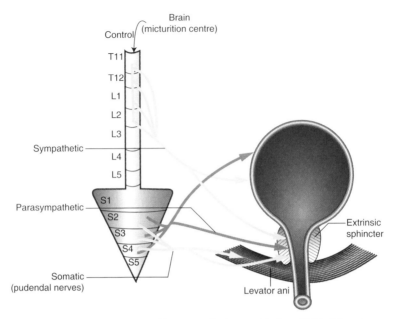

Figure 25.2 Innervation of the bladder and urethra. The sympathetic supply is from T11 to L2 and parasympathetic from S2 to S4. Somatic nerve supply is from S2 to S4 through pudendal nerves to the levator ani.

Urinary tract infections

Urinary tract infections (UTIs) are common in women and can occur at any age.

Definition

A UTI is a microbial infection, usually bacterial, which affects any part of the urinary tract. This may involve only the lower urinary tract (cystitis) or extend to the upper urinary tract (pyelonephritis), given as follows:

- Acute
  - Uncomplicated
    - Cystitis
    - Pyelonephritis
  - Complicated
    - Cystitis
    - Pyelonephritis
- Recurrent

Women are more prone to UTI than men because the female urethra is short and is close to potentially bacterially contaminated organs, namely vagina and anus. Infections can ascend from the vagina and anus easily.

Incidence

Worldwide, UTI is a common problem and occurs in 20% of adult women.

Risk factors

There are some risk factors identified (Box 25.4).

Box 25.4 Risk factors for UTI

- Sexual intercourse
- Pregnancy
- Puerperium
- Prolapse
- Oestrogen deficiency
  - Postmenopausal age
- Postoperative period

UTI, urinary tract infection.

Complicated UTI

Complicated UTI, which may be cystitis or pyelonephritis, is associated with an underlying condition as listed in Box 25.5. These conditions may lead to poor response to treatment.

Box 25.5 Underlying conditions that complicate UTI

- Diabetes
- Pregnancy
- Urinary tract obstruction/anatomical abnormality
- Hospital-acquired infection
- Renal failure/renal transplantation
- Indwelling catheter, stent

UTI, urinary tract infection.

Symptoms

The woman usually presents with typical symptoms of UTI (Box 25.6). A combination of dysuria, frequency, urgency, suprapubic pain and/or haematuria is highly suggestive of acute cystitis. Pyelonephritis presents with above symptoms and, in addition, fever, vomiting and loin pain. Renal angle tenderness may be elicited. Occasionally pyelonephritis may lead to sepsis with multiorgan dysfunction and shock.

Box 25.6 Symptoms and signs of UTI

- Cystitis
  - Frequency
  - Urgency
  - Dysuria
  - Haematuria
  - Pelvic pain
  - Fever
  - Backache
- Pyelonephritis
  - High fever with chills
  - Vomiting
  - Loin pain
  - Renal angle tenderness
  - Sepsis
  - Shock
  - Multiorgan dysfunction

UTI, urinary tract infection.

Microbiology

The usual organism is *Escherichia coli*, but infection by other Gram-negative organisms such as *Klebsiella* and *Pseudomonas* can also occur (Box 25.7).

Box 25.7 Organisms causing UTI

- *E. coli*
- *Klebsiella* sp.
- *Pseudomonas*
- *Proteus* sp.
- *Streptococcus faecalis*
- Enterococci
- *Staphylococcus saprophyticus*

UTI, urinary tract infection.

Investigations

- When typical symptoms are present and the infection is community acquired, microscopic examination of urine to demonstrate pus cells or a dipstick for nitrite is sufficient to make a diagnosis.
- Urine culture is indicated when pyelonephritis is suspected, in recurrent infections, in long-standing infections, in infection in pregnant or postmenopausal women and in postoperative and hospital-acquired infections.
- Dipstick test for nitrite can also be used. It detects infection by Enterobacteriaceae, when colony count is $>10^5$ cfu/mL.
- Ultrasonography and computed tomography to exclude obstruction or anatomical abnormalities of the urinary tract are indicated if the clinical symptoms persist after 48–72 hours of antibiotic therapy.

Management

Treatment is as listed in Box 25.8.

- Acute uncomplicated cystitis can be treated empirically with oral ciprofloxacin or levofloxacin for 3 days.
- If complicated by underlying factors, same drugs may be started and changed according to sensitivity after 48 hours. Treatment should be continued for 7 days.
- Acute uncomplicated pyelonephritis of mild or moderate severity can be treated as outpatient with empirical antibiotics while awaiting culture reports.
- Severe and complicated pyelonephritis should be treated with parenteral antibiotics, as inpatient. Duration of treatment should be 10–14 days.
- Recurrent cystitis may be treated with long-term prophylaxis, given for 6 months to 2 years.

Box 25.8 Management of UTI

- *Acute cystitis*
  - Uncomplicated
    - Empiric therapy
      - Oral nitrofurantoin 100 mg twice daily for **5–7 days**
      - (or) Oral trimethoprim/sulphamethoxazole DS 160/800 mg twice daily **for 3 days**
      - (or) Oral ciprofloxacin 250 mg twice daily **for 3 days**
      - (or) Oral norfloxacin 400 mg twice daily **for 3 days**
      - (or) Oral levofloxacin 250 mg daily **for 3 days**
  - Complicated
    - Empiric therapy
      - Oral ciprofloxacin 500 mg twice daily **for 5–10 days**
      - (or) Oral levofloxacin 750 mg twice daily **for 5–10 days**
      - Change if required, as per sensitivity
- *Pyelonephritis*
  - Mild to moderate, uncomplicated
    - Treat as outpatient
    - Empiric therapy
      - Inj. ceftriaxone 1 g IV single dose, followed by Oral ciprofloxacin 500 mg twice daily **for 7 days**
        (or) Oral levofloxacin 750 mg once daily **for 7 days**
        (or) Oral trimethoprim/sulphamethoxazole DS 160/800 mg twice daily **for 14 days**
        (or) Oral amoxicillin–clavulanate 500/125 mg **for 7 days**
    - Subsequent therapy
      - Antibiotic according to susceptibility **for 10–14 days**
  - Severe /complicated
    - Treat as inpatient
    - Empiric therapy
      - Inj. ceftriaxone 1 g IV Q6H
      - (or) Inj. cefepime 2 g IV Q12H
      - (or) Inj. piperacillin–tazobactam 3.375 mg IV Q6H
      - (or) Inj. imipenem 500 mg IV Q6H
    - Subsequent therapy
      - Antibiotics according to susceptibility **for 14 days**
- *Persistent or recurrent cystitis*
  - Oral norfloxacin 400 mg once daily **for 6 months**
  - (or) Oral trimethoprim–sulphamethoxazole (80 + 400 mg) once daily **for 6 months**

DS, double strength; *UTI*, urinary tract infection.

Prevention

Behavioural modification and other preventive measures can reduce the risk of recurrences (Box 25.9).

Box 25.9 Prevention of recurrent UTI

- Increase oral fluid intake
- Void after sexual intercourse
- Avoid holding urine for prolonged period
- Use oestrogen cream for postmenopausal women

UTI, urinary tract infection.

Urethral syndrome

Urethral syndrome usually occurs in women and is frequently misdiagnosed since it lacks precise diagnostic criteria.

Definition

Urethral syndrome (or frequency–dysuria syndrome) is defined as recurrent episodes of urethral pain during voiding with daytime frequency and nocturia in the absence of proven infection or any other pathology. It occurs mostly in women, and these women usually present with dysuria, urgency, frequency and pain in the urethra of long duration (Box 25.10).

Box 25.10 Urethral syndrome

- Occurs in 20–30% of women
- Long duration of symptoms
  - Dysuria, frequency
  - Urgency, urethral pain
- No proven infection
- Chronically inflamed urethra
- Aetiology
  - Atrophy
  - Immunological, allergic
  - Psychogenic
- Treatment
  - Urethral dilatation
  - Oestrogen cream, if postmenopausal
  - Tricyclic antidepressants

Urinary incontinence

Urinary incontinence is a distressing disorder that can affect the quality of life, but many women are unwilling to discuss it due to embarrassment.

Definition

The definition of incontinence by the International Continence Society (2002) is the complaint of involuntary leakage of urine. When leakage of urine can be demonstrated and is distressing to the patient, evaluation and treatment are necessary.

Classification

Urinary incontinence is classified into

- Stress incontinence
  - Urethral hypermobility
  - Intrinsic sphincter deficiency (ISD)
- Urgency incontinence
- Mixed incontinence
- Overflow incontinence
  - Detrusor overactivity
  - Bladder outlet obstruction
- Others
  - Functional incontinence
  - Extraurethral incontinence

Stress urinary incontinence

Stress urinary incontinence is defined as the complaint of involuntary leakage of urine with increased intra-abdominal pressure in the absence of detrusor contraction. Leakage happens on effort or exertion or on sneezing or coughing. The volume of leak is small.

- This is the most common type of urinary incontinence.
- It occurs in women of reproductive age and perimenopausal women.
- It occurs when the increased intra-abdominal pressure is not transmitted to the bladder and urethra equally. When the bladder pressure exceeds the urethral closure pressure, leakage occurs.

Pathogenesis

Stress incontinence occurs due to

- Urethral hypermobility due to damage to supports

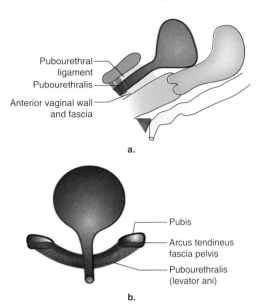

Figure 25.3 Supports of the urethra. **a.** Lateral view showing pubourethral ligament that fixes it to the pubis, the anterior vaginal wall and the fascia. **b.** Anterior view showing the pubourethralis fibres of the levator ani and the arcus tendineus fascia pelvis from which this arises.

- ISD when urethra is damaged

Urethral hypermobility Urethral support is provided by structures listed in Box 25.11. The medial fibres of the puborectalis, called the pubourethralis, form a sling around the urethra. The fibres of the levator ani arise from the arcus tendineus fascia pelvis. The anterior vaginal wall and pubourethral ligament are also important supports of the urethra (Fig. 25.3).

Box 25.11 Urethral support

- Pubourethral ligament
- Anterior vaginal wall
- Levator ani (pubourethralis)
- Arcus tendineus fascia pelvis

When there is an increase in intra-abdominal pressure, the levator ani and vaginal connective tissue contract and counter the downward-directed pressure. The pressure is equally transmitted to the bladder and urethra. When the supports are weak, the downward forces are not countered, the urethra moves downwards and there is funnelling of urethra (Fig. 25.4). The

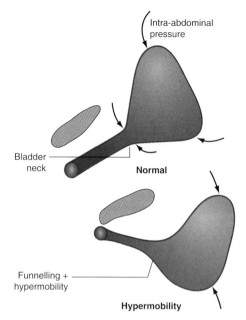

Figure 25.4 Urethral hypermobility and funnelling. In normal women, when intra-abdominal pressure increases, the urethra and bladder neck retain their position and the pressure is transmitted to urethral sphincter as well. In women with urethral hypermobility, the bladder neck and urethra move downwards and the intra-abdominal pressure causes funnelling of the upper urethra, leading to leakage of urine.

ability of urethra to close against the increased pressure is lost and leakage of urine occurs.

Intrinsic sphincter deficiency Integrity of the urethra is maintained by the epithelium, the subepithelial vascular plexus and the muscular layer consisting of smooth and striated muscles. When there is damage to the urethra due to prior surgery or trauma of delivery, leading to denervation and scarring, a lead pipe or rigid urethra results. There is loss of urethral tone, urethral closure is ineffective during increased intra-abdominal pressure and leakage occurs.

Risk factors

Several factors increase the risk of stress incontinence (Box 25.12).

There is a steady increase in the risk of stress incontinence with **age**. **Multiparity** and **vaginal delivery** can cause damage to the supports of the urethra. There is decrease in levator ani tone, descent of the urethra and funnelling. **Obesity** can cause or exacerbate stress incontinence;

Box 25.12 **Risk factors in stress urinary incontinence**

- Age
- Multiparity
- Vaginal delivery
- Obesity
- Menopause
- Chronic increase in intra-abdominal pressure
  - Chronic cough
  - Constipation
  - Occupational risk
- Smoking
- Previous surgery

there is a threefold increase in stress incontinence in obese women. **Menopausal oestrogen deficiency** leads to atrophy of connective tissue and ligaments that support the urethra. **Conditions that increase intra-abdominal pressure** such as chronic cough, constipation and smoking cause weakening of muscular and ligamentous supports and lead to pelvic organ prolapse (POP) and stress incontinence. Previous surgery causes scarring and rigid urethra with ISD.

Clinical evaluation

History
It should be thorough in order to differentiate between stress incontinence and other types of incontinence. The severity of symptoms and history of prior surgery for stress leak also helps in decision making regarding management (Box 25.13).

Physical examination
General examination and gynaecological evaluation should be performed before embarking on investigations (Box 25.14).

Demonstration of stress incontinence

- *Bladder stress test*: With the patient in dorsal or lithotomy position or standing, with the bladder comfortably full, when the patient coughs or performs Valsalva manoeuvre, leakage of urine through the urethra should be looked for. A positive test confirms stress leak.
- In patients with POP, occult stress incontinence should be checked after reducing the prolapse.
- Demonstration of stress incontinence is essential to the diagnosis.

Investigations

Simple primary care level tests are sufficient to make a diagnosis in many women (Table 25.1). Valuable information can be obtained from these tests. Advanced tests are required only in a few women.

- **Urine microscopy and culture** are essential to exclude UTI.

Table 25.1 Simple tests in urinary continence and their purpose

Test	Purpose
Urine microscopy and culture	Exclude UTI
Q-tip test	Assess urethral hyper-mobility
Postvoid residual urine measurement	Exclude overdistended bladder
Voiding diary	Assess urinary output/frequency
Bladder stress test	Assess urethral hyper-mobility

UTI, urinary tract infection.

- **Q-tip test** is performed by inserting a cotton swab in the urethra, asking the patient to perform Valsalva manoeuvre and assessing the angle of urethra (Fig. 25.5). An angle of excursion of more than 30 degrees from the horizontal indicates urethral hypermobility. However,

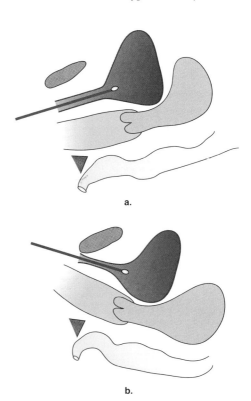

Figure 25.5 Q-tip test. a. The cotton swab inserted into the urethra remains near horizontal at rest. b. When the woman performs Valsalva manoeuvre, the tip of the swab moves upwards in women with urethral hypermobility.

this test has a poor sensitivity and is not used in current practice.

- **Postvoid residual urine** is measured by ultrasound scan or catheterization. A volume of >200 mL indicates diminished bladder contractile function usually due to neurological pathology. This evaluation is not recommended as routine in women with clinical diagnosis of stress incontinence. It is useful when outlet obstruction or overactive/neurogenic bladder is suspected.
- **Voiding diary** (or frequency volume chart) provides information about the number of voids during day and night, volume of urine voided, bladder capacity and total volume of urine output in 24 hours.

Advanced testing—Urodynamic study

Urodynamic study provides objective assessment of bladder and urethral function, and voiding function, but it is expensive and time consuming and requires special equipment. Routine urodynamic study does not improve outcome. However, it is indicated in some situations (Box 25.15).

Box 25.15 Indications for urodynamic study

- Diagnosis based on history and simple tests uncertain
- History suggestive of mixed incontinence
- Neurological dysfunction suspected
- Failed surgery for stress urinary incontinence
- Prior radiotherapy

Urodynamic study involves a battery of tests (Table 25.2). Results of urodynamic study should be interpreted with caution and correlated with clinical findings.

Management of stress incontinence

Treatment depends on the type and severity of incontinence and clinical findings and presence of comorbidity.

ISD is managed surgically. Genuine stress incontinence due to urethral hypermobility can be managed nonsurgically or surgically.

Management of stress incontinence due to urethral hypermobility

Treatment modalities of stress incontinence due to urethral hypermobility are listed in Box 25.16.

Box 25.16 Treatment modalities in stress urinary incontinence

- Lifestyle modification
- Nonsurgical management
  - Pelvic floor muscle training
  - Pessaries and urethral devices
  - Medications
- Surgical treatment
  - Vaginal
  - Abdominal
  - Laparoscopic
  - Combined

Lifestyle modification

Lifestyle changes, especially weight reduction and cessation of smoking, can reduce stress incontinence.

Nonsurgical treatment

- *Pelvic floor muscle exercises:* These are known as *Kegel exercises* and improve resting tone of the levator ani. They have been found to be better than placebo by Cochrane Review Group. The exercises may be voluntary

Table 25.2 Urodynamic studies in stress continence

Study	What it measures	Indications
Cystometry—Simple/multichannel	• Bladder pressure while filling • Detrusor activity • Urethral pressure	• Severe stress incontinence • Detrusor overactivity • Mixed incontinence
Uroflowmetry	• Urine volume voided • Detrusor pressure during voiding	• Urge incontinence • Outlet obstruction • Detrusor underactivity
Cystometrography	Vesical, urethral, abdominal pressures during voiding	• Outlet obstruction • Detrusor overactivity • Detrusor underactivity
Tests of urethral function Urethral pressure profilometry	Urethral pressure	Intrinsic sphincter deficiency
Valsalva leak point pressure	Intravesical pressure at leakage	Intrinsic sphincter deficiency

contraction of muscles or electrically stimulated. The woman is asked to tighten the pelvic floor muscles voluntarily, 8-12 contractions sustained for 8-10 seconds each, 3 times a day. Alternatively, cones may be inserted into the vagina and held in place by contracting the pelvic floor muscle.

- **Pessaries and urethral devices:** Vaginal pessaries provide support for the urethra and can decrease stress incontinence. Urethral devices are inserted into the urethra and removed before voiding. There are no randomized trials to prove their efficacy. Urinary infection can occur with urethral devices.
- **Medications:** Medications are not very effective in the management of stress incontinence. Oestrogen vaginal creams can be used in postmenopausal women. Oral oestrogen is not recommended. Duloxetine, a selective serotonin reuptake inhibitor (SSRI), has been found to be used but is only moderately effective.

Surgical management

The most effective way of curing stress incontinence is surgery. It is the choice of treatment in women with moderate to severe incontinence affecting the quality of life. Surgery elevates the bladder neck, supports the bladder neck and urethra and in some cases improves the urethral closure.

The approach may be vaginal, abdominal, laparoscopic or combined.

Vaginal procedures

These are as listed in Box 25.17.

- **Anterior colporrhaphy:** This is performed in women with cystocele and stress incontinence.

Box 25.17 Vaginal procedures in stress urinary incontinence

- Anterior colporrhaphy + Kelly stitch
  - Plication of pubovesicocervical fascia
  - Elevation of bladder neck
- Retropubic tape procedures
  - TVT
    - Midurethral
    - Attached to the anterior abdominal wall
  - TOT
    - Midurethral
    - Through obturator membrane to the thigh

TOT, transobturator tape; *TVT*, tension-free vaginal tape.

The pubovesical fascia is plicated by a series of transverse stitches and care is taken to place stitches at the level of the bladder neck. This results in elevation of the bladder neck. Failure rate is as high as 40%.

- **Tension-free vaginal tape (TVT) procedure:** This is the most common procedure used at present for stress incontinence. This can be combined with corrective surgery for POP. A tape of polypropylene mesh is placed under midurethra, passed via the retropubic space and fixed to the anterior abdominal wall just above the pubic symphysis. Studies show objective cure rate of 63-85% with very few complications (Fig. 25.6).
- **Transobturator tape (TOT) procedure:** This is a modification of TVT. Polypropylene mesh tape is placed under the midurethra and passed through the obturator membrane, avoiding the bladder and vessels in retropubic space (Fig. 25.7). The tape is fixed to the anteromedial aspect of the thigh. The results are comparable to TVT and complications such as voiding dysfunction, bladder or urethral injury are less. Therefore, TOT is preferred to TVT.
- **Midurethral slings:** Midurethral slings (TVT or TOT) are the standard of care in management of stress incontinence; other procedures are reserved for special circumstances.

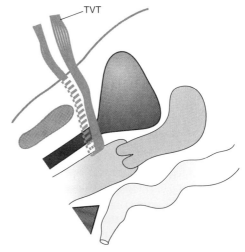

Figure 25.6 Tension-free vaginal tape (TVT) procedure. The tape of polypropylene mesh is placed under the midurethra and taken through the retropubic space to be fixed to the anterior abdominal wall.

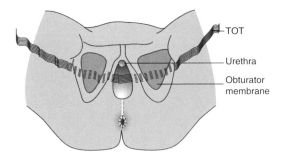

Figure 25.7 Transobturator tape (TOT) procedure. The tape is placed under the midurethra, and taken through the obturator membrane to be fixed to the thigh.

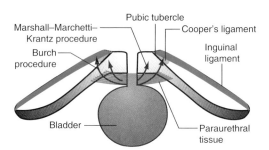

Figure 25.8 Abdominal/laparoscopic procedures. The paraurethral and paravaginal tissues are sutured to the periosteum of the posterior surface of pubis in Marshall–Marchetti–Krantz procedure and to the Cooper's ligament in Burch procedure.

Abdominal and laparoscopic procedures
These are as listed in Box 25.18.

Box 25.18 Abdominal and laparoscopic procedures

- Abdominal procedures
  - Marshall–Marchetti–Krantz procedure
    - Paraurethral tissue to the periosteum of pubis
  - Burch colposuspension
    - Paraurethral tissue to Cooper's ligament
- Laparoscopic procedures
  - Laparoscopic colposuspension
    - Paraurethral tissue to Cooper's ligament

- ***Marshall–Marchetti–Krantz procedure:*** Through a suprapubic approach, retropubic space is opened and the paraurethral tissue at the level of bladder neck is sutured to the periosteum of the posterior surface of the pubic symphysis. This procedure is used along with abdominal surgery for other gynaecological conditions (Fig. 25.8). This procedure has now been largely replaced by Burch colposuspension.
- ***Burch colposuspension:*** The approach is through the retropubic space. The paravaginal tissue at the level of bladder neck is sutured to iliopectineal (Cooper) ligament. This has been the operation of choice for stress incontinence until recently. It is now used when a woman with stress incontinence needs laparotomy/hysterectomy for other indications such as myoma or endometriosis. The long-term success rate is 70–90%.
- ***Laparoscopic colposuspension:*** In this, laparoscopic approach is used to perform a Burch

procedure. The procedure is as effective as open colposuspension, but more time consuming and needs an experienced operator.

Combined procedures
These involve abdominovaginal approach and are not commonly used now since the Burch colposuspension and TVT/TOT tape procedures are easier, more effective and safer. The procedures are listed in Box 25.19.

Box 25.19 Combined procedures in stress urinary incontinence

- Pubovaginal sling procedures
  - Proximal urethra and bladder neck to abdominal wall
- Endoscopic bladder neck suspension
  - Bladder neck to rectus sheath

- ***Pubovaginal sling procedures:*** Traditional sling procedures are known as *proximal urethral sling* or *bladder neck sling* procedures. These are performed by passing a fascial (rectus fascia or fascia lata) or polypropylene sling under the proximal urethra, at the level of the bladder neck, through a vaginal incision. The sling is attached to the rectus sheath. These procedures have a high rate of complications.
- ***Endoscopic bladder suspension:*** The proximal urethra and bladder neck are suspended by sutures passed under the urethra and fixed to the rectus sheath. The sutures are placed under cystoscopic guidance. Several procedures have been tried in the past (Pereyra's, Stamey's, etc.), but the cure rates decrease with time.

Management of intrinsic sphincter deficiency

ISD is diagnosed when the urethral closure pressure is <30 cm H_2O. Most women with failed surgery for stress incontinence are later diagnosed to have ISD.

- Management is surgical, with midurethral slings (TVT or TOT).
- Artificial sphincter is an option in women who do not respond to sling surgery.
- *Periurethral injection of bulking agents* such as bovine collagen increases urethral coaptation and is an option in older women who are not fit for surgery or those with failed midurethral sling procedures and those with scarred, fixed lead pipe urethra. The success rates are less than those with other surgical procedures.

Urge incontinence

Urge incontinence is defined as the involuntary leakage of urine accompanied by or immediately preceded by urgency. Urgency is the sudden, strong desire to pass urine that is difficult to defer. Often the woman leaks before reaching the toilet. The volume of urine lost is considerable. Frequency is more than eight voids per day.

Overactive bladder syndrome is defined as the symptom of urgency with or without urge incontinence, usually with frequency and nocturia. The most common cause of urge incontinence is detrusor overactivity. Detrusor overactivity is a diagnosis made after urodynamic testing. Overactivity may be due to neurological, psychogenic or idiopathic conditions.

The terms urge incontinence and overactive bladder are used interchangeably.

Diagnosis

Urge incontinence is the most common form of incontinence in older women. Detrusor overactivity must be differentiated from urge incontinence due to low bladder compliance in women because of previous bladder surgery or radiotherapy. Acute cystitis can also cause urgency, frequency and sometimes urge incontinence. Diagnosis is by history and investigations as given in Box 25.20.

Management

Treatment of overactive bladder is difficult and not always successful. Several approaches may have to be combined (Box 25.21).

Box 25.20 Diagnosis of urge incontinence

- Symptoms
- Past history of surgery/radiation
- Neurological problems
- Urine culture
- Voiding diary
- Cystometry
  - Detrusor activity during cystometry

Box 25.21 Management of urge incontinence/ overactive bladder

- Psychotherapy
- Bladder drill
- Biofeedback
- Medications
- Intravesical (Botox) therapy
- Surgical intervention

Bladder drill This involves voiding at scheduled times starting with a 30- to 60-minute interval. If urge to void occurs earlier, distraction methods are used to control voiding. Pelvic floor muscle training is added to control the urge to void and suppress detrusor contractions.

Biofeedback This is a form of behavioural therapy in which visual, auditory or verbal feedback is given to the patient during muscle training.

Medications Several drugs are used for the treatment of overactive bladder (Box 25.22). Vaginal oestrogens have been found to be useful in postmenopausal women. Anticholinergics are the drugs of choice. Mirabegron is a β^3 adrenoceptor agonist and is used in women who do not tolerate anticholinergics.

Box 25.22 Drugs used for the treatment of urge incontinence/overactive bladder

- Oestrogens
  - Vaginal oestrogen cream
- Anticholinergics
  - Oxybutynin
  - Tolterodine
  - Trospium
  - Solifenacin
- β^3 adrenoceptor agonist
  - Mirabegron

Intravesical therapy Capsaicin, botulinum toxin and resiniferatoxin are used as intravesical instillation in women with intractable detrusor overactivity. Effect lasts for several months.

Surgical treatment For women who do not respond to other forms of treatment and suffer from severe detrusor overactivity, surgical interventions such as augmentation cystoplasty, detrusor myectomy or urinary diversion procedures may be resorted to.

Mixed incontinence

Women with mixed incontinence have symptoms of both stress and urge incontinence. This condition should be managed initially with medical treatment for detrusor overactivity. If repeat urodynamic study reveals stress incontinence, surgical intervention with midurethral sling is warranted.

Overflow incontinence or retention with overflow

Dribbling of urine associated with a distended urinary bladder and inability to void completely is referred to as overflow incontinence. There is continuous leakage of urine or intermittent dribbling. Overflow incontinence occurs in

- Neurological conditions
- Detrusor underactivity
- Bladder outlet obstruction

Neurological conditions Neurological conditions such as spinal cord disorders, stroke and peripheral neuropathy lead to loss of bladder sensation or detrusor underactivity and give rise to overflow incontinence.

Detrusor underactivity This occurs due to inadequate contractility of detrusor muscle. This can occur in older women, due to either age or associated oestrogen deficiency. Some neurological conditions can also cause detrusor underactivity.

Bladder outlet obstruction Compression of the urethra or bladder neck can give rise to urinary retention with overflow. Urethral stricture is a common condition in older postmenopausal women. Gynaecological and obstetric conditions that can present with overflow incontinence by obstructing the urethra are listed in Box 25.23 (see Fig. 25.9).

Box 25.23 Gynaecological/obstetric causes of urinary retention

- Peripubertal
  - Haematocolpos
- Reproductive age
  - Retroverted gravid uterus
  - Ruptured ectopic gestation with pelvic haematocele
  - Cervical myoma
  - Ovarian mass
- Perimenopausal
  - Advanced POP
  - Advanced pelvic malignancy

POP, pelvic organ prolapse.

Diagnosis

Diagnosis is by history and finding a large distended bladder on examination. Thorough clinical examination is required to find out the aetiology. Imaging by ultrasonogram or magnetic resonance imaging (MRI) may be required in cases of suspected pelvic pathology. Postvoid residual urine should be measured in older women with no pelvic pathology. Some women may need urodynamic testing.

Management

Continuous bladder drainage with an indwelling catheter is usually required for neurological conditions with overflow incontinence. Underlying conditions must be evaluated and treated.

Urethral dilatation should be performed if there is stricture. Postmenopausal women may be treated with vaginal oestrogen.

If detrusor underactivity is diagnosed by urodynamic study, intermittent self-catheterization is advised. Clean catheterization and complete emptying of the bladder are important to prevent infection (Box 25.24).

Functional incontinence

Functional incontinence is the one that occurs in a woman who has normal storage and emptying functions, but has incontinence due to other conditions. The woman may find it difficult to reach the toilet in time or may experience the urge too late. The condition is common in old women, >70 years of age. The incontinence may be transient and reversible in many. The

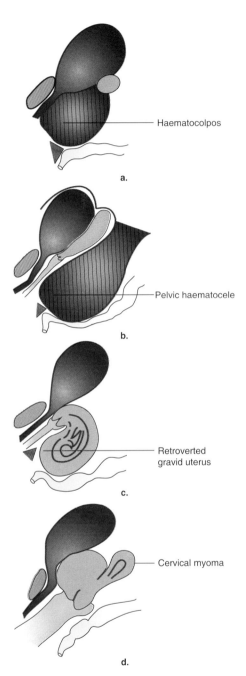

Haematocolpos

a.

Pelvic haematocele

b.

Retroverted
gravid uterus

c.

Cervical myoma

d.

Figure 25.9 Some gynaecological causes of urinary retention by compressing the urethra against the pubic bone. a. Haematocolpos. b. Large pelvic haematocele or pelvic abscess. c. Retroverted gravid uterus. d. Anterior cervical myoma.

causes can be remembered by the mnemonic DIAPPERS (Box 25.25).

Box 25.24 Diagnosis and treatment of overflow incontinence

- Diagnosis
  - History
  - Physical examination
    - Distended bladder
    - Pelvic mass/prolapse
  - Imaging
  - Postvoid residual urine
- Treatment
  - Indwelling catheter
  - Urethral dilatation
  - Treatment of the underlying condition
    - Neurological
    - Gynaecological
    - Obstetric
  - Intermittent self-catheterization

Box 25.25 Causes of functional and transient incontinence

- Delirium
- Urinary tract infection
- Atrophy
- Pharmacological
- Psychological
- Endocrinopathy
- Restricted mobility
- Stool impaction

Treatment of the underlying problem, provision of appropriate facilities, using incontinence pads, restricting fluid intake to 1 L/day and vaginal oestrogen cream for postmenopausal women are the treatment modalities recommended.

Extraurethral incontinence

When the urine escapes through abnormal openings and not through the urethra, it is known as **extraurethral incontinence**. The causes are ectopic ureter, bladder exstrophy and urinary fistulae. Ectopic ureter and bladder exstrophy are congenital abnormalities that require surgical correction. Urinary fistulae are dealt with in Chapter 26, *Urinary tract injuries, urogenital fistulas; anal sphincter injuries and rectovaginal fistulas.*

Painful bladder syndrome

Definition

Painful bladder syndrome is defined as suprapubic pain related to bladder filling, accompanied by other symptoms such as increased frequency in the absence of proven urinary infection or other obvious pathology. Urgency is also usually present. The condition is also known as **interstitial cystitis**.

Diagnosis and management

The diagnosis is by the process of exclusion. All conditions causing painful voiding such as infection, endometriosis, vulvar disease, calculi, bladder cancer, tuberculosis and urogenital atrophy must be excluded (Box 25.26).

Box 25.26 Painful bladder syndrome

- Symptoms
  - Pain on bladder filling
  - Frequency
  - Urgency
- Diagnosis
  - By exclusion of other causes
- Treatment
  - Dietary modification
  - Drugs
    - Pentosan polysulphate
    - Hydroxyzine
    - Amitriptyline
  - Intravesical instillation of drugs
  - Hydrodistension
  - Sacral root neuromodulation

Key points

- Common urological problems encountered in gynaecology include urinary tract infections (UTIs), urethral syndrome, urinary incontinence, disorders of voiding and painful bladder syndromes.
- The urinary bladder is a hollow structure. The muscle of the urinary bladder is called the detrusor muscle. The urethra has intrinsic and extrinsic sphincters.
- Women are more prone to UTI because of the short urethra, which is anatomically close to the contaminated organs such as anus and vagina.
- Typical symptoms of UTI are frequency, urgency, dysuria, haematuria and fever. The common organism causing UTI is *E. coli*. Other Gram-negative and -positive organisms may also cause infection.
- Management of uncomplicated cystitis is with norfloxacin or ciprofloxacin for 3 days.
- Urethral syndrome is defined as recurrent episodes of urethral pain during voiding in the absence of infection. It occurs in 20–30% of women and is more common in postmenopausal women. Treatment is by local oestrogen and urethral dilatation.
- Urinary incontinence may be stress incontinence, urge incontinence, mixed incontinence, overflow incontinence or functional incontinence.
- Stress incontinence is the involuntary leakage of urine with increased intra-abdominal pressure in the absence of detrusor contraction. It is common in multiparous women in association with obesity, postmenopausal status, smoking and chronic increase in intra-abdominal pressure.
- Evaluation of stress incontinence consists of urine microscopy and culture, postvoid residual urine measurements, cystometry and urodynamic studies.
- Urodynamic studies are not indicated in all women with stress incontinence. They are recommended when surgical treatment is contemplated, when there is associated pelvic organ prolapse (POP) or when there is a history suggestive of mixed incontinence.
- Initial treatment of stress incontinence may be by nonsurgical methods such as pessaries and pelvic floor training. Drugs such as imipramine and duloxetine are also used. Surgical repair may be by vaginal, laparoscopic, abdominal or combined procedures.
- Burch colposuspension has been the operation of choice in stress incontinence until recently. Vaginal procedures such as tension-free vaginal tape (TVT) and transobturator tape (TOT) procedures are currently popular.
- Urge incontinence is involuntary leakage of urine accompanied by urgency. Overactive bladder syndrome is the symptom of urgency with or without urge incontinence.
- Treatment of urge incontinence and overactive bladder is by bladder drill, psychotherapy and medications such as oxybutynin, dicyclomine, tolterodine or trospium. Intravesical botulinum, augmentation cystoplasty and detrusor myectomy are also used.
- Overflow incontinence may be due to neurogenic bladder, obstruction to the outflow of the urine, detrusor underactivity or urethral stricture.
- Urinary retention is the common problem in gynaecology. Aetiology varies with age.
- Painful bladder syndrome is usually interstitial cystitis. It is treated with drugs such as pentosan polysulphate or amitriptyline or by intravesical instillation of drugs.

Self-assessment

Case-based questions

Case 1

A 38-year-old multipara presents with a history of passage of urine on coughing for 3 years. Examination reveals a BMI of 30.

1. What details would you ask for in history?
2. What would you look for on physical examination?
3. What investigations would you ask for?
4. What is your management?

Case 2

A 30-year-old lady, mother of two children, presents with a history of inability to void for 12 hours and abdominal pain. Her last menstrual period was 45 days ago.

1. What details would you ask for in history?
2. What would you look for on examination?
3. What investigations would you order?
4. What is the management?

Answers

Case 1

1. Severity of symptom, quality of life, associated symptoms such as urgency or urge incontinence, history of cough, constipation, smoking, diabetes, history of mass descending per vaginum.
2. BMI, signs of chronic respiratory illness, mass arising from pelvis, pelvic organ prolapse. Pelvic examination to look for uterine size, descent. Demonstrable stress incontinence by bladder stress test.
3. (a) Urine culture
   (b) Pap smear
4. If there is demonstrable stress incontinence, no urge incontinence and no POP, TVT or TOT procedures

would be the treatment of choice. If there is associated POP, anterior colporrhaphy with Kelley stitch is an option. However, surgical repair of prolapse and TOT are the current recommendations.

Case 2

1. History of contraception, menstrual cycles, symptoms of pregnancy, acute abdominal pain, fainting spells. Past history of similar episodes.
2. Pallor, tachycardia, hypotension, evidence of intra-abdominal bleeding, pelvic examination for uterine size, retroversion, adnexal mass, tenderness, bogginess in POD.
3. Pregnancy test, ultrasonography.
4. (a) If the diagnosis is retroverted gravid uterus, then catheterize, leave indwelling catheter in situ, advise rest in prone position till the uterus comes to the midline and urethral kinking is relieved.
   (b) If diagnosis is pelvic haematocele due to ruptured ectopic pregnancy, then blood transfusion, laparoscopy/laparotomy.

Long-answer question

1. What is stress incontinence? Discuss the aetiology, evaluation and management of stress incontinence.

Short-answer questions

1. Gynaecological causes of urinary retention
2. Overactive bladder
3. Urodynamic studies
4. Surgical management of stress incontinence
5. Urge incontinence
6. Aetiology and management of urinary tract infections in women

26 | Urinary Tract Injuries, Urogenital Fistulas; Anal Sphincter Injuries and Rectovaginal Fistulas

Case scenario

Mrs HF, 40, underwent hysterectomy and bilateral salpingo-oophorectomy at the local hospital for extensive endometriosis 1 year ago. On the sixth postoperative day, she noticed dribbling of urine. The doctors had performed some tests and told her that there was an injury to the urinary bladder during surgery and this needed surgical repair at a tertiary centre. She had spent all her savings for her surgery and could not come immediately. But the problem was distressing; there was a smell of urine around her all the time; she had to use protective pads and had developed excoriation of the vulva. She had borrowed money and came to the hospital for treatment.

Introduction

The urinary tract is closely associated with genital tract developmentally and anatomically. Rectum and anal canal are also located just posterior to the genital tract. Therefore, the urinary tract and rectum can be damaged during gynaecological surgeries and vaginal delivery. If the injury is recognized immediately, corrective steps can be taken. But if it goes unrecognized, it can result in fistulas or other complications. With improving obstetric services, the incidence of obstetric fistulas is on the decrease, but injuries during surgical procedures do occur.

Urinary tract injuries and fistulas

Injury to the urinary tract is a dreaded complication of gynaecological surgery and obstetric procedures and often preventable.

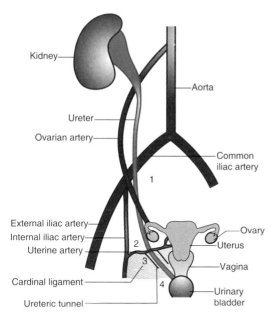

Figure 26.1 Various points at which ureter is prone to injury in gynaecological surgery. 1. At the pelvic brim, while clamping the ovarian vessels. 2. In the broad ligament while clamping the uterine vessels. 3. In the ureteric tunnel in cardinal ligament. 4. At the vault of the vagina before it enters the bladder.

Injuries to the urinary tract

Ureteric injuries

About 50% of ureteric injuries in women occur during gynaecological surgery. The course of the pelvic ureter is discussed in Chapter 1, *Anatomy of the female reproductive tract*. There are several points at which the ureter can be injured as given in Table 26.1 (see also Fig. 26.1).

The ureter has a rich blood supply, which enters from the lateral aspect in the pelvic ureter. The vessels anastomose in the adventitial sheath before entering the ureter. Devascularization takes place when the ureter is skeletonized and the adventitia is stripped.

Risk factors for ureteric injury

The risk of injury to the ureter is high in certain gynaecological conditions (Box 26.1). Injury can occur during laparoscopic surgery as well and is more likely to go unnoticed.

Table 26.1 Points at which ureter is prone to injury

Points prone to injury	Procedure during which the injury may occur
Pelvic brim	Clamping infundibulopelvic ligament
In the broad ligament	Dissection of broad-ligament myomas
Where it crosses the uterine artery	While clamping the uterine artery
In the ureteric canal	Dissection of the ureteric canal
Vaginal vault	Clamping the vaginal angle Pelvic organ prolapse
Above the uterosacral ligament	Approximation of uterosacral ligaments Moskowitz operation
All along the pelvis	Devascularization

Box 26.1 Risk factors for ureteric injury

- Pelvic malignancy
- Endometriosis
- Chronic PID
- Previous surgery
- Prior irradiation
- Obesity
- Broad-ligament tumours
- Pelvic organ prolapse
- Anomalies of the ureter

PID, pelvic inflammatory disease.

Types of ureteric injury

The types of injury are listed in Box 26.2.

Ureteric injuries diagnosed intraoperatively

Intraoperative diagnosis of ureteric injury

Intraoperative diagnosis and immediate management decreases morbidity. Methods of intraoperative diagnosis are listed in Box 26.3.

Box 26.2 Types of ureteric injury

- Crushing
- Angulation and obstruction
- Ligation
- Transection
- Cauterization
- Devascularization

- Intraoperative inspection
- Intraoperative cystoscopy
- Intravenous indigo carmine

Intraoperative inspection

This is the most important step in making a diagnosis.

If the ureter is ligated, the proximal segment dilates and the peristalsis stops.

When the ureter is transected, urine collects in the operating area. If the injury is minor, there may be no significant leakage of urine.

When ureteric injury is suspected, the ureter should be traced through its full course in the pelvis.

Intraoperative cystoscopy

Urine efflux from the ureteric orifice may be absent or slow on intraoperative cystoscopy. Almost 90% of ureteric injuries are diagnosed by cystoscopy. Partial obstruction and thermal injuries may be missed.

Intravenous administration of dye

Indigo carmine, 2.5 mL of 0.8% solution, may be injected intravenously. The dye appears in the urine within a few minutes and can easily be visualized.

Prevention

In women at high risk for ureteric injuries, the ureter should be identified before proceeding with surgery. Ureteric catheters may be placed preoperatively in select patients.

Management

Intraoperative consultation with a urologist may be required for management of ureteric injuries.

When the ureter is accidentally ligated or crushed with a clamp, placement of a stent is sufficient in most cases (Fig. 26.2).

Partial transection may also be managed with a stent.

When it is completely transected, reparative surgery is required. This depends on the level at which injury occurs (Fig. 26.3).

Management of ureteric injuries diagnosed intraoperatively is outlined in Box 26.4.

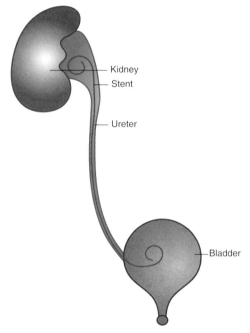

Figure 26.2 Double pigtail stent placed in the ureter for management of crush injury or after repair of transection.

- Crushing
  - Inspection for severity of injury
  - Placement of stent
- Angulation, ligation
  - Deligation, placement of stent
- Partial transection
  - Repair with placement of stenting
- Transection
  - Upper third
    - Ureteroureterostomy
    - Ureteroileal interposition
  - Middle third
    - Ureteroureterostomy
    - Ureteroileal interposition
    - Transureteroureterostomy
  - Lower third
    - Ureteroureterostomy
    - Ureteroneocystostomy
    - Vesicopsoas hitch
    - Cauterization
  - Resection and manage as per transection

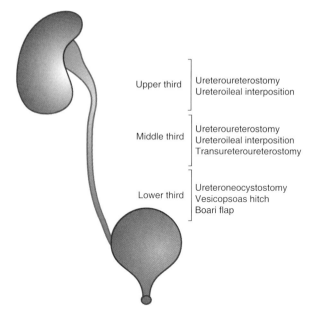

Figure 26.3 Management of transection of the ureter depends on the level at which ureter is transected, that is, in the upper third, middle third or lower third.

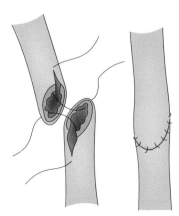

Figure 26.4 Diagrammatic representation of ureteroureterostomy. The ends are spatulated and sutured.

When transection is in upper third of the ureter, ureteroureterostomy is the procedure of choice. The cut ends can be mobilized to avoid tension and anastomosed. The ends are spatulated and sutured over an internal stent (Fig. 26.4).

When a segment of the ureter has to be resected, an ileal segment is interposed between the two cut ends of the ureter or between the ureter and the bladder (Fig. 26.5).

When middle third of the ureter is transected, ureteroureterostomy is the optimal management.

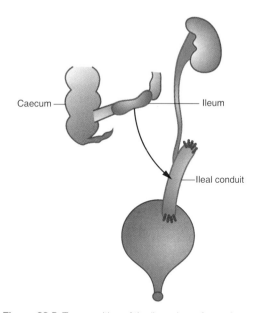

Figure 26.5 Transposition of the ileum is performed when the lower segment is not long enough to implant into the bladder without tension. A distal segment of the ileum is cut and attached to the ureter at the upper end and implanted into the bladder at the lower end.

Occasionally, transureteroureterostomy may be required, where ureter is mobilized and anastomosed to the opposite ureter (Fig. 26.6).

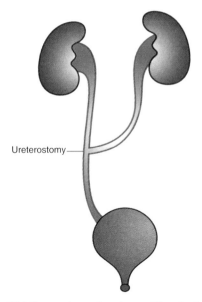

Figure 26.6 Transureteroureterostomy—When the length of the lower segment of the ureter is not adequate, the cut end is anastomosed to the ureter on the opposite side.

This procedure is not often used in current-day practice.

Boari flap is also used for extensive midureteral injuries. Boari bladder flap is fashioned with bladder wall; ureter is tunnelled in and attached to the flap (Fig. 26.7).

Injury to the lower third of ureter is most common. Transection of lower third of ureter is managed as follows:

- If 3–4 cm proximal to ureterovesical junction—Ureteroureterostomy
- If within 2 cm of ureterovesical junction—Ureteroneocystostomy
- If above two cannot be done without tension—Vesicopsoas hitch

Ureteroneocystostomy is reimplantation of ureter into the bladder. In vesicopsoas hitch, the bladder is mobilized and fixed to the psoas muscle to relieve tension (psoas hitch) after ureteroneocystostomy (Fig. 26.8).

Ureteric injuries

If not diagnosed intraoperatively, the ureteric injuries present with a variety of signs and symptoms (Box 26.5). Symptoms depend on the type of injury.

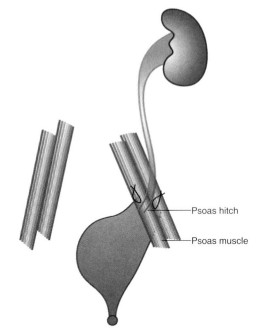

Figure 26.7 A bladder flap (Boari flap) shaped into a tube and the lower end of the ureter is attached to this to provide extra length and prevent tension.

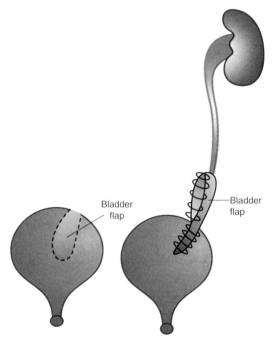

Figure 26.8 Psoas hitch procedure. The bladder is pulled up and stitched to the psoas muscle to prevent tension after ureteroneocystostomy.

Box 26.5 Signs and symptoms of ureteric injuries diagnosed postoperatively

- Flank pain
- Fever
- Sepsis
- Leakage of urine from
  - Vagina
  - Abdominal incision
- Prolonged ileus
- Abdominal pain
- Oliguria/anuria

Box 26.6 Investigations in postoperative diagnosis of ureteric injuries

- Serum creatinine
- Ultrasonogram
  - Hydronephrosis
  - Hydroureter
  - Fluid in the peritoneal cavity
- Examination of peritoneal fluid
  - Creatinine
- Computerized tomography
- Methylene blue test
  - To exclude vesicovaginal fistula excluded
- Cystoscopy and retrograde pyelography

- Transection causes leakage of urine intraperitoneally leading to sepsis, paralytic ileus and fever. Urine leaks from the abdominal incision or vagina.
- Bilateral ureteric ligation leads to anuria and renal failure. The patient may present with flank pain.
- Pyelonephritis can result from stasis of urine.
- Fistulas present with leakage of urine through the vagina during the second postoperative week.

Investigations

When ureteric injury is suspected postoperatively, evaluation of renal function and imaging to locate the site and type of injury is required (Box 26.6).

Management

This depends on the type and timing of presentation, the site of injury and the patient's condition.

Immediate treatment is to relieve obstruction and stop leakage of urine (Box 26.7).

Definitive surgery

For women with intraperitoneal or extraperitoneal leakage or obstruction, this should be undertaken as soon as the patient is stable and ready. Management of transaction and thermal injuries is the same as of intraoperatively diagnosed injuries. Very small fistulas may close with stenting. For large fistulas and when urine leaks despite stenting, surgery is required.

Injuries to the bladder and urethra

Posterior wall of the bladder lies on the anterior surface of the uterus and cervix. The trigone of

---

Box 26.7 Immediate treatment of ureteric injuries diagnosed postoperatively

- Intraperitoneal or extraperitoneal leakage/obstruction
  - Stenting
  - Percutaneous nephrostomy
- Small fistula
  - Stenting

---

the bladder, bladder neck and urethra is anterior to the vagina. Hence, the bladder and urethra can be injured in abdominal and vaginal procedures involving dissection of these structures.

Aetiology

Bladder injury and vesicovaginal fistula (VVF) occur due to several causes (Box 26.8).

Box 26.8 Causes of bladder and urethral injury and fistula

- Childhood
  - Foreign body
  - Surgery for developmental anomalies of the vagina
- Reproductive age
  - Obstetric
    - Obstructed labour
    - Operative vaginal deliveries
    - Caesarean section
    - Gynaecological surgery
  - Trauma
- Older age
  - Cervical cancer
  - Radiation
  - Gynaecological surgery

Obstetric injury

These are common in women with small pelvis and large baby or baby with anomalies. Obstructed labour and fistula formation are seen in developing countries where immediate care is not available. The bladder tissue undergoes necrosis due to prolonged pressure against the pubic bone and fistula is formed. Destructive operations on the dead foetus using sharp instruments, symphysiotomy and caesarean section late in labour with oedematous and friable bladder and deeply engaged head can cause bladder injury (Box 26.9).

Box 26.9   Obstetric causes of bladder injury and fistulas

- Obstructed labour
  - Small pelvis
  - Large baby
  - Foetal anomalies
  - Malpresentations
- Instrumental delivery
  - Destructive operations
- Caesarean section
  - Deeply engaged head
  - Oedematous bladder
  - Previous caesarean section

Gynaecological surgery

Bladder can be injured in abdominal, laparoscopic and vaginal surgeries (Box 26.10).

Risk factors for injury to bladder

Gynaecological conditions that increase the risk of bladder injury are the same as those for ureteric injuries (see Box 26.1).

Box 26.10   Gynaecological surgeries causing bladder injury

- Abdominal and laparoscopic surgeries
  - Simple hysterectomy
  - Radical hysterectomy
  - Myomectomy
  - Oophorectomy
  - Lymphadenectomy
  - Abdominal operations for prolapse
- Vaginal surgeries
  - Hysterectomy
  - Pelvic reconstructive surgery
  - Myomectomy

Intraoperative diagnosis

Intraoperatively, urine leak can be seen. If there is an indwelling catheter, leakage may not be obvious with small injuries. High index of suspicion is necessary.

Intravesical instillation of methylene blue

A total of 200–300 mL of saline mixed with few drops of methylene blue is instilled into the bladder through a catheter. Leakage of fluid stained with methylene blue helps in identification of bladder injury.

Intraoperative cystoscopy

Although routine intraoperative cystoscopy is not recommended for all pelvic surgeries, in high-risk women undergoing extensive dissection and when there is a suspicion of injury, cystoscopy is a very useful tool. The detection rate of injury increases by fivefold (Box 26.11).

Management

Small defects (<2 mm) in the bladder dome can be managed by indwelling catheter for 5–7 days (Box 26.11). Larger defects should be closed after mobilization of bladder. Bladder wall and

---

Box 26.11   Intraoperative diagnosis and management of bladder injuries

- Diagnosis
  - Urine leakage
  - Intravesical methylene blue
  - Intraoperative cystoscopy
- Management
  - Injury to bladder dome
    - Very small defects (<2 mm)
      - Expectant management
      - Indwelling catheter for 5–7 days
    - Larger defects
      - Primary closure
        - Mobilization of bladder
        - Closure of bladder and vaginal wall
        - Absorbable suture
        - Close without tension
        - In one or two layers
        - Watertight
        - Continuous drainage for 7–10 days
  - Injury to trigone
    - May involve ureters or urethra
    - Ureteric stents placed
    - Primary repair

---

vaginal wall should be closed in separate layers without tension. Continuous bladder drainage is mandatory for 7–10 days. Injuries at the trigone may involve the ureters. Hence, they should be repaired after placement of ureteric stents.

Urogenital tract fistulas

Fistulous communication between the urinary tract (ureter, bladder and urethra) and the genital tract (uterus, vagina) is the result of urinary tract injury that has not been recognized immediately and treated.

Vesicovaginal, ureterovaginal and urethrovaginal fistulas

Most urogenital fistulas are between the vagina and the urinary tract. Of these, VVFs are more common (Fig. 26.9). The cause may be gynaecological or obstetric surgery or obstructed labour, as discussed earlier. Ureterovaginal fistulas are less common.

Clinical features

Women with urogenital fistulas present with leakage of urine per vaginum (Box 26.12). This starts towards the end of the first week postoperatively. The leakage is intermittent in ureteric fistula. Long-standing fistulas are associated with excoriation of vulval skin, cystitis and vaginitis. Per speculum examination may reveal pooling of urine in the vagina and the fistula

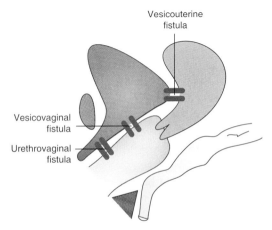

Figure 26.9 Diagrammatic representation of vesicouterine, vesicovaginal and urethrovaginal fistulas.

Vesicouterine fistula

Vesicovaginal fistula

Urethrovaginal fistula

Box 26.12 Clinical features and evaluation of urogenital tract fistulas

- Symptoms
  - Involuntary leakage of urine
    - Continuous/intermittent
- Physical examination
  - External genitalia
    - Leakage of urine
    - Excoriation
  - Per speculum examination
    - Pool of urine in vagina
    - Fistulous opening
- Investigations
  - Creatinine in the vaginal fluid
    - To exclude vaginal secretion
  - Dye test with methylene blue
    - To differentiate between ureteric and bladder fistulas
  - Urine culture
  - Cystourethroscopy
    - Site of fistula
    - Extent/size of fistula
  - IVP/RGP
    - Confirm ureteric fistula
  - MRI
    - Ureteric/urethral fistulas

IVP, intravenous pyelography; *MRI*, magnetic resonance imaging; *RGP*, retrograde pyelography.

---

may be visualized in some women with VVF. Investigations are required to assess the condition of the patient, locate the fistula, exclude the ureteric fistula and plan management.

Investigations

Dye test

This is performed by instillation of methylene blue into the bladder and inserting a tampon into the vagina. If the tampon is stained blue, it is indicative of bladder fistula. If the tampon is soaked in urine but not coloured blue, it is indicative of ureteric fistula.

Cystourethroscopy

Cystourethroscopy is essential to assess the VVFs, and size, location and proximity to ureteric orifice.

Imaging

Retrograde pyelography, intravenous pyelography and magnetic resonance imaging are useful in locating ureteric injuries.

Prognosis

Success of repair depends on several factors listed in Box 26.13.

- Size
- Site
  - Bladder
    - Bladder neck
    - Close to ureteric orifice
  - Ureter
    - Urethra
- Aetiology
  - Surgical injury
  - Malignancy
  - Radiation
- Previous failed surgery
- Scarring

Management

Surgical management

Early recognition and treatment yields the best results in urogenital fistulas.

Small fistulas detected in the immediate postoperative period may close with bladder drainage and waiting.

Long-standing and large fistulas need surgical intervention. If the tissues are healthy, immediate repair can be undertaken. Most postsurgical fistulas are repaired 6–12 weeks later. Ureteric fistulas should be repaired earlier, to prevent extensive fibrosis at the site of injury.

Preoperatively, zinc oxide cream or lanolin is used to treat local excoriation. Urinary tract infection should be treated with antibiotics.

Ureteric fistulas that occur after gynaecological surgeries are usually close to the bladder. They are managed by laparotomy, mobilization of ureter and reimplantation of ureter into the bladder. If this is not feasible, ureteroureteric anastomosis should be performed.

General surgical principles must be followed in all surgical procedures for correction of VVF (Box 26.14). VVFs may be managed by abdominal or vaginal approach (Box 26.15).

Vaginal approach is used for midvaginal and low fistulas. Most women can be treated by flap-splitting surgery in which the fistula is

Box 26.14 Surgical principles of urogenital tract fistulas

- Mobilization of bladder
- Excision of all scar tissues
- Tension-free closure
- Closure in layers
- Interposition flaps or grafts when required
- Postoperative bladder drainage

Box 26.15 Surgical management of vesicovaginal fistulas

- Vaginal procedures
  - Flap-splitting method
    - Mobilization of the vaginal and bladder flaps
    - Closure of the bladder and vagina in layers
- Latzko procedure
  - Partial colpocleisis
  - Interposition flaps/grafts
    - Labial fat pad (Martius graft)
    - Gracilis muscle graft
- Abdominal procedures
  - Transperitoneal transvesical repair
    - Bisection of the bladder
    - Repair in layers
  - Vascularized tissue grafts
    - Omental grafts
  - Urinary diversion
    - For large postradiation/malignant fistulas

excised and bladder and vaginal walls are separated by dissection and closed in layers (Fig. 26.10).

Abdominal approach is reserved for postsurgical fistulas and those in whom first surgery is not successful or fistula is large, located high up or scarred.

Urethral fistulas are more difficult to repair than vesical fistulas. Repair of urethral fistula can be vaginal or abdominal. Bladder wall can be used to construct the urethra in case of loss of a segment of urethra.

Postoperative management

This is as important as the surgical procedure. The bladder should be drained for 10–14 days. Adequate hydration ensures good urinary output. Catheter blockage should be prevented so that there is no bladder distension and tension

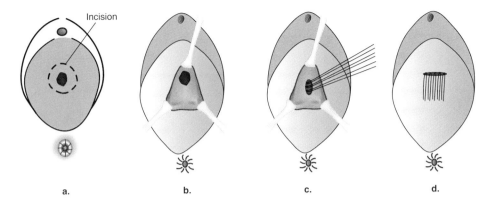

a. b. c. d.

Figure 26.10 Repair of vesicovaginal fistula by flap-splitting method. a. Incision is made around the fistula. b. The vaginal mucosa is dissected from the bladder wall. c. The bladder wall is sutured without tension. d. Vaginal wall is closed.

on the suture lines. Suprapubic catheter may be used for low fistulas.

Vesicouterine fistula

This is rare. In addition to the leakage of urine, blood in the urine (menouria) during menstruation may be present, referred to as Youssef syndrome. Management is by abdominal repair.

Anal sphincter injury and rectovaginal fistula

The rectum and the anal canal also are located in close proximity to the genital tract and are prone to injury during childbirth and gynaecological surgery. A third- or fourth-degree perineal tear that is not sutured immediately after delivery can give rise to anal incontinence. Failed repair can also lead to rectovaginal fistulas (RVFs) and anovaginal fistulas (AVFs). Passage of flatus and stools through the fistula into the vagina is the usual presenting symptom of fistula.

Anal sphincter injury

Involuntary passage of flatus and faeces, referred to as anal incontinence, is the predominant symptom of anal sphincter injury.

The most common cause is obstetric injury.

Immediate primary repair is the best treatment of anal sphincter injury, but when this

fails, the women present with incontinence and require delayed repair.

Severity of the symptoms depends on the degree of involvement of anal sphincter.

Examination reveals a tear in the lower part of the posterior vaginal wall (Fig. 26.11). The perineal body is thinned out in third-degree tear but is totally damaged in fourth-degree tears. The anal and vaginal mucosas are attached to each other with no intervening tissue.

Rectal examination is essential to assess the rectovaginal septum and anal sphincter integrity and tone.

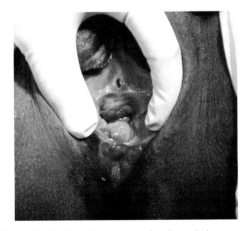

Figure 26.11 A fourth-degree perineal tear during forceps delivery in a 28-year-old lady. The anal sphincters are damaged. The patient had faecal incontinence.

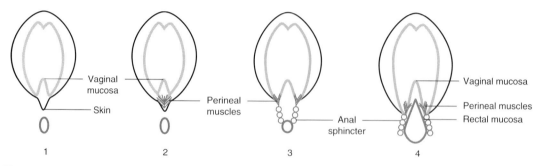

Figure 26.12 Perineal lacerations. 1. First-degree laceration involves skin and vaginal mucosa. 2. Second-degree laceration involves muscle layers as well. 3. Third-degree laceration involve the anal sphincter. 4. Fourth-degree laceration involves rectal mucosa.

Classification

Anal sphincter injury and RVFs are classified as given in Box 26.16 and Fig. 26.12. The first- and second-degree tears do not cause anal sphincter injury and will not be discussed further.

Box 26.16 Classification of anal sphincter injury and rectovaginal fistulas

- Anal sphincter injury
  - *First degree*: Perineal skin only
  - *Second degree*: Perineal skin and muscles but not the anal sphincter
  - *Third degree*: Involves anal sphincter complex
    - *3a*: <50% of external sphincter involved
    - *3b*: >50% of external sphincter involved
    - *3c*: Both internal and external sphincter involved
  - *Fourth degree*: Sphincter complex and anal mucosa involved
- Rectovaginal fistulas
  - *Low*: Vaginal opening near posterior fourchette
  - *Mid*: Vaginal opening above fourchette but below cervix
  - *High*: Vaginal opening in posterior fornix

Evaluation of anal sphincter

Preoperative evaluation of anal sphincter improves surgical outcome. The anal sphincter can be studied by different methods as listed in Box 26.17. Endoanal ultrasonography is the most commonly performed and most useful method of evaluation.

Management of anal sphincter injury

- Dietary modification and high-fibre diet can diminish symptoms and should be tried in women with minimal symptoms.

Box 26.17 Evaluation of anal sphincter

- Ultrasonography
  - Endoanal
  - Transperineal
  - Transvaginal
- Magnetic resonance imaging
- Anorectal manometry
- Pudendal nerve testing
- Electromyography
- Defaecography

- Patients must be counselled that moderate to severe degree of incontinence has a better outcome after surgical repair of anal sphincter.
- Preoperative bowel preparation is recommended (refer Chapter 33, *Preoperative preparation and postoperative management*).
- Since the operative field is likely to be soiled by faecal matter, antibiotic prophylaxis with Inj ampicillin with sulbactam 3 g intravenously along with metronidazole 500 mg is recommended.
- Transvaginal layered method of repair is the treatment of choice for third- or fourth-degree perineal tears.
- Transverse incision is made along the junction of posterior vaginal wall and anal mucosa and the vaginal and anal mucosas are dissected.
- Anal mucosa is sutured. The external anal sphincters are identified and approximated by overlap technique or end-to-end anastomosis. Perineal body is reconstructed and vaginal mucosa is trimmed and sutured (Fig. 26.13).

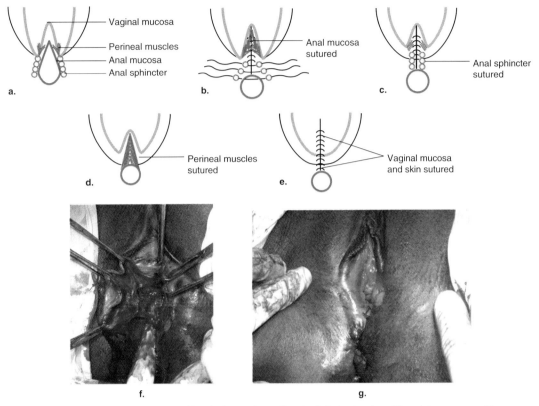

Figure 26.13 Repair of anal sphincter. a. Fourth degree laceration. b. Suturing begins with rectal mucosa. c. The anal sphincter fibres are approximated next. d. Perineal muscles sutured next. e. Finally, vaginal mucosa and skin are sutured. f. Image showing repair of anal sphincter injury. Vaginal mucosa has been dissected from the rectum. g. Repair completed. The perineal body has been reconstructed.

– Postoperatively, clear oral fluids are given for 24 hours followed by a high-fibre diet and a mild laxative for 2 weeks.

Rectovaginal fistula

RVFs usually result from failed repair of tears or fourth-degree perineal tears or, rarely, obstetric trauma. Radiation, Crohn disease and difficult hysterectomy where the cul-de-sac is obliterated by adhesions and fibrosis can also cause RVFs.

Causes are listed in Box 26.18.

Clinical features

Fistulas above the dentate line are called RVFs and those below the dentate line are called AVFs. Anal sphincter damage is usually present in AVFs.

Box 26.18 Causes of RVF

- Congenital
- Obstetric
  - Third- or fourth-degree tear
  - Median episiotomy
  - Instrumental vaginal delivery
- Gynaecological surgery
- Trauma
- Infections/inflammation
  - Diverticulitis
  - Crohn disease
- Malignancy
- Radiation

RVF, rectovaginal fistula.

The typical presentation is passage of flatus and stool through the vagina and incontinence of flatus and faeces. Rectal bleeding, diarrhoea and other symptoms of diverticulitis or Crohn disease may be present.

Vaginal and rectovaginal examinations reveal fistulous opening. Evidence of repair of perineal tear is usually present. Occasionally, there is a band of tissue separating the perineum from the fistula. Very small fistulas can be visualized by instilling air into the rectum. Endoscopy and biopsy are required if malignancy is suspected.

In women with anal sphincter injury, severity of sphincter damage should be assessed during rectal examination (Box 26.19).

Management

Surgery for RVF may be transvaginal, transanal or abdominal. Preoperative preparation is the same as for anal sphincter repair.

Transvaginal surgery is often used by gynaecologists. Very low fistulas may be converted to complete perineal tear by cutting the bridge of tissue and repaired as shown in Fig. 26.12. Low fistulas not involving the sphincter can be managed by simple fistulectomy and closure of rectal mucosa, muscularis and vaginal mucosa.

Some surgeons may do a temporary colostomy before the procedure, but this is not required in most women. Large postradiation low fistulas may require Martius graft. High fistulas are repaired transabdominally.

It is important to avoid constipation and straining in the postoperative period.

Management of RVF is summarized in Box 26.20.

Box 26.19 Clinical features and evaluation of RVF

- Symptoms
  - Incontinence of flatus and faeces
  - Passage of flatus/stool through vagina
  - Symptoms of underlying disease
- Physical examination
  - Vaginal/rectovaginal examination
    - Fistula
    - Anal sphincter tone
- Evaluation
  - Methylene blue instillation into rectum
  - Flexible endoscopy
  - Endoanal ultrasonography for sphincter integrity
  - Biopsy, if malignancy is suspected
  - Investigations for underlying disease

RVF, rectovaginal fistula.

Box 26.20 Surgical procedures for RVF

- Low RVFs
  - Transvaginal repair
    - Conversion to complete perineal tear and repair
    - Simple fistulectomy
  - Martius graft
- Mid and high RVFs
  - Abdominal repair
    - With colostomy
    - Without colostomy
    - With tissue interposition
      o Omentum
      o Rectus abdominis

RVF, rectovaginal fistula.

Key points

- Damage to the urinary tract can occur during obstetric and gynaecological surgeries. Ureter, urinary bladder and urethra are vulnerable to injury.

- The ureter is prone to injury during gynaecological surgeries at various points. These include the pelvic brim, broad ligament and ureteric canal at the vaginal vault or at the uterosacral ligament.

- The risk factors for ureteric injury are pelvic malignancies, endometriosis, chronic pelvic inflammatory disease, previous surgeries and broad-ligament tumours. The injury may be angulation, ligation, transection, cauterization, devascularization or crush injury.

- If ureteric injury is diagnosed intraoperatively, immediate repair can be performed or a stent can be inserted.

- Ureteric injuries may present postoperatively with flank pain, fever, sepsis or fistula. Immediate treatment with stenting or nephrostomy is indicated. Definitive surgery is undertaken later.

- Injuries to the bladder can occur with abdominal, laparoscopic and vaginal surgeries. When diagnosed intraoperatively, the bladder should be closed in one or two layers.

- Those who present with fistulas later should be assessed by cystourethroscopy and/or intravenous pyelography.

- The fistula may be closed by vaginal or abdominal surgery.

- Anal sphincter injury is usually caused by obstetric trauma. It presents with anal sphincter incontinence.

- Sphincter integrity should be assessed clinically and by endovaginal ultrasonography.

- Management of anal sphincter injury is by surgical repair of the perineal tear and sphincter by overlap or end-to-end anastomosis.

- Rectovaginal fistulas are divided into low, mid and high vaginal fistulas. The most common cause is the third- or fourth-degree perineal tear that has been inadequately repaired.

- Management of rectovaginal fistula is by transvaginal or abdominal repair.

Self-assessment

Case-based questions

Case 1

A 48-year-old lady underwent radical hysterectomy with lymphadenectomy for cervical cancer. Before closing, the ureters were inspected. The left ureter was found to be distended up to the uterine pedicle and there was no peristalsis.

1. What will you suspect?
2. If the ureter is found to be included in the ligature, what is the management?
3. If the ureter is trisected and ligated along with uterine vessels, what will you do?

Case 2

A 50-year-old lady underwent vaginal hysterectomy with anterior colporrhaphy, and pelvic reconstruction for pelvic organ prolapse. On the eighth postoperative day, she returned with watery discharge per vaginum.

1. What will you suspect?
2. How will you evaluate?
3. How will you manage?

Answers

Case 1

1. Ureteric ligation or angulation.
2. Remove the ligature and inspect the ureter. If the part of ureter that was ligated looks lacerated on the surface, stenting should be done.
3. Remove the ligature. Reimplant the upper end into the bladder by ureteroneocystostomy. If there is tension, perform psoas hitch operation to pull up the bladder.

Case 2

1. Vesicovaginal fistula. Must exclude ureteric fistula.
2. Per speculum examination to confirm the leakage of urine and visualize fistulous opening. Cystoscopy to look for vesicovaginal fistula. If in doubt, methylene blue dye test to exclude ureteric fistula.
3. If the fistula is small, catheterize the bladder and wait for 2–3 weeks. If the fistula is large or if urine leak continues despite catheterization, plan laparotomy and transabdominal repair.

Long-answer questions

1. How will you diagnose ureteric injury at hysterectomy? Discuss the management of intraoperative ureteric injuries.
2. What are the causes of vesicovaginal fistula? Discuss the evaluation and management of vesicovaginal fistula.

Short-answer questions

1. Diagnosis of urinary fistulas
2. Rectovaginal fistula
3. Anatomy of pelvic ureter and points at which it is prone to injury
4. Aetiology and risk factors for vesicovaginal fistula

Gynaecological Oncology

27 Preinvasive and Invasive Diseases of the Vulva and Vagina

Case scenario

Mrs HD, 60, was a mother of 5 children and grandmother of 10. She was a widow and lived with her three sons and their families. She had noticed small growth in the vulva 8 months ago but was too inhibited to discuss it with the family. Since it was painless, she thought there was nothing to worry about. However, the lesion had slowly become larger and she noticed bloodstained discharge recently. She mentioned it to her daughter-in-law who brought her at once to the hospital.

Introduction

Preinvasive and invasive diseases of the vulva are rare. Moreover, vulvar cancers do not always go through the preinvasive stages before developing into invasive cancer. Progression of preinvasive disease to malignancy is also infrequent. The incidence of preinvasive lesion is on the increase in younger women due to its association with human papillomavirus (HPV) infection.

Preinvasive disease of the vulva

Preinvasive disease of the vulva is known as vulvar intraepithelial neoplasia (VIN). These refer to the squamous intraepithelial lesions of the vulva.

Definition

VIN is the premalignant condition of the vulva where the cellular changes are limited to the epithelium but do not extend beyond the basement membrane.

Classification and terminology

- The term 'vulvar intraepithelial neoplasia' was introduced by the International Society for the Study of Vulvar Disease (ISSVD) in 1986. The current classification of VIN is given in Table 27.1 (ISSVD, 2015).
- The 2004 ISSVD classification did not include low-grade squamous intraepithelial lesions (LSILs) since they were considered a reaction to HPV infection and not premalignant lesions. However, the 2015 classification has

Table 27.1 Current classification of VIN (ISSVD, 2015)

Low-grade squamous intraepithelial lesion (flat condyloma or HPV effect)

Vulvar HSIL (corresponds to earlier VIN, usual type)

VIN, differentiated type

HPV, human papillomavirus; *HSIL*, high-grade squamous intraepithelial lesion; *ISSVD*, International Society for the Study of Vulvar Disease; *VIN*, vulvar intraepithelial neoplasia.

included LSIL since it is preferable to the term condyloma. These are caused by HPV 6 and 11.

- High-grade squamous intraepithelial lesion (HSIL) has replaced the term 'VIN usual type' and includes the warty, basaloid and mixed lesions. It is associated with high-risk HPV infection, by HPV 16, 18 and 33. Other risk factors are smoking, HIV infection and sexually transmitted infections.
- VIN differentiated is uncommon, usually associated with vulvar lichen sclerosus, not associated with HPV and occurring in older women.

Pathology

Macroscopically, the lesion may be a warty, elevated plaque that is white or red, an ulcer or a nodular lesion (Fig. 27.1). The lesions may be multifocal. Differentiated VIN is usually associated with lichen sclerosis and squamous cell hyperplasia.

Microscopically, the cells exhibit nuclear abnormalities, maturation disturbance, increase in mitotic activity and sometimes changes of HPV infection.

Symptoms

Most women with VIN are asymptomatic. Symptoms are listed in Box 27.1.

Box 27.1 Symptoms of vulvar intraepithelial neoplasia

- Asymptomatic
- Pruritus vulva
- Ulcer
- Discomfort, pain
- Warty growth
- Bleeding, discharge

Diagnosis

Diagnosis is by history, examination, colposcopy and biopsy.

- History of symptoms such as pruritus and discomfort, and history of sexually transmitted infections, genital warts and smoking are important.
- On examination, the lesions are usually multifocal and may present as ulcers, raised white or red lesions or warty condylomas.
- Colposcopy may be used, but is not as useful as it is for the diagnosis of cervical lesions. It should be performed in women with persistent lesions and persistent symptoms without obvious lesions.
- Biopsy is mandatory for diagnosis.

Management

Progression to invasive cancer occurs only in 5–10% of women. Therefore, local excision is sufficient. Management options are listed in Box 27.2.

As already mentioned, vulvar LSIL can be followed up by annual examination and colposcopy if required.

Local excision is the standard of care for vulvar HSIL and VIN differentiated. Disease-free margin of 5 mm should be obtained. Large, confluent lesions require more extensive excision and rotational flap for skin grafting.

Young women with VIN may be treated by CO_2 laser. Immune response modulators such as imiquimod are under trial.

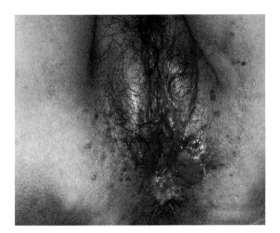

Figure 27.1 Vulvar intraepithelial neoplasia (*VIN*). 2 × 2 cm elevated plaque in the posterior aspect of the vulva.

Paget disease of the vulva

It is a predominantly intraepithelial disease. Underlying adenocarcinoma may be present. The disease occurs in older, postmenopausal women and presents with pruritus, discomfort and pain. Lesions can be extensive (Box 27.3). Management is by wide local excision with underlying dermis to exclude associated malignancy. If malignancy is present, it should be treated as a squamous cell cancer.

Invasive diseases of the vulva (vulvar cancer)

Vulvar malignancies account for 3–5% of all cancers of the female genital tract. The most common cancer of the vulva is squamous cell carcinoma. Peak incidence is found in women in their seventies. The incidence is on the rise due to increasing life expectancy of women and in younger women with HPV infection.

Risk factors

There are two types of squamous cell carcinoma with different risk factors. Type I or warty/basaloid type occurs in younger women and is HPV related, whereas type II or keratinizing type occurs in older women and is not HPV related. Type I cancers may be associated with cervical lesions.

Risk factors of the vulvar cancer are listed in Box 27.4.

Pathology

About 90% of vulvar cancers are squamous cell carcinomas (Fig. 27.2). Other histological types are very rare and are listed in Box 27.5.

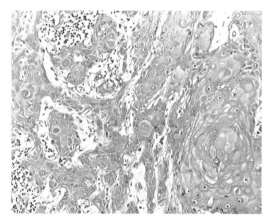

Figure 27.2 Photomicrograph showing well-differentiated keratinized malignant squamous cells and keratin pearls.

Box 27.5 Histological types of vulvar cancers

Box 27.5 Histological types of vulvar cancers

- Squamous cell carcinoma
- Basal cell carcinoma
- Adenocarcinoma
- Melanoma
- Sarcoma
- Bartholin gland tumours
  - Squamous cell carcinoma
  - Adenocarcinoma
- Undifferentiated tumours

Patterns of spread of vulvar carcinoma

The pattern in which vulvar carcinoma spreads is listed in Box 27.6.

Box 27.6 Patterns of spread of vulvar carcinoma

- Lymphatic spread
  - Inguinal and femoral nodes; iliac nodes
- Haematogenous spread
  - Distant sites including liver and lung
- Direct extension
  - Vagina, urethra and anus

The lymphatics of the vulva do not cross the midline and so unilateral vulvar malignancies are usually associated with ipsilateral femoral lymphadenopathy. However, the lymphatics of the clitoris and posterior fourchette do cross the midline. Therefore, malignant lesions from the latter sites can cause bilateral inguinofemoral nodal metastases. From the inguinofemoral nodes, they spread to the external iliac, pelvic and para-aortic nodes.

Staging of vulvar cancer

Currently used surgical staging of vulvar carcinoma is given in Table 27.2 (Fig. 27.3).

The depth of invasion is defined as the measurement of the tumour from the epithelial–stromal junction of the adjacent most superficial dermal papilla to the deepest point of invasion.

Clinical features

Symptoms and signs

Most women are asymptomatic. Pruritus is the most common symptom. The women may, in

Table 27.2 Staging of carcinoma of the vulva (FIGO, 2009)

Stage	Definition
I	Tumour confined to the vulva
IA	Lesions ≤2 cm in size, confined to the vulva or perineum and with stromal invasion ≤1.0 mm, no nodal metastasis
IB	Lesions >2 cm in size or with stromal invasion >1.0 mm, confined to the vulva or perineum, with negative nodes
II	Tumour of any size with extension to adjacent perineal structures (one-third lower urethra, one-third lower vagina, anus) with negative nodes
III	Tumour of any size with or without extension to adjacent perineal structures (one-third lower urethra, one-third lower vagina, anus) with positive inguinofemoral lymph nodes
IIIA	1. With one lymph node metastasis (≥5 mm) or 2. One to two lymph node metastasis(es) (<5 mm)
IIIB	1. With two or more lymph node metastases (≥5 mm) or 2. Three or more lymph node metastases (<5 mm)
IIIC	With positive nodes with extracapsular spread
IV	Tumour invades other regional (two-third upper urethra, two-third upper vagina) or distant structures
IVA	Tumour invades any of the following: • Upper urethral and/or vaginal mucosa, bladder mucosa, rectal mucosa, or fixed to pelvic bone • Fixed or ulcerated inguinofemoral lymph nodes
IVB	Any distant metastasis including pelvic lymph nodes

FIGO, International Federation of Gynecology and Obstetrics.

addition, have other symptoms as well (Box 27.7). The lesions may be single or multifocal, warty growths or nonhealing ulcers (Figs 27.4 and 27.5). Women may also complain of hard masses in the groin.

Clinical evaluation

History

This should focus on risk factors and symptoms (Box 27.8).

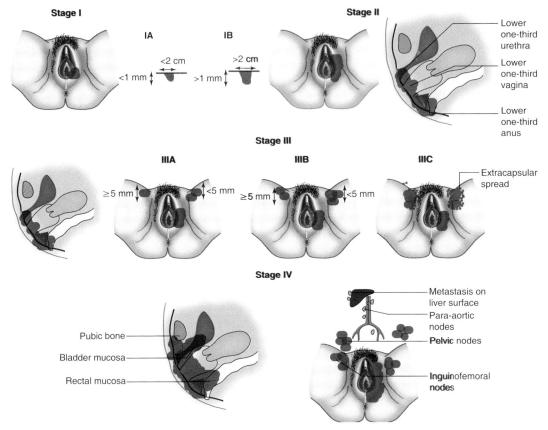

Figure 27.3 Pictorial representation of FIGO staging of vulvar cancer. **Stage IA:** Lesion ≤2 cm in size, depth of stromal invasion ≤1 mm. **Stage IB:** Lesion >2 cm in size, depth of stromal invasion >1 mm. **Stage II:** Tumour of any size with extension to adjacent perineal structures (one-third lower urethra, one-third lower vagina, anus) with negative nodes. **Stage III:** Tumour of any size with or without extension to adjacent perineal structures and positive inguinal nodes. **Stage IV:** Tumour of any size with pelvic node metastasis or involvement of bladder mucosa/rectal mucosa, pubic bone or distant metastasis. *FIGO*, International Federation of Gynecology and Obstetrics.

Box 27.7 Clinical features of vulvar carcinoma

- Symptoms
  - Long-standing pruritus
  - Bleeding, discharge
  - Pain
  - Nonhealing ulcer
  - Warty growth
  - Inguinal masses
- Signs
  - Fleshy/warty growth
  - Ulcer
  - Red or white in colour
  - Tender or painless
  - Unilateral/bilateral inguinofemoral nodes

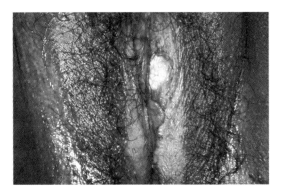

Figure 27.4 Stage I vulvar cancer. Tumour is less than 2 cm in size and is limited to vulva.

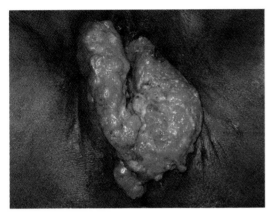

Figure 27.5 Large fungating growth, stage IV. (Patient had bilateral inguinal and pelvic node metastasis.)

Box 27.8 History in vulvar carcinoma

- Age
- Symptoms
  - Pruritus, pain, discharge, bleeding
  - Nonhealing ulcer/growth
- Past history
  - Condyloma
  - Lichen sclerosus
  - Sexually transmitted disease
- Smoking
- Immunosuppression

Physical examination

This includes examination of the lesion, assessment of extension to vagina/perineum/perianal region, and evaluation of the cervix and groin nodes (Box 27.9).

Box 27.9 Physical examination in vulvar carcinoma

- General examination
- Local lesion
  - Size
  - Location
  - Type—Warty/fleshy/ulcer
  - Extension to perineum/perianal region
- Speculum examination
  - Extension to vagina and cervix
- Extension to urethra
- Fixity to bone
- Groin nodes

Diagnosis

Diagnosis is by **wedge biopsy** from the lesion, including sufficient underlying dermis. This is performed in the outpatient clinic under local anaesthesia.

Investigations

This includes confirmation of diagnosis and evaluation of extent of the disease for planning treatment (Box 27.10). Small lesions may not require any further tests.

Box 27.10 Investigations in vulvar carcinoma

- Biopsy for confirmation of diagnosis
- Pap smear and colposcopy to assess cervix
- For large lesions
  - Cystourethroscopy
  - Proctoscopy
  - Scan/CT/MRI
    - Pelvic nodes
    - Deep infiltration of lesion
  - Positron emission tomography
    - Nodal metastasis
    - Haematogenous spread
- Advanced disease
  - Fine-needle aspiration from metastases

CT, computerized tomography; *MRI*, magnetic resonance imaging.

Prognostic factors

These are listed in Box 27.11. When diagnosed early, vulvar carcinoma has a good prognosis. Five-year survival is 90% in stage I cancer.

Box 27.11 Prognostic factors in vulvar carcinoma

- Tumour location (clitoris, posterior fourchette)
- Stage of the disease
- Lymph node metastasis
- Fixity to bone
- Local extension
- Surgical margins
- Lymphovascular space invasion
- Histology—Degree of differentiation

Sentinel node biopsy When isosulfan blue dye or radiolabelled dye is injected into the tumour, the first node that receives lymphatic drainage, called the sentinel node, can be identified intra-operatively. If biopsy of this node is negative on frozen section, a full lymphadenectomy can be omitted, thereby reducing morbidity. It is useful in small unifocal tumours with clinically nega-tive groin nodes.

Management

Treatment is mainly surgical for early stage dis-ease (Box 27.12). Postoperative adjuvant radia-tion may be required in some women. Advanced disease is treated by chemoradiation.

Box 27.12　Management of vulvar cancer

- Stage IA
  - Radical local excision
- Stage IB
  - Lateral lesions (2 cm or more from midline)
    - Radical local excision + ipsilateral inguinofemo-ral lymphadenectomy
  - Midline lesions (anterior labia minora, clitoris, posterior fourchette)
    - Radical local excision + bilateral inguinofemoral lymphadenectomy
- Stages II, IIIA
  - Radical local excision/partial vulvectomy + bilater-al inguinofemoral lymphadenectomy
- Advanced disease (IIIB–IVB)
  - Chemoradiation

Radical local excision The lesion is excised with 1 cm grossly negative margin and down to the level of inferior fascia of urogenital diaphragm.

Partial vulvectomy In women with extensive or multifocal lesions, all the involved areas have to be excised, which may include labia majora and minora, with or without clitoris and perineum. Large defects may be allowed to granulate or closed with myocutaneous flaps.

Inguinofemoral lymphadenectomy This is performed through two separate incisions, made on either groin in a line parallel to the groin crease. Superficial and deep inguinal nodes are removed. In stage IB lateral lesions, ipsilateral lymphadenectomy is sufficient. If this reveals positive nodes, contralateral lymphadenectomy should be undertaken. In women with central lesions, which may metastasise to both groins, bilateral lymphadenectomy is required.

Radiotherapy Adjuvant postoperative radia-tion is recommended for women with two or microscopically positive inguinal nodes or close or positive surgical margin. Primary radiation with chemotherapy (chemoradiation) is used for patients with advanced disease and pelvic node metastasis. Recurrent disease is also treated with radiation.

Survival

In operable cases, overall 5-year survival is about 70%. Positive groin nodes are an important prog-nostic factor and are associated with a survival of only 11%.

Preinvasive disease of the vagina

Preinvasive disease of the vagina or vaginal intraepithelial neoplasia (VaIN) usually develops in the upper third of the vagina as an extension of the cervical intraepithelial neoplasia (CIN). HPV infection is the aetiological factor. When vaginal abrasions heal, metaplastic changes occur in the vaginal mucosa and the virus enters the meta-plastic cells.

Definition

VaIN is defined as the presence of squamous cell atypia in the vaginal epithelium without invasion.

Risk factors, classification, diagnosis and treatment

- VaIN is rare, occurring in about 0.1/100,000 women. It usually occurs in postmenopausal women in the sixth decade of life.
- Infection by HPV, especially HPV 16 and 18, is the most common risk factor. It is associated with invasive or intraepithelial neoplasia of the cervix or vulva in 50–90% of patients. Smoking is also a risk factor. VaIN is often diagnosed in women who have undergone hysterectomy for CIN.
- It is classified into low-grade VaIN and high-grade VaIN.
- VaIN is usually asymptomatic and is sus-pected when Pap smear is abnormal and the cervix is normal. Speculum examination after

application of acetic acid may reveal acetowhite areas. The abnormality is usually confined to the upper one-third of vagina.

- Diagnosis is by colposcopy and biopsy.
- Low-grade lesions rarely progress to carcinoma and can be followed up with Pap smear. High-grade lesions are usually treated by surgery, which includes wide local excision and partial or total vaginectomy depending on whether the lesions are localized or multifocal. Laser ablation, loop electroexcision procedure (LEEP), topical agents and, rarely, radiotherapy have been used.

Risk factors, classification and management are summarized in Box 27.13.

In women with posthysterectomy vault lesion of high grade, excision is recommended. Before laser ablation or medical treatment in women with VaIN 3, invasive lesion must be ruled out by biopsy.

Invasive disease of the vagina (vaginal cancer)

Invasive carcinoma of the vagina is rare and accounts for 1–2% of all gynaecological cancers. If a malignant lesion in the vagina is associated with a malignant lesion in the cervix or vulva, it is considered as primary cervical or vulvar cancer. Peak incidence is in the sixth decade.

Majority of vaginal cancers extend from the cervix and are considered to be cervical cancers. When vagina and vulva are involved, they are considered to be vulvar cancers.

Risk factors

Risk factors are listed in Box 27.14.

Pathology

Upper part of the vagina develops from Müllerian ducts and is lined by columnar epithelium (*see* Chapter 1, *Anatomy of the female reproductive tract*). Lower vagina develops from sinovaginal bulbs and is lined by squamous epithelium. Later, the columnar epithelium undergoes metaplasia to squamous epithelium. The majority of cancers of the vagina are, therefore, squamous cell carcinoma (Fig. 27.6). Adenocarcinoma accounts for about 9% of all vaginal cancers.

Box 27.13 Vaginal intraepithelial neoplasia

- Occurs in postmenopausal women
- Usually in the sixth decade
- Risk factors
  - HPV infection
  - Prior hysterectomy for CIN
  - Associated CIN/VIN/invasive cancer
- Classification (2012)
  - Low-grade vaginal intraepithelial neoplasia (VaIN 1)
  - High-grade vaginal intraepithelial neoplasia (VaIN 2, 3)
- Clinical features
  - Asymptomatic
  - Abnormal Pap smear with normal cervix
  - Abnormal smear posthysterectomy for CIN
- Diagnosis
  - Speculum examination after acetic acid
  - Schiller test
  - Colposcopy
  - Biopsy
- Treatment
  - Low-grade lesion (VaIN 1)
    - Observation
    - Cytology every 6–12 months
  - High-grade lesions (VaIN 2, 3)
    - Wide local excision
    - Partial vaginectomy
    - Total vaginectomy
    - LEEP
    - Laser ablation
    - Local 5-fluorouracil cream
    - Local imiquimod cream
    - Radiotherapy

CIN, cervical intraepithelial neoplasia; HPV, human papillomavirus; LEEP, loop electroexcision procedure; VaIN, vaginal intraepithelial neoplasia; VIN, vulvar intraepithelial neoplasia.

Box 27.14 Vaginal carcinoma

- 1–2% of all gynaecological cancers
- Occurs in sixth decade
- Risk factors
  - Previous cervical cancer/CIN
  - HPV infection (high-risk serotypes)
  - Prior VaIN
  - Prior preinvasive/invasive cervical cancer

CIN, cervical intraepithelial neoplasia; HPV, human papillomavirus; VaIN, vaginal intraepithelial neoplasia.

Other cancers also occur; these are listed in Box 27.15.

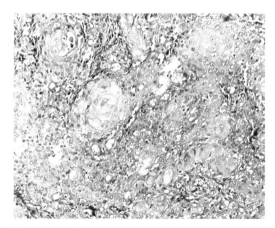

Figure 27.6 Photomicrograph showing keratin pearls characteristic of well-differentiated squamous cell carcinoma.

Box 27.16 Patterns of spread of vaginal carcinoma

- Lymphatic
  - External, internal, common iliac nodes
  - Sacral nodes
  - Inguinal nodes
  - Inferior gluteal, presacral nodes
  - Perirectal nodes
- Direct
  - Cervix
  - Vulva
  - Paracolpos
  - Bladder/urethra
  - Rectum
- Haematogenous
  - Lung, liver

Box 27.15 Pathology of vaginal cancers

- Squamous cell carcinoma
- Verrucous carcinoma
- Vaginal adenosis and DES-related tumours
  - Adenocarcinoma
  - Clear-cell adenocarcinoma
- Malignant melanoma
- Sarcoma
  - Sarcoma botryoides (rhabdomyosarcoma)
  - Malignant mixed Müllerian tumour
  - Endometrial stromal sarcoma

DES, diethylstilbestrol.

Verrucous carcinoma is a warty variant of squamous cell cancer. **Vaginal adenosis** occurs in female children exposed to diethylstilbestrol in utero. **Adenocarcinoma** and **clear-cell adenocarcinoma** arise from the areas of adenosis. **Sarcoma botryoides** occurs in infants and children and resembles a bunch of grapes.

Patterns of spread

Like all cancers, vaginal carcinoma spreads by lymphatics, direct spread and haematogenous spread (Box 27.16).

Staging

International Federation of Gynecology and Obstetrics (FIGO) staging of vaginal carcinoma is as shown in Table 27.3 (see also Fig. 27.7).

Table 27.3 FIGO staging of vaginal cancer

Stage	Definition
I	The carcinoma is limited to the vaginal wall
II	The carcinoma has involved the paravaginal tissue but has not extended to the pelvic wall
III	The carcinoma has extended to the pelvic wall
IV	The carcinoma has extended beyond the true pelvis or has involved the mucosa of the bladder or rectum; bullous oedema as such does not permit a case to be allotted to stage IV
IVA	Tumour invades bladder and/or rectal mucosa and/or direct extension beyond the true pelvis
IVB	Spreads to distant organs

FIGO, International Federation of Gynecology and Obstetrics.

Clinical features

Symptoms and signs

Vaginal bleeding is the most common symptom. Clinical features are listed in Box 27.17.

Diagnosis

Diagnosis is by **punch biopsy** and **histopathological examination**. Colposcopy is useful when a gross lesion is not visible in a woman with abnormal Pap smear.

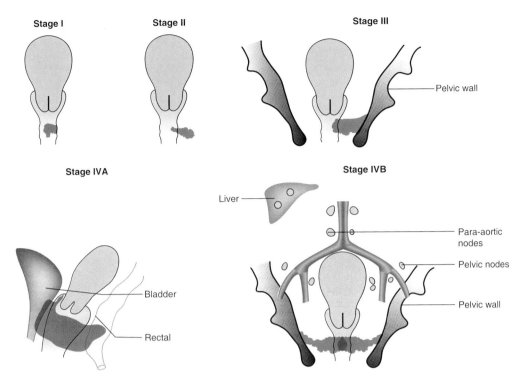

Figure 27.7 Pictorial representation of FIGO staging of vaginal cancer. Stage I: Carcinoma limited to vaginal wall. Stage II: Growth involving the subvaginal tissue, but not up to the pelvic wall. Stage III: Carcinoma extended to the pelvic wall, regional nodes (pelvic or inguinal) involved. Stage IV: Carcinoma extending to the bladder/rectal mucosa, pelvic and para-aortic nodes or distant metastasis. *FIGO*, International Federation of Gynecology and Obstetrics.

Box 27.17 Clinical features of vaginal carcinoma

- Symptoms
  - Vaginal bleeding
  - Vaginal discharge
  - Dysuria, haematuria
- Signs
  - Lesion most common in upper vagina
  - Vaginal growth
  - Ulcer

Clinical evaluation

History and physical examination

Clinical evaluation is by history and physical examination as shown in Box 27.18.

Investigations

This includes vaginal cytology, colposcopy if cytology is abnormal and no definite lesion

Box 27.18 Clinical evaluation in vaginal carcinoma

- History
  - Symptoms
    - Bleeding
      - Postmenopausal bleeding
    - Discharge/dysuria
  - Past history
    - Cervical cancer/CIN
    - HPV infection
- Physical examination
  - General examination
  - Speculum examination
    - Growth/ulcer
    - Cervical/vulvar lesion
  - Rectal examination
    - Involvement of paravaginal tissue
  - Inguinal nodes

CIN, cervical intraepithelial neoplasia; *HPV*, human papillomavirus.

is visualized, biopsy **from the lesion** for confirmation of diagnosis and investigations for staging the disease (Box 27.19). In most cases, clinical examination and biopsy would suffice. In advanced cases, nodal and distant metastasis and spread to contiguous organs should be assessed by computerized tomography/magnetic resonance imaging (CT/MRI), cystoure-throscopy and proctosigmoidoscopy.

Box 27.19 Investigations in vaginal carcinoma

- Colposcopy
- Punch biopsy
- Cystourethroscopy
- Proctosigmoidoscopy
- Chest X-ray
- CT/MRI of pelvis
- Positron emission tomography

CT, computerized tomography; *MRI*, magnetic resonance imaging.

Management

Majority of cases of vaginal cancer are treated by **radiotherapy with concurrent chemotherapy**.

Surgery is reserved for early (stage I) disease in the upper vagina (Box 27.20).

Box 27.20 Management of vaginal cancer

- Stage I
  - Upper vagina
    - Radical hysterectomy, vaginectomy, pelvic lymphadenectomy
  - Vaginal vault (posthysterectomy)
    - Vaginectomy, pelvic lymphadenectomy
  - Middle and lower third of vagina
    - Radiotherapy with concurrent chemotherapy
- Stages II–IV
  - Radiotherapy with concurrent chemotherapy (intracavitary with external radiation)
- Stage IV with fistulae
  - Pelvic exenteration

Radiotherapy is given with concurrent cisplatin. Intracavitary and external radiations are given to treat the local lesion and pelvic nodes.

Survival

A 5-year survival for stage I is about 85% and that for stages III and IV is about 58%.

Key points

- Preinvasive and invasive diseases of the vulva are rare.
- High-grade intraepithelial lesions of the vulva are due to human papillomavirus (HPV) infection.
- Vulvar intraepithelial neoplasia, differentiated type, is usually associated with lichen sclerosis or squamous cell hyperplasia.
  - Most women are asymptomatic. Others present with pruritus, ulcer, discomfort or pain.
  - Diagnosis is by biopsy. Treatment is by local excision with 5-mm free margin. Carbon dioxide laser is used in younger women.
- Paget disease of the vulva occurs in postmenopausal women. It is treated by wide local excision.
- Cancer of the vulva is usually squamous cell carcinoma. Type I cancers occur in younger women and type II in older women.
  - The most important risk factor is HPV infection.
  - The disease spreads by lymphatic, haematogenous and direct routes.
  - Most women are asymptomatic; others present with pruritus, discharge, pain or ulcer. Diagnosis is by biopsy.
  - Surgery is the treatment of choice. Radical local excision with 1-cm disease negative margin is recommended. Inguinofemoral lymphadenectomy is required for all except stage IA disease.
- Vaginal intraepithelial neoplasia (VaIN) is usually an extension of cervical intraepithelial neoplasia (CIN) and is caused by HPV infection. It is classified into low-grade and high-grade lesions and is treated by wide local excision, laser ablation or local 5-fluorouracil cream.
- Vaginal cancer is rare; most cases are extension of primary cervical or vulvar cancer. Majority of primary vaginal cancers are squamous cell carcinoma.
  - Presenting symptoms are vaginal bleeding and discharge. Diagnosis is by colposcopy and biopsy.
  - Stage I disease is treated by vaginectomy and postoperative radiation. Advanced stages are treated by chemoradiation.

Self-assessment

Case-based questions

Case 1

A 60-year-old lady presents with pruritus vulva. On examination, she has a 1.5 cm ulcer on/near the clitoris.

1. How will you proceed with clinical examination?
2. What investigations will you order?
3. If the biopsy is reported as squamous cell carcinoma, what is the management?

Case 2

A 52-year-old lady presents with bloodstained discharge per vaginum. She had undergone hysterectomy for CIN III, 3 years ago. Speculum examination reveals an area of redness at the vaginal vault but no growth or ulcer.

1. How will you proceed to evaluate this patient?
2. What is the management?

Answers

Case 1

1. Evaluation of the local lesion—Size, location, induration, extent, involvement of urethra/vagina, fixity to bone, inguinal nodes.
2. Biopsy of the ulcer for confirmation of diagnosis, U/S scan/CT pelvis to look for pelvic lymphadenopathy.

3. **(a)** Radical local excision of the lesion
   (b) If depth of invasion >1 mm, bilateral inguinofemoral lymphadenectomy since the lesion is near the clitoris

   If depth of invasion <1 mm, no lymphadenectomy is required.

Case 2

1. Since there is no obvious growth, Pap smear is the first step. If Pap smear shows VaIN/cancer, colposcopy, biopsy.
2. **(a)** If histopathology is high-grade VaIN, vaginectomy
   (b) If squamous cell carcinoma, stage I, vaginectomy with pelvic lymphadenectomy
   (c) If squamous cell carcinoma, >stage I, chemoradiation

Long-answer question

1. Discuss the classification, clinical features, diagnosis and management of carcinoma vulva.

Short-answer questions

1. Vulvar intraepithelial neoplasia
2. FIGO staging of vulvar cancer
3. Vaginal carcinoma

28 | Premalignant Diseases of the Cervix

Case scenario

Mrs NR, 32, was a civil engineer and mother of two children. She had a Pap smear at a local private clinic as part of her annual check-up. To her dismay, the smear was reported as CIN 2. She came to the tertiary centre with several questions that were bothering her—What was the implication of the report, what needed to be done next, what were the chances of her developing cervical cancer and what should she do to prevent it? She needed a sympathetic handling, counselling and evaluation.

Introduction

Cervical cancer is the second most common cancer in women in India and other developing countries. It is the most common cause of cancer deaths in women in India. Screening by Pap smear has reduced the incidence in developed countries, but implementation of this screening technique has not been successful in developing countries. About half a million new cases of cervical cancer are diagnosed globally every year and 80% of these occur in developing countries. More than 130,000 new cases occur in India annually and >75,000 die every year due to the disease. Cervical cancer is considered a public health problem and a priority in cancer control programmes by the World Health Organization (WHO). Infection with human papillomavirus (HPV) has been identified as the primary aetiological factor in cervical cancer. Invasive cervical cancer is preceded by preinvasive disease in most women. Prevention of invasive cancer is by screening, diagnosis and treatment of preinvasive diseases.

Definition

Cervical intraepithelial neoplasia (CIN) is the premalignant condition involving the uterine cervix, where the cellular abnormalities are limited to the surface epithelium and do not extend beyond the basement membrane.

Prevalence

Infection by high-risk HPV types occurs in 10–12% of women in India. The prevalence is higher in younger women and decreases as age advances. Prevalence of CIN 1 is about 3%, again higher in younger women. CIN 2 and 3 are found in 0.6% and 0.4% of population aged 30–65.

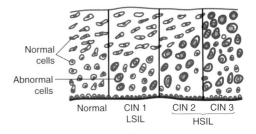

a.

Terminology

As already mentioned, in CIN, cellular changes of malignancy such as mitotic activity, proliferation of immature cells, nuclear atypia and altered nuclear/cytoplasmic ratio are seen but are limited to the surface epithelium and do not extend beyond the basement membrane.

- Terminology used in the description of premalignant lesions of the cervix has undergone a series of changes.
- In the older terminology, the cytological and histological changes were described as *mild, moderate dysplasia* and *severe dysplasia* and *carcinoma in situ*, based on the involvement of basal, intermediate and superficial cells or the full thickness of the epithelium.
- Subsequent studies demonstrated that all grades of dysplasias could progress to invasive cancer. Hence, the term *CIN* was introduced. According to the severity of cellular changes, CIN was classified into three grades: CIN 1 for mild dysplasia, CIN 2 for moderate dysplasia and CIN 3 to include both severe dysplasia and carcinoma in situ.
- Histologically, atypical changes are limited to lower one-third of epithelium in CIN 1, and extend to middle one-third in CIN 2. In CIN 3, the atypical changes are severe and extend through the entire thickness of epithelium (Fig. 28.1a–d).
- Progression from CIN 1 to CIN 3 and invasive cancer was considered a process continuum.
- Further studies demonstrated that most CIN 1 lesions regress and progression to invasive cancer occurs infrequently (1%). CIN 1 lesions are caused by HPV infection in the infectious or productive phase.
- CIN 2 and 3 lesions, on the other hand, represent high-grade lesions, and are caused by persistent HPV infection, not necessarily preceded by CIN 1, and progression to invasive cancer occurs more often (5% and 12%).

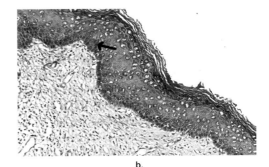

b.

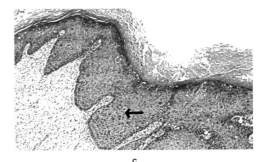

c.

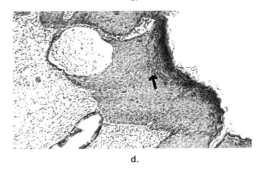

d.

Figure 28.1 Histology CIN. a. Diagrammatic depiction of histological changes in CIN. The abnormal cells are limited to the lower one-third of the epithelium in CIN 1, extend to the middle one-third in CIN 2 and occupy the entire thickness in CIN 3. b–d. Photomicrographs of CIN 1, 2 and 3. The abnormal cells are seen extending to lower, middle and upper one-third of the epithelium in b, c and d, respectively (arrows). *CIN*, cervical intraepithelial neoplasia; *HSIL*, high-grade squamous intraepithelial lesion; *LSIL*, low-grade squamous intraepithelial lesion.

- Therefore, a two-tier system was introduced for **cytology** and the terminology changed to *low-grade squamous intraepithelial lesion* (LSIL) for CIN 1 and *high-grade squamous intraepithelial lesion* (HSIL) for CIN 2 and 3. This is the **Bethesda system**, given as follows:
  - CIN   LSIL
  - CIN 2 ⎱
  - CIN 3 ⎰   HSIL
- The terms LSIL and HSIL referred to only cytological changes; histologically, the CIN terminology is still continued.
- Diagnosis of CIN 2 is often not absolutely certain. It is poorly reproducible and on further evaluation, many are reclassified as CIN 1 or CIN 3. Therefore, p16 immunostaining has been introduced to differentiate the CIN 2 lesions into
  - CIN 1 if p16 negative
  - CIN 3 if p16 positive
- Hence, in 2012, the College of American Pathologists (CAP) and American Society for Colposcopy and Cervical Pathology (ASCCP), in their consensus conference called Lower Anogenital Squamous Terminology (LAST) project, have changed the histological terminology to match the cytological terminology.
- The current terminology is as follows:
  - CIN 1 ⎱ LSIL
  - CIN 2 → p16 negative
  -       → p16 positive ⎱ HSIL
  - CIN 3
- During the transition from CIN to current terminology, the histology may be reported as LSIL (CIN 1), LSIL (CIN 2) if p16 negative, HSIL (CIN 2) if p16 positive and HSIL (CIN 3).

Aetiology and pathogenesis

To understand the pathogenesis of preinvasive cervical lesions, an understanding of the transformation zone (TZ) is essential.

The transformation zone

- Most cervical malignancies occur in the region called the TZ.

- The ectocervix and the vagina are lined by squamous epithelium and the endocervix by columnar epithelium. The junction between the two is known as the **squamocolumnar junction** (SCJ). At birth, SCJ is located on the ectocervix in most girls and this is called the **original SCJ**.
- Under the influence of oestrogens at puberty and pregnancy, the endocervix everts to expose the columnar epithelium. Glycogenization of the columnar epithelium takes place, lactobacilli colonize the epithelium and the pH becomes acidic. These changes stimulate the columnar epithelium to undergo metaplasia and convert into immature squamous and later mature squamous epithelium.
- The junction between the metaplastic squamous epithelium and the columnar epithelium is known as the **new SCJ**. The area between the original SCJ and the new SCJ, which lies more cephalad, is the **TZ** (Fig. 28.2).
- This is an area of high metaplastic activity and is vulnerable to oncogenic effects of carcinogens and most cervical cancers arise here. In postmenopausal women, the endocervical canal becomes shorter and the new SCJ moves further cephalad and lies within the endocervical canal.

Human papillomavirus and cervical cancer

It is now well accepted that cervical cancer is caused by HPV (Box 28.1). HPV infection is sexually transmitted; therefore, cervical cancer is a sexually transmitted disease (STD). HPV is a circular, double-stranded DNA virus and infects epithelial cells. More than 100 types have been identified; about 40 types infect the lower genital tract and 15 serotypes cause cervical cancer. Based on the oncogenic potential, they are classified into the following:

- ***Low-risk HPVs:*** Those that cause benign lesions. HPV 6 and 11 cause 90% of genital warts.
- ***High-risk HPVs:*** Those that cause malignant changes. HPV 16 and 18 cause 70% of cervical cancers (HPV 16—50%, HPV 18—20%); HPV 31, 33, 45, 52 and 58 cause 19% of cervical cancers.

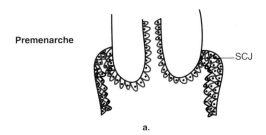

Premenarche

SCJ

a.

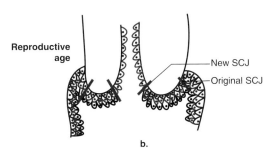

Reproductive age

New SCJ

Original SCJ

b.

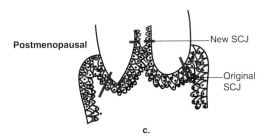

Postmenopausal

New SCJ

Original SCJ

c.

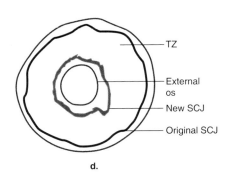

TZ

External os

New SCJ

Original SCJ

d.

Figure 28.2 Diagrammatic representation of TZ. **a.** The SCJ is on the ectocervix. **b.** The new SCJ is at the external os and the TZ is between the original and the new SCJ. **c.** The TZ extends into the cervical canal in postmenopausal women. **d.** End-on view as seen during speculum examination and colposcopy—The TZ between the original SCJ and the new SCJ. *SCJ,* squamocolumnar junction; *TZ,* transformation zone.

Cervical carcinogenesis by HPV

It occurs in four stages:

1. ***HPV infection:*** Infection by HPV occurs in >50% of women at some point in their life, the peak prevalence being at 15–25 years. The majority of HPV infections are transient and clear within 6–12 months.

2. ***HPV persistence:*** Although millions of women may be infected with the virus, persistent infection occurs only in a few.

3. ***Progression to precancerous lesion:*** Progression occurs about 10 years after infection. The virus may also enter a latent phase and re-emerge years later. The virus may persist in the cytoplasm and give rise to low-grade lesions. **When the viral DNA integrates into host cell genome, high-grade lesions develop.** This is a critical event in the development of neoplasia.

4. ***Local invasion:*** This leads to invasive cancer.

Box 28.1 Human papillomavirus

- DNA virus
- Circular, double stranded
- Exclusively infect epithelial cells
- Sexually transmitted
- More than 100 serotypes identified
- Low-risk HPVs
  - Cause genital warts
  - Seldom oncogenic
  - Predominantly HPV 6 and 11
- High-risk HPVs
  - Cause cervical, vaginal, vulvar cancer
  - Predominantly HPV 16 and 18
  - Also HPV 45, 56, 31, 33, 35, 58

HPV, human papillomavirus.

Cofactors in pathogenesis of cervical cancer

There are several cofactors involved in the progression of HPV infection to high-grade precancerous lesion and invasive cancer. These are listed in Box 28.2. Factors that increase risk of HPV infection are also risk factors for cervical cancer, though not cofactors in pathogenesis. These include early sexual activity, multiple sexual partners and multiparity. Immunosuppression due to HIV infection, immunosuppressive therapy or autoimmune disease, oral contraceptive

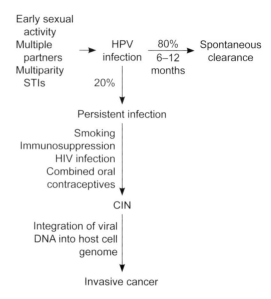

Figure 28.3 Pathogenesis of CIN and cervical cancer. *CIN*, cervical intraepithelial neoplasia; *HIV*, human immunodeficiency virus; *HPV*, human papillomavirus; *STI*, sexually transmitted infection.

use and smoking are also cofactors that promote progression to cancer.

The pathogenesis of cervical intraepithelial and invasive neoplasia is shown in Fig. 28.3.

Cytological and histological changes in squamous intraepithelial neoplasia

Cytological changes

As already discussed, CIN develops in the metaplastic epithelium of the TZ. The epithelium, due to the high mitotic activity, is vulnerable to oncogenic viruses and cofactors. The intraepithelial lesions that develop may affect the squamous or columnar cells. **Koilocytes**, which contain HPV viruses, are also seen in cytological specimens. The cellular changes consist of nuclear atypia, cellular enlargement and alteration in nuclear–cytoplasmic ratio. When these changes are mild, the lesions are described as CIN 1 or LSIL. Moderate and severe atypias are graded as CIN 2 and 3 or HSIL. The cytological and histological changes in CIN are listed in Box 28.3.

Histological changes

In addition to cellular changes such as nuclear atypia and pleomorphism, there is loss of stratification and maturation. The immature basaloid cells extend upwards to the middle and superficial layer of the epithelium.

As discussed earlier, the terms CIN 1, 2 and 3 are used to denote the level of extension of histological changes (Fig. 28.1). Currently, p16 expression is also used for risk categorization of CIN 2 lesions.

The endocervical epithelium is a monocellular layer and does not undergo similar changes. The premalignant lesion of the endocervix is **adenocarcinoma in situ**.

Prevention of intraepithelial neoplasia and cervical cancer

Primary prevention of intraepithelial neoplasia consists of creating an awareness about the risk factors among women, promoting practice of safe sex, use of condoms to prevent STDs, lifestyle modification, screening for and early treatment of premalignant lesions and HPV vaccines.

Secondary prevention is the prevention of progression of intraepithelial to invasive cancer. This consists of screening, appropriate management of preinvasive lesions and follow-up.

HPV vaccines

- Bivalent, quadrivalent and nanovalent vaccines have been developed to protect against HPV infection, genital warts and cervical cancer (Box 28.4).
- Studies have shown that they could prevent 95–100% of infections by targeted HPV types. Nanovalent vaccines cover additional 14% of HPV-associated cancers.

Box 28.4 HPV vaccines

- Bivalent (16, 18)
- Quadrivalent (6, 11, 16, 18)
- Nanovalent (6, 11, 16, 18, 31, 33, 45, 52, 58)
- Duration of action
  - 5–6 years
- Protection up to 10 years
- Age of administration (girls and boys)
  - 9–13 years
  - Catch-up vaccination
    - From 14 to 26 years in girls
    - From 14 to 21 years for boys
  - Most effective if given before the onset of sexual activity
- Dosage
  - Three doses at 0, 2 and 6 months
- Screening with cytology must continue

HPV, human papillomavirus.

- The vaccines are prophylactic, not therapeutic. Infection by HPV, if acquired before administration of vaccine, cannot be cured by the vaccine.
- There is no recommendation regarding use of vaccine after the age of 26 years.
- Currently nanovalent vaccine is recommended but if not available, one of the others can be used.
- Vaccination of men prevents genital warts and penile cancers and transmission of virus to sexual partner.
- Both quadrivalent and nanovalent vaccines can be used in boys. They should be given from 9 to 13 years, and catch-up vaccination up to 21 years.

Screening for intraepithelial and invasive cervical cancer

Screening for cervical cancer has resulted in reduction in the incidence of cervical cancer in developed countries. It is technically easy to screen for cervical cancer since

- The cervix can be easily visualized and tests performed.
- Cervical cancer goes through premalignant changes, and if the diagnosis is made at this stage, cancer can be prevented.
- There is a lag time of 10–20 years before the disease progresses from intraepithelial to invasive disease.

Several screening modalities are available, but cytology (Pap smear) is the most widely used. In resource-poor settings where Pap smear is not easily available, other methods are used. The screening modalities are listed in Box 28.5.

Cervical cytology

The abnormal cells of cervical neoplasia exfoliate and can be collected by scraping the cervix and staining the smear. Based on the severity of abnormality, it is possible to diagnose the degree of intraepithelial or invasive neoplasia. This method of screening by cytology testing was introduced by Papanicolaou and is known as the Pap smear or Pap test.

Cervical cancer screening using cytology is one of the greatest success stories. With the advent of Pap smear, incidence of cervical cancer

- Universal screening methods
  - Cytology
    - Conventional cytology (Pap smear)
    - LBC
      - Manual interpretation
      - Automated screening
  - HPV testing
- Methods for low-resource settings
  - VIA
  - VIAM
  - VILI
  - Point-of-care HPV testing

HPV, human papillomavirus; *LBC*, liquid-based cytology; *VIA*, visual inspection after acetic acid; *VIAM*, visual inspection after acetic acid with magnification; *VILI*, visual inspection after Lugol's iodine.

decreased by 60–70% in developed countries with organized screening programmes. But, in the developing countries, the results have not been so dramatic due to lack of awareness, lack of organized programmes, inadequate utilization of facilities by women, cost and so on.

Methods of cytological screening

Conventional cytology (Pap smear) Technique of Pap smear has been explained in Chapter 4, *Gynaecological history and physical examination.* The cervix is visualized after placing a bivalve speculum, and the ectocervix is scraped using an Ayre spatula and endocervix with a cytobrush (Fig. 28.4a–c). The cells are smeared on a glass slide and fixed in a 1:1 mixture of 95% ethanol and ether. Alternatively, the smears may be fixed with fixative spray. They are stained using Papanicolaou stain and examined (Fig. 28.5a–c).

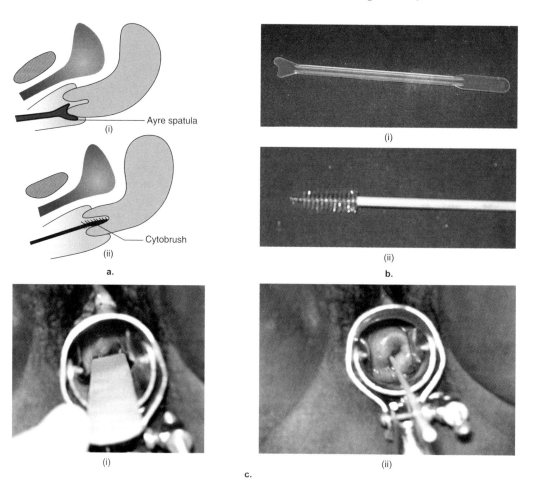

Figure 28.4 Techniques of taking Pap smear. a. Diagram of (i) spatula and (ii) cytobrush. b. Image of (i) Ayre spatula and (ii) cytobrush. c. Image of (i) Pap smear being taken with spatula and (ii) cytobrush.

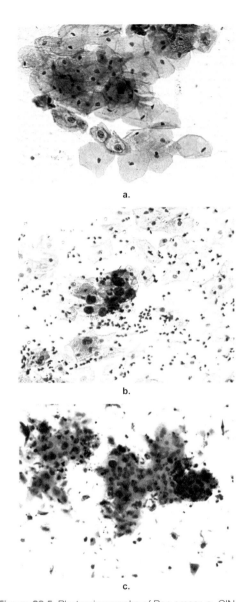

Figure 28.5 Photomicrographs of Pap smear. a. CIN 1—Two cells with enlarged nuclei and perinuclear halo are seen. b. CIN 2—One cluster of cells with enlarged nuclei with clumping of chromatin is seen. c. CIN 3—Cluster of cells with altered nuclear/cytoplasmic ratio and coarse clumping of chromatin is seen. Background contains atypical cells with pyknotic nuclei. *CIN*, cervical intraepithelial neoplasia.

Efficacy of Pap smear The Pap smear has been found to have a poor sensitivity and high false-negative rate, although the specificity of the test is high. Recent meta-analysis has shown that the sensitivity is 51%, the false-negative rate is 49% and the specificity is 98%. In order to improve the sensitivity and reduce the false-negative rate, other methods of cytological testing have been introduced.

Liquid-based cytology The cells are scraped using a special broom (Fig. 28.6), collected in a liquid medium and transported to the laboratory. It is processed; a smear of monolayer of cells is made and fixed. Drying distortion is eliminated; blood and other cells that interfere with interpretation are removed (Fig. 28.7). The residual sample can also be used for HPV testing. Liquid-based cytology (LBC) is recommended as the method of choice in the United Kingdom.

Randomized trials comparing conventional cytology and LBC have not found any difference in the cancer detection rates.

Cytology-based screening programmes have not been very successful in India and other developing countries. Some of the reasons are listed in Box 28.6.

HPV testing for cervical cancer screening

- Although HPV infection can be identified by cytology, colposcopy and histology, diagnosis of HPV infection is by HPV testing.

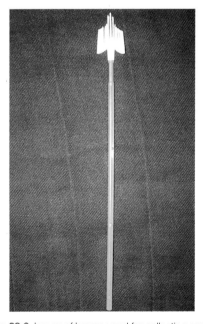

Figure 28.6 Image of broom used for collecting sample for liquid-based cytology.

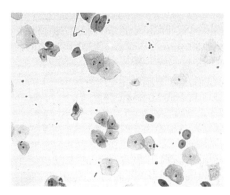

Figure 28.7 Photomicrograph of smear prepared by liquid-based cytology. Parabasal, intermediate and superficial cells are seen distinctly. There are no cellular artefacts or blood in the background.

Box 28.6 Reasons for failure of cytology-based screening programmes

- Lack of awareness
- Lack of infrastructure
- Lack of technical expertise
- Need for repeated testing
- Lack of good referral system
- Poor resources
- Poor facilities for treatment of test positives

- Tests to detect high-risk HPV DNA are commonly used. However, tests to detect mRNA are also available (Box 28.7).
- Large studies have shown that in women older than 30 years of age, HPV DNA testing is more sensitive than cytology for diagnosis of HSIL and invasive cancer including adenocarcinoma.
- In women younger than 30 years, prevalence of HPV infection is high and transient; therefore, the test has poor sensitivity and positive predictive value. Hence, the test should not be used for primary screening in women <30.
- For women >30, HPV testing may be used for
  - **Cotesting:** Along with cytology. The screening interval can be increased to 5 years.
  - **Reflex testing:** Sample is collected with cytology but performed only if cytology is equivocal.

Screening for cervical cancer in low-resource settings

Cytology and HPV testing–based screening programmes are difficult to implement in

---

Box 28.7 HPV testing for cervical cancer screening

- Detects high-risk HPVs
- DNA-based tests used often, mRNA tests available
- More sensitive than cytology alone
- <30 years of age
  - Poor specificity and positive predictive value
  - Should not be used
- >30 years of age
  - Recommended for cotesting with cytology
    - Screening intervals can be increased to 5 years
  - Reflex testing when cytology equivocal

HPV, human papillomavirus.

---

resource-poor settings. Screening strategies that are less expensive, are easy to implement and require fewer visits are more practical in low-resource settings.

Visual inspection after acetic acid

- Acetic acid, when applied to the cervix, coagulates the mucus and the areas of cells with increased chromatin density appear white. Areas of CIN, neoplasia, HPV-related changes and other abnormalities are acetowhite (Box 28.8; Fig. 28.8).
- Health workers can be trained to identify abnormal areas after application of acetic acid.
- This method has been extensively studied in developing countries including India and is currently recommended as the primary screening test for developing countries.
- Specificity of visual inspection after acetic acid (VIA) is limited (80%) and the false-positive

---

Box 28.8 Visual inspection after acetic acid for cervical cancer screening

- 3–5% freshly prepared acetic acid
- Low-grade lesions—Dull white plaques and faint borders
- High-grade lesions—Sharp borders
- Inexpensive
- Does not require expertise
- Minimal training required
- Can be performed by health workers
- Sensitivity: 79%
- Specificity: 85%
- PPV: 10–20%
- NPV: 92–97%

NPV, negative predictive value; *PPV*, positive predictive value.

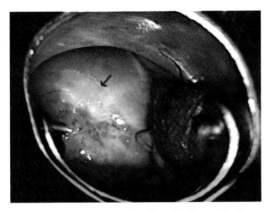

Figure 28.8 Visual inspection of cervix after application of acetic acid. Acetowhite area is indicated by arrow. Acetowhite areas indicate need for referral for colposcopy.

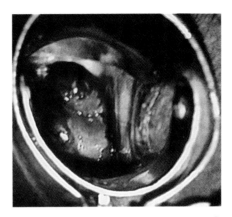

Figure 28.9 Visual inspection after Lugol's iodine. The normal areas appear mahogany brown due to glycogen content. The abnormal areas around the external os are mustard yellow.

rate is high, resulting in large number of referrals for further evaluation.

If VIA is positive, the options are as follows:

- Referral for colposcopy followed by biopsy and treatment
- Referral colposcopy and treatment based on colposcopic diagnosis (screen, see and treat)
- Immediate treatment based on VIA report (screen and treat)
- Referral for VIA with magnification (VIAM) followed by biopsy and treatment

VIA with magnification

After application of acetic acid, cervix is visualized under magnification using a handheld magnifying lens. Number of false-positives can be reduced with this technique, but the sensitivity and the specificity do not improve.

Visual inspection after Lugol's iodine

On application of iodine, normal cervical epithelium, which is rich in glycogen, stains mahogany brown (Schiller test). The abnormal areas, columnar epithelium and areas lined by immature metaplastic epithelium do not contain iodine and appear mustard yellow (Fig. 28.9). The test has the same specificity and similar advantages and disadvantages as VIA.

Point-of-care HPV testing

- The HPV tests that are routinely used in cervical cancer screening are expensive and require infrastructure for processing. Point-of-care HPV test (care HPV) is a rapid test that

identifies high-risk HPV and is less expensive. The results are available in 2.5 hours. The test is comparable to standard HPV testing and superior to VIA.
- Self-collected samples collected by the patient using a vaginal tampon, cotton swab or cytobrush can be used for HPV testing in low-resource settings where women do not have access to speculum examination.
- Combining VIA and HPV testing performed together or sequentially improves sensitivity and reduces false-positives.

Screen and treat protocols

Once the screening test is performed, those with positive tests have to be treated. Women in low-resource settings are difficult to follow up and treat. Hence, one-visit and two-visit protocols have been used to screen and treat these women.

- ***One-visit protocols:*** Screen and treat. Following screening by VIA or rapid HPV test, women who test positive are treated by cryotherapy. Compliance is better and cost is less, although overtreatment can occur with this method.
- ***Two-visit protocols:*** Screen, see and treat. Women are screened by cytology and during the second visit, women who are cytology positive are evaluated by colposcopy and treated by cryotherapy or loop electroexcision procedure (LEEP) in the same sitting. This method is not suitable for low-resource settings since colposcopy and LEEP facilities are not available.

Screening guidelines

The American College of Obstetrics and Gynecology (ACOG) and US Preventive Services Task Force (USPSTF) have published updated recommendations for cervical cancer screening in 2012 based on scientific evidence (Box 28.9).

Box 28.9 Screening guidelines (USPSTF, 2012) for cervical cancer

- Begin at age 21
- From age 21 to 29
  - Screen every 3 years with Pap smear
  - HPV testing should not be used
- From age 30 to 65
  - Screen every 5 years with Pap smear and HPV cotesting
  - Screen every 3 years with Pap smear alone
- Stop screening at 65 if previous smears are negative
- No screening is done after hysterectomy unless done for CIN 2 and 3
- Continue screening for women treated for CIN 2/3
- Conventional cytology or LBC can be used
- Women at high risk for cervical cancer must be screened more frequently

CIN, cervical intraepithelial neoplasia; HPV, human papillomavirus; LBC, liquid-based cytology; USPSTF, US Preventive Services Task Force.

Screening guidelines for low-resource settings

Since the ACOG guidelines are difficult to implement in developing countries, the WHO has recommended one smear in a lifetime at 35 years for low-resource settings. If multiple smears can be performed, screening intervals can be increased to 10 years. Even with such infrequent testing, incidence of cervical cancer can be reduced remarkably.

Reporting of cervical cytology testing—Bethesda system

The Bethesda system of reporting the cytology smears assures uniformity of reporting and provides clear guidelines for further evaluation and management. The original Bethesda system has been modified several times and the 2014 guidelines are followed now (Box 28.10).

The Bethesda system classifies squamous abnormalities into two categories as described earlier: LSIL and HSIL. LSIL includes CIN 1 and HPV-related changes, while HSIL includes CIN 2 and 3 (Box 28.10).

Box 28.10 Bethesda 2014 classification system for cervical cytology

- **Specimen type**
  - Conventional smear (Pap smear)
  - Liquid-based preparation (Pap test)
  - Other
- **Specimen adequacy**
  - Satisfactory for evaluation
  - Unsatisfactory for evaluation
- **General categorization**
  - Negative for intraepithelial lesion or malignancy
  - Other—Endometrial cells (in a woman older than 45 years)
  - Epithelial cell abnormality
- **Interpretation/results**
  - Negative for intraepithelial lesion or malignancy
  - Non-neoplastic findings (*optional to report*)
    - Non-neoplastic cellular variations
    - Reactive cellular changes associated
    - Glandular cells status posthysterectomy
  - Organisms
  - Other
  - Epithelial cell abnormalities
    - Squamous cell
      - Atypical squamous cells
        - Of undetermined significance (ASC-US)
        - Cannot exclude HSIL (ASC-H)
      - Low-grade squamous intraepithelial lesion (LSIL) (encompassing: HPV/mild dysplasia/CIN 1)
      - High-grade squamous intraepithelial lesion (HSIL) (encompassing: Moderate and severe dysplasia, CIS; CIN 2 and CIN 3)
        - With features suspicious for invasion (*if invasion is suspected*)
      - Squamous cell carcinoma
    - Glandular cell
      - Atypical
        - Endocervical cells (NOS *or specify in comments*)
        - Endometrial cells (NOS *or specify in comments*)
        - Glandular cells (NOS *or specify in comments*)
      - Atypical (level 4)
        - Endocervical cells, favour neoplastic
        - Glandular cells, favour neoplastic
      - Endocervical adenocarcinoma in situ
      - Adenocarcinoma
        - Endocervical
        - Endometrial
        - Extrauterine
        - Not otherwise specified (NOS)
- **Other malignant neoplasms (*specify*)**

ASC-H, atypical squamous cells cannot exclude high-grade lesion; ASC-US, atypical squamous cells of undetermined significance; CIN, cervical intraepithelial neoplasia; HPV, human papillomavirus; HSIL, high-grade squamous intraepithelial lesion; LSIL, low-grade squamous intraepithelial lesion.

Table 28.1 Management of women after cytology/HPV testing

Cervical cytology	HPV cotesting		
	Not done	Negative	Positive
Normal	Screen as usual	Screen as usual	Repeat cotesting after 12 months
ASC-US	HPV testing (or) repeat cytology after 1 year	Cytology-HPV cotesting after 1 year	Colposcopy
ASC-H	Colposcopy	Colposcopy	Colposcopy
LSIL	Colposcopy	Cytology-HPV cotesting after 1 year	Colposcopy
HSIL	Colposcopy	Colposcopy	Colposcopy
AGC, AGC—Favour neoplasia	Colposcopy, ECC		
AIS, adenocarcinoma	Endometrial sampling if >35 years		

AGC, atypical glandular cell; *AIS*, adenocarcinoma in situ; *ASC-H*, atypical squamous cells cannot exclude high-grade lesion; *ASC-US*, atypical squamous cells of undetermined significance; *ECC*, endocervical curettage; *HPV*, human papillomavirus; *HSIL*, high-grade squamous intraepithelial lesion; *LSIL*, low-grade squamous intraepithelial lesion.

Management after cytology or HPV testing

Since cytology–HPV cotesting is the current recommendation for women >30 years, management is based on cytology alone if HPV is not performed or both when cotesting is done. Management is based on ASCCP guidelines (2012).

Risk of progression to CIN 2 or more is the highest in HPV-positive women and lowest in HPV-negative women in all categories.

Management of women >30 years is outlined as follows and in Table 28.1:

- Normal cytology alone or normal cytology and HPV negative can be screened according to guidelines.
- Normal cytology and HPV positive should have repeat cotesting after 12 months.
- The risk of developing CIN 2 or more after atypical squamous cells of undetermined significance (ASC-US) cytology only is 6.9%, if HPV negative 1% and if HPV positive 18%. Therefore, those who are HPV positive must undergo colposcopic evaluation.
- Cytology atypical squamous cells cannot exclude high-grade lesion (ASC-H) has 35% risk of progression to CIN 2 or more. Hence, they should be evaluated by colposcopy irrespective of HPV testing.
- LSIL cytology without HPV testing needs colposcopic evaluation. However, if colposcopy is negative, repeat cotesting can be done after 1 year.

- All HSIL cytology should be evaluated by colposcopy.
- All women with the following diagnosis on smear should be evaluated by colposcopy and endocervical curettage (ECC):
  - Atypical endocervical or glandular cells (AGC)
  - Atypical endocervical or glandular cells (AGC)-favour neoplasia
  - Adenocarcinoma in situ (AIS)
  - Adenocarcinoma
- Women >35 years with AIS or adenocarcinoma, with risk factors for endometrial cancer should have endometrial sampling as well.

Colposcopy

Colposcopy is the visualization of the cervix, vagina and vulva under magnification to detect premalignant and malignant lesions. The colposcope is a magnification system with a light source, mounted on a stand (Fig. 28.10). Steps of colposcopic examination are given in Box 28.11. Saline removes mucus and discharge and makes it possible to view obvious abnormalities. On application of acetic acid, areas of high chromatin density stain white (acetowhite areas; Fig. 28.11), signifying the areas of squamous metaplasia, CIN and cancer. The new SCJ and TZ can be clearly visualized (Fig. 28.12a and b). The gland openings and abnormal vascularity become distinctly visible (Fig 28.12b and c). The abnormal areas can be well delineated with Lugol's iodine.

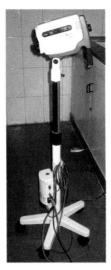

Figure 28.10　A colposcope, which is a magnification system mounted on a stand.

Box 28.11 Steps of colposcopic examination

- Place the patient in dorsal/lithotomy position
- Place colposcope 1 feet from vulva
- Insert bivalve speculum
- Focus colposcope on the cervix
- Use low power for overall visualization initially
- Shift to high power for closer visualization of lesions
- Clean with saline, remove mucus and note findings
- Apply 3% acetic acid and note findings
- Apply Lugol's iodine and note findings
- Document colposcopic findings
- Perform guided biopsy, if indicated

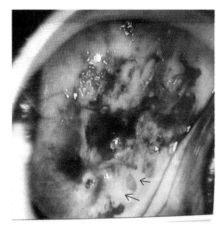

Figure 28.11　Colposcopy after application of acetic acid. The areas of squamous metaplasia are stained white (black arrows).

Colposcopy is performed in all women with abnormal cytology unless a policy of wait and watch is decided upon. It helps in localization of the lesion and in taking a directed biopsy (Box 28.12). ECC is performed whenever there is glandular cell abnormality.

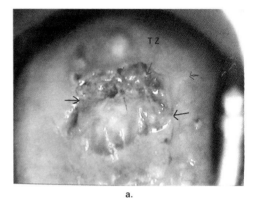

a.

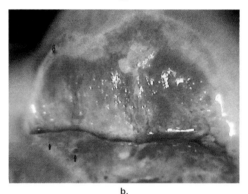

b.

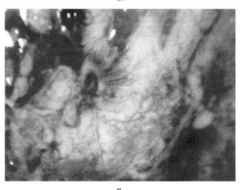

c.

Figure 28.12　Colposcopy images. a. The red columnar epithelium around the os (blue arrow), dull pink squamous epithelium (red arrow), the new SCJ (black arrows) and external os are seen. Transformation zone is marked TZ. b. Under further magnification, the gland openings in the TZ are seen (arrows). c. Mosaic pattern. The colposcopic diagnosis is CIN 2.

- Localization of lesion
- Making a diagnosis
- Taking directed biopsy
- Guiding ablative procedures

Colposcopic findings and terminology

The revised terminology by the International Federation for Cervical Pathology and Colposcopy (IFCPC), 2011, has now been adopted. The older terminology such as satisfactory and unsatisfactory colposcopy has been replaced by adequate and inadequate colposcopy, but they are not synonymous. Based on visibility, three types of SCJ and TZ are described (Box 28.13; Fig. 28.13).

Box 28.13 Colposcopic terminology

- Adequacy
  - Adequate colposcopy
    - Not obscured by inflammation, bleeding or scar
  - Inadequate colposcopy
    - Obscured by inflammation, bleeding or scar
- Squamocolumnar junction
  - Type 1
    - Completely visible
  - Type 2
    - Partially visible
  - Type 3
    - Not visible
- Transformation zone
  - Type 1
    - Entirely on the ectocervix, fully visible, can be small or large
  - Type 2
    - Has endocervical component, fully visible
  - Type 3
    - Has endocervical component, not fully visible

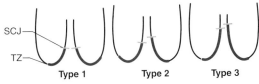

Type 1   Type 2   Type 3

Figure 28.13 Types of SCJ and TZ. Type 1—TZ and SCJ are on the ectocervix and completely visible. Type 2—The TZ extends into endocervical canal; SCJ is in the endocervical canal. TZ fully visible. Type 3—The SCJ is well into the endocervical canal; TZ extends into the canal and not fully visible. *SCJ*, squamocolumnar junction; *TZ*, transformation zone.

Typical appearance of CIN is acetowhite area with mosaic and punctation, indicating abnormal capillary distribution. These areas are also Schiller light. Colposcopic findings are graded into grade 1 (minor) and grade 2 (major) changes. Two new colposcopic signs associated with high grade lesions have been included (1) Inner border sign-a sharp acetowhite demarcation within a less opaque acetowhite area (2) Ridge sign- thick opaque ridges of acetowhite epithelium growing irregularly in the squamacolumnar juntion. The IFCPC cervical colposcopy nomenclature is given in Table 28.2.

Histological diagnosis of intraepithelial neoplasia

Following screening with cytology, HPV testing or both, colposcopy is performed as indicated. A colposcopic diagnosis of intraepithelial lesion must be confirmed by biopsy and histological examination, before definitive treatment. Histological diagnosis of squamous lesions may be LSIL or HSIL according to the LAST terminology or CIN 1, 2 or 3 according to the earlier terminology. Management is based on histological diagnosis.

Management of cervical intraepithelial neoplasia

Guidelines for the management of CIN have been developed by the ASCCP in 2012. The CIN classification of histology is used in the guidelines since p16 immunostaining is not performed and the new classification of histology is not followed globally.

Management in women <25 years is different from that in those >25 years.

Management guidelines

Management of CIN 1 (histology)

Most cases of CIN 1 regress spontaneously over time. Risk of progression to CIN 2 or more depends on

- LSIL preceded by lesser abnormalities (LSIL or ASC-US cytology)
- LSIL preceded by ASC-H or HSIL cytology

Table 28.2 2011 IFCPC cervical coloposcopy nomenclature

General assessment		• Adequate/inadequate for the reason (i.e. cervix obscured by inflammation, bleeding, scar) • Squamocolumnar junction visibility: Completely visible, partially visible, not visible • Transformation zone types 1, 2, 3	
Normal colposcopic findings		Original squamous epithelium • Mature • Atrophic Columnar epithelium • Ectopy Metaplastic squamous epithelium • Nabothian cysts • Crypt (gland) openings Deciduosis in pregnancy	
Abnormal colposcopic findings	General principles	**Location of the lesion:** Inside or outside the transformation zone, location of the lesion by clock position **Size of the lesion:** Number of cervical quadrants the lesion covers, size of the lesion in percentage of cervix	
	Grade 1 (minor)	Thin acetowhite epithelium Irregular, geographical border	Fine mosaic Fine punctation
	Grade 2 (major)	Dense acetowhite epithelium Rapid appearance of acetowhitening Cuffed crypt (gland) openings	Coarse mosaic Coarse punctation Sharp border Inner border sign Ridge sign
	Nonspecific	Leukoplakia (keratosis, hyperkeratosis), erosion Lugol's staining (Schiller test): stained/nonstained	
Suspicious for invasion		Atypical vessels **Additional signs:** Fragile vessels, irregular surface, exophytic lesion, necrosis, ulceration (necrotic), tumour/gross neoplasm	
Miscellaneous findings		Congenital transformation zone Condyloma Polyp (ectocrevical/endocervical) Inflammation	Stenosis Congenital anomaly Post-treatment consequence Endometriosis

Women >25 years of age

- If preceded by ASC-US/LSIL cytology, progression to invasive cancer is <1%. Therefore, they can be followed up with cytology/HPV cotesting at 12 months (Fig. 28.14). If cytology or HPV is positive, colposcopy is indicated.
- If preceded by ASC-H or HSIL cytology, risk of progression to cancer is higher. Management options include the following:
  - Follow-up with cotesting at 12 and 24 months and management accordingly
  - Treatment with excision procedure
  - Review of cytology, histology and colposcopy, management accordingly

Women <25 years of age

- *LSIL preceded by lesser abnormalities:* Repeat cytology at 12 and 24 months and manage accordingly.

- *LSIL preceded by HSIL/H:* Cytology and colposcopy every 6 months for 2 years. If cytology/colposcopy shows HSIL that persists for 1 year, colposcopy and biopsy are indicated.

Management of CIN 2 and 3 (histology)

Overall risk of progression to cancer is high; 5% of CIN 2 and 12% of CIN 3 progress to invasive cancer. Therefore, prompt treatment is mandatory (Fig. 28.15).

Women who have completed reproductive function

- If colposcopy is adequate and TZ is visible, excision or ablation is recommended, excision preferred.
- If colposcopy is inadequate, HSIL is recurrent or endocervical sampling reveals HSIL, excision is recommended.

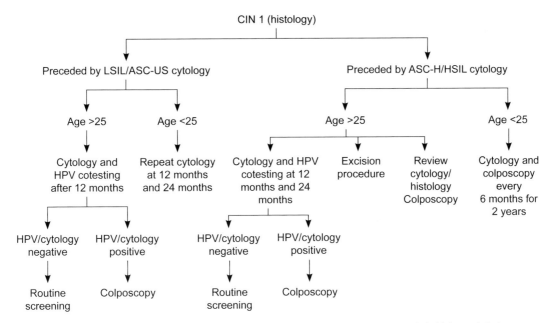

Figure 28.14 Management of CIN 1 histology. *ASC-H*, atypical squamous cells cannot exclude high-grade lesion; *ASC-US*, atypical squamous cells of undetermined significance, *CIN*, cervical intraepithelial neoplasia; *HPV*, human papillomavirus; *HSIL*, high-grade squamous intraepithelial lesion; *LSIL*, low-grade squamous intraepithelial lesion.

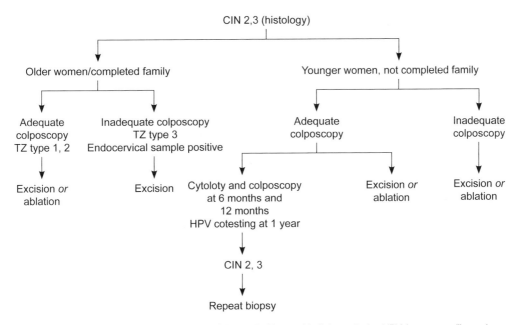

Figure 28.15 Management of CIN 2, 3 histology. *CIN*, cervical intraepithelial neoplasia; *HPV*, human papillomavirus.

430   Essentials of Gynaecology

Young women desirous of further reproductive function

- If colposcopy is adequate, options are as follows:
  - Observation with cytology and colposcopy every 6 months followed by HPV cotesting 1 year later. If HSIL persists, repeat biopsy.
  - Excision or ablation.
- If colposcopy is inadequate, immediate excision or ablation

Management of adenocarcinoma in situ (histology)

Women with AIS must undergo cold-knife conization since the lesions are in the endocervix and not visible entirely on colposcopy. Even if conization margins are negative, hysterectomy is recommended for those who have completed their family.

Treatment modalities

Currently available treatment modalities are ablative and excisional procedures (Box 28.14). Most treatments are office based.

- Efficacy is similar (90–95%) for both excision and ablation.
- Choice of method depends on the need for diagnostic specimen, availability, adverse effects, cost and desire for future childbearing.
- For high-grade lesions and endocervical lesions, excision is preferred since it provides tissue for histological confirmation and evaluation of the margins of excision.

Box 28.14 Treatment modalities for CIN

- Ablative procedures
  - Thermoablation
  - Cryotherapy
  - Carbon dioxide laser
- Excisional procedures
  - LEEP
  - Cold-knife conization
  - Carbon dioxide laser cone

CIN, cervical intraepithelial neoplasia; *LEEP*, loop electroexcision procedure.

Ablative procedures

All ablative procedures are office based and can be performed under local anaesthesia. Common

---

Box 28.15 Ablative procedures in CIN

- Specimen cannot be sent for histology
- Entire lesion and transformation zone should be visible
- Extension into endocervix should be <1.5 cm
- Prior histological confirmation of diagnosis is required

CIN, cervical intraepithelial neoplasia.

---

features of ablative procedures are given in Box 28.15.

Thermoablation

This may be performed as office procedure. Using electrocautery, the entire TZ, including the lesion, is cauterized. Depth of cauterization should be 5–7 mm to destroy the disease in the crypts. Profuse vaginal discharge is present for 3–4 weeks. Recurrence rate is slightly higher with this method. This method of treatment has been replaced by other methods now.

Cryotherapy

Cryotherapy involves freezing of the tissue followed by thawing, which leads to formation of intracellular ice crystals, resulting in expansion and rupture of cells. The freeze–thaw cycles alternate 3 minutes of freezing with 5 minutes of thawing. Carbon dioxide or nitrous oxide is used for freezing (Box 28.16). Cryoprobes are of different sizes; the probe that will cover the

---

Box 28.16 Cryotherapy in the treatment of CIN

- Refrigerant gas used
  - N_2O at −89°C
  - CO_2 at −68°C
- Two sequential freeze–thaw cycles
- Depth of destruction—5 mm
- Success rate—95%
- Treatment failure
  - Large cervix
  - Large lesion (>2 quadrants)
  - Extension into endocervical canal
- Disadvantages
  - Profuse vaginal discharge lasting for 3–4 weeks
  - Receding of SCJ into endocervical canal
- Follow-up
  - Pap smear and colposcopy at 4–6 months

CIN, cervical intraepithelial neoplasia; *SCJ*, squamocolumnar junction.

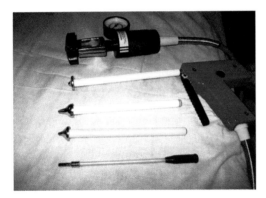

Figure 28.16 Cryoprobes of various sizes used for cryotherapy.

entire lesion should be selected (Fig. 28.16). Cryotherapy is not suitable for CIN extending to glandular crypts since depth of freezing is only 5 mm.

Laser ablation

Laser has been a popular method of treating cervical lesions (Box 28.17). CO_2 laser is used, the epithelium is vapourized, water in the cells is converted into steam and the cell is destroyed. As in cryotherapy, entire lesion should be visible.

Excisional procedures

The excision of the TZ including a portion of the endocervical canal in a cone-shaped fashion can be carried out using large loop excision, straight-wire excision or cold knife.

- These excisional procedures are all included under **conization**; the terms 'cone biopsy', 'big loop excision' and 'small loop excision' are not used (IFCPC recommendation, 2011).
- The types of excision are as follows:
  - **Type 1 excision:** Resects type 1 TZ (completely ectocervical)

Box 28.17 Laser ablation in the treatment of CIN

- Minimization of area of destruction
- No troublesome vaginal discharge
- Depth of destruction
  - 5–7 mm on the ectocervix
  - 8–9 mm around the endocervix
- Suitable for large, irregular lesions
- Success rate 95%
- Expensive equipment

CIN, cervical intraepithelial neoplasia.

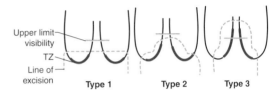

Figure 28.17 Types of excision of TZ. The line of excision should include the entire TZ. Type 1 excision resects type 1 TZ; type 2 excision resects type 2 TZ and extends into the endocervical canal; type 3 excision resects type 3 TZ; the resected tissue is cone shaped and includes significant amount of endocervical epithelium. *TZ*, transformation zone.

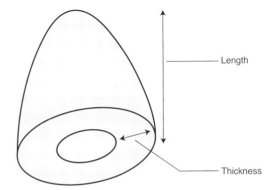

Figure 28.18 Excised specimen (conization) showing the length and thickness.

  - **Type 2 excision:** Resects type 2 TZ, includes small amount of endocervical epithelium
  - **Type 3 excision:** Resects type 3 TZ, includes longer and larger cone-shaped tissue and significant amount of endocervical epithelium (Fig. 28.17)
- The length and thickness of the excised specimen should be specified according to guidelines (Fig 28.18).
- Excisional procedures have a distinct advantage that specimen is available for histology.
- Excision by LEEP has now replaced ablative procedures since it is also an office-based procedure, is easy to perform and has very few complications.

Loop electroexcision procedure

This is also referred to as large loop excision of the transformation zone (LLETZ). This is currently the treatment of choice in most women with CIN 2 and 3 (Box 28.18). The excision is performed with a wire loop cautery, available in

Box 28.18 Loop electroexcision procedure

- Outpatient procedure
- Performed under local anaesthesia
- Wire loop cautery used
- Specimen available for histopathology
- Easy to learn
- Thermal artefact can obscure margin status

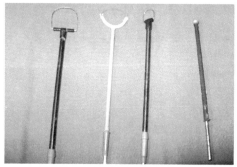

a.

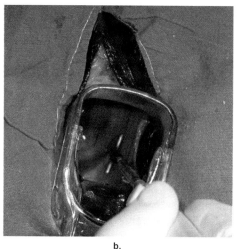

b.

Figure 28.19 Loop electroexcision procedure. a. LEEP electrodes of various sizes and rollerball electrode for haemostasis. b. LEEP procedure being performed. *LEEP*, loop electroexcision procedure.

various sizes (Fig. 28.19a and b). The lesion must be localized by colposcopy and an appropriate loop should be selected. The electrosurgical generator is set at 30–40 W power.

A straight wire may be used instead of a wire loop for performing the procedure, known as **straight-wire excision of the transformation zone (SWETZ)**.

Cold-knife conization

This refers to excision of a cone-shaped specimen from the cervix, with the base of the cone at the ectocervix and apex in the endocervical canal close to the internal os. A knife is used; the procedure requires anaesthesia and is performed in an operating room. Preoperative colposcopy determines the extent of ectocervix removed. The shape and size of tissue excised may be type 1, 2 or 3, depending on the type of TZ and extent of lesion. Conization is used only for specific indications (Box 28.19).

Box 28.19 Indications for cold-knife conization

- Lesion extending into the endocervical canal
- Histological diagnosis of AIS
- Recurrent AGC cytology
- Cytology–histology discordance
  - Cytology more severe-grade lesion
- Suspected microinvasive cancer
- Recurrent high-grade lesion
- Large lesions (>50% of cervix involved)

AGC, atypical glandular cell; *AIS*, adenocarcinoma in situ.

Procedure Steps of conization are given in Box 28.20.

Box 28.20 Steps of conization

- Spinal/general anaesthesia
- Colposcopy and application of Lugol's iodine
- Infiltration of adrenaline into the cervix
- Sutures at 3 and 9 o'clock positions
- Excision of cone using knife
- Cauterization of bleeding points
- Haemostatic pack in the vagina

The procedure is performed only in selected patients because of the immediate and late complications (Box 28.21). It should be avoided in nulliparous women as far as possible.

Laser conization

Conization may be performed using the CO_2 laser microprobe. Indications, procedure and complications are similar. It is possible to reduce the size of the cone by vapourizing the visible ectocervical lesions and excise the endocervical

Box 28.21 Complications of conization

- Immediate
  - Haemorrhage
    - Primary
    - Secondary
  - Infection
- Late
  - Cervical stenosis
  - Cervical incompetence
    - Recurrent pregnancy loss
    - Preterm labour

lesion using laser. The equipment is expensive and expertise is required for performing the procedure.

Subsequent management Conization is considered a diagnostic and therapeutic procedure. Subsequent management depends on histological examination of the margins of excised specimen. In developing countries, compliance for follow-up is poor. Further treatment has to be tailored to suit the individual. If margin is positive for CIN 3, the woman is perimenopausal or the woman is unlikely to present for follow-up, hysterectomy may be performed. Young women

and those who are likely to be regular with follow-up may be followed up with cytology and/or colposcopy (Fig. 28.20). Follow-up after negative smears should be every 6 months till two consecutive smears are negative and routine screening thereafter.

Hysterectomy

Hysterectomy is not a primary procedure for management of CIN. There are very few indications for hysterectomy in the management of preinvasive cervical disease (Box 28.22). Even after hysterectomy, follow-up with cytology is essential since vaginal vault lesions can occur after several years. Hysterectomy can be abdominal, vaginal or laparoscopic.

Box 28.22 Indications for hysterectomy in CIN

- Adenocarcinoma in situ
- CIN 3 with cone margins involved
  - Older women
  - Not reliable for follow-up
- Recurrent high-grade lesion

CIN, cervical intraepithelial neoplasia.

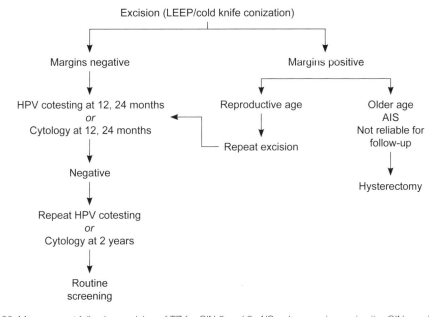

Figure 28.20 Management following excision of TZ for CIN 2 and 3. *AIS*, adenocarcinoma in situ; *CIN*, cervical intraepithelial neoplasia; *LEEP*, loop electroexcision procedure; *TZ*, transformation zone.

Key points

- Cervical cancer is the second most common cancer in women in India and more than 100,000 new cases occur every year. It is a public health problem.
- Almost all squamous cancers arise in the transformation zone, which is the area between the original and the new squamocolumnar junction.
- Premalignant lesions of the cervix are called 'cervical intraepithelial neoplasia' (CIN) in which cellular changes are confined to the epithelium but do not extend beyond the basement membrane.
- Cytological and histological terminologies of CIN have undergone several changes.
- It is now a well-accepted fact that cervical cancer is caused by human papillomavirus (HPV). The high-risk HPV 16 and 18 are associated with most invasive cancers.
- Risk factors for development of cervical cancer are high parity, early sexual activity, multiple sex partners, immunosuppression, smoking and other sexually transmitted infections.
- Screening has reduced the incidence of cervical cancer in developed countries.

- Cytology is the most popular screening test used. Sensitivity of Pap smear can be improved by liquid-based cytology. HPV cotesting with cytology is currently recommended for women >30 years.
- Visual inspection after acetic acid has been recommended for screening in low-resource settings.
- Cervical cytology is reported using the Bethesda system.
- Colposcopy is visualization of the cervix under magnification. It is the first step in the evaluation of abnormal Pap smear in most women.
- Most CIN 1 lesions regress. Only 1% of CIN 1, 5% of CIN 2 and 12% of CIN 3 lesions progress to invasive malignancy.
- Guidelines for treatment for histologically confirmed CIN have been developed.
- Treatment modalities include ablative procedures and excisional procedures. Loop electroexcision procedure is the most commonly used modality of treatment.
- Hysterectomy is not considered as primary treatment of CIN.

Self-assessment

Case-based questions

Case 1

A 40-year-old lady, multipara, presented with vaginal discharge for past 2 years and a Pap smear was taken. Pap smear revealed HSIL.

1. What is the next step in evaluation?
2. What is the management?

Case 2

A 32-year-old lady had a routine Pap smear that revealed LSIL.

1. What is the management?

Answers

Case 1

1. Colposcopy and directed biopsy.
2. If histological diagnosis is CIN 2 or 3, the TZ should be excised with LEEP. The type of excision depends on the type of transformation zone.

Case 2

1. If HPV testing is available, it should be performed. If not, colposcopy.

If HPV testing is done and is negative, cytology-HPV cotesting should be done 1 year later.

If HPV positive, colposcopy.

Long-answer questions

1. What is the epidemiology of cervical cancer? How do you diagnose and manage cervical intraepithelial neoplasia?
2. Discuss the methods of screening for cervical cancer.
3. What is cervical intraepithelial neoplasia? Discuss the management of a woman with abnormal Pap smear.

Short-answer questions

1. Pap smear
2. Screening for carcinoma cervix
3. Classification of CIN and its management
4. Colposcopy
5. Cold-knife conization
6. Human papillomavirus and its role in cervical cancer
7. HPV vaccines
8. Visual inspection of cervix after acetic acid
9. Pathogenesis and risk factors for cervical cancer
10. Loop electroexcision procedure
11. Bethesda system of reporting cervical cytology

29 | Malignant Diseases of the Cervix

Case scenario

Mrs AB, 48, came to the clinic with complaints of irregular vaginal bleeding, which was almost continuous for the past 2 months. She hailed from a village nearby, and worked as a coolie. She expected her menstruation to stop around this age and her neighbours assured her that the irregularity was a part of that process. She was married at the age of 14 and had five children, and her husband had a history of genital ulcers. She was treated by local doctor repeatedly for vaginal discharge. On further questioning, she gave a history of postcoital bleeding for the past 6 months.

Introduction

Cancer of the cervix is the third most common cancer in women worldwide and the second most common cancer in India. The disease is preventable by screening and early diagnosis and treatment is associated with good outcome. Cervical intraepithelial neoplasia (CIN; *see* Chapter 28, *Premalignant diseases of the cervix*) is the preinvasive stage of the disease. Human papillomavirus (HPV) has been identified as the causative agent in most cases.

Incidence

- Cervical cancer constitutes 13% of all cancers in women globally. It was the most common cancer in India until a few years ago.

- In the year 2008, global estimate of cervical cancer published by the World Health Organization (WHO) was 529,409 cases and 274,883 deaths. Eighty percent of the cases and deaths occur in developing countries.

- The estimates in India (2008) are 134,420 cases annually and 72,825 deaths, an incidence of 23.5/100,000. The exact incidence may be difficult to obtain because of under-reporting in rural areas.

- International data show a decline in incidence of cervical cancer in countries with successful screening programmes and early intervention. The reduction has also been attributed to epidemiological transition.

- A decrease has also been noticed in India; the reported incidence in 2014 is 20.2/100,000 for cervical cancer and 23.8 for breast cancer.

Thus, cervical cancer is now the second most common cancer in India.

- About 80–85% are squamous cell cancers and 15–20% are adenocarcinomas.
- Peak incidence in India is between 55 and 59 years. The age-specific incidence increases from 35 years.
- Mean age at diagnosis is 48 years in the West and 38 in India.

Risk factors

Risk factors for development of cervical cancer are the same as those for CIN and are listed in Box 29.1.

Pathogenesis

Cancer of the cervix is a preventable disease because it goes through preinvasive stages for several years; effective screening tests and treatment modalities are available to diagnose and treat preinvasive disease. The role of HPV infection in the pathogenesis of cervical cancer has been already discussed in Chapter 28, *Premalignant diseases of the cervix*. The HPV serotypes associated with invasive cancer are 16, 18, 31, 33, 45, 52 and 58. Of these, 70% of cases are caused by HPV 16 and 18. The infections by HPV are usually transient, but persistent infection occurs in the presence of risk factors. The HPV

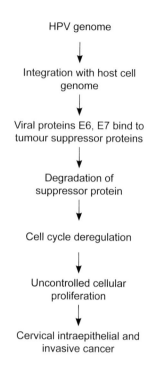

HPV genome
↓
Integration with host cell genome
↓
Viral proteins E6, E7 bind to tumour suppressor proteins
↓
Degradation of suppressor protein
↓
Cell cycle deregulation
↓
Uncontrolled cellular proliferation
↓
Cervical intraepithelial and invasive cancer

Figure 29.1 Pathogenesis of cervical cancer. *HPV, human papillomavirus.*

genome integrates with the host cell genome. The viral proteins E6 and E7 bind to tumour suppressor proteins of the host cells and cause degradation of the suppressor proteins. This leads to unregulated cell cycle, cellular proliferation and cancer. Pathogenesis of cervical cancer is shown in Fig. 29.1.

Pathology

Macroscopic appearance

Macroscopically, cervical cancers are of three types: **exophytic**, **endophytic** (infiltrative) and **ulcerative** (Fig. 29.2a and b). The exophytic growth is most common, has a typical cauliflower-like appearance and bleeds on touch. The macroscopic features of all the three types are given in Box 29.2.

Microscopic appearance

The predominant type is **squamous cell carcinoma** (SCC), comprising 75–80% of cervical cancers (Fig. 29.3a and b) arising from the

- Exophytic
  - Irregular growth (cauliflower-like)
  - Vascular
  - Fungating
- Endophytic
  - Barrel-shaped
  - Stony hard
- Ulcerative
  - Large ulcers
  - Indurated

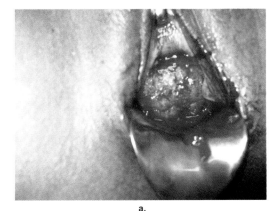

a.

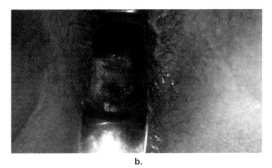

b.

Figure 29.2 Macroscopic appearance of cervical cancer. a. Large exophytic cancer—Cauliflower-like, friable growth arising from the cervix, filling the vagina. There is contact bleeding following insertion of speculum. b. Ulcerative growth—Large ulcer involving the entire cervix, which also bleeds on touch.

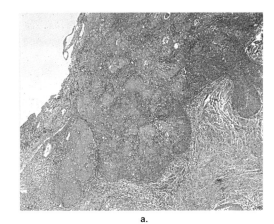

a.

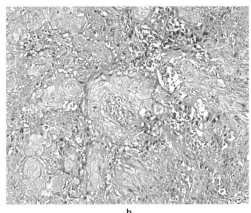

b.

Figure 29.3 Microscopic appearance of squamous cell carcinoma. a. Photomicrograph shows cervix infiltrated by tumour composed of nests of squamous cells. b. Photomicrograph of the same slide, under high power, shows nests of malignant squamous cells with keratin pearls.

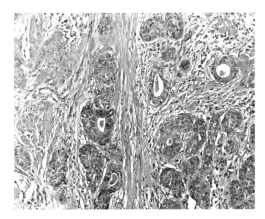

Figure 29.4 Photomicrograph of adenocarcinoma. Malignant glandular cells are seen infiltrating the stroma of the cervix.

ectocervical squamous epithelium. Fifteen to twenty percent are **adenocarcinomas** (Fig. 29.4) arising from the columnar epithelium of the endocervix. Histological types of cervical cancers are listed in Box 29.3. The other types mentioned in the box are rare and constitute about 5% of all cervical cancers.

Box 29.3 Histological types of cervical cancer

- Squamous carcinoma
  - Large cell tumours
    - Keratinizing
    - Nonkeratinizing
  - Small cell tumours
    - Poorly differentiated
    - Anaplastic
- Adenocarcinoma
  - Endocervical
  - Endometrioid
  - Minimal deviation
  - Papillary villoglandular
  - Serous
  - Clear cell
  - Mesonephric
- Mixed cervical carcinomas
  - Adenosquamous
  - Glassy cell
  - Adenoid cystic
  - Adenoid basal epithelioma
- Neuroendocrine tumours of the cervix
  - Large cell
  - Small cell
- Other malignant tumours
  - Sarcomas
  - Lymphomas

Box 29.4 Patterns of spread of cervical cancer

- Direct extension
  - Vagina
  - Uterine corpus
  - Parametrium
  - Pelvic side wall
  - Bladder
  - Rectum
  - Ovary (rare, <1%)
- Lymphatic spread
  - Primary nodes
    - Paracervical
    - Parametrial
    - Internal iliac
    - External iliac
    - Obturator
    - Sacral
  - Secondary nodes
    - Common iliac
    - Para-aortic
    - Inguinal
    - Left supraclavicular (scalene)
- Haematogenous spread
  - Liver
  - Lungs
  - Bone

Squamous cell cancers may be large cell keratinized, nonkeratinized or small cell tumours. Keratinization and epithelial pearl formation are absent in poorly differentiated tumours. Adenocarcinomas are of several types and are classified according to the type of epithelium. Mucinous carcinoma is the most common. Mixed carcinomas are rare. Neuroendocrine tumours are aggressive and have a poor prognosis.

Histological grading

Histologically, according to the presence of keratinization, mitotic activity and nuclear pleomorphism, cervical cancers are divided into grades 1, 2 and 3 (well differentiated, moderately differentiated and poorly differentiated, respectively) tumours. The association between histological grading and prognosis is not clear-cut.

Patterns of spread

Like other malignancies of the genital tract, cervical cancer spreads by **direct extension**, and **lymphatic** and **haematogenous spread** (Box 29.4).

Direct spread upwards and downwards results in involvement of the uterine corpus and vagina, respectively. Extension to the parametrium can extend to the pelvic wall. Ureteric obstruction usually occurs and may result in hydroureteronephrosis and renal failure (Fig. 29.5). It was believed that lymphatic spread first occurs to the paracervical region and parametrium followed by obturator, external and interiliac nodes and then to the secondary nodes. However, subsequent studies have shown that the initial spread can occur to any of the pelvic or even the para-aortic nodes (Fig. 29.6). The left scalene node is usually involved in very advanced disease.

The incidence of lymph node involvement increases with stage of disease (Table 29.1) and forms the basis for the type of surgery and extent of node dissection.

By haematogenous spread, the tumour metastasizes to liver, lungs and bone. Haematogenous spread usually occurs in advanced disease.

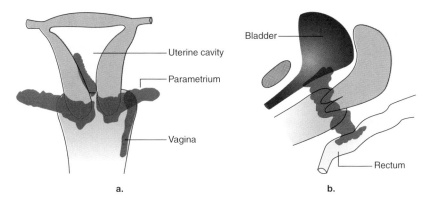

Figure 29.5 Diagram depicting direct spread of cervical cancer. **a.** Upwards to the uterine corpus, downwards to the vagina, laterally to the parametria. **b.** anteriorly to the bladder and posteriorly to the rectum.

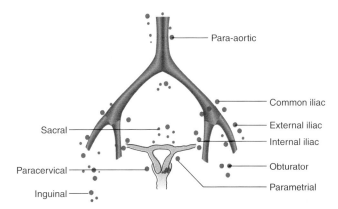

Figure 29.6 Lymphatic spread of cervical cancer to pelvic, para-aortic, inguinal and left supraclavicular nodes.

Table 29.1 Incidence of lymph node metastasis by stage		
Stage	Pelvic nodes (%)	Para-aortic nodes (%)
IA1	0.5–1	0
IA2	7	<1
IB	16	8
IIA	25	10
IIB	32	20
III	45	30
IV	55	40

Lymphovascular space invasion

This is one of the prognostic factors. The tumour cells invade the capillaries and lymphatic channels. When lymphovascular space invasion (LVSI) is present, even when the disease is staged as early, more radical treatment and adjuvant therapy are required.

Staging

Staging of cervical cancer is **clinical** because it is predominantly a disease of poor-resource settings where imaging and surgical staging may not be feasible or cost-effective. International Federation of Gynecology and Obstetrics (FIGO) staging (2008) is given in Table 29.2 (see also Fig. 29.7). The term **early stage disease** is used for stages IA, IB and IIA and locally **advanced disease** for stages IIB–IVA. Carcinoma in situ is not included in FIGO staging.

Tumour, nodes and metastasis (TNM) staging has been created by American Joint Committee on Cancer but is not commonly used.

Table 29.2	FIGO staging of cervical cancer (2008)
Stage I	The carcinoma is strictly confined to the cervix (extension to the corpus should be disregarded)
IA	Invasive carcinoma, which can be diagnosed only by microscopy, with deepest invasion <5.0 mm and largest extension <7.0 mm. Vascular space involvement, venous or lymphatic, does not affect classification
IA1	Measured stromal invasion of <3.0 mm in depth and horizontal extension of <7.0 mm
IA2	Measured stromal invasion of >3.0 mm and not >5.0 mm and horizontal extension of <7.0 mm
IB	Clinically visible lesions limited to the cervix uteri or microscopic lesions greater than stage IA*
IB1	Clinically visible lesion <4.0 cm in greatest dimension
IB2	Clinically visible lesion >4.0 cm in greatest dimension
Stage II	Cervical carcinoma invades beyond the uterus, but not to the pelvic wall or to the lower third of the vagina
IIA	Without parametrial invasion
IIA1	Clinically visible lesion <4.0 cm in greatest dimension
IIA2	Clinically visible lesion >4.0 cm in greatest dimension
IIB	With obvious parametrial invasion
Stage III	The tumour extends to the pelvic wall and/or involves the lower third of the vagina and/or causes hydronephrosis or nonfunctioning kidney
IIIA	Tumour involves the lower third of the vagina, with no extension to the pelvic wall
IIIB	Extension to the pelvic wall and/or hydronephrosis or nonfunctioning kidney
Stage IV	The carcinoma has extended beyond the true pelvis or has involved (biopsy proven) the mucosa of the bladder or rectum. A bullous oedema of the bladder, as such, does not permit a case to be allotted to stage IV
IVA	Spread of the growth to adjacent organs
IVB	Spread to distant organs, including peritoneal spread, supraclavicular, mediastinal, para-aortic nodes, lung, liver or bone

FIGO, International Federation of Gynecology and Obstetrics.
*All macroscopically visible lesions are allotted to stage IB.

The standard staging procedure includes the following (accepted by FIGO):

- Per speculum, bimanual pelvic and rectal examination to assess size of tumour, vaginal extension and parametrial invasion are mandatory.
- Cervical biopsy, endocervical curettage or conization is required for confirmation of diagnosis, if not clinically obvious.
- Preoperative colposcopy in early stage disease helps in identifying CIN III changes in the upper vagina, which determines the size of the vaginal cuff to be removed.
- Cystoscopy and proctoscopy are performed in all women with advanced disease for extension to bladder and rectum. Hysteroscopy is used to detect extension to uterus and in endocervical lesions.
- Intravenous pyelography (IVP) is used to detect hydroureteronephrosis and chest X-ray for lung metastasis.

Other modalities used to determine extent of disease

Accurate assessment of parametrial infiltration, nodal metastasis, tumour volume and distant metastasis is not possible by clinical staging alone. Other modalities are, therefore, used in many centres when these are available. Imaging, especially magnetic resonance imaging (MRI), is encouraged for pretreatment evaluation and planning the appropriate management. However, it should be remembered that the results of these tests **do not alter the FIGO staging**. Once assigned, the stage remains the same.

The modalities used are listed in Table 29.3.

- IVP is necessary in women with clinical parametrial infiltration. When ureteric obstruction is diagnosed, the disease is upstaged to stage III even if parametrial disease does not extend to pelvic side wall. As already mentioned, this can be used in FIGO staging. Most centres now use computed tomography (CT) or MRI for evaluation of urinary tract.
- Transvaginal ultrasonography may be helpful in identifying bulky disease that is not clinically obvious (endophytic). Disease extension to uterine corpus, pyometra, associated gynaecological pathology such as myoma or ovarian cyst can also be diagnosed by ultrasonography (Fig. 29.8).

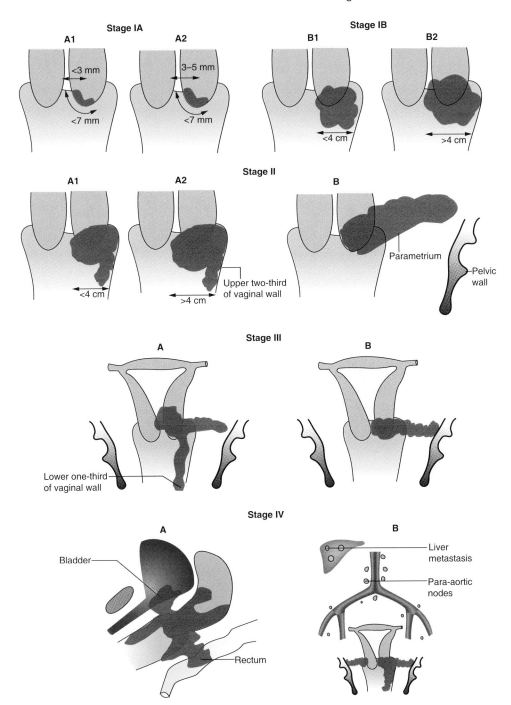

Figure 29.7 FIGO staging of cervical cancer. **Stage IA1:** Stromal invasion <3 mm depth and <7 mm horizontal extension. **Stage IA2:** Stromal invasion 3–5 mm depth and <7 mm horizontal extension. **Stage IB1:** Visible lesion <4 cm in greatest dimension. **Stage IB2:** Visible lesion >4 cm in greatest dimension. **Stage IIA1:** Extension to upper 2/3rd of vagina, <4 cm in greatest dimension. Stage IIA2: Extension to upper 2/3rd of vagina, >4 cm in greatest dimension. **Stage IIB:** Extension to parametrium but not up to pelvic wall. **Stage IIIA:** Extension to lower third of vagina. **Stage IIIB:** Extension to pelvic wall. **Stage IVA:** Spread to adjacent organs (bladder and rectum). **Stage IVB:** Distant metastasis to para-aortic nodes and liver. *FIGO*, International Federation of Gynecology and Obstetrics.

Table 29.3 Other modalities for staging

Test	Uses
Imaging	
Ultrasonography	• Tumour volume, hydroure-teronephrosis
	• Liver metastasis
	• Associated gynaecological pathology
CT scan	• Lymph node metastasis
	• Hydroureteronephrosis
	• Hepatic and other distant metastasis
MRI	• Parametrial infiltration
	• Lymph node metastasis
	• Tumour volume
	• Hydroureteronephrosis
	• Vaginal extension
PET scan	• Lymph node metastasis
	• Other metastasis
PET/CT	Lymph node metastasis
Procedures	
Flexible sigmoidos-copy	Large bowel involvement
Sentinel node biopsy	Lymph node involvement

CT, computed tomography; *MRI*, magnetic resonance imaging; *PET*, positron emission tomography.

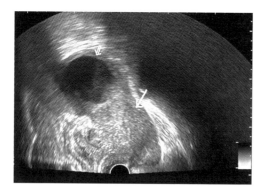

Figure 29.8 Transvaginal ultrasonogram showing a large growth in the cervix (arrow) and uterus with pyometra (double arrow).

- CT scan is useful for visualization of enlarged lymph nodes, liver, urinary tract and skeletal metastasis (Fig. 29.9). The primary lesion in the cervix can also be visualized, but parametrial infiltration cannot be accurately assessed.
- MRI is the imaging modality of choice in women with early stage disease where there

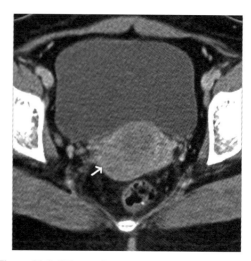

Figure 29.9 CT scan shows the cervix expanded with growth. Parametrial infiltration is not clearly evident. *CT*, computed tomography.

is suspicion of parametrial infiltration (Fig. 29.10). It can identify nodes <1 cm in size, tumour volume, parametrial extension, extension to uterine corpus and vagina more accurately and has a higher sensitivity.
- Positron emission tomography (PET) identifies microscopic metastasis in nodes. This is especially useful for evaluation of para-aortic nodes for extended-field radiation.
- Sentinel node biopsy for detection of micro-metastasis is being evaluated. Studies have found it to be more sensitive than imaging.
- Sigmoidoscopy may be performed in women with large tumours with extensive metastasis. However, with increasing use of MRI, sigmoidoscopy, cystoscopy and IVP are used much less often now.

Surgical staging

Since prediction of para-aortic lymph node metastasis is not accurate with clinical staging, surgical staging has been resorted to in clinically advanced disease. This may be performed laparoscopically or by laparotomy (Box 29.5). When nodal metastasis is present, this may be debulked, and extended-field radiation may be given. The benefit of surgical staging when MRI and PET/CT scan are available is controversial. Surgical staging is not recommended as a routine.

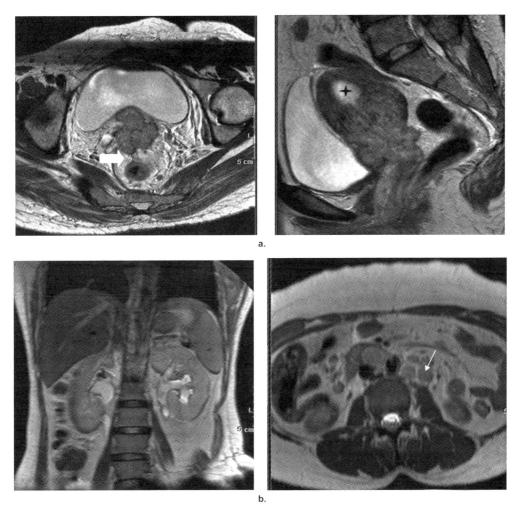

Figure 29.10 MR images of cervical cancer stage IVB. **a.** T2 axial and sagittal images of the pelvis. Mass in the cervix infiltrates the mesorectum (arrow) and the lower uterine body with mild hydrometra (asterisk). Bilateral parametrial infiltration and shortening also present. **b.** T2 coronal section in the same patient, showing bilateral hydroureteronephrosis on. T2 axial section shows multiple para-aortic nodes (arrow). *MR*, magnetic resonance.

Box 29.5 Surgical staging in cervical cancer

- Purpose
  - To identify lymph node metastasis
  - To debulk nodal disease
- Route
  - Laparoscopy
  - Laparotomy
    - Transperitoneal
    - Extraperitoneal
- Disadvantages
  - Bowel complications

Tumour markers

Serum SCC antigen is elevated in squamous cell cancer of the cervix. Its role is being evaluated especially in early stage disease, to decide on adjuvant radiation.

Clinical features

Cervical cancer usually occurs in multiparous women between 35 and 65 years of age, mean age being 38 in India. Many women with early stage disease are asymptomatic.

Symptoms

Classic symptom of cervical cancer is abnormal uterine bleeding, which may be intermenstrual, postmenopausal or, in sexually active women, postcoital bleeding. When the growth enlarges and fungates, foul-smelling vaginal discharge is common. Occasionally, uncontrolled bleeding occurs when the ulcerative growth erodes a vessel. Vaginal discharge is also a common symptom. Discharge may be bloodstained and/ or foul-smelling in case of fungating infected growth. Advanced disease that infiltrates the nerves can give rise to pelvic pain and pain radiating down the sciatic nerve distribution. Obstruction to lymphatics and veins causes pedal oedema. When tumour infiltrates the bladder or rectum, fistulae may form, giving rise to urinary or faecal incontinence. The symptoms are listed in Box 29.6.

Signs

Characteristic signs of cervical cancer are listed in Box 29.7. The cervical lesion may be exophytic, endophytic or ulcerative. The tumour is very vascular and bleeds on touch during speculum examination and bimanual examination.

Box 29.6 Symptoms of cervical cancer

- Asymptomatic
- Cachexia
- Abnormal uterine bleeding
  - Intermenstrual bleeding
  - Postmenopausal bleeding
  - Postcoital bleeding
  - Continuous bleeding
  - Uncontrolled profuse bleeding
- Vaginal discharge
  - Foul-smelling
  - Bloodstained
- Pain
  - Pelvic pain
  - Low back pain
  - Pain radiating down the posterior thigh
- Pedal oedema
- Urinary symptoms
  - Haematuria
  - Urinary incontinence
- Faecal incontinence

Box 29.7 Signs in cervical cancer

- Cervical lesion
  - Exophytic growth
    - Cauliflower-shaped
    - Fungating
    - Bleeding on touch
    - Friable
    - Fixed
    - Indurated
  - Endophytic growth
    - Barrel-shaped, hard
  - Ulcerative lesion
    - Ulcer, induration
- Vaginal extension of tumour
- Uterus
  - Normal/enlarged
  - Tender in case of pyometra
- Parametrial infiltration

Exophytic tumours are also friable and tumour tissue may be found on the examining finger. Parametrial infiltration can be felt on rectal examination. Uterus is usually normal in size, and may be uniformly enlarged and tender when there is pyometra. This is seen in postmenopausal women or when the growth is endophytic, obstructing the cervical canal.

Clinical evaluation

History

Cervical cancer is almost always a clinical diagnosis, confirmed by biopsy. The purpose of clinical evaluation is to make a diagnosis, stage the disease and plan management. Clinical evaluation starts with history, which should focus on all relevant details (Box 29.8).

Physical examination

A thorough physical examination including general, systemic and pelvic examination, as given in Box 29.9, is mandatory. Clinical staging should also be completed during physical examination.

Diagnosis

- Pap smear is not necessary when an obvious growth is visible. **Biopsy** is the first step. A

- Age
  - 35–65, mean age 38
- Parity
  - Multipara
- Loss of appetite and weight
- Past history
  - Age at first intercourse
  - Multiple sexual partners
  - STIs, immunosuppression, COC use
- Symptoms
  - Instrumental/postcoital/postmenopausal bleeding
  - Discharge, pain
  - Other symptoms as listed in Box 29.6

COC, combined oral contraceptive; *STI*, sexually transmitted infection.

Box 29.9 **Physical examination in cervical cancer**

- General examination
  - Cachexia
  - Pallor
  - Pedal oedema
  - Supraclavicular and inguinal nodes
- Systemic examination
  - Pulmonary metastasis
- Abdominal examination
  - Enlarged uterus, tenderness
  - Ascites
  - Hepatomegaly
- Speculum examination
  - Growth on the cervix
    - Type—Exophytic/endophytic/ulcerative
    - Bleeding on touch
    - Friability
    - Fixity/induration
  - Vaginal extension
  - Rectal examination
    - Parametrial infiltration
    - Rectal mucosa
  - Rectovaginal examination
    - Infiltration of rectovaginal septum

punch biopsy should be taken from the edge of the lesion to avoid necrotic tissue, using a cervical punch biopsy forceps (Fig. 29.11).
- If a lesion is not visible as in stage I disease and the woman is being evaluated for abnormal cytology, colposcopy and directed biopsy or cone biopsy is required. Indications for

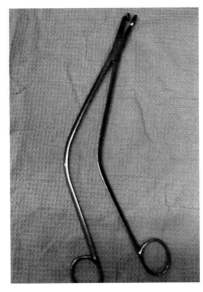

Figure 29.11 Cervical punch biopsy forceps. This is used to take a biopsy from the growth on the cervix.

cone biopsy are discussed in Chapter 28, *Premalignant diseases of the cervix.*
- An expanded barrel-shaped cervix with endophytic lesion indicates the need for an endocervical curettage as well.

Management

Pretreatment evaluation

In women with early disease, parametrial infiltration and vaginal extension are usually assessed by clinical examination. If there is a doubt regarding parametrial infiltration, MRI is useful. Ultrasonography should be performed when there is uterine/adnexal enlargement. In case of suspicious nodes on MRI, PET is used to exclude nodal disease.

All women with clinically advanced disease require MRI or cystoscopy, proctoscopy and IVP. If clinical staging indicated advanced disease (IIB or more) and chemoradiation is planned, complete blood count, liver and renal function tests should be ordered. MRI/CT scan/PET is performed in selected cases to assess para-aortic node metastasis.

Pretreatment evaluation is summarized in Box 29.10.

Treatment

The two main modalities of treatment are **surgery** and **radiotherapy**. Surgery is limited to early stage disease, but radiotherapy can be used in all stages.

Treatment of early stage disease

Stage IA

Stage IA1

- *Microinvasive carcinoma:* Invasive carcinoma that can be diagnosed only by microscopy is staged as IA. It is also called **preclinical carcinoma**. Stage IA1 has a depth of invasion of <3 mm and breadth of <7 mm.
- Women with microinvasive cancer are asymptomatic and are diagnosed during evaluation of abnormal cytology. **Conization** is mandatory for diagnosis of microinvasive carcinoma.
- The incidence of pelvic lymph node metastasis in this stage is 0.5–1%. Therefore, the recommended treatment is simple hysterectomy. Vaginal cuff should be removed if colposcopy shows intraepithelial changes at the upper vagina.
- Conization is sufficient in young women desirous of further childbearing, provided the cone margins are free.

Stage IA2

- Tumours with a depth of invasion of 3–5 mm and breadth of <7 mm are staged as stage IA2.

The reported incidence of pelvic node metastasis is about 7%. Local recurrences occur in 2.9–3.4%.
- The recommended surgery is modified radical hysterectomy (type II hysterectomy) and pelvic lymphadenectomy.
- Women who wish to preserve fertility may be treated with radical trachelectomy and laparoscopic pelvic lymphadenectomy.

Women with stage IA disease who are not candidates for surgery due to severe comorbidities may be treated by radiotherapy.

Management of stage IA cervical cancer is given in Fig. 29.12.

Stages IB and IIA

Stage IB tumours are still confined to the uterus. When the tumour is <4 cm, it is staged as IB1, and when >4 cm, as IB2. Stage IIA are cancers with vaginal extension to upper two-third but no parametrial infiltration, subdivided into IIA1 when the tumour is <4 cm and IIA2 when >4 cm.

Treatment options for stages IB1 and IIA1 are similar and are discussed together in the following. Stage IB2 and IIA2 diseases have higher incidence of pelvic node metastasis and recurrence rate and will be discussed later.

Stages IB1 and IIA1

Women with stage IB1 and IIA1 diseases can be treated by radical hysterectomy (type III) with pelvic lymphadenectomy (Wertheim hysterectomy) or radiotherapy since both have the same cure rate. Oophorectomy is not essential in cervical cancer since ovarian metastasis occurs only in 0.5% of women. Advantages and disadvantages of both modalities of treatment have to be considered before making a decision.

In young women who desire fertility, have stage IB1 disease and in whom the tumour is <2 cm in size, radical trachelectomy and pelvic lymphadenectomy can be performed. Several successful pregnancies have been reported after this procedure, but cervical incompetence is a known complication.

Advantages and disadvantages of radical surgery and radiotherapy Intraoperative and postoperative complications such as haemorrhage, ureteric and vascular injury, infection and thromboembolism are more with surgery. Radiotherapy is associated with more long-term bowel and bladder problems, which occur in about 8% of patients. Vaginal shortening and

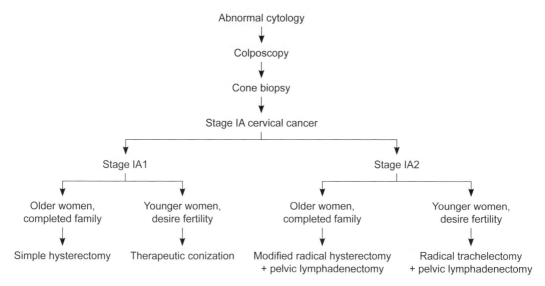

Figure 29.12 Management of stage IA cervical cancer.

stenosis that occur following radiation give rise to dyspareunia and coital difficulties. Advantages and disadvantages of radical surgery and radiotherapy are given in Table 29.4.

Table 29.4 Advantages and disadvantages of radical surgery and radiotherapy	
Radical surgery	**Radiotherapy**
Ovaries can be preserved	Ovaries are irradiated Partial preservation with transposition
No vaginal narrowing/ shortening	Vaginal stenosis common
Sexual function can be preserved	Dyspareunia/difficulty in coitus common
More immediate complications • Haemorrhage • Ureteric injury • Vascular injury • Thromboembolism • Infection • Lymphocyst formation	Very few immediate complications • Nausea, vomiting • Diarrhoea
Few late complications	More late complications • Radiation proctitis • Radiation cystitis • Vaginal stenosis • Fistula formation
Difficult in women with comorbidities • Obesity • Ischaemic heart disease • Poor functional status	Indicated in women with comorbidities

Criteria for decision making in stages IB1 and IIA1

Surgery is the treatment of choice in premenopausal or immediate postmenopausal women with tumours <4 cm, with no associated medical complications. Older, obese women with associated medical complications are treated with radiotherapy. If radiotherapy is decided upon, chemotherapy is administered concomitantly (chemoradiation).

Factors that are taken into account for decision making regarding surgery/radiotherapy are listed in Box 29.11.

Box 29.11 Criteria for decision making in stages IB1 and IIA1
• Age • Menopausal status • Stage of disease • Size of tumour (<4 cm) • Comorbidities   – Obesity   – Poor functional status   – Older age   – Uncontrolled diabetes/hypertension

Stages IB2 and IIA2

Tumours >4 cm in size have a higher incidence of lymph node metastasis and a higher chance of local, regional and distant recurrences. Although several modalities of treatment have been considered, concurrent chemotherapy with radiation (chemoradiation), similar to advanced stage disease, is the treatment of choice in these patients.

Treatment of advanced disease

Stages IIB–IVA

These are referred to as advanced stage disease since the disease has extended to the parametrium and adjacent organs. Choice of treatment is radiation therapy with concomitant chemotherapy (chemoradiation). Survival rates are low and recurrence rates are high in this group of patients.

Stage III

The management of stage III is same as that of stages IIB–IVA.

Stage IVB

This stage has a poor prognosis due to distant metastasis. Palliative radiotherapy and/or palliative chemotherapy should be used to treat these women.

Treatment of stages IB–IV is summarized in Box 29.12.

Box 29.12 Treatment of cervical cancer stages IB–IV

- Stage IB1　　Radical hysterectomy with pelvic lymphadenectomy *or* chemoradiation
- Stage IB2　　Chemoradiation
- Stage IIA1　 Radical hysterectomy with pelvic lymphadenectomy *or* chemoradiation
- Stage IIA2　 Chemoradiation
- Stage III　　 Chemoradiation
- Stage IVA　　Chemoradiation
- Stage IVB　　Palliative radiation *or* palliative chemotherapy

---

Surgical procedures

Hysterectomy

Simple hysterectomy (type I) This is also called extrafascial hysterectomy. The uterus and cervix

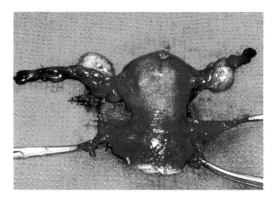

Figure 29.13 A specimen removed by radical hysterectomy; uterus, cervix, tubes, ovaries and parametria are seen.

are removed along with the fascia covering the anterior surface of the uterus and cervix, but not the parametrium or paracervical tissue.

Modified radical hysterectomy (type II) This is otherwise known as extended hysterectomy. The uterus, cervix and cuff of the vagina are removed along with the parametrium and paracervical tissue medial to ureters. The uterine artery is ligated where it crosses the ureter, the ureter is deroofed in the cardinal ligament and retracted laterally and the parametrium up to that point is removed.

Radical hysterectomy (type III) The uterus, cervix, cuff of the vagina, parametria up to the pelvic sidewall and paracervical tissue are removed. The uterine artery is ligated at its origin from the internal iliac, the ureters are dissected and mobilized to enable the removal of the entire parametria and paracolpos (Fig. 29.13).

The three types of hysterectomies are shown in Fig. 29.14.

Pelvic lymphadenectomy

This involves removal of parametrial nodes, obturator, internal iliac, external iliac, sacral and common iliac nodes (Fig. 29.15).

Nerve-sparing radical hysterectomy

Bladder, bowel and sexual dysfunctions are common following radical hysterectomy. Careful dissection of uterosacrals and parametrium to preserve the hypogastric plexus to avoid these complications is known as nerve-sparing radical hysterectomy.

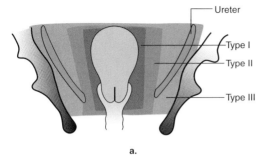

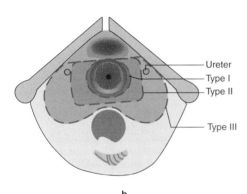

Figure 29.14 Diagrammatic representation of the types of hysterectomy. a. Frontal view. b. Cross-sectional view. The innermost line indicates type I, the middle line type II and the outer line type III.

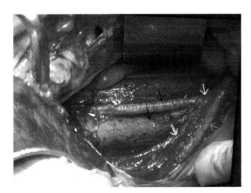

Figure 29.15 Pelvic lymphadenectomy. The external iliac artery (black arrow), vein (black double arrow), bifurcation of common iliac artery (white arrow) and internal iliac artery (white double arrow). The ureter is seen crossing the common iliac at its bifurcation (blue arrow).

Complications of radical hysterectomy

The intraoperative and postoperative complications are listed in Box 29.13.

Box 29.13 Complications of radical hysterectomy

- Intraoperative
  - Haemorrhage
  - Injury to
    - Blood vessels
    - Ureter
    - Bladder
    - Bowel
    - Obturator nerves
- Postoperative
  - Immediate
    - Haemorrhage
    - Infection
      - Peritonitis
      - Urinary tract infection
    - Paralytic ileus
    - Atelectasis/pneumonia
    - Venous thrombosis
    - Embolism
    - Urinary fistulas
  - Late
    - Bladder dysfunction
    - Sexual dysfunction
    - Lymphedema

Radical trachelectomy

This involves the removal of cervix almost up to the internal os along with the paracervical tissue (Fig. 29.16).

- The surgery can be performed vaginally or abdominally, although vaginal route is the preferred route.

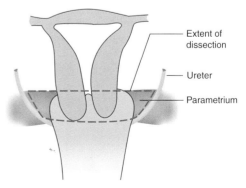

Figure 29.16 Diagrammatic representation of radical trachelectomy. Ectocervix and parametrium medial to ureter are removed (indicated by dotted line).

- The ureters are deroofed and the paracervical tissue medial to the ureter is removed on both sides along with the cervix. The uterus is reattached to the vagina.
- Lymphadenectomy is performed laparoscopically. Women who undergo this procedure will need a cerclage during pregnancy.
- Cervical stenosis, miscarriage and preterm labour are the known complications, but successful pregnancies occur in almost 30% of women.
- The criteria for radical trachelectomy are as follows:
  - Young women, desirous of fertility preservation
  - Tumour confined to cervix, <2 cm in size
  - No parametrial invasion (on MRI)

Radiotherapy

Radiotherapy is a common modality of treatment used in management of cervical cancer.
This may be

- Primary chemoradiation
- Postoperative adjuvant radiation

The type of radiation may be

- External radiation
- Intracavitary radiation or brachytherapy

Primary radiation

This is used for stages IB2, IIB2 and all advanced stages. This is also the treatment of choice in women who are not candidates for radical surgery.

- A CT, MRI or PET may be used for planning radiation.
- For calculation of dose of radiation, two points are used (Fig. 29.17).
  - **Point A:** 2 cm above the external os and 2 cm lateral to the cervical canal. Theoretically this corresponds to the point where the uterine artery and ureter cross.
  - **Point B:** 3 cm lateral to point A (5 cm lateral to the cervical canal). This corresponds to the obturator nodes at the pelvic side wall.
- The total dose is 80–85 Gy at point A and 50–65 Gy at point B.
- External radiation delivers uniform dose of radiation to the tumour and entire pelvis. It is administered in fractions, 5 days/week for 5 weeks.

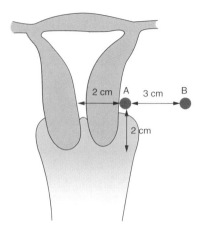

Figure 29.17 Points A and B used in radiotherapy. Point A is 2 cm above the external os and 2 cm lateral to the cervical canal. Point B is 3 cm lateral to point A.

- Intracavitary radiation is delivered using a tandem inserted into the uterus and vaginal ovoids inserted into the vagina (Fig. 29.18). The tandem and ovoids are inserted under anaesthesia and the radioactive source is loaded later.
- Intracavitary radiation delivers maximum dose to the tumour, parametrium and paravaginal tissue, and the radiation diminishes towards the lateral pelvic wall.
- The dose is delivered as follows:
  - Low-dose rates (LDRs) over 36–48 hours using caesium-137 as radioactive source (or)
  - High-dose rates (HDRs) over two to three visits as outpatient treatment using iridium-192 as radioactive source
- External radiation is usually administered first, to shrink the tumour. Intracavitary radiation is administered later.

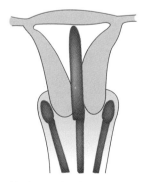

Figure 29.18 Uterine tandem inserted into the uterine cavity and vaginal ovoids used for intracavitary radiation.

Adjuvant radiation

This is indicated in women with

- Stromal invasion—Superficial and deep
- LVSI
- Positive surgical margins
- Positive lymph nodes
- Microscopic parametrial involvement

External radiation is used for postoperative adjuvant radiotherapy. A dose of 50 Gy is delivered to the pelvis.

Extended-field radiation

The field of radiation is extended upwards to cover the para-aortic nodes. The complications are more with this because the abdominal structures also receive irradiation. This is required in women with para-aortic node involvement.

Combined modalities

Chemoradiation

Chemoradiation is the concomitant administration of chemotherapy along with radiotherapy. **This is the treatment of choice in cervical cancer.** The synergistic action of the two types of therapies gives better results. Chemotherapy also acts as a radiosensitizer. The drug used is cisplatin 40 mg/m^2, administered weekly for 4 weeks. This has become the standard of care in the treatment of cervical cancer stages IB2 and IIA2–IVA. The schedule of chemoradiation for cervical cancer is given in Box 29.14.

Box 29.14 Chemoradiation for cervical cancer

- Chemotherapy
  - Cisplatin 40 mg/m^2 weekly for 4 weeks
- External radiation
  - Started along with chemotherapy
  - Daily for 5 days/week, total 5 weeks (25 fractions)
- Intracavitary radiation
  - LDR
    - Radioactive source: Caesium-137
    - Duration: 36–48 hours
  - HDR
    - Radioactive source: Iridium-192
    - Once a week for 2–3 weeks
- Total dose
  - Point A: 80–85 Gy
  - Point B: 55–65 Gy

HDR, high-dose rate; *LDR*, low-dose rate.

Neoadjuvant chemotherapy

Chemotherapy administered before hysterectomy is referred to as neoadjuvant chemotherapy. This shrinks the tumour and makes surgery feasible. This is one of the treatment options in locally advanced cervical cancer, where the tumour is bulky. Neoadjuvant chemotherapy followed by surgery is not superior to chemoradiation.

Prognostic factors

The disease-free and overall survival depends on several prognostic factors. These are listed in Box 29.15.

Box 29.15 Prognostic factors in cervical cancer

- FIGO stage of tumour
- Histological type
- Grade of tumour
- Size of tumours (<4 cm/>4 cm)
- Lymph node metastasis
- LVSI
- Molecular markers
- Age of the patient
- Functional status
- Comorbidities

FIGO, International Federation of Gynecology and Obstetrics; *LVSI*, lymphovascular space invasion.

Survival

Five-year survival for various stages of the disease is given in Table 29.5.

Table 29.5 Five-year survival in cervical cancer

Stage	Five-year survival (%)
IA	95–100
IB	80–88
IIA	64–68
IIB	40–45
III	18–39
IV	14–18

Post-treatment surveillance

Patients should be followed up every 3 months for 3 years, every 6 months for 2 years and yearly thereafter. At each visit, complete clinical evaluation and Pap smear should be performed. Radiological evaluation is required when any abnormality is detected.

Adenocarcinoma

- Adenocarcinomas constitute 15–20% of cervical cancers. They arise from the endocervical glandular epithelium.
- Like the squamous cancers, 70–80% are caused by HPV.
- Macroscopically, they are usually endophytic growths and the ectocervix may look normal. Pelvic and rectal examination reveals a ballooned-out cervix. Adenocarcinomas can also present as exophytic growths similar to squamous cell cancer.
- Microscopically, several histological variants are known to occur, but they are rare.
- Microinvasive adenocarcinomas are defined as adenocarcinomas with depth of invasion <5 mm. The lesions can be multifocal, and, therefore, hysterectomy is recommended.
- Adenocarcinomas were believed to be more radioresistant than squamous cell cancers, but studies have shown that when treatment is the same as for squamous cell cancers, the survival is similar.
- Therefore, adenocarcinomas are currently treated the same way as squamous cell cancers, stage for stage.

Cervical cancer in pregnancy

Cervical cancer is the most common gynaecological cancer in pregnancy. The foetus has to be taken into consideration while making decisions regarding diagnostic and therapeutic procedures. Also, some complications of

Table 29.6 Safety and complications of procedures in cervical cancer in pregnancy

Procedure	Safety/complications
Diagnosis	
Colposcopy	Safe
Biopsy	Increased bleeding
Endocervical curettage	Rupture of membranes
Conization	Increased risk of miscarriage
Imaging	
Ultrasonography	Safe
CT scan	Foetal radiation
MRI	Safe
Treatment	
Surgery	Increased bleeding
Radiotherapy	• Abortion • Foetal death
Chemotherapy	• Abortion • Congenital malformations • Foetal death

CT, computed tomography; *MRI*, magnetic resonance imaging.

surgical intervention are more when the woman is pregnant. Vaginal bleeding may be the presenting symptom or the diagnosis may be made by routine cervical cytological screening. The safety and complications of procedures used for diagnosis and treatment in pregnant women are listed in Table 29.6.

CIN needs colposcopic evaluation. High-grade squamous intraepithelial lesion (HSIL) can be followed up with repeat colposcopy. Cone biopsy and further management are deferred till postpartum period. Punch biopsy may be performed if invasive cancer is suspected.

Management of invasive cancer in pregnancy is depicted in Fig. 29.19. Chemoradiation in early pregnancy results in foetal death and spontaneous expulsion. Close to term, classical caesarean section is recommended since vaginal delivery and lower segment section are associated with more blood loss. Vaginal delivery is also associated with a higher risk of recurrence of tumour and episiotomy site metastasis.

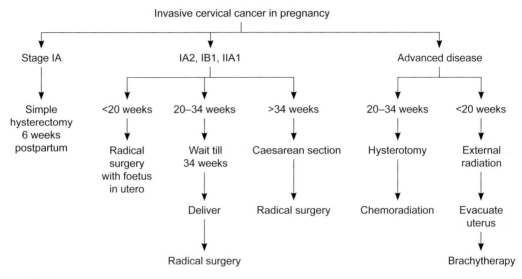

Figure 29.19 Management of invasive cancer in pregnancy.

Key points

- Cervical cancer is the second most common cancer in women worldwide and the most common cancer in India and in other developing countries.

- The risk factors are the same as those for cervical intraepithelial neoplasia.

- Human papillomavirus (HPV) infection is causative in most cases of cervical cancer. The HPV genome integrates into the cervical cell genome and causes malignant change.

- Macroscopically, the cancer may be exophytic, endophytic or ulcerative. Exophytic growth is most common and has atypical cauliflower-like appearance and bleeds on touch.

- Squamous cell carcinoma comprises 80–85% of all cervical cancers and 15–20% are adenocarcinomas.

- Cervical cancer spreads by direct spread, lymphatic spread and haematogenous spread.

- Staging of cervical cancer is clinical and is as recommended by International Federation of Gynecology and Obstetrics (FIGO) in 2008.

- Imaging and other procedures cannot be used to modify staging.

- Predominant symptoms of cervical cancer are abnormal uterine bleeding in the form of intermenstrual bleeding, postcoital bleeding or postmenopausal bleeding and vaginal discharge. Classic signs are growth, bleeding on touch, friability and fixity.

- Diagnosis is by history, physical examination and biopsy. Pretreatment evaluation includes imaging and other investigations depending on the stage of the disease.

- Treatment of microinvasive carcinoma is by therapeutic conization or simple hysterectomy depending on the age of the patient and desire for fertility.

- Stage IA2 is treated by modified radical hysterectomy and pelvic lymphadenectomy.

- Stages 1B1 and IIA1 can be treated with radical hysterectomy and pelvic lymphadenectomy or chemoradiation.

- Stages IB2 and IIA2 are treated with chemoradiation since nodal metastasis and recurrence rates are higher when tumour is >4 cm in size.

- Stages IIB, III and IV are treated with chemoradiation.

- Primary radiotherapy is usually given as combination of intracavitary and external radiations.

- Five-year survival is 95–100% in stage IA but drops to 14–18% in stage IV.

- Cervical cancer is the most common gynaecological cancer in pregnancy. Treatment depends on the stage of disease and gestational age.

Self-assessment

Case-based questions

Case 1

A 40-year-old lady presents with postcoital bleeding. Her body mass index is 26 and she has no other medical problem.

1. What details will you ask for in history?
2. How will you evaluate this lady?
3. If the diagnosis is cervical cancer stage IB1, what is the management?

Case 2

A 52-year-old lady presents with postmenopausal bleeding. Examination reveals stage IIB cervical cancer.

1. How will you proceed to evaluate her?
2. What is the management?
3. How will you administer radiotherapy?

Answers

Case 1

1. (a) History—Parity, age at marriage, multiple sexual partners, contraception, history of STDs
   (b) Duration of symptoms, history of intermenstrual bleeding, vaginal discharge, pelvic pain, low backache
2. (a) Physical examination—General examination (pallor, supraclavicular/inguinal nodes, pedal oedema)
   (b) Abdominal examination—Uterine mass, tenderness
   (c) Speculum examination—Growth, characteristics of the growth—Bleeding on touch, friability, induration, size of the growth, vaginal extension
   (d) Bimanual pelvic examination—Uterine size, vaginal involvement
   (e) Rectal examination—Parametrial infiltration
   (f) Investigations—Punch biopsy from the no-necrotic area of the growth

3. Since she has early stage disease—Haemoglobin, blood sugar, creatinine, chest X-ray, MRI to exclude parametrial invasion, if in doubt.

   Since she is young, has stage IB1 disease and has no comorbidities—Radical hysterectomy and pelvic lymphadenectomy with preservation of ovary.

Case 2

1. (a) History—Duration of symptoms, amount of bleeding, vaginal discharge
   (b) Examination—Pallor, supraclavicular/inguinal nodes, hepatomegaly, size of the growth, vaginal extension, parametrial infiltration
   (c) Investigations—Punch biopsy from the margin of the growth, IVP to exclude ureteric obstruction, chest X-ray, complete blood count, creatinine, liver function tests, blood sugar
2. Since the stage of the disease is IIB, treatment is chemoradiation.
3. Chemoradiation—External radiation 5 days/week for 5 weeks along with cisplatin 40 mg/m^2 weekly for 4 weeks followed by intracavitary irradiation by LDR for 36–48 hours. Total dose to point A, 85 Gy and to point B, 65 Gy.

Long-answer questions

1. What are the clinical features of carcinoma cervix? Discuss the staging of cervical cancer and outline the management of stage IB of carcinoma cervix.
2. Discuss the aetiology, clinical features and management of carcinoma cervix.

Short-answer questions

1. FIGO staging of carcinoma cervix
2. Clinical features of cervical cancer
3. Management of stage IA cervical cancer
4. Radiotherapy in cervical cancer

30 | Premalignant and Malignant Diseases of the Uterus

Case scenario

Mrs VK, 65, was a retired college professor, who lived in a metropolitan city and spent 6 months in a year with her only daughter in the United States. She was a diabetic for 10 years and hypertensive, and had dyslipidaemia. She was also obese, with a body mass index (BMI) of 42. (She weighed 110 kg.) She was advised weight reduction, diet, exercises and lifestyle modification, none of which she followed. She noticed small amount of vaginal bleeding 1 month ago but ignored it. The bleeding recurred, was moderate in quantity this time, and she came for evaluation to the hospital.

Introduction

Premalignant diseases of the endometrium occur in perimenopausal or even younger women, but about 10% of postmenopausal women with bleeding have endometrial cancer. Postmenopausal bleeding, therefore, is always a cause for concern. The bleeding occurs most often due to some pathology in the genital tract and endometrial cancer must be excluded. The disease, if diagnosed early, has a good prognosis.

Premalignant disease of the uterus

Complex endometrial hyperplasia with atypia is considered a premalignant lesion since it can precede or occur along with endometrial carcinoma.

Endometrial hyperplasia

Endometrial hyperplasia is characterized by proliferation of the endometrial glands. It results from excess or unopposed oestrogen action on the endometrium.

Incidence

Global incidence of endometrial hyperplasia is 130/100,000 women years. Exact incidence in India is not known. The incidence is increasing due to increase in obesity.

Risk factors

Endometrial hyperplasia can occur with chronic anovulatory cycles in young women and perimenopausal women. In postmenopausal women, it can occur with unopposed oestrogen therapy, oestrogen-secreting tumours or tamoxifen therapy. Risk factors for endometrial hyperplasia are the same as those for endometrial carcinoma (Box 30.1).

Box 30.1 Risk factors for endometrial hyperplasia

- Chronic anovulation
- Polycystic ovarian syndrome
- Obesity
- Unopposed oestrogen therapy
- Tamoxifen therapy
- Oestrogen-secreting tumours of the ovary
- Lynch syndrome

Classification

Based on the natural history of the lesions, cytological and architectural features, the World Health Organization (WHO) has classified endometrial hyperplasia as given in Table 30.1.

Table 30.1 Classification of endometrial hyperplasia

Type of hyperplasia	Progression to cancer (%)
Simple hyperplasia without atypia	1
Complex hyperplasia without atypia	3
Simple hyperplasia with atypia	8
Complex hyperplasia with atypia	29

Microscopic features

The microscopic features of endometrial hyperplasia are described in Table 30.2. The features are shown in Figs 30.1 and 30.2.

Clinical features

The peak incidence of endometrial hyperplasia is between ages 40 and 55. Simple hyperplasia is more common than hyperplasia with atypia. Young women with hyperplastic endometrium present with periods of amenorrhoea followed by prolonged and profuse bleeding. Perimenopausal women present with a

Table 30.2 Microscopic features of endometrial hyperplasia

Type of hyperplasia	Microscopic features	
	Glands	Stroma
Simple without atypia	Increased, cystically dilated	Abundant
Complex without atypia	Closely packed, complex pattern	Scanty
General features of atypia	• Increased nuclear/cytoplasmic ratio • Irregular shape and size of nuclei • Loss of polarity	
Simple with atypia	• Cystically dilated	Abundant
Complex with atypia	• Closely packed, crowding, complex pattern • Features of atypia	Scanty

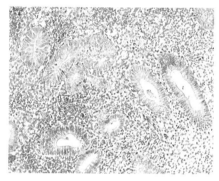

Figure 30.1 Photomicrograph showing endometrium with complex hyperplasia without atypia. There is crowding of glands with back-to-back arrangement but no nuclear/cytoplasmic changes.

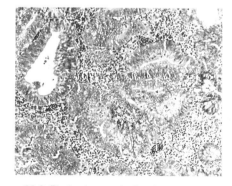

Figure 30.2 Photomicrograph showing endometrium with complex hyperplasia with atypia. The hyperplastic changes are more pronounced with marked crowding of glands. In addition, there are nuclear stratification and mitoses, which are characteristics of atypia.

similar history and older women present with postmenopausal bleeding.

Diagnosis

Endometrial hyperplasia may be suspected in women with a typical history. Vaginal ultrasound

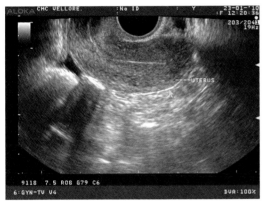

a.

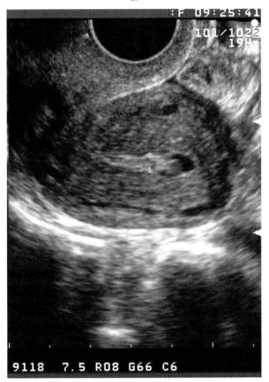

b.

Figure 30.3 Transvaginal ultrasonographic pictures of (a) a postmenopausal woman showing normal, thin, atrophic endometrium, thickness 2 mm; and (b) a woman with postmenopausal bleeding showing endometrial thickness of 9 mm indicating endometrial hyperplasia.

reveals thickened endometrium (Fig. 30.3). Final diagnosis is by histological examination of endometrial tissue, obtained by endometrial sampling or curettage. Methods of evaluation of the endometrium are discussed later in this chapter.

Management

Management depends on the type of hyperplasia and the age of the patient (Fig. 30.4).

- Progestins, given in high doses, are effective in reversing hyperplastic changes with or without atypia.
- Hyperplasia without atypia at all ages is treated with progestin therapy. Medroxyprogesterone acetate (MPA), combined oral contraceptive pills, micronized progesterone or levonorgestrel intrauterine system (LNG-IUS) may be used.
- Duration of treatment is 6 months. Endometrial biopsy is not required to assess response.
- Hyperplasia with atypia is usually complex. Associated carcinoma may be present in 40% of women. If this is diagnosed on endometrial sampling, a curettage should be performed before proceeding with treatment.
- Hysterectomy is the treatment of choice in women who have completed family.
- In younger women, desirous of further childbearing, progestins may be used. MPA, megestrol acetate or LNG-IUS may be used.
- Sampling of the endometrium every 3 months is mandatory to assess response.
- Duration of treatment is 9 months for those with atypia.
- Other drugs such as aromatase inhibitors, gonadotropin-releasing hormone (GnRH) analogues and danazol have been tried in management of endometrial hyperplasia but are not recommended for routine use.

Malignant diseases of the uterus

Malignant diseases of the uterus include endometrial carcinoma and uterine sarcoma.

Endometrial carcinoma

Endometrial cancer is the third most common gynaecological cancer in the developing world where cervical cancer is more common.

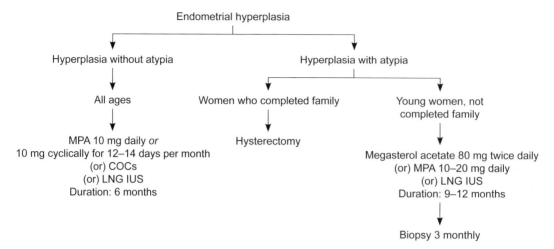

Figure 30.4 Management of endometrial hyperplasia. *COC*, combined oral contraceptive; *LNG-IUS*, levonorgestrel intrauterine system; *MPA*, medroxyprogesterone acetate.

It is primarily a disease of the postmenopausal woman, usually occurring in sixth and seventh decades of life; 75% of cases occur after 50 years of age. The disease has a lower mortality rate than other gynaecological cancers due to early presentation.

Incidence

Globally, the incidence of endometrial cancer is 25.4/100,000 women/year; mortality is 4.5/100,000 women/year. It is 4.5/100,000 women/year in India according to some authors. The prevalence of endometrial cancer is increasing globally due to increase in life expectancy, use of postmenopausal hormone replacement therapy and increase in obesity in the population.

It is predominantly a disease of the older, postmenopausal women. The mean age at diagnosis is 63 years. Majority of the cases occur between 55 and 75 years.

Classification

Endometrial cancers are of two types, type I and type II. The pathogenesis and clinical behaviour are different in the two types of cancers (Table 30.3).

Risk factors

Several risk factors have been identified, the most important being **unopposed oestrogen action on the endometrium** (Box 30.2). Most risk factors act through this mechanism.

Table 30.3 Type I and type II endometrial cancers

Type I	Type II
Grade 1 or 2 endometrioid	Grade 3 endometrioid or nonendometrioid
Constitutes 80%	Constitutes 20%
Occurs in	Occurs in
• Younger women	• Older women
• Caucasian	• Nonwhites
• Nullipara	• Multipara
• Obese	• Nonobese
Oestrogen dependent	Nonoestrogen dependent
COCs and smoking protective	Smoking not protective
Favourable prognosis	Poor prognosis
PTEN, *K-ras* mutations	*p53* mutations

COC, combined oral contraceptive; *PTEN* and *p53*, tumour suppressor genes.

Obesity is a common cause of endogenous oestrogen production. The adrenal androstenedione is aromatized to oestrone in peripheral adipose tissue. Although oestrone is a weak oestrogen when it is unopposed by progesterone as in anovulatory cycles, which are common in obese women, endometrial hyperplasia and carcinoma can occur.

Polycystic ovarian syndrome and **anovulatory infertility** are associated with anovulation and hyperoestrogenic state.

- Age: 55–75 years, mean age 63 years
- Postmenopausal
- Race: Caucasian
- Prolonged/unopposed oestrogen
  - Obesity
  - Nulliparity
  - Polycystic ovarian syndrome
  - Early menarche
  - Late menopause
  - Anovulatory infertility
  - Postmenopausal oestrogen therapy
  - Oestrogen-secreting ovarian tumours
- Tamoxifen therapy
- Diabetes, hypertension
- Hereditary
  - HNPCC syndrome
- Germline mutations
  - *PTEN*
  - *p53*
  - *BRCA1*

HNPCC, hereditary nonpolyposis colorectal cancer; *PTEN p53* and *BRCA1*, tumour suppressor genes.

Nulliparity, **early menarche** and **late menopause** are associated with prolonged, uninterrupted menstrual cycles, which is also a risk factor. Oestrogen-secreting tumours such as granulosa cell tumours and thecoma are rare causes.

Postmenopausal oestrogen replacement therapy is a risk factor; therefore, oestrogen should never be prescribed without progesterone in women with intact uterus.

Tamoxifen, used in postmenopausal women with breast cancer, has an oestrogenic effect on the endometrium and can cause endometrial polyp, hyperplasia and carcinoma. Routine screening with vaginal ultrasound is not recommended since tamoxifen causes subepithelial stromal hypertrophy and, therefore, increases endometrial thickness. But when bleeding occurs in women on tamoxifen, they should be evaluated.

Diabetes and **hypertension** are known risk factors presumably because of their association with obesity and increased peripheral oestrone production.

Hereditary factors play a role as well. Women with Lynch II syndrome [hereditary nonpolyposis colorectal cancer (HNPCC)] and those with germline mutations (*PTEN*, *p53*) and *BRCA1* are also at an increased risk.

Screening

Routine screening for endometrial cancer is not cost-effective and is not recommended.

Only 50% of endometrial cancers have malignant cells in Pap smear. Therefore, this cannot be used as a screening test.

Presence of normal endometrial cells in Pap smear in postmenopausal women (not on hormone therapy) warrants further evaluation. However, normal endometrial cells, which are usually reported on cytology in asymptomatic premenopausal women >40 years, are of little significance. Abnormal endometrial cells in Pap smear are associated with 25% risk of malignancy.

Screening by transvaginal sonography and endometrial sampling is expensive and is recommended for only high-risk women, such as those with a family history of Lynch II syndrome.

Pathology

Macroscopic appearance

Endometrial cancer may be a malignant polyp or growth in the uterine cavity. It may be seen extending to the cervix or myometrium (Fig. 30.5a and b). Pyometra may be present.

The most common histopathological type is adenocarcinoma. There are several other histological types, listed in Box 30.3.

- Endometrioid adenocarcinoma
  - Variant with squamous differentiation
  - Villoglandular variant
  - Secretory variant
  - Ciliated variant
- Mucinous carcinoma
- Serous carcinoma
- Clear cell carcinoma
- Squamous cell carcinoma
- Mixed cell carcinoma
- Undifferentiated carcinoma

About 80% of the tumours are of the endometrioid type, **type I** (Fig. 30.6). There are variants in this type with squamous differentiation, villoglandular configuration, secretory and ciliary. They behave like endometrioid tumour and have a favourable prognosis. The glands are back

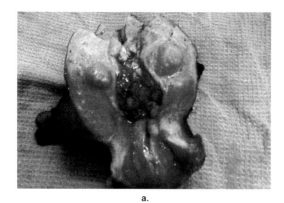

a.

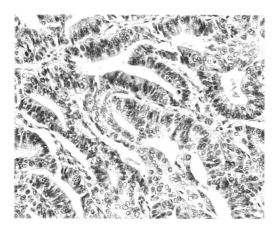

b.

Figure 30.5 Gross appearance of endometrial cancer. a. Growth limited to the cavity with no gross myometrial invasion. b. Large growth filling the cavity, extending to the cervix with myometrial invasion.

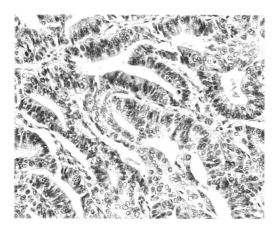

Figure 30.6 Microscopic appearance of endometrial adenocarcinoma. Endometrial glands are lined by cells with increased mitotic activity and pseudostratification of nuclei.

to back with very little stroma. Cells are well differentiated.

Type II cancers include serous carcinomas and clear cell carcinomas. They are high grade and aggressive, and have a poor prognosis.

Serous carcinomas have a papillary architecture with marked nuclear atypia. Clear cell tumours have tubular, papillary or solid architecture. Lymphovascular space invasion (LVSI) and nodal and distant metastasis are frequently seen.

Histological grading

The degree of differentiation is an important pathological feature that determines prognosis and management. The poorer the differentiation, the more is the risk of lymph node metastasis. According to the grading system proposed by International Federation of Gynecology and Obstetrics (FIGO) in 1989, endometrial cancers are divided into three grades (Table 30.4). This grading is applicable to all endometrioid cancers and other tumours of good prognosis.

Table 30.4 Histological grading of endometrial cancer

Grade	Definition
Grade 1 (well differentiated)	<5% of a nonsquamous or nonmorular solid
Grade 2 (moderately differentiated)	6–50% of a nonsquamous or nonmorular solid growth pattern
Grade 3 (poorly differentiated)	>50% of a nonsquamous or nonmorular solid growth pattern

Hormone receptors in endometrial cancer

Oestrogen and progesterone receptors are found in endometrial cancer cells. They are prognostic indicators irrespective of the grade of the tumour. Patients with positive hormone receptors have better survival and respond better to hormone therapy.

Patterns of spread of endometrial cancer

Endometrial cancer is generally slow to spread. It spreads by various routes, as given in Box 30.4.

Box 30.4 Spread of endometrial cancer

- Direct extension
- Lymphatic spread
- Haematogenous spread
- Retrograde transtubal spread

By **direct spread**, endometrial cancer extends into the myometrium and serosa, to the cervix, tubes, broad ligament, bowel, bladder and other pelvic structures.

Lymphatic spread occurs along the uterine vessels to the internal, external and common iliac and para-aortic nodes. Along the branches of the ovarian vessels, the tumour spreads directly to para-aortic nodes. Rarely, it can spread to inguinal nodes via the lymphatics that run along the round ligament.

Haematogenous spread is to lungs, liver, brain, bone and other sites.

Retrograde transtubal spread occurs through the tubes to the peritoneal cavity and ovaries.

Myometrial invasion is an important prognostic factor since lymph node metastasis increases with depth of invasion. In grade 1 tumours with no myometrial invasion, pelvic nodal involvement is seen in 1% of women and para-aortic involvement in <1% of women.

Staging of endometrial cancer

Staging of endometrial cancer is surgical. Clinical staging significantly understages the disease and is used only in women who are not fit for surgery. FIGO staging of endometrial cancer (2009) is given in Table 30.5 (Fig. 30.7).

Clinical features

Symptoms and signs

The most common presentation of endometrial cancer is **postmenopausal bleeding**. Abnormal uterine bleeding in perimenopausal women should always be viewed with suspicion. This may be intermenstrual bleeding, periods of amenorrhea followed by heavy bleeding and frequent menstruation. Symptoms and signs are listed in Box 30.5.

Advanced stages with ovarian metastasis may simulate ovarian malignancy with ascites, hepatomegaly and omental caking.

Clinical evaluation

History

History of conditions causing prolonged oestrogen action and abnormal uterine bleeding in women in postmenopausal age group can raise the clinical suspicion of endometrial cancer in many patients (Box 30.6).

Table 30.5 FIGO staging of carcinoma endometrium (2008)

Stage I	Tumour confined to the corpus uteri
IA G1 2 3	No or less than half myometrial invasion
IB G1 2 3	Invasion equal to or more than half of the myometrium
Stage II G1 2 3	Tumour invades cervical stroma, but does not extend beyond the uterus
Stage III	Local and/or regional spread of the tumour
IIIA G1 2 3	Tumour invades the serosa of the corpus uteri and/or adnexae
IIIB G1 2 3	Vaginal and/or parametrial involvement
IIIC	Metastases to pelvic and/or para-aortic lymph nodes
IIIC1 G1 2 3	Positive pelvic nodes
IIIC2 G1 2 3	Positive para-aortic lymph nodes with or without positive pelvic lymph nodes
Stage IV	Tumour invades bladder and/or bowel mucosa and/or distant metastases
IVA G1 2 3	Tumour invasion of bladder and/or bowel mucosa
IVB G1 2 3	Distant metastases, including intra-abdominal metastases and/or inguinal lymph nodes

FIGO, International Federation of Gynecology and Obstetrics; *G*, histological grade.
Endocervical glandular involvement is considered Stage I.
Positive peritoneal cytology must be reported separately and without changing the stage.

Box 30.5 Symptoms and signs of endometrial carcinoma

- Symptoms
  - Abnormal uterine bleeding
    - Postmenopausal bleeding
    - Intermenstrual bleeding
    - Frequent menstruation
    - Periods of amenorrhoea and heavy bleeding
  - Abnormal vaginal discharge
- Signs
  - Enlarged uterus
  - Tumour
  - Pyometra

Physical examination

This should be done systematically as mentioned in Box 30.7.

The uterus is usually bulky, but a grossly enlarged uterus indicates rapidly growing

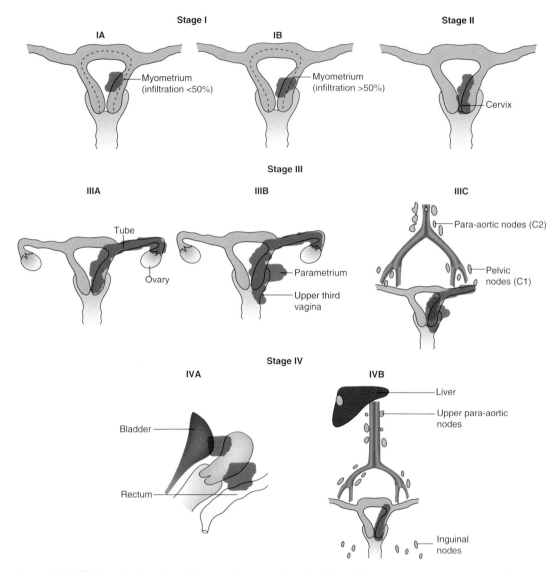

Figure 30.7 FIGO staging of endometrial cancer. **Stage IA:** Growth with <50% myometrial invasion. **Stage IB:** Growth invading >50% myometrium. **Stage II:** Growth invading cervical stroma. **Stage IIIA:** Growth involving serosa of uterus and adnexa. **Stage IIIB:** Tumour extends to vagina and /or parametrium. **Stage IIIC1:** Metastasis to pelvic nodes; C2: Metastasis to para-aortic nodes. **Stage IVA:** Tumour involves the bladder and/or bowel mucosa. **Stage IVB:** Distant metastasis including inguinal nodes. *FIGO,* International Federation of Gynecology and Obstetrics.

undifferentiated tumour such as papillary serous or clear cell carcinoma (Fig. 30.8). Irregular uterine enlargement can be due to associated myomas. Uniformly enlarged uterus that is tender may be filled with pus (pyometra).

Differential diagnosis

Other causes of postmenopausal bleeding are listed in Box 30.8. Benign conditions and

oestrogen therapy are more common causes of bleeding, but in a postmenopausal woman with bleeding, malignancy must be excluded.

Diagnosis

Histopathological examination of biopsy specimen is the gold standard for diagnosis of endometrial cancer. But evaluation usually begins with transvaginal ultrasonography (Box 30.9).

Box 30.6 History in endometrial carcinoma

- Age: >45 years
- Parity: Nulliparous
- Symptoms
- Past history
  - Anovulatory cycles
  - Early menarche
  - Late menopause
- Family history
  - HNPCC
  - Breast cancer
- Medical conditions
  - Diabetes
  - Hypertension
  - Obesity
- Medications
  - Oestrogen therapy
  - Tamoxifen

HNPCC, hereditary nonpolyposis colorectal cancer.

Box 30.7 Physical examination in endometrial carcinoma: General

- Body mass index
- Blood pressure
- Breast examination
- Lymph nodes
  - Inguinal
  - Supraclavicular
- Abdominal examination
  - Uterine enlargement
  - Ascites
  - Hepatomegaly
- Per speculum examination
  - Bleeding
  - Pap smear
- Pelvic examination
  - Uterine enlargement
  - Tenderness
  - Adnexal mass

Box 30.8 Causes of postmenopausal bleeding

- Endometrial cancer
- Cervical cancer
- Oestrogen therapy
- Atrophic endometrium
- Endometrial polyp
- Endometrial hyperplasia
- Atrophic vaginitis
- Oestrogen-producing ovarian tumours
- Sarcomas of the uterus

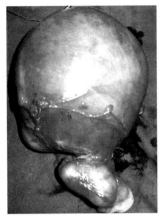

a.

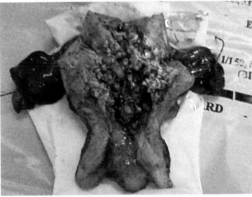

b.

Figure 30.8 Surgical specimen of uterus with endometrial cancer. a. Uniformly enlarged uterus. b. Cut section of the uterus showing the tumour filling the uterus and invading the myometrium.

Box 30.9 Investigations in endometrial carcinoma

- Transvaginal ultrasonography
  - Endometrial thickness
  - Size and shape of the uterus
  - Endometrial polyp
  - Pyometra
  - Ovarian mass
- Sonosalpingography
  - Endometrial polyp and growth
- Endometrial tissue for histology
  - Office biopsy (Pipelle)
  - Dilatation and curettage (fractional)
- Hysteroscopy
  - Growth
  - Polyp

- The initial evaluation of postmenopausal bleeding is much debated. Endometrial biopsy and transvaginal ultrasound are the two main modalities available.

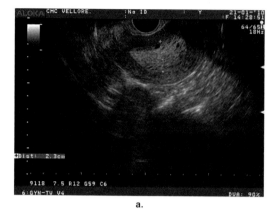

a.

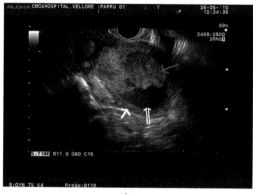

b.

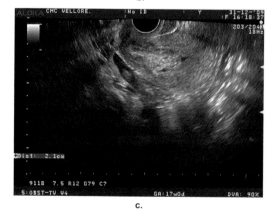

c.

Figure 30.9 Ultrasonographic findings in postmenopausal bleeding. a. Endometrial thickness of 2.3 cm with echogenic tumour in the cavity. b. Uterus enlarged, myometrium thinned out (arrow), large tumour in the cavity (red arrow) and pyometra (double arrow). c. Endometrial thickness of 2.1 cm. The hyperechoic area is surrounded by anechoic rim—Endometrial polyp.

- Most clinicians choose **transvaginal ultrasound** as the first step (Fig. 30.9). An endometrial thickness of >5 mm in postmenopausal women has a sensitivity of 90% and specificity of 50% for diagnosis of endometrial cancer. Endometrial polyps and pyometra can also be diagnosed by ultrasonography.
- If a polyp is found, hysteroscopy and polypectomy may be performed, but if there is a growth or endometrial thickness is >5 mm, fractional dilatation and curettage (D&C) is required.
- **Sonosalpingography** is helpful in women with suspected polyps on ultrasonogram but is not used as a routine in the diagnosis of endometrial cancer.
- **Endometrial sampling** is an outpatient procedure performed using **Pipelle** (Fig. 30.10) or Endocell. Sensitivity of this procedure is 99% and specificity is 98%. But in a woman with a high index of suspicion, if the result is negative or inconclusive, or if tissue is inadequate, D&C is mandatory.
- Endometrial sampling with Pipelle is an outpatient procedure and requires no cervical dilatation or anaesthesia.
- Endometrial sampling is indicated in
  - Women with postmenopausal bleeding
  - Postmenopausal women on oestrogen therapy
  - Women with HNPCC syndrome
  - Premenopausal women with abnormal bleeding with risk factors such as chronic anovulation, polycystic ovary syndrome (PCOS), obesity and metabolic syndrome
- D&C should be performed in the following situations:
  - Recurrent bleeding with endometrial sampling negative
  - Recurrent bleeding with endometrial thickness <5 mm
  - Complex atypical hyperplasia

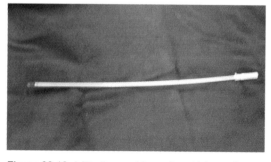

Figure 30.10 A Pipelle, used for endometrial sampling.

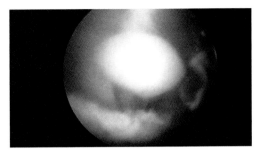

Figure 30.11 Endometrial polyp visualized through hysteroscope in a 60-year-old woman with postmenopausal bleeding.

- When performing D&C, endocervical sample should be taken first followed by endometrial curettage and sent for histological examination separately. This is known as fractional curettage and is performed to rule out endocervical extension of endometrial cancer or a primary endocervical cancer.
- **Hysteroscopy** is useful when polyps are seen on ultrasonogram or when D&C is negative in a patient in whom the index of suspicion is high (Fig. 30.11).

Management

Pretreatment evaluation

Once the diagnosis of endometrial cancer is made, pretreatment evaluation is required to assess the fitness for surgery, feasibility of surgery, extent of spread and other comorbid conditions (Box 30.10).

- Routine preoperative blood tests are performed to exclude diabetes, dyslipidaemia and anaemia. Chest X-ray is mandatory to look for pulmonary metastasis and evaluate the cardiorespiratory status.
- Ultrasonography is useful in determining the extent of the disease, although it is not as sensitive as computed tomography (CT) scan or magnetic resonance imaging (MRI).
- MRI is an excellent tool for assessment of myometrial invasion, parametrial extension and nodal metastasis (Fig. 30.12). It is not recommended as a routine, but is useful in women who are clinically diagnosed to have advanced disease or type II disease, or who are not good candidates for surgery. MRI may also be used when primary endocervical cancer is suspected or when decision regarding lymphadenectomy is difficult.

Box 30.10 Pretreatment evaluation in endometrial carcinoma

- Haemoglobin
- Blood sugar
- Serum creatinine
- Lipid profile
- Chest X-ray
  - Metastasis
- Abdominal and pelvic ultrasonography
  - Ascites
  - Liver metastasis
  - Pelvic/para-aortic lymphadenopathy
  - Myometrial invasion
  - Extension to cervix
  - Ovarian metastasis
- CT/MRI
  - Type II disease
  - Advanced disease
    - Myometrial invasion
    - Extent of disease
- CA 125

CA 125, a protein tumour marker; *CT*, computed tomography; *MRI*, magnetic resonance imaging.

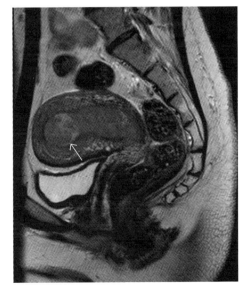

Figure 30.12 MRI of a woman with endometrial cancer. T2 sagittal section—The endometrial cavity is distended with isointense mass filling it. There are areas of myometrial infiltration (arrow). *MRI*, magnetic resonance imaging.

- CA 125, a tumour marker, used in epithelial ovarian cancer, is elevated in advanced stages. Estimation of CA 125 may be used to determine extrauterine spread and follow-up in women with advanced disease.

Treatment of endometrial cancer

Treatment is based on age and general condition of the patient, stage of disease and grade of tumour. Surgical staging is mandatory in all women. This can be performed by laparotomy or laparoscopy. Steps of surgical staging are outlined in Box 30.11.

Box 30.11 Steps of surgical staging in endometrial carcinoma

- Adequate abdominal incision (preferably vertical)
- Peritoneal washings for cytology
- Exploration of pelvis and abdomen
- Extrafascial hysterectomy
- Bilateral salpingo-oophorectomy
- Open the uterus
  - Assess the size and site of tumour
  - Depth of myometrial invasion
  - Cervical extension
- Lymphadenectomy (pelvic? Para-aortic)
- Advanced stage
  - Cytoreductive surgery

- There is a controversy regarding pelvic lymphadenectomy in early stage of endometrial cancer.
- Currently lymphadenectomy is recommended in all women except those with preoperative diagnosis of grade 1 tumours, <2 cm in size and <50% myometrial invasion. In these women, the incidence of lymph node metastasis is low (Box 30.12).
- There is controversy regarding para-aortic lymphadenectomy as well. Since para-aortic lymphadenectomy is associated with high morbidity, some authors recommend pelvic lymphadenectomy but only enlarged para-aortic nodes are removed. Others recommend pelvic and para-aortic lymphadenectomy whenever lymphadenectomy is indicated.
- Infracolic omentectomy should be performed in women with serous and clear cell histology.

Box 30.12 Situations where selective lymphadenectomy can be omitted

- Stage IA, grade 1, tumour <2 cm in size
- (With) non–clear cell or nonserous histology

- Irrespective of tumour grade or stage, they also require lymphadenectomy.
- Part of resected tumour tissue should be sent for hormone receptor status in all women.
- Sentinel node biopsy is still investigational in endometrial cancer.
- Women with stage II disease (cervical extension) are also managed with simple hysterectomy and lymphadenectomy.
- Advanced disease should be managed by cytoreductive surgery.

Laparoscopic and vaginal surgeries

Vaginal and laparoscopic surgeries are associated with less postoperative morbidity, early ambulation and better wound healing. Since most women with endometrial carcinoma are obese, these approaches may be preferable in women with stage IA, grade 1 disease where lymphadenectomy is not required. Surgeons who have the expertise in laparoscopic pelvic and para-aortic lymphadenectomy may perform the entire procedure laparoscopically even in women with more advanced disease.

Postoperative adjuvant therapy

Modalities of adjuvant therapy are given in Box 30.13.

Box 30.13 Postoperative adjuvant therapy in endometrial carcinoma

- Radiotherapy
  - Vaginal brachytherapy
  - External radiation
    - Pelvic radiation
    - Extended-field radiation
    - Whole abdominal radiation
- Chemotherapy

Radiotherapy

Vaginal vault is a common site of recurrence even in women with disease that is confined to the uterus. This can occur by direct spread or by lymphatic route.

Vaginal brachytherapy is vault radiation administered through the vagina. It reduces the vault recurrence from 15% to 1–2%.

External pelvic radiation reduces pelvic node recurrences in women who are at high risk. This includes women with cervical extension, adnexal involvement, grade 3 tumours and deep myometrial invasion.

Extended-field radiation includes pelvic, common iliac and para-aortic nodes. Women with gross disease confined to the pelvis but found to have histologically positive para-aortic nodes are candidates for extended-field radiation.

Whole abdominal radiation is required in women with stage III and IV disease. The entire abdomen is irradiated shielding the kidneys. Gastrointestinal and haematological toxicities are common with whole abdominal radiation.

Choice of adjuvant therapy

Based on the stage of disease at surgery, histo-pathology, risk of recurrence and other factors, women with endometrial cancer are categorized into the following three groups:

- *Low risk*: Stage IA, grade 1 or 2, no lympho-vascular space involvement, endometrioid histology.
- *Intermediate risk*: Stage IA, grade 3, stage IB, grade 1, 2 or 3, and stage II, LVSI, non–clear cell and serous. They are subdivided into low intermediate risk and high intermediate risk based on the following risk factors:
  - Deep myometrial invasion
  - Grade 2 or 3 histology
  - LVSI
  High intermediate risk includes
  - Age >70 years with one risk factor
  - Age 50–69 with two risk factors
  - Age 18–50 with three risk factors
  Low intermediate risk includes
  - All other intermediate-risk categories
- *High risk*: Stage III or IV, clear cell and serous cancers of any stage

The choice of postoperative adjuvant therapy is based on risk category (Table 30.6). These guidelines are not rigid and each centre may have protocols that differ slightly.

- Patients with low-risk disease and low-risk intermediate disease have a low incidence of locoregional recurrence. Hence, no adjuvant therapy is indicated.
- Patients with high-risk intermediate disease have a higher risk of locoregional recurrence. Hence, adjuvant radiotherapy is recommended. Pelvic radiation, compared to vaginal brachytherapy, is associated with a higher risk of early and late complications and no

Table 30.6 Postoperative adjuvant therapy in endometrial carcinoma

Stage	Adjuvant Therapy
• Low risk	No adjuvant therapy, observation
• Intermediate risk	
– Low intermediate risk	No adjuvant therapy, observation
– High intermediate risk	Vaginal brachytherapy *or* external pelvic radiation
• High risk	
– Serous carcinoma	
▪ Stage I, limited to endometrium	Vaginal brachytherapy
▪ Stages IA and B	Chemoradiation
▪ Stage II	Chemoradiation
– Clear cell carcinoma	
▪ Stages I and II	Vaginal brachytherapy
– Stage III serous and clear cell	Chemotherapy *or* pelvic radiation
– Stage IVA serous and clear cell	Chemotherapy
– Stage IVB serous and clear cell	Palliative treatment

additional overall survival. Hence, vaginal brachytherapy is recommended.

- Women with serous carcinoma must receive adjuvant therapy. Stage I disease limited to endometrium may be treated with brachytherapy. However, for stage I disease with myometrial invasion and stage II disease, concurrent chemotherapy and pelvic radiation (chemoradiation) is recommended.
- Clear cell carcinomas do not benefit from chemotherapy. Hence, vaginal brachytherapy is used as adjuvant therapy.
- Women with stage III disease, irrespective of histology, should receive adjuvant chemotherapy. Some centres treat them with pelvic radiation.
- Stage IVA disease may be difficult to resect completely. Women with stage IVA disease should receive postoperative chemotherapy.
- Survival in stage IVB disease is poor. Hence, palliative treatment is recommended.

Chemotherapy

Indications for chemotherapy have been already discussed. Recurrent cancer has been treated with chemotherapy with varying degree of response. Drugs used are listed in Box 30.14.

- Cisplatin/carboplatin
- Paclitaxel
- Doxorubicin
- Cyclophosphamide

Usually a combination of carboplatin and paclitaxel is used.

Hormone therapy

Progesterone therapy can be used in advanced and recurrent endometrial cancers that are progesterone receptor positive. In recurrent disease, tamoxifen and other third-generation selective oestrogen receptor modulators (SERMs) are also being tried.

The dosage used is MPA 200 mg daily orally. This has to be continued indefinitely. Megestrol acetate 40 mg four times daily (oral) is also an option.

Fertility-preserving treatment in endometrial cancer

Occasionally, endometrial cancer is encountered in young nulliparous women who wish to preserve reproductive function. Fertility-preserving treatment with progestin alone is an option in these women (Box 30.15).

- The criteria for fertility sparing treatment are as follows:
  - Endometrioid tumours
  - Stage IA, limited to the endometrium
  - Grade 1 histology
- Myometrial invasion should be excluded by MRI, histology confirmed by endometrial sampling.
- Oral MPA 600 mg daily or megestrol acetate 40 mg four times daily may be used.
- Endometrial biopsy should be performed 3 months after starting treatment. If there is no response, the dose may be increased. If there is no response after 6–9 months, hysterectomy should be proceeded with.
- If there is response, biopsy is repeated every 3 months till two consecutive biopsies are negative. Patient may then be allowed to conceive.

Prognostic factors

Prognosis depends on several factors as listed in Box 30.16. Tumours with diploid DNA content

- Young women, desiring fertility preservation
- Endometrioid tumours
- Stage IA limited to endometrium
- Grade 1 histology
- Tumour <2 cm
- Preoperative MRI mandatory
- MPA 600 mg daily orally
- Repeat biopsy every 3 months
  - If no response
    - Increased dose
    - Repeat biopsy every 3 months
    - Hysterectomy if no response in 6–9 months
  - If response
    - Treatment continued till three consecutive biopsies negative

MPA, medroxyprogesterone acetate; *MRI*, magnetic resonance imaging.

Box 30.16 Prognostic factors in endometrial carcinoma

- Age
- Histological type
- Histological grade
- Stage of tumour
- Size of tumour
- Type of carcinoma
- Histology
- Depth of myometrial invasion
- Lymphovascular space invasion
- Cervical extension
- Adnexal involvement
- Lymph node metastasis
- Peritoneal cytology
- Hormone receptor status

have relatively early stage disease and are well-differentiated tumours and have a good prognosis.

Survival

Endometrial cancer presents early with vaginal bleeding; therefore, most cases are stage I or II at diagnosis. Prognosis is generally good. Five-year survival rates are given in Table 30.7.

Uterine sarcoma

Sarcomas comprise <5% of all uterine tumours. Most sarcomas occur in the perimenopausal or

Table 30.7 Five-year survival for each surgical stage in endometrial carcinoma

Stage	Survival (%)
IA	91
IB	91
II	80
IIIA	66
IIIB	50
IIIC	57
IVA	25
IVB	20

postmenopausal age. Prolonged menopausal hormone therapy (MHT) and pelvic radiation increase the risk of uterine sarcoma (Box 30.17). Prognosis is poor and adjuvant treatment has not shown a clear benefit.

Box 30.17 Uterine sarcomas

- <5% of all uterine tumours
- Occur in perimenopausal or postmenopausal women
- Risk increased with
  - Prior pelvic radiation
  - MHT for >5 years
- Treatment: Surgery and adjuvant therapy
- Poor prognosis

MHT, menopausal hormone therapy.

Classification

There are several histological types of uterine sarcoma and an elaborate WHO classification is available, which is beyond the scope of this book.

Uterine sarcomas may be broadly divided into the following two categories:

1. **Pure**, which has only mesodermal elements
2. **Mixed**, which has mesodermal and epithelial elements

- Each category is further subdivided into **homologous** and **heterologous** tumours. Homologous tumours contain mesodermal elements that are normally present in the uterus such as smooth muscle. Heterologous

tumours contain mesodermal elements that are not normally present in the uterus such as striated muscle and cartilage (Box 30.18). Pure heterologous tumours are rare.

- The common uterine sarcomas are leiomyosarcomas, carcinosarcomas (malignant missed Müllerian tumours), endometrial stromal sarcomas and undifferentiated sarcomas.

Box 30.18 Broad classification of uterine sarcomas

- Pure
  - Homologous
    - Leiomyosarcomas
    - Endometrial stromal sarcomas
    - Undifferentiated endometrial sarcoma
  - Heterologous
    - Rhabdomyosarcomas
    - Chondrosarcomas
- Mixed
  - Carcinosarcoma (mixed Müllerian tumour)
  - Adenocarcinoma
  - Adenomyoma

Staging and treatment

Endometrial sarcomas are also staged surgically. FIGO has staged leimyosarcomas and endometrial stromal sarcomas in 2009. Sarcomas have a propensity for early haematogenous spread. General principles of treatment are outlined in Box 30.19. Response to adjuvant radiation is poor. Adjuvant chemotherapy may be beneficial in a few women.

Box 30.19 Treatment of uterine sarcomas

- Primary treatment
  - Abdominal total hysterectomy with BSO
- Adjuvant therapy
  - Radiation therapy
  - Chemotherapy
    - Doxorubicin
    - Docetaxel
    - Cisplatin
    - Ifosfamide

BSO, bilateral salpingo-oophorectomy.

Key points

- Premalignant lesion of the endometrium is endometrial hyperplasia. Malignancy can be carcinoma or sarcoma.

- Risk factors for endometrial hyperplasia and carcinoma are conditions that cause hyperoestrogenism, such as chronic anovulation, polycytic ovarian syndrome, obesity, oestrogen-secreting tumours of the ovary and postmenopausal oestrogen therapy. Tamoxifen also increases the risk.

- Endometrial hyperplasia can be simple or complex, with or without atypia. Complex hyperplasia with atypia is considered premalignant since risk of progression is 29%.

- Young women with hyperplasia present with prolonged bleeding after periods of amenorrhoea. Older women present with perimenopausal or postmenopausal bleeding.

- Diagnosis of endometrial hyperplasia is by endometrial sampling and histological examination of the specimen.

- Management of endometrial hyperplasia depends on the type of hyperplasia and the age of the patient. Simple hyperplasia can be managed with combination oral contraceptive pills in women of all age groups. Complex hyperplasia is usually managed with hysterectomy. Young women desirous of retaining reproductive function can be treated with megestrol acetate or medroxyprogesterone acetate with close follow-up by endometrial sampling.

- Endometrial cancer is the third most common gynaecological cancer in developing countries.

- In addition to the hyperoestrogenic conditions, hereditary nonpolyposis colorectal cancer syndrome and germline mutations are also risk factors in endometrial cancer.

- There are several histological types, but endometrioid adenocarcinoma is the most common. Histological grading is an important feature that determines staging and management.

- Endometrial cancer spreads by lymphatic, haematogenous and direct spread.

  - Staging is surgical and is as recommended by International Federation of Gynecology and Obstetrics in 2009.

  - The most common symptom is abnormal uterine bleeding, which may be postmenopausal, perimenopausal or just acyclic. Vaginal discharge may be present in some. Uterus may be normal or enlarged.

  - Diagnosis is by histopathological examination of the biopsy specimen. Transvaginal ultrasonography may be used to measure endometrial thickness and exclude pyometra before biopsy. Hysteroscopy and guided biopsy are indicated when endometrial polyp is suspected.

  - Preoperative evaluation by MRI is useful for assessment of myometrial invasion and nodal metastasis.

  - Staging laparotomy, total abdominal hysterectomy (TAH), bilateral salpingo-oophorectomy (BSO) and selective pelvic and para-aortic lymphadenectomy are the treatments of choice. Lymphadenectomy may be omitted in stage IA, grade 1 tumours less than 2 cm in size.

  - Postoperative adjuvant radiotherapy consists of vault radiation, pelvic radiation or chemoradiation depending on the stage of the disease.

  - Progestins are used in advanced and recurrent disease, progesterone receptor–positive tumours.

  - Five-year survival is 91% in stage I, but drops to 20% in stage IV.

- Uterine sarcomas may be pure or mixed, homologous or heterologous. Leiomyosarcoma and endometrial stromal sarcoma, carcinosarcoma and undifferentiated endometrial sarcoma are the most common.

- Treatment is by TAH and BSO followed by adjuvant chemotherapy or radiotherapy.

Self-assessment

Case-based questions

Case 1

A 45-year-old nulliparous lady presents with irregular cycles, bleeding for 10–15 days every 2–3 months for 3 years.

1. What details will you ask for in history?
2. What will you look for on clinical examination?
3. What investigations will you order?

4. If the diagnosis is complex hyperplasia with atypia, what is the management?

Case 2

A 54-year-old mother of one child presents with postmenopausal bleeding.

1. How will you clinically evaluate?
2. What investigations will you order?

3. If the diagnosis is stage I endometrial adenocarcinoma grade 2, no LVSI, what is the management?
4. What adjuvant therapy will you use?

Answers

Case 1

1. Age at menarche, history of anovulatory bleeding, diabetes, hypertension, polycystic ovarian syndrome, family history of uterine cancer, colonic cancer.
2. **(a)** General examination—BMI, pallor, blood pressure
   (b) Abdominal and pelvic examination—Uterine size, adnexal mass
3. Pipelle endometrial aspiration.
4. Since the risk of malignancy is high, D&C to exclude invasive cancer, abdominal/vaginal/laparoscopic hysterectomy.

Case 2

1. **(a)** History—Amount of bleeding, frequency
   (b) Predisposing factors—Oestrogen therapy, PCOS, age at menarche, age at menopause, diabetes, hypertension, family history of uterine/colonic cancer
   (c) Examination—Blood pressure, BMI, enlarged uterus, adnexal mass

2. **(a)** Transvaginal ultrasonography—Endometrial thickness, polyp, adnexal mass
   (b) D&C
3. Surgical staging, total abdominal hysterectomy, BSO, peritoneal washing, selective pelvic and para-aortic lymphadenectomy.
4. If the stage is IA, grade 1, 2 (low risk)—No adjuvant therapy.

   If stage IB, grade 2 (low intermediate risk)—No adjuvant therapy.

Long-answer questions

1. Discuss the pathology, clinical features and management of endometrial carcinoma.
2. What are the causes of postmenopausal bleeding? Discuss the management of a 55-year-old lady with stage II endometrial cancer.

Short-answer questions

1. Endometrial hyperplasia
2. FIGO staging of endometrial cancer
3. Management of endometrial hyperplasia
4. Adjuvant therapy in endometrial cancer
5. Postmenopausal bleeding

31 | Malignant Diseases of the Ovary and Fallopian Tube

Case scenario

Mrs AB, 52, was a postmenopausal lady living in a small town with her two sons who were attending college. Her husband was a bank officer and worked in a city 150 km away. Mrs AB had noticed vague ill health, abdominal bloating, loss of appetite and early satiety for the past 6 months. She was busy taking care of the children and her husband was away, so she had not taken the problems seriously. She noticed that her abdomen looked bigger than usual. Her husband had come home 2 days ago and noticed that she had lost a lot of weight, looked ill and her abdomen was markedly distended. Fearing the worst, he had brought her to the hospital for treatment.

Introduction

Ovarian cancer is the second most common gynaecological cancer. Several types of neoplasms can arise from the ovary. Most cases are diagnosed late because effective screening methods are not available. Therefore, it is the most common cause of gynaecological cancer mortality. Newer therapeutic modalities are under trial, but survival has not improved significantly.

Classification

Ovarian cancers are broadly classified into three groups according to their tissue of origin (Fig. 31.1):

- Epithelial cancers (70%)
- Germ cell tumours (5–10%)
- Sex cord-stromal tumours (15–20%)

In addition to these primary tumours, metastatic tumours constitute (5%) of all ovarian tumours.

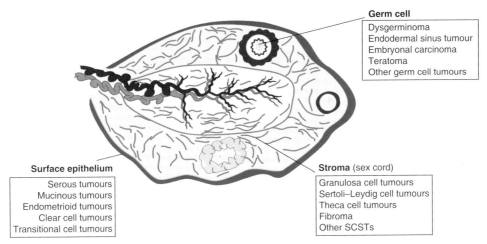

Germal cell
Dysgerminoma
Endodermal sinus tumour
Embryonal carcinoma
Teratoma
Other germ cell tumours

Surface epithelium
Serous tumours
Mucinous tumours
Endometrioid tumours
Clear cell tumours
Transitional cell tumours

Stroma (sex cord)
Granulosa cell tumours
Sertoli–Leydig cell tumours
Theca cell tumours
Fibroma
Other SCSTs

Figure 31.1 Diagrammatic representation of origin of ovarian tumours. The epithelial tumours arise from the surface epithelium, germ cell tumours from the germ cells in the ovarian follicles and the SCSTs from the stroma of the ovary. *SCST*, sex cord-stromal tumours.

Epithelial cancers are the most common. High-grade serous carcinoma resembles fallopian tube carcinoma and peritoneal carcinoma closely in histology and clinical behaviour. Hence, it is now believed that these cancers originate from the fallopian tubes.

Epithelial carcinoma of the ovary, fallopian tube and peritoneum

Although ovarian cancer is common, primary tubal and peritoneal carcinomas were considered rare. However, with better understanding of pathogenesis, high-grade serous epithelial cancer and peritoneal cancer are now known to arise from fallopian tube and exhibit similar clinical behaviour. Therefore, epithelial carcinomas of the ovary, fallopian tube and peritoneum are now considered as one clinical entity. Staging and management of these cancers are also similar.

Incidence of carcinoma of the ovary, fallopian tube and peritoneum

Epithelial ovarian cancer (EOC) is a disease of the older women, mean age at diagnosis being 60, but it can occur at any age. About 40% of EOCs occur at >70 years of age and 70% are at stage III or IV at diagnosis. Overall, 5-year survival

is about 20%. There is a geographic variation in incidence. Women in North America have a much higher risk than those in Africa and Japan.

The age-standardized incidence rate for ovarian cancer in various registries varies from 0.9 to 8.4/100,000 person-years. Globally, there were 239,000 cases diagnosed in 2012. The incidence in developing countries is 9.4/100,000 and mortality rate is 5.1/100,000. EOC is the most common. The incidence rises with age. It is 0.2–1.4/100,000 at <20 years and 47–57/100,000 at >70 years. The lifetime risk of developing ovarian cancer is 1.4–1.9%.

Incidence of fallopian tube carcinoma was considered very low. However, recent studies have shown that high-grade serous ovarian carcinomas arise from the fallopian tube. Similarly, peritoneal carcinoma was also considered to be rare until recently.

Risk factors for epithelial ovarian cancer

Several factors increase the risk of ovarian cancer; some play a causative role, and others are associations. Risk factors for tubal and peritoneal cancers are not clearly defined but have been found to be the same in general.

- **Incessant ovulation** is considered to be an important aetiological factor. This explains the increased risk in nulliparous women and women with infertility, early menarche and late menopause. Multiparous women and those who breast-feed have a reduced risk for the same reason.

- **Prolonged use of ovulation-inducing drugs** such as clomiphene has also been implicated.
- **Exposure of ovarian cells to high gonadotropin milieu** also plays a role in the causation of ovarian cancer.

Risk factors for EOCs are listed in Box 31.1.

Box 31.1 Risk factors for EOC

- Older age group
- Nulliparity
- Infertility
- Early menarche
- Late menopause
- White race
- Endometriosis/PID
- PCOS
- Genetic factors
  - *BRCA* gene mutation
  - Lynch syndrome (HNPCC syndrome)
- Diet rich in animal fat
- Perineal exposure to talc
- Obesity

EOC, epithelial ovarian cancer; *HNPCC,* hereditary nonpolyposis colorectal cancer; *PCOS,* polycystic ovarian syndrome; *PID,* pelvic inflammatory disease.

Genetic factors in epithelial ovarian cancer

About 5–10% of ovarian cancers are associated with genetic factors. There are two types of hereditary ovarian cancers:

1. Germline mutations of *BRCA1* and *BRCA2*
2. Hereditary nonpolyposis colorectal cancer (HNPCC; Lynch II) syndrome

- Mutations in the *BRCA1* and, to a lesser extent, *BRCA2* genes are responsible for most hereditary breast–ovarian cancers. Lifetime risk of ovarian cancer with *BRCA1* mutation is 35–40% and with *BRCA2* is 13–23%. *BRCA1*-associated cancers occur earlier. *BRCA2*-associated cancers have a better prognosis.
- *BRCA1* mutation is also a risk factor for tubal and peritoneal carcinomas.
- HNPCC syndrome is a less common genetic cause of ovarian cancer. It is associated with endometrial, urogenital, ovarian and gastrointestinal cancers. Ovarian cancer in this group also occurs earlier.

- The risk of carrying a gene for ovarian cancer increases with the number of relatives with the same cancer. When two first-degree relatives are affected, the possibility of carrying an affected gene is 35–40%.

Screening for epithelial ovarian cancer

Most ovarian cancers are diagnosed at an advanced stage because there is no effective screening method available and early ovarian cancer is a silent disease. Routine screening has not been found to be effective in decreasing mortality. Methods that have been used are listed in Box 31.2.

Box 31.2 Screening methods for EOC

- Routine yearly pelvic examination
- TVS
- Tumour markers
  - CA 125
  - HE4
  - CA-19-9, CA-15-3
- Proteomic patterns
- Multimodal screening

EOC, epithelial ovarian cancer; *HE4,* human epididymis protein; *TVS,* transvaginal ultrasonography.

Routine pelvic examination has a low sensitivity for diagnosis of ovarian cancer.

Transvaginal ultrasonography (TVS) is used extensively to differentiate between benign and malignant tumours of the ovary (Fig. 31.2a–d). Ultrasonographic characteristics of malignancy are listed in Box 31.3. Due to neovascularization of malignant tissue, the blood flow is increased and the resistance is low. This can be measured using Doppler and the resistance index calculated. Ovarian volume of >20 cm^3 in premenopausal women and >10 cm^3 in postmenopausal women are considered abnormal. Ultrasonography has a high sensitivity but low specificity for diagnosis of early ovarian cancer.

Tumour markers in epithelial ovarian cancer

CA 125

- **It is a glycoprotein** tumour marker secreted by the ovarian cancer cells. Normal level is <35 U/mL.

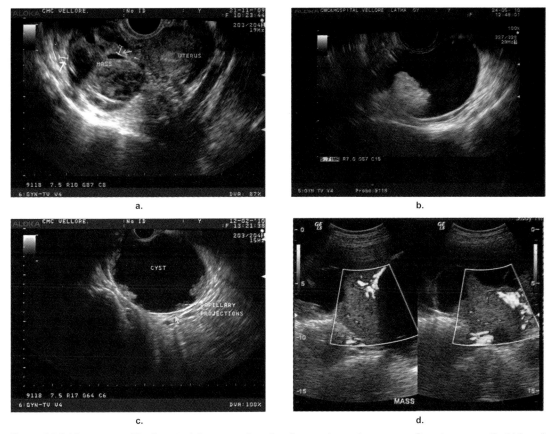

Figure 31.2 Ultrasonographic characteristics suggestive of malignancy in ovarian mass. a. Complex mass with thick wall (white arrow) and thick septae (coloured arrow). b. Cyst with solid area within. c. Cyst with papillary excrescences within. d. Cyst with increase in vascularity.

Box 31.3 Ultrasonographic characteristics of malignancy in ovarian mass

- Ovarian volume >10 cm^3
- Solid/complex (solid and cystic)
- Multiloculated
- Thickness of cyst wall (>3 mm)
- Septal thickness (>2 mm)
- Bilateral
- Papillary excrescences
- Increase in vascularity
- Doppler resistance index <0.40

- The test has a high false-positive rate because conditions causing peritoneal irritation increase the level of CA 125. Levels are elevated in other benign conditions such as endometriosis, pelvic inflammatory disease (PID), recent surgery, tuberculosis and myoma and malignancies of the breast, lung, pancreas and colon.
- A cut-off value of 35 U/mL is used in postmenopausal women, but in premenopausal women, a cut-off value of 200 U/mL is recommended.
- The test is more useful in monitoring response to treatment in women with ovarian cancer and in diagnosis of recurrence.
- Used alone, the test lacks specificity and the sensitivity is about 50%. The test is combined with TVS in multimodal screening.
- Serial estimation of CA 125 has been found to be more useful than a single value for screening. This is used in **risk of ovarian cancer algorithm (ROCA)**. Compared to annual screening by transvaginal sonography alone, serial CA 125 measurements (ROCA) followed by TVS had a better positive predictive value.

Human epididymis protein

It is a tumour marker that has been found to have the same sensitivity as CA 125. A combination of CA 125 and human epididymis protein (HE4) is used in **risk of ovarian malignancy algorithm (ROMA)**, which is used to calculate risk of ovarian cancer. The patients are categorized into low risk and high risk based on ROMA. This has been found useful in postmenopausal women.

Proteomic patterns

These are proteins and protein fragments that circulate in the blood indicating early changes caused by genetic mutations. Their use as markers of ovarian cancer is being studied. Evaluation of six analytes and CA 125, known as **OvaSure blood test**, has been found to have a high sensitivity and specificity.

Multimodal screening

Using a combination of CA 125 and ultrasonography improves the sensitivity and specificity. Usefulness of this multimodal screening in general population is being studied. Using a combination of age, menopausal status, CA 125 and ultrasonography, various indices have been developed for calculating the risk of malignancy. The UK Collaborative Trial of Ovarian Cancer Screening (UKCTOCS), a large randomized trial evaluating multimodal screening, showed a significant reduction in mortality.

Genetic testing is indicated in women with a family history of EOC. A pedigree analysis is mandatory. Clear guidelines are available for testing for *BRCA1* and *BRCA2*. Current recommendation is that all women with EOC, fallopian tube or peritoneal cancer who are younger than 70 should undergo genetic testing. Women in the family identified as at high risk should undergo counselling and tested for *BRCA1* and *BRCA2*.

Recommendations for screening

Routine screening of women at low risk is not currently recommended. In women with familial cancer syndromes, genetic testing is the first step. For those with positive genetic test, screening with pelvic examination, CA 125 and TVS every 6 months beginning at age 30 years is recommended by some but no increase in survival has been found. Hence, for high-risk women, chemoprophylaxis and early risk–reducing salpingo-oophorectomy are recommended.

Box 31.4 Prevention of EOC

- Oral contraceptives
- Prophylactic bilateral salpingo-oophorectomy
- Tubal ligation
- Hysterectomy

EOC, epithelial ovarian cancer.

Prevention

In women who are at a high risk for EOC, prophylaxis is indicated. Methods used are listed in Box 31.4.

- **Chemoprevention** with combined oral contraceptives (COCs) is a proven method of prevention and the protective effect persists for 10 years or more after stopping the medication. There is a 50% reduction of ovarian cancer risk when COCs are used for 5 years.
- **Prophylactic salpingo-oophorectomy** is recommended at >35 years of age after these women complete their family. This procedure reduces the *BRCA*-related risk by 90%.
- **Hysterectomy** is mandatory in women with HNPCC syndrome. In women with breast–ovarian cancer syndrome, the role of hysterectomy is not yet proven. This may be considered in older women along with salpingo-oophorectomy.
- A reduction in risk of endometrioid cancer has been found with **tubal ligation**. Endometrioid cancer is thought to arise from endometrial cells transported to ovary through the tube by retrograde menstruation.

Pathogenesis of epithelial ovarian, tubal and peritoneal cancer

The pathogenesis of EOC has been better understood over the years.

- The surface of the ovary is lined by a single layer of coelomic epithelium or modified mesothelium. These cells can undergo metaplasia into Müllerian epithelium. Lining cells of tube and endometrium, transported during menstruation to the ovarian surface, may also develop into Müllerian epithelium and line the ovarian surface. Müllerian inclusions develop beneath the ovarian surface during repair after ovulation. Epithelial cancers that arise from ovarian surface can have their origin from any of these cells.

- Currently, it has been shown that some of the epithelial cancers can also arise from the lining cells of the fimbrial end of the fallopian tube.
- Therefore, according to their tissue of origin, EOCs are classified into the following:
  - *Type I:* Cancers that arise from surface epithelium or Müllerian inclusions. They are slow-growing tumours, present at early stage and include low-grade serous, mucinous, endometrioid and clear cell tumours.
  - *Type II:* Cancers that arise from the fimbrial end of the fallopian tube or peritoneum are high grade and progress rapidly. They are more common than type I and present in advanced stages. They are also associated with p53 and *BRCA1* mutations.

Hence, cancer of the ovary, fallopian tube and peritoneum are now considered a single entity and are staged by the same International Federation of Obstetrics and Gynecology (FIGO) system.

The most common EOC is the serous type (75–80%).

Classification of epithelial ovarian, fallopian tube and peritoneal cancer

- Based on molecular genetic analysis and immunohistochemistry, the epithelial ovarian, tubal and peritoneal carcinomas are classified as shown in Box 31.5.

Pathology

Macroscopic appearance

Malignant epithelial tumours vary in size. They are cystic with solid areas or are predominantly solid (Fig. 31.3a and b). Papillary excrescences may be present on the surface and within the tumour (Fig. 31.4a and b); haemorrhage and necrosis are common. Mucinous tumours can be very large (Fig. 31.5). Malignant tumours are very vascular.

Microscopic appearance

Histological features (Figs 31.6 and 31.7) and the frequency of occurrence of the common epithelial tumours are listed in Table 31.1.

Box 31.5   Classification of carcinoma of the ovary, fallopian tube and peritoneum

- Type I
  - Slow growing
  - Early stage at diagnosis
  - Arises from
    - Coelomic epithelium
    - Müllerian epithelium
    - Endometrial cells
    - Müllerian inclusions
  - Includes
    - LGSC
    - Endometrioid tumours
    - Clear cell tumours
    - Mucinous tumours
- Type II
  - Rapidly going
  - Poor prognosis
  - Late stage at diagnosis
  - Arises from
    - Fallopian tube
    - Peritoneum
    - Ovarian surface epithelium
  - Includes
    - HGSC
    - Transitional cell (Brenner) tumours*
    - Undifferentiated tumours#

HGSC, high-grade serous tumour; *LGSC*, low-grade serous tumour.

*Brenner (transitional cell) cancers are considered a subset of HGSCs.

#Undifferentiated carcinoma is rare and is considered to be a HGSC with little or no differentiation.

- Histological features are similar to their cells of origin. Low-grade serous tumour (LGSC) and high-grade serous tumour (HGSC) are differentiated by the degree of nuclear atypia, mitotic activity and cellular differentiation.
- Mucinous tumours arise from Walthard inclusions and the cells resemble lining cells of the endocervix and gastrointestinal tract.
- Clear cell tumours have cells with hobnail appearance and stroma is characteristically hyalinized.
- Endometrioid tumours arise from endometrial cells that reach the ovary through retrograde menstruation, and histological features are the same as endometrial cells.

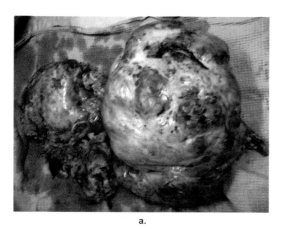 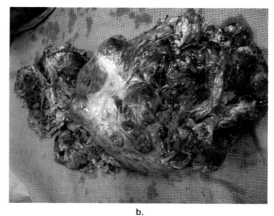

a.   b.

Figure 31.3 Mucinous cystadenocarcinoma. a. Ovarian tumour with cystic and solid areas. b. Cut section of the same tumour shows haemorrhage, cystic filled with mucin and solid areas.

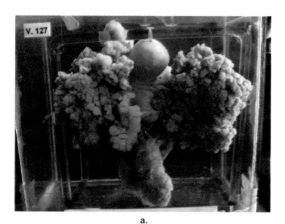

a.

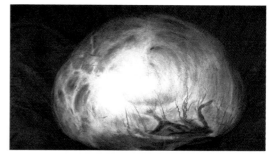

Figure 31.5 Large mucinous tumour. Blood vessels are seen on the surface indicating a vascular tumour.

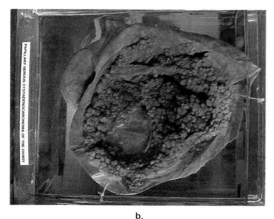

b.

Figure 31.4 Serous carcinoma of the ovary. a. Specimen of uterus and ovaries covered with papillary excrescences. b. Papillary projections within the cyst on cut section.

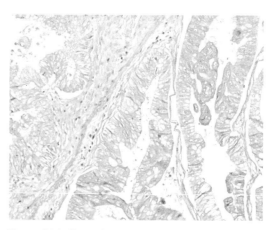

Figure 31.6 Photomicrograph showing tumour with cystic spaces lined by tall, mucin-secreting columnar cells—Mucinous cystadenocarcinoma.

Table 31.1 Histological features and frequency of occurrence of common epithelial tumours

	Cellular type	Other features	Frequency of occurrence (%)
Low-grade serous	• Tubal epithelium • Ovarian surface epithelium	• Psammoma bodies • Uniform nuclei, low mitotic activity	<5
Mucinous	Walthard cell nests	Mucin-secreting cells, resemble endocervical, gastric cells	3
Endometrioid	Endometrial cells	Well-differentiated, villoglandular cells	10
Clear cell	Müllerian epithelium	• Clear and hobnail cells • Hyalinized stroma	10
High-grade serous	• Tubal epithelium • Peritoneum • Ovarian surface epithelium	• Papillary, glandular, solid • Marked cytological atypia • High mitotic activity	70

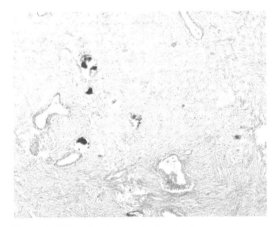

Figure 31.7 Photomicrograph showing tumour with cystic spaces lined by cuboidal cells—Serous cystadenocarcinoma.

Secondary tumours of the ovary

Ovaries are a common site of metastasis in breast cancers and gastrointestinal cancers. Spread to ovary may be transcoelomic or haematogenous. The secondary tumours are known as **Krukenberg tumours**. These are bilateral, solid and mobile with bosselated surface. Microscopically, signet ring cells are characteristic of these tumours. Non-Krukenberg secondaries also occur.

Histological grade of EOC

According to the degree of differentiation, EOCs are classified into three histological grades (Box 31.6). This is based on nuclear pleomorphism and architectural features. Histological grade is

an important prognostic factor and is taken into consideration while planning treatment.

Box 31.6 Histological grade of EOC

- Grade I: Well differentiated
- Grade II: Moderately differentiated
- Grade III: Poorly differentiated

EOC, epithelial ovarian cancer.

Patterns of spread of epithelial cancer of the ovary, fallopian tube and peritoneum

The predominant method of spread is by exfoliation of malignant cells into the peritoneal cavity that is deposited on the surface of various intra-abdominal organs. The cells are carried by peritoneal fluid as it circulates. Other routes of spread are as for other cancers of the genital tract (Box 31.7).

Staging of epithelial cancer of the ovary, fallopian tube and peritoneum

Epithelial cancer of the ovary, fallopian tube and peritoneum is staged surgically. Laparotomy is mandatory for appropriate staging of the disease. Staging by FIGO (2014) is given in Table 31.2 and diagrammatically depicted in Fig. 31.8.

- Grade of tumour and histological type should be recorded.

Table 31.2 FIGO staging of epithelial cancer of the ovary, fallopian tube and peritoneum (2014)

Stage I	Tumour limited to the ovaries or fallopian tubes
Stage IA	Tumour limited to one ovary (capsule intact) or fallopian tube; no tumour on ovarian or fallopian tube surface; no malignant cells in ascites or peritoneal washings
Stage IB	Tumour limited to both ovaries (capsules intact) or fallopian tubes; no tumour on ovarian or fallopian tube surface; no malignant cells in ascites or peritoneal washings
Stage IC	Tumour either stage IA or IB, but with any of the following
Stage IC1	Surgical spill
Stage IC2	Capsule ruptured before surgery or tumour on ovarian or fallopian tube surfaces
Stage IC3	Malignant cells in the ascites or peritoneal washings
Stage II	Tumour involving one or both ovaries or fallopian tubes with pelvic extension (below the pelvic brim) or peritoneal cancer
Stage IIA	Extension and/or implants on the uterus, fallopian tubes/ovaries
Stage IIB	Extension to other pelvic intraperitoneal tissues
Stage III	Tumour involves one or both ovaries or fallopian tubes, or peritoneal cancer, with cytologically or histologically confirmed spread to the peritoneum outside the pelvis and/or metastasis to the retroperitoneal lymph nodes
Stage IIIA	Positive retroperitoneal lymph nodes and/or microscopic metastasis beyond pelvis
Stage IIIA1	Positive retroperitoneal nodes only (cytologically or histologically proven)
Stage IIIA1(i)	Metastasis <10 mm in greatest dimension
Stage IIIA1(ii)	Metastasis >10 mm in greatest dimension
Stage IIIA2	Microscopic extrapelvic (above the pelvic brim) peritoneal involvement, with or without positive retroperitoneal lymph nodes
Stage IIIB	Macroscopic peritoneal metastasis beyond pelvis up to 2 cm in greatest dimension, with or without positive retroperitoneal lymph
Stage IIIC	Macroscopic peritoneal metastasis beyond pelvis more than 2 cm in greatest dimension (includes extension of tumour to capsule of liver and spleen without parenchymal involvement of either organ), with or without positive retroperitoneal lymph nodes (includes extension to capsule of liver or spleen)
Stage IV	Distant metastasis (excludes peritoneal metastasis)
Stage IVA	Pleural effusion with positive cytology
Stage IVB	Parenchymal metastases and metastases to extra-abdominal organs (including inguinal lymph nodes and lymph nodes outside the abdominal cavity). Includes parenchymal liver metastasis

FIGO, International Federation of Obstetrics and Gynecology.

Box 31.7 Patterns of spread of epithelial tumour of the ovary, fallopian tube and peritoneum

- Transcoelomic
  - Surfaces of intra-abdominal organs
  - Omentum
  - Undersurface of diaphragm
  - Peritoneal surfaces
- Lymphatic spread
  - Para-aortic up to the level of renal vessels
  - Internal iliac, external iliac, obturator
  - Inguinal
- Direct spread
  - Uterus, tubes, rectosigmoid, pelvis
- Haematogenous
  - Liver, lung, brain

- Ovarian, fallopian tube and peritoneal cancers are staged together. The primary site of origin should be noted.
  - If intraepithelial or invasive lesion is found in the tube, it is considered fallopian tube primary.
  - If there is no lesion in the tube and at least 0.5 cm of tumour is within ovarian parenchyma, it is ovarian primary.
  - If neither of the above is applicable, it is primary peritoneal carcinoma.

Clinical features of epithelial cancer of the ovary, fallopian tube and peritoneum

Symptoms

- EOC usually occurs in the sixth decade. Majority of women are asymptomatic. However, some

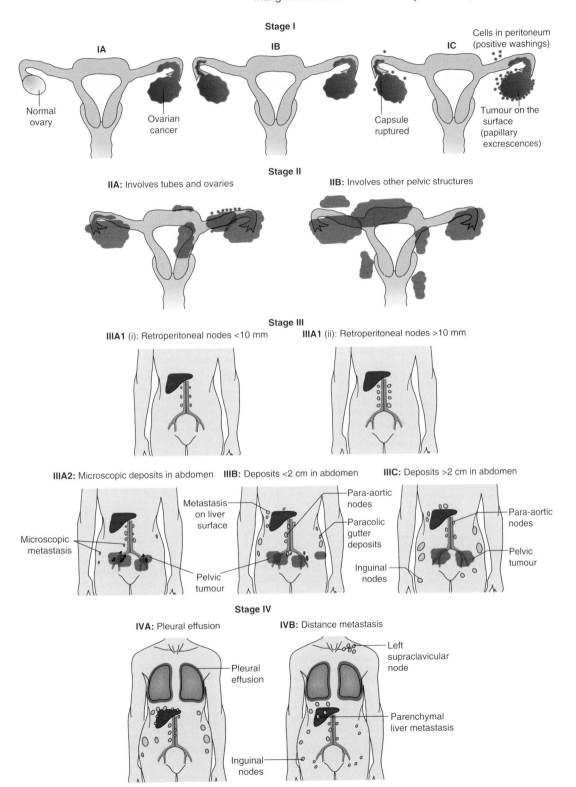

Figure 31.8 FIGO staging of ovarian cancer. *FIGO,* International Federation of Obstetrics and Gynecology. *See* Table 31.8 for an explanation of different stages.

symptoms are commonly reported by many women with early stage EOC. The **symptom index** includes the following if they are new symptoms and occur >12 times/month:
- Abdominal discomfort/pain
- Abdominal swelling/bloating
- Difficulty in eating

- When ascites or pleural effusion develops, women present with massive abdominal distension and dyspnoea. Compression of the bladder or rectum by the ovarian mass results in urinary frequency or bowel symptoms. Occasionally, women present with irregular menses or postmenopausal bleeding (Box 31.8).
- Profuse watery vaginal discharge, known as **hydrops tubae profluens**, is said to be pathognomonic of tubal cancer.
- Classical triad of fallopian tube cancer includes vaginal discharge, pelvic pain and bleeding/adnexal mass and occurs in 15% of women.

Box 31.8 Clinical features of epithelial cancer of the ovary, fallopian tube and peritoneum

- Symptoms
  - Asymptomatic
  - Symptom index
    - Abdominal pain
    - Abdominal distension/bloating
    - Difficulty in eating/feeling full
  - Weight loss
  - Abdominal mass
  - Urinary frequency
  - Irregular menses/postmenopausal bleeding
  - Vaginal discharge
  - Dyspnoea
  - Nausea/constipation
- Signs
  - Lymphadenopathy
  - Ascites
  - Lower abdominal mass
  - Omental cake
  - Adnexal mass
  - Nodules in the pouch of Douglas

Signs

A mass may be palpable in the lower abdomen, which is hard and fixed. Omental deposits forming omental cake can be felt in the upper abdomen or at the level of the umbilicus. Smaller

ovarian masses may not be palpable abdominally. Ascites is common and is due to intraperitoneal (IP) metastatic disease. On pelvic examination, the ovaries are enlarged and hard; fixed and secondary deposits may be felt as nodules in the pouch of Douglas.

Clinical evaluation

History

History (Box 31.9) and physical examination are important for arriving at a diagnosis.

Box 31.9 History

- Age
- Parity
- Symptoms
- Past history
  - Infertility
  - Endometriosis
  - Age at menarche/menopause
- Family history
  - Cancers of ovary/uterus/breast/colon

Physical examination

This should be thorough and systematic as shown in Box 31.10. Examination may reveal a cachexic lady with a grossly distended abdomen in case of advanced stage of the disease (Fig. 31.9). Lymphadenopathy must be looked for with special attention to left supraclavicular nodes. An upper abdominal mass or a mass arising from the pelvis is usually felt on examination. The location of the mass, size, shape, consistency, margins and mobility must be noted. Malignant tumours are large, hard, solid or partly solid and fixed. Margins may be ill defined due to ascites. Upper abdominal mass is usually an omental cake. Presence of large-volume ascites may make the palpation difficult.

Further evaluation

Early stage disease

Confirmation of diagnosis of ovarian/tubal/peritoneal cancer can be established only by laparotomy. However, women with early stage disease and adnexal mass without other clinical signs of malignancy need further evaluation before proceeding with surgery (Box 31.11).

Box 31.10 Physical examination

- General examination
  - Weight/body mass index
  - Lymphadenopathy
    - Supraclavicular
    - Inguinal
- Breast examination
- Abdominal examination
  - Ascites
  - Mass arising from the pelvis
    - Size, shape, consistency, margins, mobility
  - Upper abdominal mass
    - Size, shape, consistency, margins, mobility
  - Hepatosplenomegaly
- Pelvic examination
  - Adnexal mass
    - Size, location, mobility, consistency
- Rectovaginal examination
  - Rectal mucosa
  - Extraluminal mass

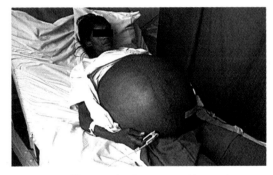

Figure 31.9 Photograph of a woman with grossly distended abdomen due to ascites and large ovarian tumour.

Box 31.11 Further evaluation in early stage disease

- Ultrasonography
  - Tumour morphology
  - Nodal disease
  - Ascites
  - Extent of intraperitoneal spread
- Doppler flow studies—Resistance index
- CA 125
  - >35 U/mL postmenopausal
  - >200 U/mL premenopausal

Ultrasonography

This is the first step in the evaluation. **Abdominal** and **transvaginal sonography** should be performed. Ultrasonographic features of malignancy are given in Box 31.3 (see Figs 31.10–31.12).

- In addition to the tumour characteristics, morphology of the other ovary, enlarged para-aortic nodes, ascites and metastasis to other intra-abdominal viscera can be evaluated by ultrasonography.
- Large deposits in the subdiaphragmatic space, disease in the lesser sac and omental cake can be detected.
- In premenopausal women, tumours of <8 cm without other features of malignancy and normal CA 125 can be followed up and re-evaluated 2 months later. Surgery can be considered if the tumour increases in size or does not regress.
- In postmenopausal women, a cut-off size of 5 cm is recommended.
- Ovarian volume of >20 cm^3 in premenopausal women and >10 cm^3 in postmenopausal women is an indication for further evaluation.

Doppler flow studies

In malignant tumours, there is neovascularization. The newly formed vessels lack muscle layer, and, therefore, the resistance is low. This can be measured using Doppler. Increased vascularity with low resistance index indicates malignancy.

CA 125

CA 125 levels are useful in differentiating benign from malignant lesions. The sensitivity is high in postmenopausal women, but in premenopausal women, other conditions can also lead to elevated levels, as already discussed.

It is also useful for early diagnosis of recurrence and response to therapy. High levels are indicative of advanced-stage disease and, therefore, poor prognosis.

Advanced-stage disease

Clinical examination may be sufficient to arrive at a diagnosis in women with advanced-stage disease. However, evaluation of extent of disease and assessment of operability are essential. Other causes of ascites and pelvic mass should also be ruled out. Ultrasonography, computed

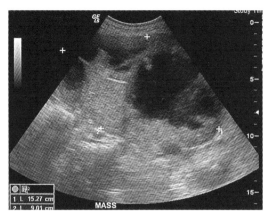

Figure 31.10 Ultrasonogram shows a complex ovarian mass with solid and cystic areas.

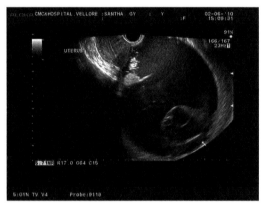

Figure 31.11 Ultrasonogram shows a large cyst with solid papillary projection within and smaller locules within.

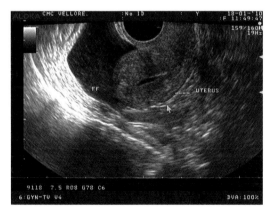

Figure 31.12 Ultrasonogram shows ascitic fluid in the pouch of Douglas.

Box 31.12 Further evaluation—Advanced-stage disease

- Ultrasonography
  - Details of the tumour
  - Involvement of adjacent organs
  - Ascites
  - Metastasis (>2 cm)
    - Under surface of the diaphragm
    - Liver parenchyma
    - Lesser sac
    - Omentum
    - Surface of bowel
    - Para-aortic/pelvic nodes
- CT
  - Detects disease 1.5–2 cm
- MRI
  - Detects disease >1 cm
- PET/CT
  - Metastatic disease
- Paracentesis
- Fine-needle aspiration cytology/biopsy

CT, computed tomography; *MRI*, magnetic resonance imaging; *PET*, positron emission tomography.

tomography (CT) and/or magnetic resonance imaging (MRI) may be used to determine the extent of the disease (Box 31.12). CT or MRI is used when there is large volume of ascites and extensive disease. For the diagnosis of retroperitoneal and IP metastasis in ovarian cancer, CT is an excellent modality (*see* Chapter 5, *Imaging in gynaecology*; Figs 31.13a and b and 31.14a and b). MRI can pick up smaller nodes. Positron emission tomography (PET)/CT is also useful in detecting metastatic disease. However, if surgical exploration is planned, either CT or MRI is usually sufficient.

If the tumour is considered inoperable and neoadjuvant chemotherapy (NACT) is being considered as a treatment option, diagnosis should be confirmed. This is done by aspiration of ascitic fluid to look for malignant cells or by fine-needle aspiration biopsy of the mass under ultrasound guidance.

Differential diagnosis

Early stage cancer must be differentiated from other pelvic masses and benign ovarian lesions.

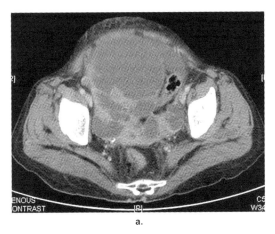
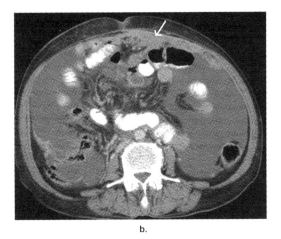

a.   b.

Figure 31.13 CT scan with oral and intravenous contrast. **a.** Bilateral cystic and solid masses in the adnexa with enhancement of the solid areas. **b.** Ascites and omental thickening (arrow), referred to as 'omental cake'. *CT*, computed tomography.

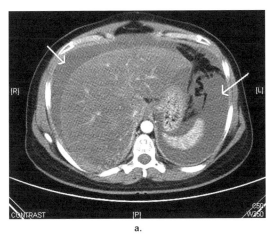
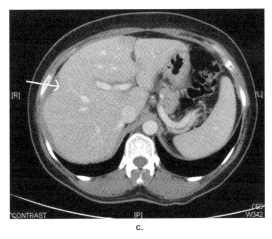

a.   c.

Figure 31.14 CT scan. **a.** Upper abdomen with ascitic fluid (arrows). **b.** Metastatic deposits on the surface of the liver causing indentation on the surface (arrow). *CT*, computed tomography.

In women with advanced-stage disease, other causes of ascites and lower abdominal masses should be excluded (Box 31.13).

Imaging and CA 125 are useful in differentiating other ovarian masses from ovarian malignancy. Liver function tests, carcinoembryonic antigen (CEA), gastroscopy, colonoscopy and mammography are required in women with ascites and pelvic masses to rule out primary gastrointestinal or breast tumours and liver disease.

Preoperative evaluation

Once the diagnosis of ovarian malignancy is established, surgery is the mainstay of

management. Preoperative workup is given in Box 31.14. If extensive surgery is anticipated, 2 units of blood-packed cells should be kept ready. Anticoagulation and prophylactic antibiotics should be administered as discussed in Chapter 33, *Preoperative preparation and postoperative management.*

Management of epithelial ovarian, tubal and peritoneal cancers

Most women with EOC, tubal and peritoneal cancers are managed by primary surgery for

- Early stage disease
  - Functional ovarian cysts
  - Benign ovarian tumours
  - Tubo-ovarian mass
    - PID
    - Tuberculosis
  - Endometriosis
  - Subserous myoma
  - Pelvic kidney
- Advanced-stage disease
  - Abdominal tuberculosis
  - Liver disease
  - Secondary tumours
    - Breast
    - Bowel
    - Pancreas
    - Stomach
  - Fallopian tube carcinoma

PID, pelvic inflammatory disease.

Box 31.14 Preoperative workup

- Routine blood tests
  - Haemoglobin
  - Complete blood count
  - Liver function tests
  - Plasma glucose
- Chest X-ray
- ECG

ECG, electrocardiogram.

staging and cytoreduction, followed by adjuvant therapy. A group of patients with advanced disease in whom optimal cytoreduction is not considered feasible are treated by NACT followed by surgery. Therefore, the management can be

- Early stage disease
  - Primary surgery followed by adjuvant chemotherapy
- Advanced disease
  - Primary surgery followed by adjuvant chemotherapy
  - NACT followed by cytoreductive surgery

Surgical staging

The goals of primary surgery in early and advanced ovarian cancer are to stage the disease

Box 31.15 Steps of surgical staging

- General anaesthesia
- Vertical midline incision
- Ascitic fluid or peritoneal washing for cytology
- Examination of the ovaries and pelvis
- Systematic exploration of all organs
- Multiple biopsies
- TAH with BSO
- Infracolic omentectomy
- Pelvic and para-aortic lymphadenectomy

BSO, bilateral salpingo-oophorectomy; *TAH*, total abdominal hysterectomy.

and resect as much tumour as possible. Steps of staging laparotomy are given in Box 31.15.

- Vertical incision allows exploration of all organs and access to upper abdomen.
- Ascitic fluid should be aspirated and sent for cytology. If no ascites is present, 50–100 mL of saline should be instilled into the pelvis, abdomen, subdiaphragmatic space and paracolic gutters using a rubber catheter and the fluid should be aspirated.
- The ovaries should be inspected for signs of malignancy (Box 31.16).

Box 31.16 Examination of the ovarian tumour

- Size, shape
- Consistency—Cystic/solid/mixed
- Papillary excrescences
- Rupture of capsule
- Fixity to surrounding structures
- Bilateral tumour
- Vascularity
- Spread to uterus/tubes/bladder/bowel/pelvis

- Systematic exploration of other organs is mandatory for staging and assessment of operability. This is done in a clockwise fashion, starting with the caecum and moving towards ascending colon, hepatic flexure, right kidney, liver, gallbladder, right hemidiaphragm, spleen, transverse colon, lesser sac, splenic flexure, descending colon, sigmoid, rectum, small bowel, omentum and para-aortic nodes.
- In women with no obvious stage IIIB/IIIC or IV disease, biopsies should be taken from suspicious areas, paracolic gutters, diaphragm,

pelvic walls and bowel surfaces. Random biopsies must be taken if there are no suspicious areas.

- Posterior peritoneum should be opened and retroperitoneum explored for pelvic and para-aortic lymph nodes. Pelvic and para-aortic lymph node sampling should be performed even in women with stage I disease because microscopic deposits in the nodes will upstage the disease.

Management of early-stage epithelial ovarian, fallopian tube and peritoneal cancer

Outline of management for patients with stage I and II ovarian/tubal/peritoneal cancer is given in Box 31.17. Even when the disease appears to be confined to ovaries, microscopic metastasis has been found in the lymph nodes, peritoneum and subdiaphragmatic area. A thorough surgical staging is, therefore, mandatory.

Box 31.17 Management of early stage disease

- Surgical staging
- Total abdominal hysterectomy
- Bilateral salpingo-oophorectomy
- Infracolic omentectomy
- Pelvic and para-aortic lymph node sampling
- Multiple peritoneal biopsies

Adjuvant therapy in early stage disease

Chemotherapy is the accepted adjuvant therapy in ovarian cancer. Based on the prognosis, early stage tumours are categorized into low risk and high risk (Table 31.3). Adjuvant therapy is recommended in all except stage I low-risk disease.

Table 31.3 Risk categorization in early stage disease

Low risk	High risk
Stage IA/B	Stage IC, Stage II
Non–clear cell tumours	Clear cell tumours
Grade 1 or 2	Grade 3
No dense adhesions	Dense adhesions
Diploid tumour	Aneuploid tumour

Adjuvant therapy in early stage disease is as given in Box 31.18. Combination of carboplatin and paclitaxel is recommended, based on several randomized trials:

Box 31.18 Adjuvant therapy in early stage disease

- Stage I, low risk   No adjuvant therapy
- Stage I, high risk   Three to six cycles of chemotherapy
- Stage II   Three to six cycles of chemotherapy

- Paclitaxel IV 175 mg/m^2
- Carboplatin IV 350–600 mg/m^2 [corresponds to area under the curve (AUC), 5–6, depends on glomerular filtration rate]
- The two drugs to be administered once in 3 weeks for three to six cycles

Radiotherapy was used in the past for treatment of ovarian cancer but had been stopped because of side effects. However, recent trials on women with stage IC and II clear cell and endometrioid cancers have shown survival benefit with pelvic and abdominal radiation. This is being evaluated further.

Fertility-sparing treatment in early stage disease In young women with stage IA or B, grade 1 disease, who desire fertility, unilateral oophorectomy or bilateral ovarian cystectomy is an option. The uterus and ovaries are generally removed after childbearing.

Laparoscopic surgery Laparoscopic surgery is now being increasingly used in early ovarian cancer. Care must be taken to avoid spill of tumour. If exploration of abdomen and staging are inadequate, conversion to laparotomy is required. Laparoscopic surgery should be performed by an experienced laparoscopic surgeon.

Management of advanced-stage epithelial ovarian, fallopian tube and peritoneal cancer

About 70% of women have stage III or IV disease at diagnosis. Integrated multidisciplinary approach with the involvement of a surgical and medical oncologist, radiologist, pathologist and palliative care specialist is required in these women.

Staging laparotomy and primary cytoreductive surgery followed by postoperative adjuvant chemotherapy is the current recommendation for treatment of advanced-stage disease. However, this may not be feasible in all patients and may increase morbidity. An alternative approach is NACT followed by surgery and postoperative chemotherapy for few more cycles.

The decision for primary surgery versus NACT is taken after complete evaluation including imaging. Factors that make cytoreduction difficult are as follows:

- Involvement of liver parenchyma
- Bowel involvement, infiltration of small bowel mesentery
- Diffuse peritoneal carcinomatosis
- Large, fixed tumour
- Upper abdominal disease including involvement of pancreas and lesser sac
- Poor general condition of the patient, including age, comorbidities and performance status

If primary surgery is considered feasible, surgical staging should be proceeded with.

Primary cytoreductive surgery

Women with advanced-stage disease have large tumour deposits in the lesser sac, subdiaphragmatic area, liver surface and surface of bowels with large retroperitoneal nodes and omental cake. They also have large-volume ascites.

Debulking of the tumour is recommended for various reasons, namely:

- The large tumour and deposits are poorly vascularized and chemotherapeutic agents do not reach adequate concentrations in these tissues.
- Large tumours also contain more cells in the resting phase, which do not respond to chemotherapy.
- Cells in the small residual masses are faster growing and respond better to chemotherapy.
- With smaller tumour volume, less number of cycles of chemotherapy may be required.
- Removing tumour tissue enhances the immune system.
- Cytoreductive surgery reduces ascites, improves gastrointestinal function and relieves symptoms.

The goal of primary cytoreductive surgery is to remove all the primary tumour and metastatic disease, if possible, so as to reduce the residual tumour to optimal status (Box 31.19).

- If there is no grossly visible disease after surgery, it is **complete cytoreduction**.

Box 31.19 Primary cytoreductive surgery

- Total hysterectomy
- Bilateral salpingo-oophorectomy if feasible
- Infracolic omentectomy
- Removal of as much tumour as possible
- Retroperitoneal lymphadenectomy

- If the residual tumour masses are <1 cm, it is considered as **optimal cytoreduction**. Patients whose tumour is completely removed or cytoreduced to <1 cm have the best overall survival.
- If the residual tumour masses are >1 cm, it is **suboptimal cytoreduction**. The prognosis is poorer in these women.
- Removal of metastatic tumour may involve bowel resection, partial hepatectomy or splenectomy.
- Instruments such as cavitron ultrasonic surgical aspirator (CUSA) and argon beam coagulator may be required for removal of subdiaphragmatic disease.
- All grossly enlarged and suspicious retroperitoneal (pelvic and para-aortic) nodes must be removed.
- If cytoreduction is optimal and IP chemotherapy is planned, the port should be placed.
- Blood loss, operating time and morbidity are higher with this surgery. It must be performed by surgical oncologists in whose hands it is feasible in 70–90% of cases.

Adjuvant therapy in advanced-stage disease

All women with advanced-stage disease must be given adjuvant chemotherapy as detailed later in this chapter.

Neoadjuvant chemotherapy

- As already discussed, primary cytoreduction to optimal residual tumour volume is difficult to achieve in some advanced cancers. Assessment of residual volume is most often inaccurate.
- In women with advanced-stage cancer, large-volume ascites, cachexia and poor performance status, mortality associated with primary surgery is 1.8–2%. Morbidity is also higher and this may delay initiation of chemotherapy.
- A significant reduction in postoperative gastrointestinal complications, infections and pulmonary complications has been found with NACT.

- Indications
  - Advanced-stage ovarian cancer
    - Age >70 years, weight loss >10–15%
    - Large, bulky upper abdominal disease
    - Omentum replaced by tumour
    - Tumour extending to spleen
    - >2 cm tumour in small-bowel mesentery
    - Cancer coating the diaphragm
    - Massive ascites and pleural effusion
- Advantages
  - Rapid subjective improvement
  - Subsequent surgery easier, less morbidity
  - Less postoperative complications
  - Best test for chemosensitivity

- Indications and advantages of NACT are given in Box 31.20.
- Confirmation of diagnosis and histology is mandatory before proceeding with NACT. This is done by
  - Abdominal paracentesis and examination of ascetic fluid
  - Fine-needle aspiration of tumour
  - Tru-Cut biopsy of tumour
- After confirming the diagnosis and assessment of extent of the disease by CT/MRI, three cycles of chemotherapy with combination of intravenous (IV) carboplatin and paclitaxel are administered.
- The patient is reassessed after three cycles with CA 125, clinical examination and imaging. Cytoreductive surgery is performed when there is reasonable chance of optimal cytoreduction. If the situation warrants, this may be done after four or five cycles of chemotherapy.
- The tumour masses usually become smaller and mobile, ascites and pleural effusion regress and surgery is easier.
- Three more cycles of chemotherapy are given postoperatively.
- Progression of tumour during NACT indicates chemoresistant disease and optimal cytoreduction is not feasible. The tumour masses should be treated with second-line chemotherapy.

Chemotherapy in ovarian cancer

Various randomized trials have compared the efficacy of the drugs available, dosage and combinations. The results are as follows:

- Combination chemotherapy is superior to single-agent chemotherapy.
- A platinum analogue must be included in the combination. Carboplatin has less gastrointestinal effects, nephrotoxicity, neurotoxicity and ototoxicity than cisplatin and is equally effective. However, it can cause myelosuppression.
- Addition of paclitaxel to carboplatin improves the response rates. Hence, combination of carboplatin and paclitaxel is the standard of care in EOC, tubal and peritoneal cancers.
- Combination of cisplatin and paclitaxel is recommended for IP therapy.

Recommended dosage and routes of administration

- *Optimally cytoreduced stage III*: A combination of IV and IP chemotherapy is recommended. This results in increased overall and progress-free survival.
- The regimen used in stage III optimally cytoreduced patients is six cycles of
  - IV paclitaxel (135 mg/m^2 over 24 hours) on day 1
  - IP cisplatin (100 mg/m^2 in 1 L of normal saline) on day 2
  - IP paclitaxel (60 mg/m^2) on day 8
- *Suboptimally cytoreduced advanced-stage disease*: IV paclitaxel 175 mg/m^2 with carboplatin AUC 5 or 6 or 350–450 mg/m^2 is currently recommended.
- Dose-dense therapy with weekly paclitaxel and 3-weekly carboplatin has a better outcome in these women except in those with clear cell or mucinous tumours.

IV chemotherapy is easy to administer and is given every 3 weeks for six to eight cycles depending on response and toxicity. This route of administration is used in all women.

IP chemotherapy is administered through a specially designed port. The dose of drug delivered to the tumour is higher since it reaches the tumour directly. However, this method of administration is not useful in large-volume residual disease. Toxicity is higher. It is, therefore, useful in women with stage III disease who have optimal cytoreduction.

Angiogenesis inhibitors in ovarian, tubal and peritoneal cancer

Molecular targeted therapy with angiogenesis inhibitors is being tried in the treatment of advanced disease. Addition of angiogenesis inhibitor, bevacizumab, in advanced-stage disease improves outcome. The drug may be used concurrently or after chemotherapy. It is also used in recurrent disease.

Assessment of response to adjuvant therapy

This is done clinically, radiologically and using tumour markers (Box 31.21).

Box 31.21 Assessment of response to therapy

- Clinical evaluation
  - In suboptimally debulked patients
  - Size of residual tumour
  - Mobility
  - New lesions
- Radiological assessment
  - Ultrasonography
  - CT
  - MRI
- CA 125
  - Serial estimations
  - Response to therapy
  - Early diagnosis of relapse
- PET/CT
  - Small, radiologically undetectable lesions

CT, computerized tomography; *MRI*, magnetic resonance imaging; *PET*, positron emission tomography.

Subsequent management

This depends on response to adjuvant chemotherapy. Patients may have complete response, partial response, persistent disease or progression of disease during chemotherapy (Box 31.22).

Box 31.22 Subsequent management after adjuvant chemotherapy

- Complete response
  - Follow-up
- Partial response
  - Continue the same chemotherapy for three more cycles
  - (or) Switch to second-line chemotherapy
- Stable disease
  - Switch to second-line chemotherapy
- Progression of disease
  - Switch to second-line chemotherapy

Management of patients with complete response These women are considered to be in remission. However, 80% of women with stage III or IV in remission will relapse within 5 years and ultimately die of the disease. Maintenance or consolidation chemotherapy has not been found to be useful. These women are, therefore, followed up clinically, radiologically and with CA 125.

Management of patients with partial response Continuing the same chemotherapy for a total of nine cycles is an option. Toxicity increases with increasing the number of cycles of the therapy. Women who do not respond adequately within 6 months of therapy have a poor prognosis, may not respond to further therapy and relapse early. Switching to second-line chemotherapy is also an option.

Management of patients with stable and progressive disease These patients have a poor prognosis. Second-line chemotherapy can be tried, but response is variable.

Second-look surgery

This was considered the gold standard for confirming response to chemotherapy and identifying residual disease (Box 31.23). This may be by laparotomy or laparoscopy.

Box 31.23 Second-look surgery in epithelial ovarian, tubal and peritoneal cancer

- Performed after completion of chemotherapy
- Steps
  - Peritoneal washing
  - Thorough inspection of organs
  - Multiple biopsies
- No residual disease—Stop chemotherapy
- Microscopic residual disease—Continue chemotherapy
- Macroscopic residual disease—Secondary cytoreduction
- No survival benefit
- Additional morbidity
- Not recommended except in research setting

Interval cytoreductive surgery

In some women with advanced-stage disease, extensive disease makes it impossible to perform cytoreductive surgery. In this situation, removal of part of the tumour, biopsy or suboptimal cytoreduction is performed and the abdomen is closed. After three cycles of combination chemotherapy, interval cytoreduction surgery is performed.

This is also performed after NACT in women with inoperable disease at diagnosis. Three more cycles of chemotherapy are given postoperatively. Trials show that overall survival is better than in the group with no interval surgery.

Secondary cytoreductive surgery

This has limited place in the management of ovarian cancer. This is usually performed when there is gross recurrent or residual disease after completion of chemotherapy. Since these patients have poor prognosis, generally there is no benefit in terms of overall survival. In patients with recurrence after a treatment-free interval of 24 months, some survival benefit was demonstrated, but the procedure is not recommended as a routine.

Second-line chemotherapy

These are the agents used in platinum-resistant patients. The drugs used are listed in Box 31.24.

> **Box 31.24 Agents used in second-line chemotherapy of ovarian cancer**
>
> - Docetaxel
> - Topotecan
> - Liposomal doxorubicin
> - Gemcitabine
> - Etoposide
> - Ifosfamide
> - Tamoxifen

Other treatment modalities

These are listed in Box 31.25.

> **Box 31.25 Other treatment modalities**
>
> - Immunotherapy
> - Hormone therapy
> - Gene therapy
> - High-dose chemotherapy with autologous bone marrow transplantation
> - Radiation therapy

Radiation therapy has been used in early stage cancer and in patients with recurrence with variable results. Other methods of treatment are still experimental.

Prognostic factors

As in other cancers, prognosis depends on the stage of the disease at diagnosis and type and

> **Box 31.26 Prognostic factors in epithelial ovarian, tubal and peritoneal cancer**
>
> - FIGO stage
> - Histological type
> - Histological grade
> - Diploid/aneuploid tumours
> - Age of the patient
> - Size of the tumour
> - Residual disease after surgery
> - Ascites
> - Performance status of the patient
> - Intraperitoneal rupture of the tumour
> - Tumour spill
> - Pretreatment CA 125 levels
>
> FIGO, International Federation of Obstetrics and Gynecology.

grade of tumour in addition to other factors. Prognostic factors are listed in Box 31.26.

Survival

Overall survival in EOC is about 45%, which is much less than that in endometrial or cervical cancers. Five-year survival for advanced-stage disease is low and most women die of the disease (Box 31.27).

> **Box 31.27 Survival in epithelial ovarian cancer by FIGO stage**
>
> - Stage I: 80–90%
> - Stage II: 60–70%
> - Stage III: 30–35%
> - Stage IV: 15–20%
>
> FIGO, International Federation of Obstetrics and Gynecology.

Borderline epithelial tumours of the ovary (tumours of low malignant potential)

Epithelial tumours with cellular features of malignancy but without stromal invasion are referred to as **borderline tumours** or **tumours of low malignant potential** (LMP). Their biological behaviour is also intermediate between that of benign and malignant tumours.

- Borderline tumours constitute 10–15% of epithelial tumours. Risk factors are the same as for invasive cancer.
- They often occur in younger women who have not completed reproductive function.
- Mucinous, serous, endometrioid and clear cell tumours can present as borderline tumours. They are most often serous or mucinous tumours.
- In women with mucinous tumours, pseudomyxoma peritonei can occur.
- Serous and mucinous borderline tumours can present with stromal invasion, defined as 5 mm in linear extent or 10 mm² in area, known as **microinvasive carcinoma**. Prognosis is uncertain, but these may be associated with areas of invasive tumour or represent the premalignant stage.
- Even when the primary tumour is borderline, metastasis lesions may reveal noninvasive or invasive histology. Extraovarian invasive disease has a poorer prognosis.

Clinical features of borderline epithelial tumours

Borderline tumours often present as adnexal mass. Sonographic features and tumour markers are not useful for diagnosis of these tumours. Diagnosis is by laparotomy and histological evaluation of the tumour. Frozen section has a low sensitivity for diagnosis. The clinical features of borderline epithelial tumours are listed in Box 31.28. Staging is the same as for EOC.

Box 31.28 Clinical features of borderline tumours (LMP)

- Occur in younger women (forties)
- Asymptomatic/mass/distension
- Vary in size, can be large
- Staging same as for invasive cancer
- Cannot be distinguished from malignant tumours preoperatively

LMP, low malignant potential.

Management of borderline epithelial tumours

- Laparotomy and surgical staging is required in all women.
- Stage I tumours in young women can be treated by unilateral oophorectomy.

- Older women and those with stage II–IV disease require hysterectomy, bilateral salpingo-oophorectomy (BSO), omentectomy and cytoreductive surgery.
- In women with advanced-stage disease, and invasive implants, adjuvant chemotherapy has been recommended, but it does not reduce recurrence.

Malignant germ cell tumours of the ovary

Benign and malignant tumours can arise from the germ cells of the ovary. The most common germ cell tumour is cystic teratoma, which is a benign disease of the ovary and fallopian tube. About 20–25% of all ovarian tumours are germ cell tumours and 3% of these are malignant. Epidemiology and other characteristics of germ cell tumours are given in Box 31.29.

Box 31.29 Epidemiology and characteristics of malignant germ cell tumours

- Constitute 5% of all ovarian malignancies
- 3% are malignant
- 70% occur before age 20
- Majority are stage I at diagnosis
- Mostly unilateral
- Grow rapidly
- Very chemosensitive
- Very good prognosis

Classification

The WHO classification of germ cell tumours (2014) is given in Box 31.30.

Histogenesis

The primordial germ cells migrate from the yolk sac through the dorsal mesentery to the genital ridge. Dysgerminomas and embryonal carcinomas arise from these primitive germ cells. Dysgerminoma does not have the potential to differentiate further. But embryonal carcinomas have cells that are totipotent and can differentiate into embryonic tissues such as ectoderm, endoderm and mesoderm and into extraembryonic tissues such as yolk sac and trophoblasts (Fig. 31.15).

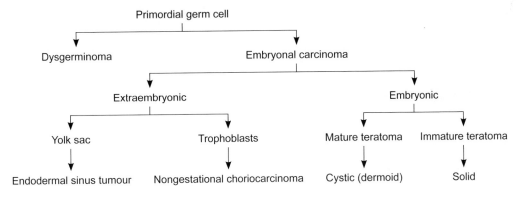

Primordial germ cell

Dysgerminoma   Embryonal carcinoma

Extraembryonic   Embryonic

Yolk sac   Trophoblasts   Mature teratoma   Immature teratoma

Endodermal sinus tumour   Nongestational choriocarcinoma   Cystic (dermoid)   Solid

Figure 31.15 Histogenesis of germ cell tumours.

Box 31.30 WHO classification of germ cell tumours

- Primitive germ cell tumours
  - Dysgerminoma
  - Endodermal sinus (yolk sac) tumour
  - Embryonal carcinoma
  - Polyembryoma
  - Nongestational choriocarcinoma
  - Immature teratoma
  - Mature teratoma
    - Solid
    - Cystic (dermoid cyst)
  - Mixed germ cell tumours
- Monodermal teratomas and highly specialized tumours
  - Thyroid tumours (struma ovarii)
  - Carcinoid tumours
  - Neuroectodermal tumours
  - Squamous cell and adenocarcinomas
  - Sarcomas
  - Sebaceous tumours

Table 31.4 Tumour markers in germ cell tumours

Tumour	AFP	hCG	LDH
Dysgerminoma	–	±	+
Embryonal carcinoma	+	+	–
Endodermal sinus tumour	+	–	–
Choriocarcinoma	–	+	–
Immature teratoma	±	–	–
Polyembryoma	±	+	–
Mixed tumours	±	±	–

AFP, α-fetoprotein; *hCG*, human chorionic gonadotropin; *LDH*, lactic dehydrogenase.

Tumour markers

Tumour markers secreted by germ cell tumours are given in Table 31.4. Placental alkaline phosphatase (PLAP) is also produced by dysgerminoma. Measurement of these is useful in diagnosis, assessment of response to therapy and follow-up.

Risk factors

The most common malignant germ cell tumour is dysgerminoma. The known risk factor for the development of this tumour is a dysgenetic gonad. The risk is increased in dysgenesis containing Y-chromosome—Turner mosaic, Klinefelter syndrome, androgen-insensitivity syndrome, and pure and mixed gonadal dysgenesis.

Pathology

Germ cell tumours are solid tumours or contain solid and cystic areas (Fig. 31.16). Cut section has a solid, uniform, tan appearance in dysgerminoma (Fig. 31.17) and variegated appearance with areas of haemorrhage and necrosis in endodermal sinus tumour.

Germ cell tumours are unilateral tumours, except dysgerminomas, which are bilateral in 15% of the cases. The salient pathological features of the three most common germ cell tumours (dysgerminoma, endodermal sinus tumour and immature teratoma) are given in Table 31.5. Other germ cell tumours are rare. Dysgerminoma has a characteristic histological appearance similar to seminoma and consists of sheets of uniform, round cells and leucocytic infiltration (Fig. 31.18).

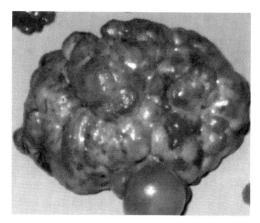

Figure 31.16 Large, solid, lobulated tumour in a 21-year-old lady—Immature teratoma.

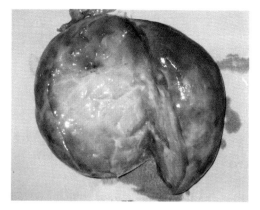

Figure 31.17 Solid tumour in a 16-year-old girl. Cut section of a solid tumour with a uniform, tan appearance—Dysgerminoma.

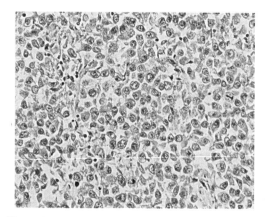

Figure 31.18 Photomicrograph of the same tumour (as in Fig. 31.17) showing monotonous round cells—Dysgerminoma.

Table 31.5 Pathology of common germ cell tumours		
Dysgermi-noma	**Endodermal sinus tumour**	**Immature teratoma**
Most common	Third most common	Second most common
5% from dysgenetic gonad	Very rapid growth	Rapid growth
15–20% bilateral	Always unilateral	Rarely bilateral
Gross appearance		
Solid, bosselated	Cystic areas of necrosis	Large, lobulated or rounded
Microscopic appearance		
Large, round, clear cells	Schiller–Duval bodies	Mixture of tissues
Extensive infiltration with leucocytes, plasma cells	Cystic spaces lined by flattened epithelium	Neuroectoderm predominates
		Graded 1–3 based on immature neural element
Age group		
<20 years	Prepubertal	<20 years
Stage at diagnosis		
70% Stage I	65% Stage I	50–60% Stage I

Clinical features

Germ cell tumours occur predominantly in young girls younger than 20 years of age, sometimes premenarcheal. Acute abdominal pain is common and is due to necrosis, haemorrhage, torsion or rupture. About 25% are asymptomatic, while others present with abdominal mass, distension or other symptoms listed in Box 31.31. Examination reveals a solid lower abdominal mass, with or without ascites and metastasis to other areas.

Investigations

In many asymptomatic young girls, germ cell tumours are diagnosed incidentally on ultrasonography. Any solid tumour on ultrasonography in this age group should arouse suspicion of a germ cell tumour (Fig. 31.19). Other investigations are listed in Box 31.32.

Box 31.31 Clinical features of germ cell tumours

- Age: 10–20 years
- Symptoms
  - Asymptomatic
  - Acute abdominal pain
  - Lower abdominal mass
  - Rapid increase in size
  - Abdominal distension
  - Menstrual irregularities
- Signs
  - Weight loss
  - Lymphadenopathy
  - Pleural effusion
  - Ascites
  - Lower abdominal solid mass

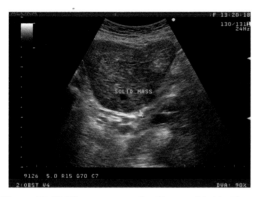

Figure 31.19 Ultrasonogram of a 19-year-old girl with a pelvic mass showing a solid tumour—Germ cell tumour.

Box 31.32 Investigations in germ cell tumours

- Ultrasonography
  - Complex ovarian mass
  - Low resistance index on Doppler
- Tumour markers
  - α-Fetoprotein
  - hCG
  - LDH
- Karyotyping if prepubertal

hCG, human chorionic gonadotropin; *LDH*, lactic dehydrogenase.

Management

Surgery

Primary treatment is surgical. However, since the disease occurs mostly in young girls, conservative surgery is the norm. Adequate surgical staging is essential (Box 31.33). In young girls where

Box 31.33 Surgical management of germ cell tumours

- Adequate incision
- Peritoneal washing
- Exploration of abdominal organs
- Young girls, reproductive function desired, any stage
  - Unilateral oophorectomy
  - Frozen section
  - Contralateral ovary inspected, biopsy if required
  - Pelvic and para-aortic lymphadenectomy
  - Peritoneal and omental biopsies
- Reproductive function not desired, >stage I
  - Bilateral salpingo-oophorectomy
  - Hysterectomy
  - Infracolic omentectomy
  - Pelvic and para-aortic lymphadenectomy
  - If not feasible
    - Cytoreductive surgery

conservative surgery is planned, frozen section should be sent for diagnosis. Careful inspection and palpation of contralateral ovary and biopsy of suspicious areas is mandatory if frozen section is reported as dysgerminoma since it is the only germ cell tumour that can be bilateral.

Adjuvant therapy

Patients with stage IA dysgerminomas and stage IA, grade 1 immature teratomas do not need adjuvant therapy. For all other stages and other tumours, adjuvant therapy is by platinum-based combination chemotherapy, since germ cell tumours are extremely chemosensitive. Currently recommended combination is bleomycin, etoposide and cisplatin (BEP) for three cycles.

Survival

As already mentioned, prognosis in germ cell tumours is good. Survival rates are given in Box 31.34.

Box 31.34 Survival in germ cell tumours

- Dysgerminoma
  - Stage I: 95%
  - Stages II–IV: 85%
- Endodermal sinus tumour
  - Stage I: 80%
  - Stages II–IV: <10%
- Immature teratoma
  - Stage I: 90%
  - Stages II–IV: 75%

Sex cord-stromal tumours

These are tumours derived from the mesenchyme of the ovaries, which include cells surrounding the oocytes and secreting ovarian hormones. The tumours contain granulosa/theca cells or Sertoli–Leydig cells and other indifferent cells. About 5–8% of all ovarian tumours belong to this category. The tumours are classified by the WHO (2014) as given in Box 31.35.

Box 31.35 Classification of sex cord-stromal tumours

- Pure stromal tumours
  - Fibroma/fibrosarcoma
  - Thecoma
  - Sclerosing stromal tumour
  - Leydig cell tumour
  - Steroid cell tumour
- Pure sex cord tumours
  - Granulosa cell tumour
  - Adult type
  - Juvenile type
  - Sertoli cell tumour
  - Sex cord tumour with annular tubules
- Mixed sex cord-stromal tumours
  - Sertoli–Leydig cell tumours
  - Sex cord-stromal tumours, NOS

NOS, not otherwise specified.

Clinical features and management

- The two malignant sex cord-stromal tumours are granulosa cell tumours and Sertoli–Leydig cell tumours.
- They are slow-growing tumours and recurrences occur as late as 30 years after surgery, but mean duration is 6 years.
- Surgery is the mainstay of treatment. Since most women have stage I disease at diagnosis, unilateral salpingo-oophorectomy is sufficient. The prognosis in stage I is excellent and 5-year survival is 90%.
- In women who have completed family or have advanced-stage disease, hysterectomy and BSO are performed.
- Adjuvant platinum-based chemotherapy is recommended in women with stage I with large tumour, high mitotic index (>10/high-power field), tumour rupture, surface tumour and stage II–IV disease.

- Granulosa cell tumours and Sertoli–Leydig cell tumours secrete **inhibin A and B**, and this is used as a tumour marker.

Granulosa cell tumour

Clinical features and management of granulosa cell tumours are summarized in Box 31.36. Granulosa cell tumours are of two types: **adult** and **juvenile**. They secrete oestrogen. Adult granulosa cell tumour usually presents with abnormal uterine bleeding or postmenopausal bleeding and may be associated with endometrial hyperplasia/carcinoma. Juvenile tumour may present as precocious puberty. Grossly, they are solid tumours or contain some cystic areas (Fig. 31.20).

Box 31.36 Clinical features and management of granulosa cell tumour

- Can be adult or juvenile type
- Secretes
  - Oestrogen
  - Inhibin A and B
- Presents with
  - Postmenopausal bleeding
  - Endometrial hyperplasia/carcinoma
  - Precocious puberty
- 90% unilateral and stage I at diagnosis
- Stage I, young women
  - Unilateral salpingo-oophorectomy
- Stages II–IV, women who completed family
  - Hysterectomy, bilateral salpingo-oophorectomy

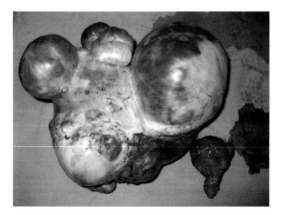

Figure 31.20 Tumour with solid and cystic areas in a 52-year-old lady with postmenopausal bleeding—Granulosa cell tumour.

Sertoli–Leydig cell tumour

Sertoli–Leydig cell tumours secrete androgen and cause hirsutism and virilization. They usually present at an early stage. About 15–20% are malignant. Clinical features and management of Sertoli–Leydig cell tumours are listed in Box 31.37.

Box 31.37 Clinical features and management of Sertoli–Leydig cell tumour

- Mean age at occurrence — 30 years
- Secretes
  - Androgens
  - Inhibin A and B
- Presents with
  - Hirsutism, virilization
- Unilateral
- >90% stage I at diagnosis
- Young, Stage I
  - Unilateral salpingo-oophorectomy
- Older, Stage II–IV
  - Hysterectomy, bilateral salpingo-oophorectomy

Adjuvant therapy in sex cord-stromal tumours

Adjuvant chemotherapy with BEP is recommended for women with stage I disease with high-risk factors—Large size, capsule rupture, tumour on the surface, high mitotic activity and positive peritoneal washing. All women with stage II–IV tumours also require chemotherapy. Inhibin levels can be used to monitor response and recurrence in granulosa cell tumours.

Other sex cord-stromal tumours

Thecomas

These are oestrogen-secreting, solid, benign tumours. They occur in older postmenopausal women and present with bleeding/pelvic mass. Treatment is surgical resection of the tumour.

Gynandroblastoma

Gynandroblastomas contain well-differentiated Sertoli and granulosa cells. These tumours are rare and can produce androgens, oestrogen or both. Most tumours are benign.

Key points

- Ovarian cancer is the second most common cancer of the female genital tract. Ovarian malignancies are classified into epithelial, germ cell and sex cord-stromal tumours.

- Epithelial ovarian, tubal and peritoneal cancers are now grouped together since they have the same pathogenesis and histology.

- Epithelial ovarian cancer occurs in older women and has an overall 5-year survival of about 20%.

- Risk factors are nulliparity, infertility, family history of breast or ovarian cancer and a diet rich in animal fat.

- Routine screening of ovarian cancer is not recommended. Screening of high-risk women is by transvaginal ultrasonography, tumour markers and genetic testing. A multimodal screening is recommended.

- Epithelial cancers of the ovary/tube and peritoneum are classified into type I and type II. Type II tumours are also known as high-grade serous carcinomas.

- According to the degree of differentiation, epithelial cancers of the ovary, tube and peritoneum are divided into three histological grades. They are staged according to the International Federation of Obstetrics and Gynecology (FIGO) recommendations.

- Epithelial ovarian/tubal/peritoneal cancers spread by transcoelomic, lymphatic, direct and haematogenous spread.

- Malignant epithelial tumours of the ovary, tube and peritoneum are asymptomatic in majority of women. They may present with weight loss, abdominal distension, loss of appetite and dyspnoea. Examination may reveal ascites, lymphadenopathy, abdominal mass, omental cake and nodules in the pouch of Douglas.

- Diagnosis is by ultrasonography, Doppler flow studies and CA 125. Further evaluation with computed tomography (CT)/magnetic resonance imaging (MRI) may be required for detection of nodal and distended metastasis.

- All women with epithelial ovarian, tubal and peritoneal cancers require staging laparotomy. Ascitic fluid should be taken for peritoneal cytology; ovaries and other organs should be inspected and multiple biopsies should be taken. Total abdominal hysterectomy (TAH) with bilateral salpingo-oophorectomy (BSO), infracolic omentectomy, pelvic and para-aortic lymphadenectomy should be performed whenever possible. When this is not feasible, cytoreductive surgery should be performed.

- Women with early stage disease are characterized into high risk and low risk. Those with high-risk disease should be given adjuvant chemotherapy.

- All women with advanced-stage disease require adjuvant chemotherapy. Combination of faclitaxel and carboplatin is used. Response to treatment is

(Continued)

Key points (Continued)

assessed by clinical evaluation, imaging and CA 125 levels.

- In selected women, primary chemotherapy followed by interval cytoreductive surgery may be undertaken.

- Second-look surgery is not recommended as a routine. Second-line chemotherapy is used for women with resistant and recurrent disease.

- Epithelial ovarian tumours with cellular features of malignancy but without stromal invasion are classified as borderline tumours. They are managed by laparotomy and unilateral oophorectomy in young women. Older women require hysterectomy and BSO. Adjuvant therapy does not improve survival.

- About 20–25% of all ovarian tumours are germ cell tumours and 3% are malignant. Germ cell tumours are classified according to the WHO classification. They occur in young girls younger than 20 years of age.

- The tumour markers secreted by germ cell tumour are α-fetoprotein (AFP), human chorionic gonadotropin (hCG) and lactic dehydrogenase (LDH).

- Malignant germ cell tumours are predominantly solid, present with acute lower abdominal pain or mass and increase rapidly in size.

- Ultrasonography, Doppler flow studies and estimation of tumour markers are required to confirm the diagnosis.

- Dysgerminoma is the most common germ cell tumour. It is bilateral in 15–20% of cases. Therefore, careful inspection of the other ovary is required during conservative surgery.

- Diagnosis and management are same as for other germ cell tumours. Prognosis is very good. Primary treatment is surgical. In young girls, unilateral oophorectomy and frozen section for confirmation of diagnosis are recommended. If reproductive function is not desired and the disease is more advanced than stage I, hysterectomy, BSO, omentectomy and pelvic and para-aortic lymphadenectomy are recommended.

- All germ cell tumours are chemosensitive. Adjuvant chemotherapy consists of a combination of bleomycin, etoposide and cisplatin.

- Sex cord-stromal tumours constitute about 5–8% of all ovarian tumours. Granulosa cell tumours, thecoma–fibroma, Sertoli–Leydig cell tumours and gynandroblastomas belong to this category.

- Sex cord-stromal tumours have a low malignant potential, present at stage I and have a good prognosis. Unilateral salpingo-oophorectomy is sufficient in most. Those with advanced-stage disease require hysterectomy and BSO.

Self-assessment

Case-based questions

Case 1

A 40-year-old lady, nulliparous, comes for a gynaecological check-up. On clinical examination, she is found to have an adnexal mass of 6 cm.

1. What details will you ask for in history?
2. How will you proceed to evaluate her?
3. Ultrasonography reveals a complex mass of 6 × 7 cm with resistance index of 0.2; CA 125 is 165 U/mL. What is the management?

Case 2

A 58-year-old lady presents with abdominal distension, discomfort and dyspnoea. On examination, she has a hard lower abdominal mass and ascites.

1. What details will you ask for in the history?
2. How will you proceed to examine her?
3. What investigations will you order?
4. What is the management?

Answers

Case 1

1. (a) Age at menarche, history of treatment for infertility, endometriosis, family history of breast, ovarian, endometrial cancers
   (b) Symptoms—Abdominal discomfort, weight loss, loss of appetite, bladder/bowel symptoms
2. (a) Clinical examination
      (i) General examination—Breast, lymphadenopathy
      (ii) Abdomen—Ascites
      (iii) Pelvic examination—Size of the mass, fixity, tenderness, nodules in POD
   (b) Investigations—Vaginal and abdominal ultrasonography and CA 125, and Doppler flow study
      Ultrasonography—To reveal size of the mass, cystic or solid, multiloculated, septal thickness, thickness of the cyst wall, papillary projections, bilaterality, ascites, lymph nodes
      Doppler flow study—For resistance index
      Elevated CA 125 suggests a malignant tumour.

3. Complex mass of 6 × 7 cm with a low resistance index is suggestive of malignancy. CA 125 is also elevated, making the probability of malignancy higher. The patient, therefore, needs staging laparotomy.
   (a) Preoperative evaluation—Routine tests
   (b) Staging laparotomy. Since the patient is 40 years old, hysterectomy, bilateral salpingo-oophorectomy, infracolic omentectomy, pelvic and para-aortic lymph node sampling and multiple biopsies
   (c) Adjuvant therapy—If stage IA/B, grade 1 or 2, no adjuvant therapy

If stage IC or stage IA/B, grade 3 or stage II—Chemotherapy with carboplatin and paclitaxel for three to six cycles.

Case 2

1. (a) Parity, in]fertility, age at menarche and menopause
   (b) Duration of symptoms, weight loss, loss of appetite, bladder/bowel symptoms
   (c) Family history of breast, ovarian, endometrial, colon cancer
2. (a) General examination—Lymph nodes (supraclavicular, inguinal), breast, respiratory system for pleural effusion, abdomen for ascites, hepatosplenomegaly, mass, omental cake
   (b) Pelvic examination—To look for mass, nodules in POD
   (c) Rectovaginal examination—To inspect rectal mucosa
3. (a) Ultrasound scan—To evaluate the extent of the disease, CA 125 as baseline for follow-up
   (b) Chest X-ray—To look for pleural effusion, ECG as routine preoperative workup
   (c) Other routine preoperative investigations
   (d) CT scan to assess feasibility of primary surgery
   (e) If disease found in upper abdomen and the patient considered for neoadjuvant chemotherapy, para-

centesis for cytology and/or fine-needle aspiration cytology of the mass
4. (a) Staging laparotomy, TAH, BSO and infracolic omentectomy, if feasible. If not, cytoreductive surgery.
   (b) Postoperative chemotherapy with carboplatin and paclitaxel every 3 weeks for six cycles. Assess clinically, with ultrasonogram/CT/MRI and CA 125 for response. Decide regarding further management.
   (c) If decided on neoadjuvant therapy, chemotherapy for three cycles followed by surgery and postoperative chemotherapy for three or more cycles.

Long-answer questions

1. Discuss the clinical features, diagnosis, staging and management of malignant epithelial ovarian, tubal and peritoneal cancer
2. Discuss the clinical features and management of ovarian germ cell tumours.

Short-answer questions

1. Dysgerminoma
2. Granulosa cell tumour
3. Solid (immature) teratoma of ovary
4. Signs and symptoms of malignant ovarian tumour
5. CA 125
6. Tumour markers in ovarian cancer
7. Role of imaging in the management of malignant ovarian tumours
8. Screening for ovarian cancer
9. FIGO staging of epithelial ovarian, tubal and peritoneal cancer
10. Germ cell tumours of the ovary

32 | Gestational Trophoblastic Disease

Case scenario

Mrs VR, 25, married for 8 months, presented with a history of vaginal bleeding during the third month of her pregnancy. She had excessive vomiting and had consulted a local doctor and was given medications. She had been advised an ultrasonography since the doctor suspected that all was not well with the pregnancy. Mrs VR noticed some vesicles along with the bleeding and was worried. Her mother realized that something was wrong and brought her for a consultation.

Introduction

When the trophoblast of the placenta undergoes abnormal proliferation, it results in molar pregnancy, which is a benign condition. However, malignant changes may ensue. This group of disorders that develop from the placental trophoblast are referred to as gestational trophoblastic disease (GTD). When diagnosed early and treated appropriately, prognosis is good.

Definitions

The term GTD is used to describe a group of tumours derived from placental trophoblastic tissue. This includes hydatidiform mole and gestational trophoblastic neoplasias (GTNs).

GTN is the term applied to a subset of GTDs that are locally invasive and have the capability to metastasize outside the uterus. This includes all GTDs except hydatidiform mole, given as follows:

- Invasive mole
- Choriocarcinoma
- Placental site trophoblastic tumour (PSTT)
- Epithelioid trophoblastic tumour (ETT)

GTDs secrete human chorionic gonadotropin (hCG), which serves as a reliable tumour marker. They have a good prognosis.

Incidence

There is wide variation in the reported incidence of GTD—From 1/1000 in North America and

Europe to 12/1000 in India and Indonesia. The difference in incidence may be due to socioeconomic and nutritional factors. Incidence is highest in the Southeast Asian countries.

Risk factors

Risk factors associated with GTD are listed in Box 32.1.

Box 32.1 Risk factors in gestational trophoblastic disease

- Maternal age
  - <20 years
  - >35 years
- Obstetric history
  - Previous abortion
  - Previous hydatidiform mole
- Race
- Vitamin A deficiency
- Use of combined oral contraceptive pills
- Low socioeconomic status

Hydatidiform mole

Proliferation and hydropic degeneration of the chorionic villi give rise to the typical vesicles characteristic of hydatidiform mole. This is of two types:

- Complete mole
- Partial mole

Complete hydatidiform mole

Complete mole is far more common than partial mole.

Pathology

Placenta consists of three types of trophoblasts: syncytiotrophoblasts, cytotrophoblasts and intermediate trophoblasts. **Syncytiotrophoblasts** are highly differentiated cells and secrete hCG. **Cytotrophoblasts** are primitive trophoblasts, polygonal in shape with mitotic activity. They do not secrete hCG. **Intermediate trophoblasts** invade the decidua, myometrium and blood vessels. They secrete hCG, but not to the same extent as syncytiotrophoblasts.

The pathological features of complete mole are given in Box 32.2. The villi that become

---

Box 32.2 Pathological features of complete hydatidiform mole

- Macroscopic
  - Vesicular, 'grape-like' appearance
- Microscopic
  - Hydropic degeneration of chorionic villi
  - Proliferation of trophoblasts
  - Absence of foetal tissues
- Diploid karyotype—Paternally derived

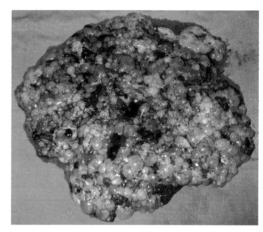

Figure 32.1 Hydatidiform mole. Note the classic grape-like oedematous villi.

oedematous give rise to the classic grape-like appearance, filling the uterine cavity (Fig. 32.1). They secrete large amounts of hCG. Microscopic examination reveals characteristic trophoblastic proliferation and hydropic degeneration of the villi (Fig. 32.2). Foetal tissues are not present.

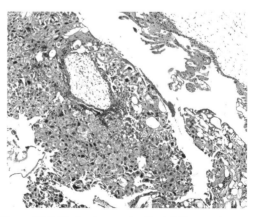

Figure 32.2 Photomicrograph of hydatidiform mole revealing characteristic features of trophoblastic proliferation and hydropic degeneration of villi.

Clinical features

Clinical features depend on the gestational age at which diagnosis is made, size of the uterus and serum hCG levels.

Symptoms

In the past, when ultrasonography was not available or was not used liberally, diagnosis of hydatidiform mole was made only when the patient presented with symptoms of miscarriage. Anaemia, large uterus, large theca lutein cysts, pre-eclampsia and hyperemesis were common. But with routine and liberal use of ultrasonography in the recent years, most cases are diagnosed early, by 12 weeks. Symptoms of hydatidiform mole are given in Box 32.3.

Box 32.3 Symptoms of hydatidiform mole

- Vaginal bleeding
- Passage of vesicles
- Anaemia
- Hyperemesis gravidarum
- Pre-eclampsia
- Thyrotoxicosis
- Respiratory symptoms
  - Trophoblastic embolization
  - Thyroid storm

Vaginal bleeding is the most common symptom. **Passage of vesicles** is pathognomonic but occurs rarely. **Anaemia** is uncommon when diagnosis is made early and bleeding has not been profuse or prolonged. **Hyperemesis** and **pre-eclampsia** have been attributed to the high levels of hCG but are infrequent now. hCG stimulates the thyroid gland and causes elevation of thyroxin levels. Very few women, however, present with symptoms of **hyperthyroidism**, but when this is present, anaesthetic complications must be anticipated.

Trophoblastic embolization can occur during or after evacuation of mole. This manifests clinically as chest pain, dyspnoea and tachypnoea. Rales are heard on auscultation and chest X-ray reveals diffuse infiltration.

Signs

Signs of hydatidiform mole are described in Box 32.4. **Uterus is larger than gestation** in 30% of women, corresponds to gestation in 50% and is smaller in 20%. Large uterus is associated

---

Box 32.4 Signs of hydatidiform mole

- Pallor
- Signs of pre-eclampsia
  - Elevated blood pressure
  - Proteinuria
- Signs of hyperthyroidism
  - Tachycardia
  - Tremor
- Uterus larger than gestation
- Absence of foetal parts
  - External ballottement
  - Foetal heart sounds
- Doughy consistency
- Vaginal bleeding
- Ovarian cysts on pelvic examination

---

with markedly elevated levels of hCG. **Theca lutein cysts** develop due to stimulation of ovaries by hCG. Large (>6 cm) cysts are associated with high levels of hCG. They usually regress after evacuation of the mole when hCG levels decrease. Persistence of the cysts is suggestive of continued high levels of the hormone probably due to invasive mole or choriocarcinoma. Pre-eclampsia, when it occurs, develops early (<20 weeks). Hyperthyroidism occurs late in pregnancy and when hCG levels are very high.

Diagnosis

- A diagnosis of hydatidiform mole is made by history and clinical examination if the pregnancy is >16–18 weeks. History of previous molar pregnancy and symptoms such as vaginal bleeding and hyperemesis gravidarum, if present, should arouse suspicion. Physical examination may reveal vaginal bleeding, uterus larger than period of gestation and theca lutein cysts.
- However, most women present with bleeding earlier in pregnancy and diagnosis is made by ultrasonography. Ultrasonographic features of complete hydatidiform mole are listed as follows (Fig. 32.3):
  - Complex, echogenic intrauterine contents with cystic anechoic spaces, known as **snowstorm appearance**
  - Absence of foetal parts
  - Absence of amniotic fluid
  - Theca lutein cysts (Fig. 32.4)
- *Elevated β-hCG levels*: Serum hCG levels are much higher than in normal pregnancy. Pre-evacuation hCG levels are >100,000 mIU/mL

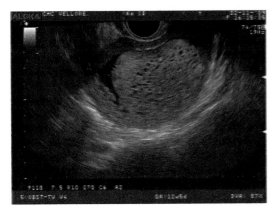

Figure 32.3 Ultrasonographic appearance of hydatidiform mole—Complex, echogenic intrauterine contents with cystic spaces giving rise to 'snowstorm appearance'.

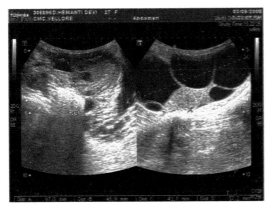

Figure 32.4 Ultrasonographic appearance of theca lutein cysts—Bilateral multiloculated cysts.

in 30–40% of molar pregnancies. The levels are also raised in multifoetal pregnancy; therefore, ultrasonographic confirmation of diagnosis is mandatory. Serum hCG values are useful for follow-up and diagnosis of GTN.

- Determination of ploidy by flow cytometry is useful in differentiating partial mole (which is triploid) from complete mole (which is diploid). This may be required in early pregnancy when histological features are not conclusive. Immunostaining for protein that is expressed by maternal gene also helps in the diagnosis.

Management
Evacuation of mole

Hydatidiform mole has to be evacuated. Haemoglobin should be estimated and packed

cells kept ready. Suction evacuation is the method of choice. Blood pressure must be controlled and precautions taken to manage a thyroid storm, if it occurs. Serum β-hCG levels must be estimated. Steps of this procedure are given in Box 32.5.

Box 32.5 Steps of suction evacuation

- Packed cells kept ready
- Regional/general anaesthesia
- Large-bore needle for IV access
- Cervix dilated to 10–12 mm
- Evacuation with suction cannula
- Oxytocin infusion 20 units in 1 L of saline
- Uterine curettage to ensure completion

IV, intravenous.

There is a concern that uterine contractions may force the trophoblastic tissues into the venous sinuses and cause embolization. Therefore, oxytocin infusion should be started only after the evacuation is begun and prostaglandins for cervical ripening must be avoided.

Hysterectomy

Hysterectomy is occasionally performed with mole in situ for older women, >40 years of age. Ovaries are usually retained. Hysterectomy eliminates the possibility of invasive mole and reduces risk of GTN. Metastatic trophoblastic neoplasia can occur even after hysterectomy; follow-up is mandatory.

Gestational trophoblastic neoplasia after evacuation of mole

GTN occurs in nearly 20% of women with complete mole. About 15% develop locally invasive disease and 4–5% develop metastatic disease. Risk factors for development of GTN are listed in Box 32.6.

Box 32.6 Risk factors for development of GTN

- Uterus larger than gestation
- Pre-evacuation hCG >100,000 mIU/mL
- Theca lutein cysts >6 cm in size
- Age >40 years

GTN, gestational trophoblastic neoplasia; *hCG*, human chorionic gonadotropin.

Partial hydatidiform mole

These reveal lesser degree of trophoblastic proliferation and hydropic degeneration than complete mole and contain foetal tissue. Clinically, they are often misdiagnosed as incomplete abortion. Histological features of partial mole are listed in Box 32.7.

Box 32.7 Histological features of partial hydatidiform mole

- Focal trophoblastic proliferation
- Focal hydropic degeneration and villous oedema
- Presence of foetal tissue
- Triploid karyotype

Clinical presentation of partial mole is also different (Box 32.8). Most women present with vaginal bleeding. Ultrasonography may reveal cystic spaces in the placental tissue, but diagnosis may be difficult (Fig. 32.5). The usual diagnosis is missed abortion and the molar changes may be diagnosed only on histological examination.

Box 32.8 Clinical features of partial hydatidiform mole

- Vaginal bleeding
- Uterus appropriate for gestational age
- No hyperemesis/pre-eclampsia/hyperthyroidism
- No theca lutein cysts
- Ultrasonography
  - Cystic spaces in the placenta
  - Reduced amniotic fluid
  - Foetus with growth restriction
  - Increased transverse diameter of the gestational sac
- Usually diagnosed on histopathology
- hCG elevation not marked
- Progression to GTN in 2–4%

GTN, gestational trophoblastic neoplasia; *hCG*, human chorionic gonadotropin.

Prophylactic chemotherapy

Chemotherapy given after evacuation of complete mole can prevent GTN. This has been tried in high-risk women who are not compliant with hCG surveillance and has been shown to reduce the incidence of GTN. Both methotrexate and actinomycin D may be used. However, use of prophylactic chemotherapy is controversial and

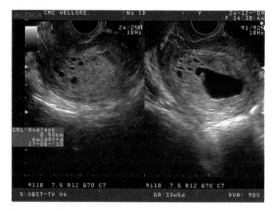

Figure 32.5 Ultrasonographic appearance of partial mole showing cystic spaces in the placental tissue and gestational sac with foetal pole.

is not universally recommended. It may have a role in women with multiple high-risk factors.

Postmolar follow-up

Hyperthyroidism and hypertension, if present, usually regress after evacuation of mole. Theca lutein cysts regress in 2–3 months.

Serum β-hCG serves as a sensitive test for surveillance after evacuation of mole. Postmolar follow-up is given in Box 32.9. The earlier recommendation was to continue weekly hCG measurements till β-hCG is normal for 3 consecutive weeks and continue surveillance for 6 months after that. But it has been found that after a single normal level of β-hCG, progression to GTN is

---

Box 32.9 Postmolar follow-up

- Serum β-hCG
- 48 hours after evacuation
  - Weekly thereafter
  - Continued till levels <5 mIU/mL (nondetectable) for 2 weeks
  - Monthly for 6 months
- Pelvic examination every 2 weeks
  - Uterine size
  - Size of theca lutein cysts
- Chest X-ray if β-hCG plateaus or rises
- Contraception till hCG levels normalize and remain so for 6 months
  - Combined oral pills
  - DMPA

DMPA, depot medroxyprogesterone acetate; *hCG*, human chorionic gonadotropin.

unlikely. Therefore, surveillance and contraception can be discontinued when a single value of β-hCG is undetectable or <2 mIU/mL.

Quiescent gestational trophoblastic disease

In some women, low levels (<200 mIU/mL) of hCG persist for several months after evacuation of mole. It is indicative of a small active focus of syncytiotrophoblast cells. About 10% will develop active GTN; therefore, close follow-up is essential. However, quiescent GTN is not an indication for chemotherapy.

A variant of β-hCG, known as **hyperglycosylated hCG (hCG-H)**, may be used to differentiate between quiescent and active GTN. This is produced by the invasive cytotrophoblasts during implantation and in GTN. It is more sensitive and specific for the diagnosis of GTN and a rising level indicates development of active disease.

Diagnosis of gestational trophoblastic neoplasia following hydatidiform mole

Since most cases of GTN occur during postmolar surveillance, certain criteria are used for diagnosis (Box 32.10). Tissue diagnosis is seldom obtained.

Further evaluation and management of GTN is discussed later in this chapter.

> **Box 32.10 Criteria for the diagnosis of postmolar trophoblastic neoplasia**
>
> - Plateau of hCG lasting for four measurements, over a period of 3 weeks or longer, that is, days 1, 7, 14, 21
> - Rise of hCG >10% on three consecutive weekly measurements, over a period of 2 weeks or longer, that is, days 1, 7, 14
> - Persistence of detectable levels of hCG for >6 months
> - Histological diagnosis of choriocarcinoma
>
> *hCG*, human chorionic gonadotropin.

Contraception

If pregnancy occurs during follow-up, the associated increase in β-hCG can interfere with detection of GTN. Therefore, contraception should be

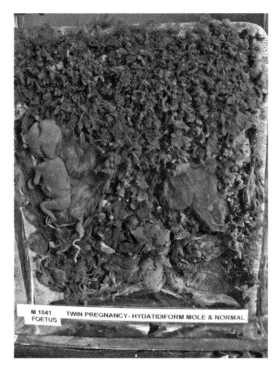

Figure 32.6 Specimen of molar pregnancy with coexisting foetus. Well-formed foetus is seen along with classic grape-like molar tissue.

advised during this period. Intrauterine devices, though reliable, can cause irregular bleeding and are not suitable. Combined oral contraceptive pills or depot medroxyprogesterone acetate (DMPA) is recommended.

Molar pregnancy with coexisting foetus

In a twin pregnancy, one can be a complete mole and the other a normal foetus (Fig. 32.6). This situation is rare, but live births of normal foetus are known. Complications associated with this are listed in Box 32.11.

> **Box 32.11 Complications in molar pregnancy with coexisting foetus**
>
> Increased risk of
> - Spontaneous abortion
> - Chromosomal anomalies
> - Pre-eclampsia
> - Foetal growth restriction

Gestational trophoblastic neoplasia

The locally invasive and metastatic subtypes of GTD are known as GTNs. Invasive mole and choriocarcinoma are common, but PSTT and ETT are rare. Majority of GTNs occur after a complete mole, but they may also occur after partial mole, normal pregnancy, miscarriage or termination of pregnancy. Invasive mole and choriocarcinoma are associated with high levels of hCG, but PSTT and ETT have low hCG levels.

Since the diagnosis of GTN is made on the basis of clinical presentation, elevated β-hCG and evidence of metastases on imaging, tissue for histology is seldom obtained. Therefore, a definitive histological diagnosis of the type of GTN is not made in most cases.

GTN can occur during the following:

- Molar pregnancy (50%)
- Miscarriage
- Tubal pregnancy
- Normal term or preterm pregnancy

Risk factors

Risk factors for development of GTN after hydatidiform mole have already been discussed (Box 32.6).

Invasive mole

An invasive mole is the most common GTN. It is locally invasive but metastasizes in 5% of cases. Invasive mole always develops after a complete or partial mole.

Pathology

Hydropic villi are present. The proliferating cytotrophoblasts and syncytiotrophoblasts invade the myometrium and serosa, and occasionally extend to the parametrium and vaginal wall. Preservation of villi with trophoblasts extending into the myometrium is the characteristic feature of invasive mole.

Other features are listed in Box 32.12.

Box 32.12 Invasive mole

- Trophoblastic invasion of
  - Myometrium
  - Serosa
  - Parametrium
  - Uterine vessels
  - Vagina
- Always originates from complete or partial mole
- Presents with
  - Vaginal bleeding
  - Enlarged uterus
  - Elevated β-hCG
- Complications
  - Uterine perforation
- Intraperitoneal haemorrhage
  - Profuse vaginal bleeding
  - Sepsis

hCG, human chorionic gonadotropin.

Choriocarcinoma

This is the next common trophoblastic neoplasia and constitutes about 30–40% of the trophoblastic neoplasia cases. This can be locally invasive and metastasize. Choriocarcinoma can develop after term pregnancies, molar pregnancies, abortions or ectopic pregnancies. It is an aggressive tumour and metastasizes rapidly.

Pathology

- **Macroscopic appearance:** Choriocarcinoma appears as highly vascular, dark red or blackish mass with haemorrhage (Fig. 32.7). The growth can be seen extending to the myometrium.
- **Microscopic appearance:** The tumour is composed of sheets of anaplastic cytotrophoblasts and syncytiotrophoblasts but is characterized by the absence of chorionic villi. There is necrosis and haemorrhage. The tumour extends into the myometrium (Fig. 32.8). The metastatic lesions are also haemorrhagic, dark red or black and well circumscribed.

Patterns of spread

Early haematogenous spread is characteristic of choriocarcinoma (Table 32.1). Pulmonary metastasis is the most common. Metastasis to vagina giving rise to suburethral nodules, other pelvic organs, liver and brain also occurs through the haematogenous route.

Placental site trophoblastic tumour

This is a rare tumour that develops from extra-villous, intermediate trophoblasts (Box 32.13). It is locally invasive but can metastasize. Serum hCG levels are low, but the syncytiotrophoblasts secrete human placental lactogen. PSTT occurs more often following nonmolar pregnancy or miscarriage.

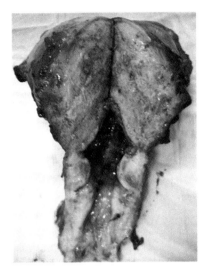

Figure 32.7 Uterus with choriocarcinoma; the tumour appears dark red with haemorrhage.

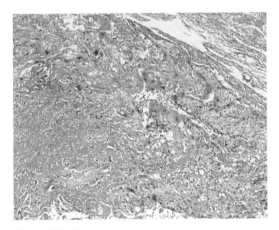

Figure 32.8 Microscopic appearance of choriocarcinoma—Trophoblastic proliferation with infiltration into myometrium and absence of chorionic villi.

> **Box 32.13 Placental site trophoblastic tumour**
>
> - Arises from intermediate trophoblasts
> - More common after normal pregnancy
> - Locally invasive
> - Metastasizes late
> - β-hCG not elevated
> - Does not respond to chemotherapy
> - Treatment of choice is hysterectomy
>
> hCG, human chorionic gonadotropin.

Epithelioid trophoblastic tumour

Only few cases of epithelioid tumours have been reported. This tumour also arises from syncytiotrophoblasts, but is histologically distinct from PSTT. Serum hCG levels are low and diagnosis is usually late. It is locally invasive but can metastasize.

Staging of gestational trophoblastic neoplasia

The currently accepted staging is the one recommended by the International Federation of Obstetrics and Gynecology (FIGO) (Table 32.2; Fig. 32.9).

Risk factor scoring

The prognostic scoring system developed by the World Health Organization (WHO) in 1983 has been modified by FIGO and is currently recommended (Table 32.3).

- A score of 0–6 is low-risk disease and can be managed by monotherapy.
- A score of ≥7 is high-risk disease and requires combination chemotherapy.

Table 32.1 Haematogenous spread in choriocarcinoma

	Frequency (%)
Lung	80
Vagina	30
Pelvis	20
Liver	10
Central nervous system	10
Others	
Spleen	<5
Kidney	<5
Gastrointestinal tract	<5

Table 32.2 FIGO staging of GTN

Stage I	Disease confined to the uterus; persistent elevation of serum β-hCG
Stage II	GTN extends outside of the uterus but is limited to the genital structures (adnexa, vagina, broad ligament)
Stage III	GTN extends to the lungs, with or without known genital tract involvement
Stage IV	All other metastatic sites (brain, liver)

FIGO, International Federation of Obstetrics and Gynecology; GTN, gestational trophoblastic neoplasia; hCG, human chorionic gonadotropin.

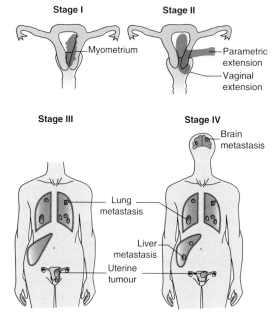

Figure 32.9 FIGO staging of GTN. **Stage I:** Disease confined to the uterus. **Stage II:** Disease extends outside of the uterus but is limited to the genital structures (adnexa, vagina, broad ligament). **Stage III:** Disease extends to the lungs, with or without known genital tract involvement. **Stage IV:** Disease extends to all other metastatic sites (brain, liver). FIGO, International Federation of Obstetrics and Gynecology; GTN, gestational trophoblastic neoplasia.

FIGO staging and risk factor scoring (2002) for GTN

The combination of FIGO staging and risk factor scoring is currently used for management of GTN. Women with stage I usually have a low-risk score and most women in stage IV have a high-risk score. Therefore, it is most useful in stages

Table 32.3 FIGO risk scoring system

	Scores			
	0	**1**	**2**	**4**
Age (years)	<40	≥40	—	—
Antecedent pregnancy	Mole	Abortion	Term	—
Interval months from index pregnancy	<4	4–6	7–12	≥13
Pretreatment serum β-hCG (mIU/mL)	$<10^3$	10^3– $<10^4$	10^4–$<10^5$	$≥10^5$
Largest tumour size (including uterus)		3–<5 cm	≥5 cm	
Site of metastases	Lung	Spleen, kidney	Gastrointestinal	Liver, brain
Number of metastases	—	1–4	5–8	>8
Previous failed chemotherapy	—	—	1 drug	≥2 drugs

FIGO, International Federation of Obstetrics and Gynecology; hCG, human chorionic gonadotropin.

II and III. The stage is represented by Roman numeral (I–IV), followed by a colon and the risk score in Arabic numerals (e.g. FIGO stage II: 9).

Clinical features

- GTN that develops during follow-up after evacuation of hydatidiform mole is usually diagnosed when serum β-hCG levels do not normalize as expected. The criteria are given in Box 32.10. These women may have irregular vaginal bleeding or amenorrhoea, enlarged uterus, persistent theca lutein cysts or vaginal nodules.
- When GTN develops after an interval or following a miscarriage or normal pregnancy, symptoms depend on the stage of the disease.

Nonmetastatic disease

Disease confined to the uterus can be asymptomatic. Theca lutein cysts persist due to persistently elevated hCG. Clinical features are given in Box 32.14.

Metastatic disease

Symptoms and signs of metastatic disease depend on the site of metastasis (Table 32.4). They can also be asymptomatic. Pulmonary

Box 32.14 Clinical features of nonmetastatic GTN

- Asymptomatic
- Vaginal bleeding
- Amenorrhoea
- Uterine enlargement
- Persistent theca lutein cysts
- Purulent vaginal discharge
  - Sepsis
- Intraperitoneal bleeding
  - Uterine perforation

GTN, gestational trophoblastic neoplasia.

Table 32.4 Clinical features of metastatic GTN

Site of metastasis	Symptoms
Lungs	• Cough, haemoptysis, dyspnoea, chest pain • Pulmonary hypertension
Vagina	• Asymptomatic • Profuse bleeding
Liver	• Asymptomatic • Capsular rupture and haemorrhage • Jaundice, epigastric pain
Brain	• Convulsions, focal neurological deficits

GTN, gestational trophoblastic neoplasia.

lesions are most common. In addition to cough and haemoptysis, they can also lead to secondary pulmonary hypertension. Vaginal metastases are very vascular and bleed profusely, if biopsied. They are often located suburethrally. Liver metastasis occurs late and is more common in GTN following term pregnancy. Hepatic lesions can stretch the capsule and cause capsular rupture resulting in intraperitoneal bleeding. Brain metastasis is also seen when there is delay in diagnosis and causes convulsions and focal neurological deficits depending on their location. Liver and brain metastases are usually associated with lung and pelvic metastasis.

Clinical evaluation

When GTN is diagnosed on the basis of elevated hCG following molar pregnancy, the patient should be evaluated to determine the extent of the disease, presence or absence of metastases, stage of the disease and risk factor scoring.

History

History should focus on antecedent pregnancy, symptoms and their duration and prior treatment, if any (Box 32.15).

Box 32.15 History in GTN

- Age
- Symptoms
- Duration of symptoms
- Interval from antecedent pregnancy
- Antecedent pregnancy
  - Mole
  - Miscarriage
  - Term pregnancy
  - Ectopic gestation
- Prior treatment
  - Evacuation of mole
  - Hysterectomy
  - Chemotherapy
    - Single agent
    - Combination

GTN, gestational trophoblastic neoplasia.

Physical examination

General, systemic and pelvic examinations are mandatory (Box 32.16).

Box 32.16 Physical examination in GTN

- General examination
  - Pallor
- Respiratory system
  - Respiratory rate
  - Rales on auscultation
- Central nervous system
  - Level of consciousness
  - Focal neurological deficits
- Abdominal examination
  - Hepatomegaly, tenderness
  - Uterine enlargement
  - Intraperitoneal bleeding
    - Guarding
    - Rigidity
- Speculum examination
  - Suburethral/vaginal nodules
  - Bleeding
- Bimanual examination
  - Uterine size
  - Theca lutein cysts

GTN, gestational trophoblastic neoplasia.

Investigations

When the disease is suspected on the basis of symptoms, estimation of serum β-hCG is the first step in diagnostic evaluation.

Serum β-hCG

The levels of serum β-hCG may be very high in choriocarcinoma. Pretreatment value is of prognostic significance and should be documented.

Imaging

Diagnosis of uterine tumour and metastases is by **imaging** (Box 32.17). The uterine lesion can be detected on **ultrasonography**. The tumour choriocarcinoma and invasive mole are very vascular and the tumour may be seen infiltrating the myometrium (Fig. 32.10). **Chest X-ray** is used for diagnosis and counting the number of pulmonary metastases (Fig. 32.11). This should be performed in all patients with GTN. **Computed tomography** (CT) may be useful, but findings on CT are not used for scoring. Abdominal and hepatic lesions are evaluated by ultrasonography or CT as required. **Magnetic resonance imaging** (MRI) or CT can be used for diagnosis of brain lesions (Fig. 32.12). **Positron emission tomography** (PET)/**CT** is useful when MRI/CT does not reveal metastasis but β-hCG is elevated.

Pretreatment investigations

All women with GTN need chemotherapy. Pretreatment investigations to evaluate liver and

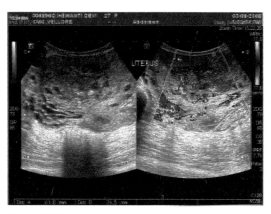

Figure 32.10 Ultrasonography shows tumour in the uterine cavity infiltrating the myometrium. The tumour is very vascular, a characteristic feature of choriocarcinoma.

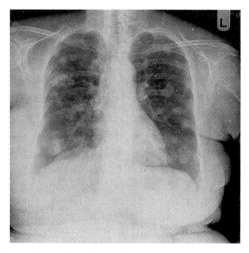

Figure 32.11 Chest X-ray of a lady with choriocarcinoma showing multiple rounded opacities consistent with 'cannon ball' secondaries.

renal functions and complete blood are mandatory (Box 32.18). Baseline serum β-hCG level must also be documented.

Box 32.17   Methods used for diagnosis of metastases

- Ultrasonography of abdomen and pelvis
  - Uterine lesions
  - Theca lutein cysts
  - Hepatic metastases
- Chest X-ray
  - Diagnosis of lung metastases
  - Number of lesions
- CT thorax
  - Pulmonary micrometastases
- CT abdomen
  - Hepatic and intra-abdominal lesions
- CT/MRI brain (if pulmonary metastasis present)
  - Brain metastases

CT, computed tomography; *MRI*, magnetic resonance imaging.

Box 32.18   Pretreatment investigations in GTN

- Haemoglobin
- Complete blood count
- Liver function tests
- Renal function tests

GTN, gestational trophoblastic neoplasia.

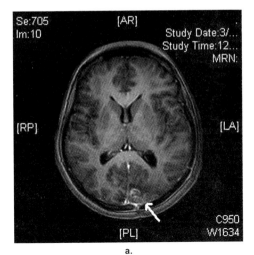

a.

b.

Figure 32.12 Magnetic resonance imaging showing brain secondaries in choriocarcinoma. a. Post-gadolinium T1W images showing cluster of ring-enhancing lesions in the left occipital lobe (arrow). b. T2W axial section showing well-defined lesions that have a T2 hypointense rim and perilesional oedema in the left occipital lobe (arrow).

Endometrial curettage

Histological diagnosis of choriocarcinoma is not required for initiation of treatment. Invasive mole cannot be diagnosed by endometrial curettage. Moreover, curettage is associated with a risk of perforation and haemorrhage.

Endometrial curettage may be required for diagnosis of PSTT and ETT. In women who present with symptoms suggestive of GTN and low hCG levels, these should be suspected and curettage should be performed. High index of suspicion is necessary to make a diagnosis.

Management of GTN

Chemotherapy is the mainstay of management of GTN. Women who have low-risk GTN by the risk scoring system are treated with single-agent chemotherapy and those with high-risk GTN are treated with multiagent therapy. Hysterectomy is warranted in some situations in the management of GTN.

Hysterectomy

Hysterectomy followed by adjuvant single-agent chemotherapy may be considered as first choice in women with low-risk disease who do not desire fertility. Hysterectomy reduces the total dose of chemotherapy required. Other indications are given in Box 32.19.

Box 32.19 Indications for hysterectomy

- Women with low-risk GTN who do not desire fertility
- Perforating mole with intraperitoneal haemorrhage
- Uncontrolled vaginal bleeding
- Chemoresistant disease confined to the uterus
- Placental site trophoblastic tumour
- Epithelioid trophoblastic tumour

GTN, gestational trophoblastic neoplasia.

Management of low-risk GTN

Low-risk disease includes the following:

- Women with a WHO risk score of 1–6
  - Almost all women with stage I disease
  - Women with stage II/III with WHO score 1–6

As discussed earlier, hysterectomy should be considered in older women who do not desire fertility. This should be followed by chemotherapy.

Treatment of low-risk disease is by single-agent chemotherapy. Methotrexate and actinomycin D are the commonly used chemotherapeutic agents.

Methotrexate

Methotrexate is the drug of choice. It is effective and well tolerated.

- Folic acid is required for the synthesis of thymidine and purine, which are essential for the synthesis of DNA and RNA. Methotrexate is a folic acid antagonist and acts by inhibiting enzyme folic acid reductase, which is required for folic acid metabolism. It acts on the rapidly dividing cells. Folinic acid, which has the same action as folic acid and is not inhibited by methotrexate, is used to reduce its toxicity (Box 32.20).
- Randomized trials have proved the efficacy of intramuscular (IM) and intravenous methotrexate in the management of GTN. Oral preparation, which was popular earlier, is not used any more. When the drug is used in high dose, folinic acid is administered alternating with methotrexate (folinic acid rescue) to prevent toxicity. Dosage and administration are given in Table 32.5.
- Liver function tests and complete blood count should be monitored during treatment with high-dose regimens. Methotrexate should be withheld if the liver enzymes are elevated or the total leucocyte count and platelet count fall.
- Remission rate is 80% with methotrexate. Response rates are similar with all regimens. However, most centres use the 8-day methotrexate with folinic acid rescue regimen or weekly IM dosing.

Box 32.20 Methotrexate

- Most common drug used for treatment of GTN
- Folic acid antagonist
- Inhibits DNA and RNA synthesis
- Inhibits rapidly dividing cells
- Adverse effects
  - Gastrointestinal mucositis
    - Diarrhoea
    - Stomatitis
    - Nausea
  - Alopecia
  - Bone marrow suppression
  - Hepatotoxicity

DNA, deoxyribonucleic acid; *GTN*, gestational trophoblastic neoplasia; *RNA*, ribonucleic acid.

Table 32.5 Methotrexate—Dosage and administration

Dose	Frequency	Route of administration
30–50 mg/m²	Weekly	IM
1 mg/kg, days 1, 3, 5, 7, alternating with folinic acid 0.1 mg/kg, days 2, 4, 6, 8	Every 2 weeks	IM
0.4 mg/kg/day for 5 days	Alternate weeks	IM
100 mg/m²	Every 2 weeks	IV infusion

IM, intramuscular; *IV*, intravenous.

Actinomycin D

This is the second-line drug used in the treatment of GTN. Studies have shown that it is as effective as methotrexate. It is usually used when there is no response to methotrexate. Toxicity is higher. Dosage, route of administration and side effects are given in Box 32.21.

Box 32.21 Actinomycin D

- As effective as methotrexate in GTN
- More toxic
- Dosage
  - 9–13 µg/kg/day IV × 5 days every 2 weeks
  - 1.25 mg/m² IV bolus every 2 weeks
- Adverse effects
  - Alopecia
  - Nausea
  - Nephrotoxicity

GTN, gestational trophoblastic neoplasia; *IV*, intravenous.

Management of low-risk GTN is summarized in Box 32.22. Serum β-hCG should be monitored weekly until three consecutive values are normal. Contraception should be continued. If there is no response to therapy, switching to alternative drugs is indicated (Box 32.22). Other drugs that have been used are oral etoposide and 5-fluorouracil. Response to therapy is usually good, fertility is preserved and cure rate is 100%.

Box 32.22 Management of low-risk GTN

- Consider hysterectomy if fertility is not desired
- Chemotherapy with single-agent methotrexate/actinomycin D
- Weekly serum β-hCG
- Monitor liver functions and complete blood count
- If hCG levels plateau or rise, switch to alternative drugs
- If methotrexate resistant, switch to actinomycin D
- If actinomycin resistant, switch to methotrexate
- Continue till three consecutive hCG values are normal
- Continue monitoring and contraception for 12 months
- Cure rate is 100%

GTN, gestational trophoblastic neoplasia; hCG, human chorionic gonadotropin.

Management of high-risk GTN

High-risk GTN includes patients with risk score of 7 or more:

- Women with stage IV disease
- Women with stage II/III disease with WHO score ≥7

Aggressive therapy with multiagent chemotherapy is warranted in these women. The multidrug regimen consists of etoposide, methotrexate, actinomycin D, cyclophosphamide and vincristine with folinic acid rescue (EMA-CO; Table 32.6). Each course is given for over 8 days and next course started on day 15.

Multiagent chemotherapy is toxic, and the toxicity includes alopecia, stomatitis, gastrointestinal mucositis and myelosuppression. Alternative regimens including platinum and etoposide are under trial for resistant cases.

Remission rate with EMA-CO is 78%, the regimen is well tolerated and fertility rate following treatment is high. Hence, it is used as the primary treatment for high-risk GTN.

Management of metastases

Patients with metastatic disease may require surgical intervention to remove chemoresistant disease or control haemorrhage. Brain metastasis is treated by radiation. These are listed in Table 32.7.

Table 32.6 Multiagent chemotherapy for high-risk GTN

Day	Drug	Dosage
1	Etoposide	100 mg/m^2 IV over 30 minutes
	Methotrexate	100 mg/m^2 IV bolus followed by 200 mg/m^2 IV over 12 hours
	Actinomycin D	0.5 mg IV bolus
2	Etoposide	100 mg/m^2 IV over 30 minutes
	Actinomycin D	0.5 mg IV bolus
	Folinic acid	15 mg oral Q12H for four doses
8	Cyclophosphamide	600 mg/m^2 IV
	Vincristine	1.0 mg/m^2 IV

GTN, gestational trophoblastic neoplasia; IV, intravenous.

Table 32.7 Management of metastases

Site	Intervention	Indication
Vagina	• Packing • Wide local excision • Local radiation • Arterial embolization	Profuse bleeding
Lung	Pulmonary wedge resection	Chemoresistant disease
Liver	Intra-arterial chemotherapy	Chemoresistant disease
	Partial hepatic resection	
	Arterial embolization	Haemorrhage
Brain	Whole brain irradiation	Chemoresistant disease

Management of women with high-risk disease is summarized in Box 32.23. Surveillance and contraception should be continued for 24 months since late recurrences can occur. Complete remission is achieved in 75–80% of women.

Survival

GTN has a good prognosis with 100% complete remission rates in low-risk disease. With multiagent therapy, survival rate in high-risk disease is

Box 32.23 Management of high-risk GTN

- Multiagent chemotherapy
  - EMA-CO every 2 weeks
- Monitor serum hCG weekly
- Monitor response by serum β-hCG
  - Response: >10% decline
  - Plateau: ±10% change
  - Resistance: <10% rise
- Switch to alternative regime if resistant
- Monitor till three consecutive hCG values are normal
- Monthly hCG till 12 consecutive nondetectable levels
- Contraception for 24 months
- Management of chemoresistant metastases
  - Surgery
  - Radiation
  - Selective arterial embolization

EMA-CO, etoposide, methotrexate, actinomycin D, cyclophosphamide and vincristine with folinic acid rescue; *GTN*, gestational trophoblastic neoplasia; *hCG*, human chorionic gonadotropin.

about 80–90%. When brain metastasis is present, survival reduces to 50–60%.

Pregnancy after GTD

Contraception should be advised for all women with molar pregnancy and GTN as already discussed. There is a 1–2% risk of having a repeat molar pregnancy after a complete or partial mole. Therefore, ultrasonography should be performed in the first trimester. Outcome of pregnancies after chemotherapy for GTN has been found to be normal.

Management of PSTT and ETT

These do not respond well to chemotherapy. Hence, hysterectomy followed by combination chemotherapy (EMA-CO) is the recommended treatment. Prognosis in metastatic disease is poor.

Key points

- The term gestational trophoblastic disease is used to describe a group of tumours derived from placental trophoblastic tissue. This includes hydatidiform mole, invasive mole, choriocarcinoma and placental site trophoblastic tumour.

- The term gestational trophoblastic neoplasia (GTN) is used to describe tumours that are locally invasive and have the capability to metastasize. This includes invasive moles, choriocarcinoma, placental site trophoblastic tumour and epithelioid trophoblastic tumour.

- All gestational trophoblastic tumours secrete human chorionic gonadotropin (hCG).

- Risk factors for gestational trophoblastic disease are maternal age, previous hydatidiform mole, race, low socioeconomic status and use of combined oral contraceptive pills.

- Hydatidiform mole occurs due to proliferation and hydropic degeneration of chorionic villi.

- The typical presenting symptoms of hydatidiform mole are vaginal bleeding, passage of vesicles, hyperemesis gravidarum, anaemia and pre-eclampsia. Clinical examination reveals a uterus that is larger than gestation with or without theca lutein cyst of the ovary. Signs of pre-eclampsia may be present. Foetal parts are absent and there may be vaginal bleeding.

- Diagnosis of hydatidiform mole is by symptoms, signs, serum β-hCG levels and ultrasonography.

- Management of hydatidiform mole is by suction evacuation.

- Risk factors for GTN are large uterus, hCG more than 100,000 mIU/mL, theca lutein cysts more than 6 cm and age greater than 40 years.

- Since GTN may occur in 20% of women following hydatidiform mole, follow-up is mandatory.

- Partial mole has features of hydatidiform mole along with foetal tissue.

- Postmolar follow-up consists of serial estimation of serum β-hCG, pelvic examination and chest X-ray. Contraception with combined oral contraceptive pills or depot medroxyprogesterone acetate (DMPA) is recommended.

- GTN may be local invasive or metastatic. Invasive mole is the most common. It presents with vaginal bleeding and elevated β-hCG.

- Choriocarcinoma develops after term pregnancies, molar pregnancies, abortions or ectopic pregnancies. It spreads by haematogenous route.

- Staging of GTN according to International Federation of Obstetrics and Gynecology (FIGO) is into stages I, II, III and IV. Prognostic scoring system by the World Health Organization (WHO) is used for management.

- Ultrasonography, chest X-ray, computed tomography (CT) of the abdomen/thorax and magnetic resonance imaging (MRI) of the brain are used for evaluation and staging of GTN.

- Chemotherapy with methotrexate is the mainstay of management of low-risk GTN. Actinomycin D may be used as an alternative.

- Combination chemotherapy is used for the management of high-risk GTN.

- Monitoring for 12–22 months is required after treatment of GTN.

Self-assessment

Case-based questions

Case 1

A 25-year-old lady with previous normal delivery of a healthy child presents with 10 weeks' amenorrhoea and excessive vomiting and minimal vaginal bleeding. On examination, her uterus is 14 weeks' size. Pregnancy test is positive.

1. How will you evaluate her?
2. If the diagnosis is hydatidiform mole, what is the management?
3. How will you follow up this patient?

Case 2

A 38-year-old lady, mother of three children, presents with irregular vaginal bleeding. She gives a history of a molar pregnancy 8 months ago.

1. How will you evaluate her?
2. If her serum β-hCG is 12,000 mIU/mL, uterus is normal size, lutein cysts are 6 × 6 cm and chest X-ray shows two coin-shaped lesions, what is the FIGO stage and risk score?
3. How will you manage her?

Answers

Case 1

1. Since the uterus is larger than the dates and she has hyperemesis and bleeding, perform ultrasound scan to exclude twins/hydatidiform mole.

   If molar pregnancy is diagnosed, clinical evidence of hyperthyroidism should be looked for. Blood pressure should be checked. Serum β-hCG and Hb should be asked for.

2. Packed cells should be available. Suction curettage is the treatment of choice. The material should be sent for histopathology.

3. (a) At discharge:
    (i) Serum β-hCG 48 hours after suction curettage
    (ii) U/S scan for size of theca lutein cysts
    (iii) Chest X-ray
    (iv) Combine OC pills
    (v) Counsel regarding follow-up

   (b) Follow-up:
    (i) Weekly β-hCG, pelvic examination once in 2 weeks till levels are <5 mIU/mL
    (ii) Contraception till then
    (iii) Evaluate for GTN if hCG levels plateau or rise

Case 2

1. (a) History—Symptoms, previous chemotherapy
   (b) Clinical examination—Pallor, vaginal metastases, uterine size, lutein cysts, examination of respiratory and nervous systems
   (c) Serum β-hCG, chest X-ray, complete blood count, liver function tests, renal function tests, ultrasonography of abdomen and pelvis for uterine size, theca lutein cysts, disease in pelvis and abdomen
   (d) If chest X-ray shows metastases, CT brain
2. FIGO stage III, risk score 5, low-risk group.
3. Since she is 38 years old and has three children, option of hysterectomy should be discussed.

   Single-agent chemotherapy with weekly IM methotrexate or IV with folinic acid rescue on alternate days should be given either as primary treatment or as adjuvant to hysterectomy.

   Treatment continued till serum hCG levels are normal for 3 consecutive weeks.

   Follow-up continued for 6 months. Contraception with combined OC pills if hysterectomy is not performed.

Long-answer questions

1. Describe the signs, symptoms and management of vesicular mole.
2. Discuss the diagnosis and management of gestational trophoblastic neoplasia.

Short-answer questions

1. Staging and prognostic scoring of gestational trophoblastic neoplasia
2. Invasive mole
3. Chemotherapy in gestational trophoblastic neoplasia
4. Follow-up after evacuation of hydatidiform mole
5. Clinical features of hydatidiform mole

Section 7

Operative
Gynaecology

33

Preoperative Preparation and Postoperative Management

Case scenario

Mrs BV, 56, was evaluated for postmenopausal bleeding at a private hospital. She was diagnosed to have endometrial cancer and was advised staging laparotomy, hysterectomy and pelvic node dissection. Mrs BV was obese, diabetic and asthmatic. She was considered high risk for anaesthesia and referred to our hospital for further management.

Introduction

Optimal outcome of any surgical procedure depends on several factors such as appropriate selection of procedure, skill of the surgeon and anaesthetist, adequate and thorough preoperative evaluation and postoperative management. In addition to evaluating the patient for surgery, preoperative preparation involves allaying the patient's anxiety and obtaining informed consent. It also reduces the chance of unanticipated situations during surgery.

Goals of preoperative preparation

The goals of preoperative preparation are listed in Box 33.1.

Box 33.1 Goals of preoperative preparation

- Identify risk factors
  - Medical
  - Surgical
- Modify risk factors
- Obtain specialist consultations
- Plan
  - Appropriate anaesthesia
  - Surgical steps
  - Postoperative management
- Educate the patient
- Find out the patient's preferences
- Obtain informed consent

Preoperative evaluation

Preoperative evaluation includes history, physical examination and investigations. These have been discussed in detail in the various chapters for the specific gynaecological conditions.

History

Additional details in history that are required prior to surgery are given in Box 33.2.

Box 33.2 History

- Age
- Parity
- Obstetric and gynaecological history
- Medical history
  - Cardiovascular diseases
  - Pulmonary conditions
  - Neuromuscular conditions
  - Diabetes and endocrine disorders
  - Haematological conditions
- Medications
- Allergies
- Previous surgery
  - Anaesthesia
  - Type of surgery
  - Complications
- Family history
  - Haemorrhagic conditions
  - Anaesthetic complications
  - Other inherited conditions

Age is an important factor since older patients have a higher prevalence of diabetes mellitus, hypertension and organ dysfunction. Electrolyte disturbances, fluid overload, drug-induced renal failure and excessive response to sedation are common in older women. Coexisting **medical conditions** must be evaluated thoroughly, if required, by a specialist, to avoid intraoperative and postoperative complications. Patients who have had **previous surgery** may have adhesions. Previous anaesthetic problems can recur. Several **medications** interfere with anaesthesia. **Family history** may reveal unsuspected conditions such as scoline apnoea or bleeding disorders. **Allergies** to drugs must be noted and the suspected groups of drugs avoided.

Physical examination

The patient must be examined for signs of cardiovascular or respiratory disease or other medical disorders and fitness for anaesthesia (Box 33.3).

Gynaecological evaluation should be aimed at planning the route of surgery, determining the

---

Box 33.3 Physical examination for preoperative evaluation

- Vital signs
- General examination
  - BMI
  - Pallor
- Examination of various systems
  - Cardiovascular
  - Pulmonary
  - Neurological
- Abdominal examination
  - Scars
  - Size of the mass
- Pelvic examination
  - Size of the uterus/mass
  - Mobility
- Per rectal examination
  - Extension of disease to rectal lumen
  - Pouch of Douglas

BMI, body mass index.

---

need for special investigations and anticipating and avoiding complications.

Calculating the body mass index (BMI) is important since obese women need special instruments and positioning. Also, administration of general/regional anaesthesia is difficult and fluid management can pose problems. Lean patients withstand blood loss poorly and need expert fluid management. On evaluation, abnormalities of various systems must be investigated further. Presence of scars, size and mobility of the mass helps in decision regarding the route of surgery. Pelvic examination should be repeated prior to surgery even if it has been performed in the clinic earlier, in case the findings have changed. Extension of disease to rectum or colon may necessitate bowel preparation.

Investigations

Important determinants of the choice of investigations are age of the patient, presence of comorbidities, nature and extent of disease, and extent of surgical procedure to be performed. If the patient has no risk factors, is premenopausal and is <50 years, only minimum investigations are required. If a woman is older and postmenopausal, but no other risk factors are present, few additional tests are needed (Boxes 33.4 and 33.5). Pretest counselling is mandatory before ordering screening tests for blood-borne viruses.

Box 33.4 Routine preoperative investigations

- Low risk, premenopausal
  - Haemoglobin
  - Urinalysis
  - Blood sugar
  - Serum creatinine
  - Blood-borne virus screen
- Low risk, postmenopausal, >50 years
  - All the above tests
  - ECG

ECG, electrocardiography.

Box 33.5 Additional preoperative investigations

- Diabetes: HbA1C, plasma glucose
- Hypertension: Chest X-ray
- Cardiac disease: Chest X-ray, echocardiography
- Pulmonary disease: Pulmonary function tests
- Prior/current hepatic disease ⎫
- Extensive malignancy ⎭ Prothrombin time, platelets Liver function test
- Ureteric obstruction ⎫
- Extensive malignancy ⎭ Contrast-enhanced CT with arterial, venous and delayed phase
- Suspected adhesions ⎫
- Infiltration to other organs ⎭ CT scan/MRI
- Prolapse: Urine culture
- Renal failure: Electrolytes, creatinine
- Thyroid dysfunction: Free T4 and TSH

CT, computed tomography; *MRI*, magnetic resonance imaging; *T4*, thyroxine concentration; *TSH*, thyroid-stimulating hormone.

Routine urinalysis, electrolytes, liver function tests, tests for haemostasis, electrocardiography and chest X-ray are *not* recommended in healthy young adults.

Additional investigations to assess fitness for surgery are required if the patient is diabetic or hypertensive, or has other comorbidities. If the patient has extensive malignancy, ureteric or bowel involvement is suspected or adhesions are anticipated, additional investigations are necessary.

Anaesthesia evaluation

This is mandatory for all preoperative patients. Surgical risk is assigned using American Society

Table 33.1 ASA physical status classification

ASA class	Class definition
I	A normal healthy patient
II	A patient with mild to moderate systemic disease
III	A patient with severe systemic disease that substantially limits activity but is not incapacitating
IV	A patient with severe systemic disease that is a constant threat to life
V	A moribund patient who is not expected to survive for 24 hours with or without operation
VI	A declared brain-dead patient whose organs are being removed for donor purposes

ASA, American Society of Anesthesiologists.

of Anesthesiologists (ASA) physical status classification (Table 33.1).

Based on this classification, the method of anaesthesia, postoperative pain relief and patient-controlled analgesia (PCA) must be decided and discussed with the patient. Need for intensive care unit (ICU) care postoperatively should be anticipated and decided on.

Preoperative preparation

Antimicrobial prophylaxis

- Most minor procedures such as endometrial biopsy, cervical biopsy and laparoscopy are clean procedures, and prophylactic antimicrobials are not recommended.
- Gynaecological surgeries where vagina is opened or the peritoneal cavity is entered through the vagina are considered 'clean contaminated' and prophylactic antimicrobials are recommended to prevent surgical site infection (Box 33.6).
- Single dose of antibiotic, administered within 1 hour before the surgery, provides adequate blood levels at the onset and throughout the procedure.
- One of the **cephalosporins** is the drug of choice. Metronidazole with levofloxacin or gentamicin or a combination of clindamycin and gentamicin is recommended in patients who are sensitive to penicillin.
- When there is frank sepsis with pus in the pelvis/peritoneal cavity, antibiotic therapy with a

Box 33.6 Prophylactic antimicrobial indications

- Indications
  - Vaginal hysterectomy
  - Abdominal/laparoscopic hysterectomy
  - Pelvic reconstructive surgery
  - Dilatation and evacuation
- Timing
  - At induction of anaesthesia
- Dosage
  - Single dose
  - Dose to be repeated if
    - Duration >3 hours
    - Blood loss >1.5 L
- Choice of antibiotics
  - Cefazoline 1–2 g IV single dose
  - (or) Cefoxitin 2 g IV single dose

combination to cover Gram-negative, Gram-positive and anaerobic organisms is instituted preoperatively and continued for an appropriate length of time.

- In women with cardiac valvular disease, infective endocarditis prophylaxis should be given.

Thromboprophylaxis

- Venous thromboembolism (VTE) and pulmonary embolism (PE) are a major cause of mortality after gynaecological surgery. Prophylaxis against thromboembolism is an integral part of preoperative preparation.
- This is decided based on the risk stratification by American College of Chest Physicians (ACCP), 2012, which divides patients into very low-, low-, moderate- and high-risk groups. Risk of VTE in the various risk categories is given in Box 33.7.
- Risk factors include age (>40, >60, >75), BMI, sepsis, associated pulmonary or cardiac diseases, type of surgery, presence of malignancy, bed rest and immobilization, family history of thrombophilias, past history of VTE and pelvic/hip fracture.
- Patients should not be hospitalized unless absolutely necessary, till the day prior to surgery, and should be asked to continue normal activities.
- Medications such as oral contraceptive (OC) pills, oestrogens and tamoxifen must be discontinued at least 1 month prior to surgery. Alternatively, thromboprophylaxis can be instituted for women on these medications.

Box 33.7 Risk of VTE in various risk categories

Risk category	Estimated risk of VTE (%)
Very low	<0.5
Low	1.5
Moderate	3.0
High	6.0

VTE, venous thromboembolism.

- Thromboprophylaxis may be started 12 hours prior to surgery and continued till the patient is well ambulated. Mechanical methods such as compression stockings and intermittent sequential pneumatic compression are used to prevent venous stasis in the calf muscles, which is a major cause of VTE.

Recommended prophylaxis for the various risk groups is given in Box 33.8.

Box 33.8 Recommended thromboprophylaxis

Very low risk	• No anticoagulation • Early ambulation
Low risk	Intermittent pneumatic compression (or) Graduated compression stockings
Moderate risk	LMWH (or) Low-dose UFH (or) Intermittent pneumatic compression
High risk	LMWH (or) Low-dose UFH *plus* intermittent pneumatic compression

LMWH, low-molecular-weight heparin; *UFH*, unfractionated heparin

Drugs used for thromboprophylaxis

Low-molecular-weight heparin (LMWH) and unfractionated heparin (UFH) are used for thromboprophylaxis.

Low-molecular-weight heparin LMWH is the drug of choice. It can be given once daily and does not require monitoring. The risk of thrombocytopaenia is low. Subcutaneous administration of enoxaparin 40 mg once daily is started 12 hours prior to surgery and continued for 3–5 days or till the patient is well ambulated. Other LMWHs can also be used.

Unfractionated heparin This is usually given in a dose of 5000 units. It is usually begun 2 hours prior to surgery and continued 12 hourly. It is less expensive and effective but requires twice-daily dosing and monitoring of platelet count.

Management of medical comorbidities

- **Diabetes mellitus:** For all patients with diabetes going for elective surgery, it is preferable to get the HbA1C down to <8% before taking up for surgery. Patients with diabetes mellitus who are well controlled on oral hypoglycaemic agents can continue these up to the night before surgery. On the morning of surgery, the patient needs to be started on IV dextrose saline with added short-acting insulin, and the capillary blood sugars should be monitored hourly so as to titrate the dose of insulin to maintain blood sugar in the range of 100–160 mg/dL. Oral antidiabetics can be restarted as soon as the patient is started on oral fluids.
- **Hypertension:** It is important to get the blood pressure readings down to 120/80 to 130/85 mmHg in patients going for elective surgery. While this is being achieved, serum creatinine and electrolytes need to be monitored and optimized.
- **Obesity:** Obesity is a risk factor for deep vein thrombosis and PE. Intubation and spinal/epidural anaesthesia may be difficult. Wound healing may be delayed. For elective surgery, preoperative weight optimization is advisable. Thromboprophylaxis is mandatory.

The patient's **medication list** should be reviewed and appropriate adjustments made. Drugs such as aspirin and oestrogen must be discontinued and oral anticoagulants should be changed to heparin.

Bowel preparation

Routine bowel preparation is not recommended. When extensive bowel adhesions are anticipated and bowel entry is a possibility, bowel preparation with polyethylene glycol (PEG) electrolyte solution or sodium phosphate and oral neomycin was recommended until recently. But there is no conclusive evidence of benefit from bowel preparation according to *Cochrane Database of Systematic Reviews.* It is now believed that faeces is important for colonic healing and continuing

normal diet till a few hours before anaesthesia minimizes postoperative ileus and helps early feeding. Preoperative enema is, however, helpful in anal sphincter repair procedures since it delays the passage of stools and allows initial healing.

Blood transfusion

In women who are anaemic, treatment with oral iron will raise the haemoglobin in a few weeks. But if surgery is required immediately, **transfusion of packed cells** is required to bring the haemoglobin up to 8 g%.

Two or more units of packed cells should be cross-matched and available for use intraoperatively if blood loss of more than 30% of blood volume is anticipated. Single-unit transfusions are not used as there is no benefit and there are recognized complications of needless transfusion.

Autologous transfusion is another option where blood is collected from the patient preoperatively and transfused intraoperatively or postoperatively. This is rarely required in gynaecological surgery, except when extensive surgeries such as retroperitoneal node dissection or exenteration are considered. Patient's haemoglobin must be >11 g% and the last collection should be >72 hours before surgery.

Other preoperative preparations are listed in Box 33.9.

Box 33.9 Preoperative preparation

- Correct anaemia
  - Oral iron therapy
  - Transfusion
- Stop medications that increase blood loss
  - Hormones
  - Anticoagulants
  - Aspirin, clopidogrel
- Treat urinary infection
- Consider vaginal oestrogen in postmenopausal women

Informed consent

It is important to discuss the details of diagnosis, options for management, type of surgery, route of surgery, type of anaesthesia, possible complications and other risks with the patient. In premenopausal women, if there is definite indication for oophorectomy such as endometriosis, malignancy or pelvic inflammatory disease, the patient should be informed about the problems of oestrogen deprivation and need for replacement. In women who are postmenopausal, option of oophorectomy must be discussed (Box 33.10).

Box 33.10 Informed consent: Issues to be discussed

- Surgical procedure
  - Diagnosis
  - Treatment options
  - Type and route of surgery
  - Type of anaesthesia
  - Possible complications
- Premenopausal women
  - Need for oophorectomy
  - Postoperative hormone therapy
- Postmenopausal women
  - Option of oophorectomy
- Postoperative period
  - Indwelling catheter
  - Pain relief
  - Ambulation
  - Care of the wound
  - Duration of hospital stay

Postoperative management

Postoperative management consists of supportive care to maintain homeostasis, prevention of complications, pain relief, early recognition and management of complications (Box 33.11).

Box 33.11 Components of postoperative management

- Monitoring
- Fluid and electrolyte management
- Diet
- Pain control
- Ambulation
- Care of the surgical site
- Management of complications

Postoperative monitoring

The patient should be monitored closely in the immediate postoperative period, every hour for the first 4 hours or till the vital signs stabilize and then every 4 hours for 24 hours (Box 33.12).

Box 33.12 Postoperative monitoring

- Pulse
- Blood pressure
- Respiratory rate
- Level of consciousness
- Intake/output
- Obvious bleeding
  - Surgical wound
  - Vagina

Fluid and electrolyte management

Daily requirement of a normal postoperative patient is about 35–40 mL/kg/day, including replacement of insensible loss. About 1 mEq/kg/day of sodium and potassium is required. Therefore, 125 mL/hour of 5% dextrose saline or Ringer lactate with 20 mEq/L of potassium chloride is administered for the first 24 hours. Fluid requirement changes with several factors (Box 33.13). Urine output should be 30 mL/hour. If there is oliguria, it is important to determine whether it is prerenal and increase the intravenous fluids.

Box 33.13 Factors determining fluid requirement

- Vomiting/gastric aspirate
- Bowel distension
- Haemorrhage
- Urine output
- Oral intake
- Insensible loss

Diet

Most patients can have a normal meal 6 hours after vaginal surgery, simple abdominal procedures such as hysterectomy and laparoscopic surgery. Early feeding has been shown to be beneficial.

Pain control

Postoperative analgesia is usually started after surgery, but pre-emptive analgesia that is started earlier prevents nociceptive stimulation of the brain. This has been shown to provide overall better pain control. Methods used to reduce pain are given in Box 33.14. Nonsteroidal anti-inflammatory drugs (NSAIDs) such as diclofenac should be used with caution in the elderly as there is a risk of renal failure.

Box 33.14 Methods used for pain control

- Pre-emptive analgesia
  - NSAIDs started preoperatively
  - Local anaesthetic injection at incision site
- Patient-controlled analgesia
  - Intravenous
  - Epidural
- Peripheral nerve blocks
  - Transverse abdominis plane block
- Intravenous/intramuscular narcotics
  - Inj fentanyl 0.2 µg/kg IV hourly
  - Inj morphine 8 mg IM 4–6 hourly

IM, intramuscular; *NSAID*, nonsteroidal anti-inflammatory drug.

For injection into the incision site, 0.25% bupivacaine is used. PCA may be intravenous narcotics or epidural narcotics. The patient controls the frequency of administration by the preprogrammed pump. The total dose and duration of analgesia required are less with PCA. Intravenous or intramuscular narcotics given 4–6 hourly are used infrequently now.

Ambulation

Early ambulation ensures early return of bowel motility, facilitates voiding and prevents VTE.

Care of the surgical site

Epithelialization of the wound occurs in 24–48 hours and is complete by 5 days. The dressing can be removed after 48 hours. Sutures can be removed by day 6 for transverse incisions and day 8 for vertical incisions.

Management of complications (intraoperative and postoperative)

The common intraoperative and postoperative complications are listed in Box 33.15.

Box 33.15 Intraoperative and postoperative complications

- Haemorrhage
  - Intraoperative
  - Postoperative
- Infections
  - Surgical site
  - Vaginal cuff cellulitis/abscess
  - Peritonitis
  - Urinary tract
  - Respiratory
  - Septicaemia
- Venous thromboembolism and pulmonary embolism
- Urinary complications
  - Retention
- Gastrointestinal complications
  - Paralytic ileus
  - Small bowel obstruction
- Injuries
  - Urinary tract
  - Bowel

Haemorrhage

Haemorrhage that occurs during surgery is referred to as **primary haemorrhage**. It occurs in 1–2% of abdominal and vaginal hysterectomies. Incidence is more in radical hysterectomy, pelvic lymphadenectomy, exenteration procedures and where there are adhesions due to endometriosis or pelvic inflammatory disease.

Intraoperative haemorrhage

- This is managed by pressure, haemostatic stitches, hypogastric artery ligation and/or packing. The bleeding vessel should be identified and isolated before placing a clamp or ligature in order to avoid injuring the ureter, especially during hysterectomy.
- Venous bleeding is more difficult to manage but can be controlled by pressure. Rents in larger veins such as iliac veins can be closed with 6-0 or 8-0 Prolene.
- If bleeding vessel is difficult to dissect free, hypogastric artery ligation can be performed. Packing is resorted to if all attempts fail and is seldom required in gynaecological surgery (Box 33.16).

Postoperative haemorrhage

- Postoperative bleeding is usually diagnosed by tachycardia, hypotension, reduction in urinary

Box 33.16 **Management of haemorrhage**

- Intraoperative
  - Isolation and ligation of the vessel
  - Haemostatic sutures
  - Pressure
  - Ligation of hypogastric arteries
  - Packing
- Postoperative
  - Diagnosis
    - Tachycardia
    - Hypotension
    - Oliguria
    - Tachypnoea
    - Abdominal distension
      - Ultrasonogram/CT scan
    - Serial haematocrit
  - Management
    - Early laparotomy
    - Pelvic arterial embolization

CT, computed tomography.

output and abdominal distension. Monitoring during the immediate postoperative period is essential for prompt diagnosis of haemorrhage.
- Bleeding should be diagnosed early, before hypovolaemic shock and coagulation abnormalities set in. High index of suspicion is required.
- Ultrasound scan may reveal intra-abdominal haemorrhage and serial haematocrit confirms the diagnosis.
- Re-exploration and haemostasis, hypogastric artery ligation and pelvic arterial embolization are options for management. Monitoring in intensive care may be required.

Hypovolaemic shock

- Treatment of haemorrhagic or hypovolaemic shock consists of restoration of intravascular volume with intravenous fluids, blood or blood products and control of haemorrhage.
- Resuscitation begins with infusion of normal saline followed by colloids while awaiting blood or packed cells.
- Central venous pressure should be monitored. Inotropics are not useful in hypovolaemic shock.
- Patients may be in disseminated intravascular coagulation; hence, platelet count, prothrombin time, activated partial thromboplastin time (aPTT) and fibrinogen should be checked and appropriate blood products infused.

- Laparotomy should be performed without delay and bleeding controlled.

Infection

The first sign of postoperative sepsis is **fever**. Postoperative fever is defined as temperature of 38°C after the first 24 hours on two occasions at least 4 hours apart. Infection usually presents as **cellulitis** around the vaginal cuff. **Haematoma** at the vaginal vault may get infected and an abscess can form. When infection spreads intraperitoneally, it results in general peritonitis and interloop abscesses and/or subdiaphragmatic abscesses. **Urinary infection** and **pneumonia** are also common causes of postoperative fever. **Septicaemia** is a known complication. Patients with **VTE** can have fever. Rarely previously unrecognized endocrine abnormalities such as **occult thyrotoxicosis** may cause fever and tachycardia.

Clinical evaluation in postoperative infection

The patient should be clinically evaluated to locate the site of infection (Box 33.17). If the patient is asymptomatic, surgery is uncomplicated and temperature is not persistently elevated, she can be observed for 24–48 hours before proceeding with investigations.

Box 33.17 **Clinical evaluation of postoperative fever**

- History
  - Fever with chills
  - Cough
  - Dysuria
  - Diarrhoea/tenesmus
  - Vaginal discharge
  - Calf muscle pain
- Clinical examination
  - Tachycardia
  - Hypotension
  - Respiratory symptoms and signs
  - Abdomen
    - Tenderness
    - Rigidity
    - Mass
  - Surgical wound
  - Calf muscle tenderness
  - Pelvic/rectal examination
    - Induration
    - Mass
    - Abscess

Investigations in postoperative infection

Investigations should be based on the patient's symptoms and clinical findings (Box 33.18).

Box 33.18   Investigations in postoperative infection

- Complete blood count
- Urine culture and sensitivity
- Ultrasonography
  - Transabdominal
  - Interloop abscess
  - Subdiaphragmatic abscess
  - Kidneys
  - Transvaginal
  - Vault haematoma
  - Pelvic abscess
- Chest X-ray
- Lower limb Doppler study

Management of postoperative infection

This depends on the site of infection (Box 33.19).

Box 33.19   Management of postoperative infection

- Urinary tract infection
  - Antibiotic therapy
- Respiratory infection
  - Antibiotic therapy
  - Chest physiotherapy
- Surgical wound infection
  - Open sutures to drain pus
  - Sterile dressing
- Vaginal cuff cellulitis
  - Antibiotics
  - Tab. augmentin 625 mg twice daily × 5 days
  - Tab. metronidazole 400 mg thrice daily × 5 days
- Pelvic abscess
  - Drainage through vagina
- Peritonitis
  - Intravenous fluids
  - Nasogastric suction
  - Antibiotics
- Intraperitoneal abscess
  - Ultrasound-guided drainage if single
  - Laparotomy and drainage if multiple

Deep vein thrombosis (DVT) and pulmonary embolism

This may present as deep vein thrombosis or PE (Box 33.20).

Box 33.20   Venous thromboembolism

- Deep vein thrombosis
  - Symptoms and signs
    - Involves unilateral lower limb
    - Swelling
    - Pain
    - Erythema
    - Positive Homans sign
  - Diagnosis
    - Doppler
- Pulmonary embolism
  - Symptoms and signs
    - Tachypnoea
    - Chest pain
    - Hypoxia
  - Diagnosis
    - Chest X-ray
    - Arterial blood gas
    - VQ scan
    - Spiral CT/CT pulmonary angiogram

CT, computed tomography; *VQ*, ventilation perfusion.

The patient usually has pain and swelling of the lower limb with positive Homans sign. Diagnosis of DVT is by venous Doppler. Tachypnoea and chest pain are symptoms of PE. Confirmation with chest X-ray, ventilation perfusion (VQ) scan, spiral CT pulmonary angiogram and immediate treatment is mandatory.

Management of DVT and PE

Deep vein thrombosis and PE are treated by intravenous UFH or subcutaneous LMWH. After anticoagulation is achieved, which usually takes 3–4 days, oral anticoagulants are started, usually warfarin. This must be continued for 6 months. UFH therapy should be monitored by aPTT.

Urinary complications (urinary retention)

Most gynaecological surgeries involve mobilizing the bladder, blunt or sharp dissection of the bladder base and resultant denervation of the bladder. Placement of indwelling bladder catheter prior to surgery is the routine practice. The catheter is removed on the second postoperative day following simple surgeries such as abdominal and vaginal hysterectomy and laparoscopic surgery but may be left for 48–72 hours if there has been extensive dissection or repair of a large cystocele. Urinary retention following removal of the catheter is a common problem. Placement of vaginal packs to control bleeding increases the risk of retention. Management is by recatheterization, treatment of urinary infection and bladder training, if required.

Gastrointestinal complications

Postoperative ileus is usually due to hypokalaemia or peritonitis but can also occur after bowel handling during surgery and opioid analgesics. The distension occurs during the first 48–72 hours and may be associated with fever. Bowel sounds are absent. Plain radiograph of the abdomen reveals distension of small and large bowel down to the rectum. **Small bowel obstruction** is generally due to adhesion formation and occurs 5–7 days after surgery. The patient has abdominal distension with borborygmi and brisk, high-pitched tinkling sounds in case of obstruction. Usually only distended small bowel loops with multiple air–fluid levels are seen on plain radiograph of the abdomen (Table 33.2).

Treatment of paralytic ileus is by intravenous fluids, potassium replacement and antibiotics if there is peritonitis. Patients with bowel obstruction should also be managed conservatively, but those who do not respond require laparotomy and release of adhesions.

Injuries

Urinary tract injuries are dealt with in Chapter 26, *Urinary tract injuries, urogenital fistulas; anal sphincter injuries and rectovaginal fistulas*. **Injuries to small** or **large bowel** occur when there are extensive adhesions and dissection of large or small bowel is required. If recognized intraoperatively, small bowel rents can be closed

Table 33.2 Paralytic ileus and small bowel obstruction

	Paralytic ileus	Small bowel obstruction
Symptoms and signs	• Abdominal distension • Absent bowel sounds	• Abdominal distension • Brisk, tinkling bowel sounds
Aetiology	• Electrolyte disturbances • Intraoperative bowel handling • Opioid analgesia • Prolonged surgery • Peritonitis	Postoperative adhesions
Diagnosis		
Plain X-ray abdomen	Distended small and large bowel loops with multiple air–fluid levels	Distended small bowel loops with multiple air–fluid levels
Management	• IV fluids • Potassium replacement • Antibiotics in peritonitis	• IV fluids • Potassium replacement • Surgery, if no response

IV, intravenous.

immediately. Large bowel injury or devascularization may need defunctioning colostomy and closure of the rent. The colostomy is closed after 6–12 weeks after performing a distal colonogram. Bowel injuries that are not recognized at surgery present with abdominal distension and signs of peritonitis. Septicaemia and septic shock can occur rapidly. Immediate diagnosis and laparotomy, in addition to antibiotics and management of shock, are essential.

Key points

- Preoperative evaluation, preparation for surgery and appropriate postoperative management are important for optimal outcome of any surgery.
- The goals of preoperative preparation are to identify risk factors, obtain specialist consultations, plan the appropriate anaesthesia and surgery, educate and counsel the patient and obtain informed consent.
- Preoperative evaluation consists of detailed history, physical examination and ordering appropriate investigations.
- Anaesthesia evaluation is mandatory. Surgical risk is assigned using American Society of Anesthesiologists physical status classification.
- Surgeries in which the vagina is opened or peritoneal cavity is entered through the vagina are considered 'clean contaminated' and antibiotics should be given.
- Single-dose antibiotic administered within 1 hour prior to surgery is adequate. One of the cephalosporins is recommended.
- Risk stratification is used for administration of thromboprophylaxis.

(Continued)

Key points *(Continued)*

- Diabetes, hypertension and other medical conditions should be evaluated and brought under control.

- Anaemia should be corrected. If blood loss of more than 30% of blood volume is anticipated, 2 or more units of packed cells should be cross-matched and kept ready.

- Informed consent should be obtained prior to surgery. Surgical procedure should be performed. Need for oophorectomy, postoperative pain management and risk of complications must be discussed with the patient.

- Close postoperative monitoring is required to diagnose bleeding, hypotension or sepsis early.

- Fluid and electrolyte management, diet, ambulation and surgical site care are important components of postoperative management.

- Postoperative bleeding is diagnosed by tachycardia, hypotension, reduced urinary output and abdominal distension. Ultrasonography may clinch the diagnosis. Blood transfusion, laparotomy and ligation of the bleeding vessel or internal iliac artery may be required.

- Fever may be the first indication of sepsis. Tachycardia and hypotension indicate septicaemia.

- Urinary tract and respiratory infections are common and can be treated with antibiotics. Peritonitis, pelvic and interloop or subdiaphragmatic abscesses require imaging and appropriate therapy.

- Deep vein thrombosis and pulmonary embolism need evaluation with X-ray, ventilation perfusion (VQ) scan or spiral computerized tomography (CT). Treatment is by intravenous unfractionated heparin or subcutaneous low-molecular-weight heparin.

- Paralytic ileus must be differentiated from bowel obstruction. Intravenous fluids and antibiotics are required in both. Bowel obstruction may require re-exploration by laparotomy.

Self-assessment

Case-based questions

Case 1

A 56-year-old lady is diagnosed to have endometrial carcinoma. Abdominal hysterectomy and bilateral salpingo-oophorectomy with selective pelvic and para-aortic lymphadenectomy are planned. Her BMI is 30. She is a diabetic on metformin and asthmatic on inhalers.

1. What will you look for on clinical examination?
2. What problems do you anticipate in the intraoperative and postoperative periods?
3. What investigations will you order?
4. What is the preoperative preparation?

Case 2

A 48-year-old lady had abdominal hysterectomy and bilateral salpingo-oophorectomy for endometriosis. Six hours after surgery, she was found to be restless; pulse rate was 120/minute and blood pressure 110/60.

1. What will you suspect?
2. What will you look for on clinical examination and what investigations will you order?
3. What is your management?

Answers

Case 1

1. (a) General examination—Breathlessness, respiratory rate
   (b) Respiratory system—Rhonchi, crepitations
   (c) Abdomen—Mass
   (d) Pelvic examination—Size of uterus, adnexal mass

2. (a) Intraoperative—Problems during intubation due to obesity, hyperglycaemia, bronchospasm, haemorrhage, VTE
   (b) Postoperative—Hyperglycaemia, electrolyte imbalance, paralytic ileus, VTE, wound breakdown, infection

3. Routine investigations, plasma glucose, HbA1C, pulmonary function tests.

4. (a) Consultation—With anaesthetists, pulmonologist and diabetologist
   (b) Discussion with the patient about possible complications and counselling her regarding early ambulation, breathing exercises
   (c) Thromboprophylaxis, compression stockings intraoperatively; adequate control of blood sugar

Case 2

1. Haemorrhage.
2. Clinical examination—Pallor, abdominal distension, shifting dullness, vaginal bleeding, bleeding from surgical site.
   Investigations—Serial haematocrit 2-hourly, ultrasound of abdomen.
3. (a) If diagnosis is confirmed, no vaginal bleeding—Relaparotomy, religate the bleeding stump.
   (b) If vaginal bleeding is present, examine under anaesthesia; attempt to ligate the bleeding vessel at the vaginal angle. If unsuccessful, relaparotomy.

Long-answer questions

1. Discuss the preoperative preparation and postoperative management of a 60-year-old lady with diabetes, hypertension and bronchial asthma.

2. Discuss the evaluation and management of postoperative haemorrhage following radical hysterectomy and pelvic lymphadenectomy.

Short-answer questions

1. Primary haemorrhage
2. Thromboprophylaxis for gynaecological surgery
3. Role of prophylactic antibiotics for gynaecological surgery
4. Posthysterectomy pelvic abscess
5. Postoperative pulmonary embolism
6. Postoperative pain control
7. Postoperative urinary retention

34 | Gynaecological Surgery

Case scenario

Mrs VA, 35, came to the clinic for a second opinion regarding a surgical procedure she had been advised. She had gone to her local general practitioner with a history of mass descending per vaginum. She had a 5-year-old girl and was keen on having another child. She was concerned that surgical treatment of prolapse may involve removing her uterus or reduce her chances of conception in some way. She wanted to know if surgery was necessary, and if so, what would be the nature of the surgery, nature of anaesthesia and postoperative complications that she should anticipate. She wanted to discuss all this before making a decision.

Introduction

Gynaecological surgical procedures can be performed vaginally, abdominally or through the endoscopic approach. Vaginal approach is unique to pelvic surgery and has many advantages over abdominal approach. Endoscopic surgical procedures can be performed with a laparoscope or hysteroscope.

Preoperative preparation

Before surgery, it is important to discuss with and explain to the patient the details of the procedure to be performed and the possible risks, and obtain consent.

Consent

Informed consent is mandatory before all surgical procedures. This has been discussed in Chapter 33, *Preoperative preparation and postoperative management.* The indication for the surgery, possible complications, details of anaesthesia, postoperative management, time to resumption of daily activities, anticipated time of return to work and possible need to avoid sexual intercourse must be discussed.

Documentation

Indications, details of anaesthesia, details of the procedure, intraoperative complications, estimated blood loss, intraoperative consultations and frozen section reports should be documented.

Vaginal surgical procedures

Many simple vaginal surgical procedures can be performed as outpatient. Major procedures require admission and general or spinal anaesthesia.

Office procedures

Several minor gynaecological diagnostic and therapeutic procedures through the vaginal approach are performed as office procedures under paracervical block combined with intravenous sedation or oral analgesic (Box 34.1). Major vaginal procedures require admission to hospital and general or regional anaesthesia.

Patient position and preparation

The patient should be asked to empty the bladder prior to the procedure. Most vaginal surgeries are performed with the patient in dorsal lithotomy position. The limb is flexed at the hip and knee, abducted and externally rotated at the hip, and legs are supported by stirrups (Fig. 34.1). This position provides adequate exposure of the perineum. The perineum and vagina should be cleaned with an antiseptic (povidone iodine) and draped with sterile drapes. Antibiotic prophylaxis with oral doxycycline 100 mg 30 minutes before the procedure is recommended for dilatation and curettage (D&C).

Analgesia

Oral analgesic is given before the procedure and paracervical block or intravenous analgesia may be used during the procedure.

Preparation, position and analgesia are summarized in Box 34.2.

Cervical punch biopsy

Indications This is done when colposcopy reveals cervical intraepithelial neoplasia (CIN)

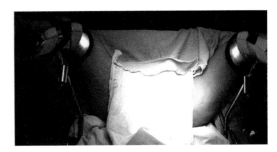

Figure 34.1 Dorsal lithotomy position—The thighs are flexed, abducted and externally rotated. Knees are flexed and supported by stirrups. This is the position of choice for vaginal surgeries.

II/III lesion or in frank invasive cervical cancer and a biopsy confirmation is sought prior to definitive treatment. It is usually done using a cervical punch biopsy forceps under colposcopic guidance.

Instruments Cusco bivalve speculum and cervical punch biopsy forceps are used for this procedure. These instruments are shown in Figs 4.10 and 29.11, respectively.

Procedure

- Cervix is exposed with Cusco bivalve speculum.
- Three percent to 5% acetic acid is applied to cervix and colposcopy is performed to localize the lesions.
- Biopsy with cervical punch biopsy forceps is taken from the abnormal area.
- Vagina is packed.

Complications Haemorrhage from biopsy site can occur but is usually prevented by packing.

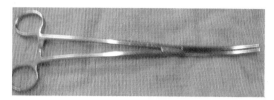

Figure 34.2 Uterine packing forceps. This is used to hold the pedicle of cervical polyp and twist it off.

Cervical polypectomy

Indication The indication is polyp arising from ectocervix or endocervix.

Instruments The instruments used are Cusco speculum, uterine packing forceps or Kelley clamp.

Procedure This procedure is performed to remove cervical polyps arising from ectocervix or endocervical canal. After the cervix is exposed with Cusco speculum, the polyp is grasped with an Allis clamp or uterine packing forceps (Fig. 34.2) and twisted till it breaks off at the pedicle.

Complications Usually there are no complications. Occasionally, there may be bleeding from the base of the pedicle, which can be controlled by packing.

Loop electroexcision procedure

The procedure is also known as large loop excision of the transformation zone (LLETZ). This is an excisional procedure performed in women with CIN II/III. Conization can also be performed by loop electroexcision procedure (LEEP). The endocervical lesion is removed with a loop with smaller diameter, while ectocervical lesion is removed with a larger loop.

Indications for loop electroexcision procedure

- CIN II/III on colposcopy
- Upper limit of the lesion clearly visible
- Lesion occupying <50% of the cervix

Instruments A plastic bivalve speculum is used to avoid accidental electrical burns to vagina. The LEEP electrodes are available in various sizes (Fig. 34.3). The surgeon assesses the size of the lesion and selects an appropriate electrode. A rollerball electrode is used to achieve haemostasis after the procedure.

Procedure

- Cervix is exposed with bivalve speculum.

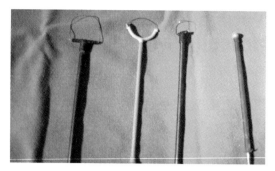

Figure 34.3 Wire loops of various sizes used for LEEP procedure. *LEEP*, loop electroexcision procedure.

- Abnormal area is delineated using acetic acid or Lugol's iodine.
- Adrenaline diluted with saline to 1:200,000 is infiltrated into the cervix circumferentially to cause vasoconstriction and thereby reduce bleeding.
- LEEP electrode of an appropriate size is chosen.
- An appropriate cutting current is set to avoid charring and thermal artefact.
- The electrode is moved from left to right or below upwards to gently resect the abnormal area. Movement above downwards should be avoided since bleeding from the area above will obscure visibility (Fig. 34.4). With experience, it is easy to identify the thickness of the tissue to be removed.
- The excision is of three types:
  - *Type 1 excision:* Resects type 1 TZ (completely ectocervical)
  - *Type 2 excision:* Resects type 2 TZ, includes small amount of endocervical epithelium
  - *Type 3 excision:* Resects type 3 TZ, includes longer and larger cone-shaped tissue

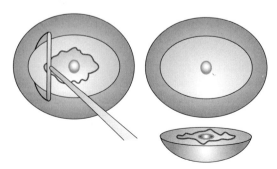

Figure 34.4 LEEP procedure—The transformation zone and the abnormal area are excised in one sweep from side to side. *LEEP*, loop electroexcision procedure.

and significant amount of endocervical epithelium
- The raw area is cauterized with rollerball cautery. Alternatively, Monsel paste may be used to arrest bleeding if it is trivial.
- Vagina is packed.

Complications Haemorrhage and removal of excess of cervical tissue are known complications.

Endometrial biopsy

This can be performed without dilating the cervix. It is a diagnostic procedure.

Indications The indications for endometrial biopsy are given in Box 34.3.

Box 34.3 Indications for endometrial biopsy

- Infertility
  - Confirm ovulation
  - Rule out tuberculosis
  - Diagnosis of LPD
- Endometrial hyperplasia
  - Diagnosis
  - Assessment of response to therapy
- Genital tuberculosis
  - Diagnosis
  - Assessment of response to treatment

LPD, luteal phase defect.

Instruments The instruments used are shown in Fig. 34.5a. Endometrial biopsy curette (Novak curette; Fig. 34.5b) can be generally introduced without cervical dilatation. The exceptions are some postmenopausal and nulliparous women with tightly closed os.

Procedure

- The patient is positioned and analgesia administered.
- Pelvic examination should be performed to assess the size and shape of uterus and whether it is anteverted or retroverted.
- Posterior vaginal wall is retracted with Sims speculum.
- Anterior lip of cervix is held with vulsellum.
- Uterine sound is inserted to measure uterocervical length (Fig. 34.5c).
- Endometrial biopsy curette is inserted and biopsy is taken from anterior or posterior wall by scraping with the curette.
- Specimen is fixed in formalin.

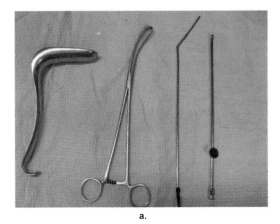

a.

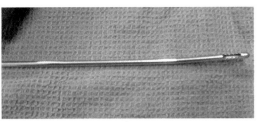

b.

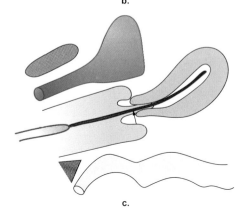

c.

Figure 34.5 Endometrial biopsy. a. Sims speculum, vulsellum, uterine sound and endometrial biopsy curette (from left to right). Sims speculum is used to retract vaginal walls, vulsellum is used to hold the anterior or posterior cervical lip and uterine sound is used to measure the uterocervical length. Endometrial biopsy curette is used to take endometrial biopsy. This does not require cervical dilatation. b. Magnified view of endometrial biopsy curette. c. Measuring the uterocervical length using uterine sound. The length is marked by an arrow.

Complications Uterine perforation, which can occur during introduction of the uterine sound or curette, is a rare complication.

Dilatation and curettage

This procedure involves dilatation of the cervix using a series of graduated metal dilators followed by curettage of the uterine cavity.

Indications These are listed in Box 34.4.

Instruments In addition to the speculum, vulsellum and uterine sound, Hegar dilators and a sharp-edged curette are used for this procedure (Fig. 34.6a and b). The dilators are numbered from 1 to 16, the numbers indicating their diameter in millimetres.

Procedure

- Vaginal wall is retracted, cervix held with vulsellum and uterus sounded.
- The cervix is gradually dilated using Hegar dilators up to size 8 (Fig. 34.6c).
- The curette is introduced and the endometrial cavity is curetted thoroughly (Fig. 34.6d).
- Specimen is fixed in formalin.

Complications Uterine perforation can occur during dilatation of the cervix if undue force is used, the uterine walls are soft or the length of the uterus is misjudged.

Fractional curettage This procedure is a modification of D&C where the endocervix is curetted before dilating the cervix, the cervix is dilated and the endometrial cavity is then curetted. The

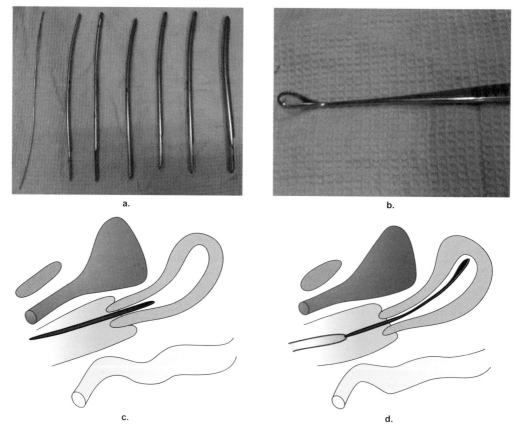

a. b. c. d.

Figure 34.6 Dilatation and curettage. a. Hegar dilators. They are used for gradual dilatation of cervix. The size of the dilator indicates the diameter in millimetres. b. Curette. Sharp and blunt curettes are used to curette the endometrial cavity. c. Diagrammatic representation of cervical dilatation. d. Endometrial curettage after dilatation.

endocervical and endometrial samples are sent in different containers to the lab. In the past, when preoperative staging of endometrial cancer was a routine practice, this procedure was used to exclude extension of tumour to endocervix. Current staging of endometrial cancer is surgical and this procedure is not used now.

Endocervical curettage The endocervix is curetted with a small sharp curette, but the cervix is not dilated and endometrial cavity is not curetted. This is done to obtain endocervical sample in women with cytological diagnosis of atypical glandular cells of unknown significance (AGUS), adenocarcinoma in situ (AIS) and adenocarcinoma.

Endometrial thermal ablation (or thermal balloon ablation)

In this procedure, the endometrium is destroyed by heat. A balloon filled with water, which is gradually heated, is accurately placed within the uterine cavity. The procedure is described in detail in Chapter 7, *Abnormal uterine bleeding.*

Major vaginal surgical procedures

These are performed under general or regional anaesthesia. Preoperative preparation for major procedures is discussed in Chapter 33, *Preoperative preparation and postoperative management.* All vaginal surgeries discussed in the following are performed with the patient in dorsal lithotomy position.

Cold knife conization

In this procedure, a cone-shaped area of cervix with the base at the ectocervix and apex at the level of the internal os is removed using a knife.

Indications These are listed in Box 34.5.

Instruments Instruments used are the same as those for office procedures—Sims speculum, vulsellum, Allis clamps, uterine sound, knife with number 15 blade, diathermy with rollerball electrode and sutures.

Procedure

- Bladder is catheterized and emptied and pelvic examination is performed.

Box 34.5 Indications for conization

- Large lesions (>50% of cervix involved)
- Lesion extending into endocervical canal
- Recurrent high-grade lesion
- Suspected microinvasive cancer
- Histological diagnosis of adenocarcinoma in situ
- Recurrent atypical glandular cells on cytology
- Cytology–histology discordance
  - Lesion of greater severity shown by cytology

- Posterior vaginal wall is retracted with Sims speculum.
- Cervix is painted with acetic acid or Lugol's iodine.
- Anterior lip of cervix is held with vulsellum.
- Two haemostatic sutures at 3 and 9 o'clock positions are used to occlude the descending cervical artery (Fig. 34.7).
- Adrenaline diluted with saline to 1:200,000 is infiltrated into the cervix circumferentially. This reduces bleeding during the procedure.
- Endocervical curettage is performed.
- Incision is made on the ectocervix around the abnormal area with a 2- to 3-mm margin using knife with number 15 blade.
- Incision is deepened to the desired depth with the knife directed towards the endocervical canal (Fig. 34.8).
- Cone-shaped cervical tissue is removed (Fig. 34.9). Haemostasis is achieved by rollerball cautery.
- Vagina is packed and the pack is left in place for 48 hours.

Complications These are listed in Box 34.6.

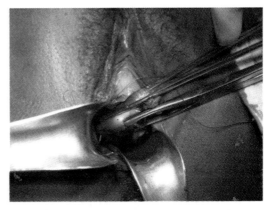

Figure 34.7 Haemostatic suture at 9 o'clock position on the lateral aspect of the cervix to occlude the descending cervical artery prior to conization.

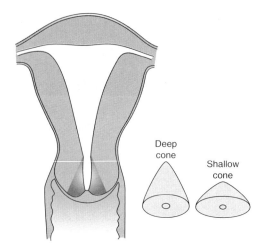

Figure 34.8 Diagram showing deep and shallow cone.

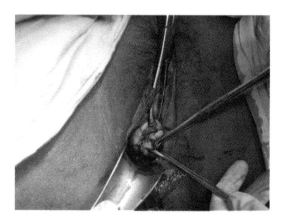

Figure 34.9 Conization: Cone-shaped tissue has been dissected out from the cervix.

Box 34.6 Complications of cold knife conization

- Immediate
  - Haemorrhage
  - Infection
- Delayed
  - Cervical stenosis
  - Cervical incompetence

Vaginal hysterectomy

It is the removal of the uterus through the vagina. The most common indication is pelvic organ prolapse (POP). It is easier to perform vaginal hysterectomy when there is descent of cervix, but this route of hysterectomy is an option even when there is no descent. Vaginal hysterectomy has several advantages over abdominal approach and according to *Cochrane* review and recommendations, vaginal hysterectomy should be performed whenever it is feasible and when no contraindications are present. Advantages of vaginal hysterectomy are listed in Box 34.7.

Box 34.7 Advantages of vaginal hysterectomy

- Decrease in
  - Intraoperative blood loss
  - Postoperative pain
  - Paralytic ileus
- Early ambulation
- Early return to normal activity
- Reduced hospital stay
- No incisional hernia

Indications These are listed in Box 34.8.

Box 34.8 Indications for vaginal hysterectomy

- Pelvic organ prolapse
- Benign diseases of the uterus
  - Uterine myoma <12 weeks' size
  - Adenomyosis
  - AUB/endometrial hyperplasia
  - CIN III/microinvasive cervical cancer

AUB, abnormal uterine bleeding; *CIN*, cervical intraepithelial neoplasia.

Contraindications It is difficult to remove a large uterus through the vagina unless the uterus is bisected or the myoma is morcellated. Adhesions of the uterus to bowel or pelvic wall due to endometriosis or chronic pelvic inflammatory disease (PID) can also make the surgery difficult. Contraindications are listed in Box 34.9. Most are relative contraindications. Prior to vaginal hysterectomy, laparoscopic assessment

Box 34.9 Contraindications to vaginal hysterectomy

- Large uterus >12 weeks' size when size not reducible
- Endometriosis
- Chronic pelvic inflammatory disease
- Previous laparotomy
- Ovarian mass
- Genital malignancy

and release of adhesions may facilitate the procedure. Uterus larger than 12 weeks' size may be difficult to remove vaginally, but size can be reduced by morcellation or enucleation of myoma and bisection of the uterus. In women with malignancy, abdominal approach is preferred unless lymphadenectomy is performed laparoscopically.

Instruments These are shown in Fig. 34.10. The three clamps used are as follows:

- Straight or Spencer Wells clamps for cardinal and uterosacral ligaments
- Heaney clamps for uterine vessels
- Kelley clamps for round ligament, tube and ovarian ligaments

In addition to these clamps, Sims speculum, vulsellum, Allis clamps and other instruments used in general surgical procedures are required. These instruments are used in all vaginal surgical procedures and will not be described under each procedure.

Procedure of vaginal hysterectomy in pelvic organ prolapse

Initial preparation

- Antibiotic prophylaxis, single dose as discussed in Chapter 33, *Preoperative preparation and postoperative management*
- General or regional anaesthesia
- Dorsal lithotomy position
- Pelvic examination under anaesthesia (extent of POP, size and mobility of uterus reassessed under anaesthesia and appropriate reconstructive surgery planned)
- Bladder catheterized

Procedure

Images of steps of vaginal hysterectomy are given in Fig. 34.11.

- Posterior vaginal wall is retracted with Sims speculum; cervix is held with vulsellum and pulled down.
- Adrenaline with 1:200,000 dilution is infiltrated into submucosal tissue of the anterior vaginal wall to make dissection easier and reduce bleeding.
- A curvilinear incision is made on the anterior vaginal wall at the level of the bladder sulcus just below the level of vaginal rugae.

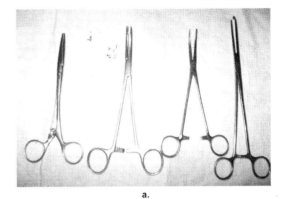

a.

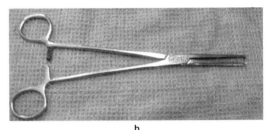

b.

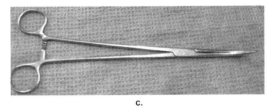

c.

Figure 34.10 Instruments for hysterectomy. a. Used for vaginal and abdominal hysterectomy; from left to right are Spencer Wells clamp, Heaney clamp, Kelley clamp and Allis clamp. The straight or Spencer Wells clamp is used for clamping cardinal ligament and uterosacral ligament. The Heaney clamp is used for uterine vessels. The Kelley clamp is used to clamp the tube, utero-ovarian ligament and round ligament. Long Allis clamps are used for holding the vaginal walls during dissection and closure, holding the pubococcygeus muscle during perineorrhaphy and getting a firm hold on other tissues. b. Kocher clamp. This can be used in place of Spencer Wells clamp or Allis clamp. c. Magnified view of Kelley clamp.

- From the centre of the curvilinear incision another vertical incision is made and extended vertically upwards in the midline in the form of an inverted T over the cystocele to just below the external urethral meatus. The vaginal flaps are dissected from the bladder by sharp dissection.

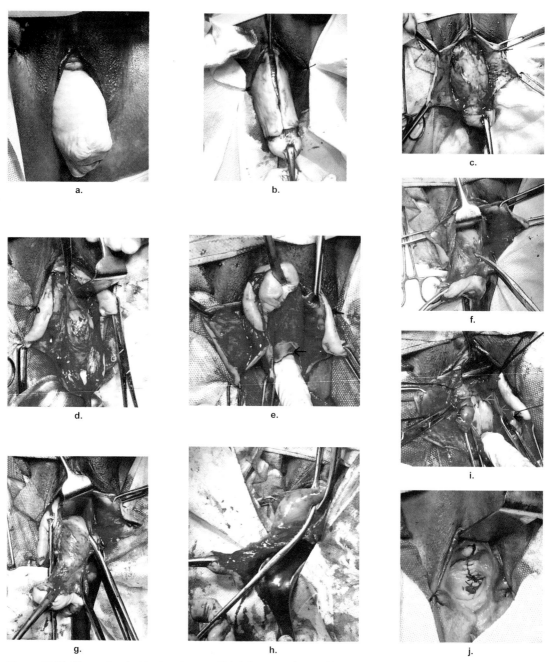

Figure 34.11 Steps of vaginal hysterectomy. **a.** Third-degree prolapse with cystocele and enterocele. **b.** Inverted 'T'-shaped incision has been made on the anterior vaginal wall **c.** The vaginal walls have been dissected and bladder is exposed. **d.** Bladder has been pushed up. The uterovesical peritoneum has been opened. **e.** Posterior vaginal wall has been dissected. Pouch of Douglas has been opened (arrow). **f.** Cardinal and uterosacral ligaments are clamped together by straight clamp. **g.** Uterine vessels have been clamped. **h.** The round ligament, tube and ovarian ligament have been clamped. **i.** The specimen of uterus has been removed. Suture has been taken through vaginal wall (black arrow), uterosacral ligaments (blue arrow) and posterior peritoneum (green arrow) to perform McCall culdoplasty. **j.** Vaginal wall has been sutured.

- Vesicocervical ligaments are cut. Bladder is pushed up to reveal the uterovesical peritoneum. The peritoneum is opened.
- Another curvilinear incision is made on posterior vaginal wall at the level of the attachment of uterosacral ligaments to cervix and this incision is extended to join the anterior incision to complete the circle. Posterior vaginal wall is dissected from the cervix to expose the peritoneum of the pouch of Douglas. Peritoneum is opened. The uterus is now held in place by the lateral ligaments.
- The cardinal and uterosacral ligaments are clamped with two straight or Spencer Wells clamps, cut between the clamps and ligated on both sides.
- Similarly, the uterine vessels are clamped with two Heaney clamps, cut between clamps and ligated on both sides.
- The round ligament, ovarian ligament and fallopian tube are clamped together as a single stump using Heaney or Kelley clamps, cut and ligated. The uterus is removed.
- The ovaries are removed only when indicated and this is more difficult in vaginal hysterectomy than in abdominal hysterectomy. The infundibulopelvic ligaments are clamped and the ovaries are removed separately after completing the hysterectomy.
- The excess cul-de-sac peritoneum is excised.
- Pelvic reconstructive procedures are performed as given in the following.

Pelvic reconstructive surgery

This is usually performed after vaginal hysterectomy but can also be done individually, depending on the nature and extent of pelvic relaxation.

Repair of anterior vaginal wall prolapse

Anterior vaginal wall prolapse or cystocele can be a central or paravaginal defect. These are repaired by anterior colporrhaphy or site-specific repair.

Anterior colporrhaphy

Repair of the central defect by plication of the pubovesicocervical fascia is called anterior colporrhaphy.

Procedure

- When the procedure is performed without hysterectomy, the same inverted 'T'-shaped incision is made on the anterior vaginal wall, vaginal flaps are dissected away from the bladder and the bladder is exposed. The lateral dissection should continue up to the pubic rami. Bladder pillars are cut and the bladder is pushed up.
- Pubovesicocervical fascia is plicated by taking interrupted stitches on the fascia from the patient's left to right (Fig. 34.12a–c).
- Three or more rows of stitches are placed one below the other and tied to close the defect and support the bladder. These stitches serve to elevate the bladder to its normal anatomical position.

Site-specific repair

Procedure

- Lateral dissection is continued beyond the pubic rami.
- Cave of Retzius is entered and the arcus tendineus fascia is palpated.
- Pubovesicocervical fascia is sutured to arcus tendineus fascia pelvis by three or four sutures on either side to recreate the lateral sulci.

Repair of posterior vaginal wall prolapse—McCall culdoplasty

Repair of enterocele by fixing the vaginal vault to uterosacral ligaments and approximating the uterosacral ligaments is known as McCall culdoplasty. This also prevents future vaginal vault prolapse by supporting the vaginal vault.

Procedure

- The cut and ligated ends of the uterosacral ligaments are identified and held with Allis clamps.
- A suture is taken through the vaginal vault from outside in on the patient's left side, and then through the left uterosacral ligament. This is continued as a series of bites through the serosa of the anterior rectosigmoid, and then through the right uterosacral ligament and brought out through the vaginal vault on the right side (Fig. 34.13).

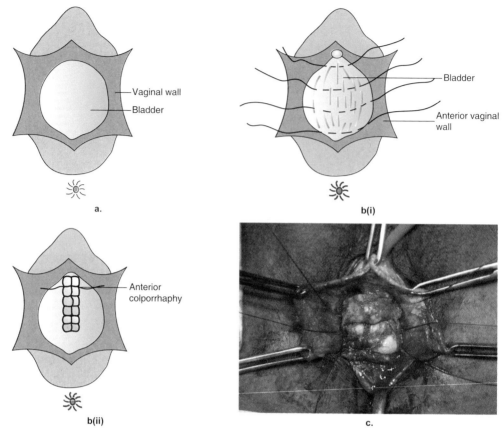

Figure 34.12 Diagrammatic representation of anterior colporrhaphy. **a.** The anterior vaginal wall is dissected away from the bladder. **b.** (i and ii) Vesicocervical fascia is plicated by series of transverse sutures placed one below the other. **c.** Photomicrograph of anterior colporrhaphy. Series of sutures have been placed through the vesicocervical fascia.

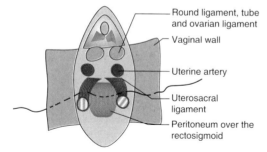

Figure 34.13 Diagrammatic representation of McCall culdoplasty. The stitch is taken through the vaginal wall, left uterosacral ligament, peritoneum on the anterior surface of the rectum, right uterosacral ligament and vaginal wall on the right side.

- When the suture is tied, the uterosacrals are brought together and fixed to the vaginal vault.

- The above-mentioned procedures are performed and excess vaginal wall is excised. Vaginal vault is closed. Vagina is packed. Catheter is left in place for 24–48 hours.

Repair of rectocele and deficient perineum

This is performed through a separate incision made on the posterior vaginal wall.

Procedure

- A transverse incision is made along the mucocutaneous junction of the posterior fourchette.
- The incision is extended as inverted 'T' on the posterior vaginal wall up to the upper limit of rectocele.
- Posterior vaginal flaps are reflected by dissecting the rectum from the vaginal wall.
- Repair is proceeded with.

Repair of rectocele

This may be by posterior colporrhaphy or site-specific repair.

Posterior colporrhaphy

Repair of rectocele by plicating the rectovaginal fascia is termed posterior colporrhaphy.

Procedure

- The rectovaginal fascia visible on the surface of the rectum is plicated by transverse sutures from the patient's left to right (Fig. 34.14).
- Series of two or three sutures are placed one below the other and later tied to reconstruct the fascia and support the rectal wall.

Site-specific repair

Identifying the exact nature and site of posterior vaginal wall defect and repairing it is known as site-specific repair.

Procedure

- The defects in rectovaginal fascia may be transverse defects at different levels, identified by rectal examination, and the fascia repaired at the specific site of damage in site-specific repair. The damaged ends of fascia retract upwards and downwards. These are brought together by sutures (Fig. 34.15).

Perineorrhaphy

Reconstruction of perineal body is called perineorrhaphy. This should be done very carefully as overzealous correction can lead to narrowing of introitus and dyspareunia.

Procedure

- The posterior part of the pubovaginalis muscle can be identified on the sides. These are approximated by one or two sutures (Fig. 34.16).

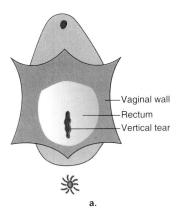
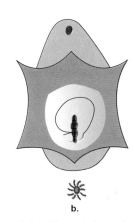

Figure 34.14 Diagrammatic representation of rectocele repair (posterior colporrhaphy). a. The posterior vaginal wall has been dissected away from the rectum. b. The central defect in the rectovaginal fascia is identified and the fascia is plicated.

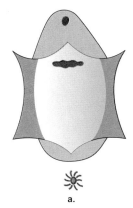
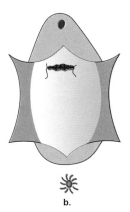

Figure 34.15 Diagrammatic representation of site-specific repair of posterior vaginal wall defect. a. The transverse defect at a higher level is identified. b. Defect repaired by suturing the separated ends of the rectovaginal fascia.

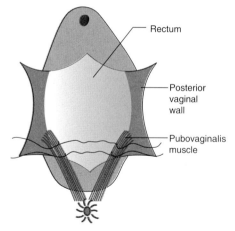

Figure 34.16 Diagrammatic representation of perineorrhaphy. Posterior vaginal wall has been dissected from the rectum. The pubococcygeus muscles are visible. These are brought together and the muscles of the perineal body are sutured to reconstruct the perineal body.

- The retracted ends of the muscles forming the perineal body (superficial and deep perineal muscles) are approximated.
- Vaginal incision is closed.
- Skin is sutured.

Complications These are listed in Box 34.10.

Box 34.10 Complications of vaginal hysterectomy and pelvic reconstructive procedures

- Immediate complications
  - Haemorrhage
    - Primary
    - Secondary
  - Infection
    - Urinary tract infection
    - Cuff cellulitis
    - Vaginal vault abscess
    - Peritonitis
  - Injury to adjacent organs
    - Bladder
    - Small bowel
    - Rectum
    - Ureter
    - Urethra
  - Thrombosis and pulmonary embolism
- Late complications
  - Dyspareunia
  - Recurrence of prolapse

Sacrospinous colpopexy

This is the suturing of the vaginal vault to sacrospinous ligament to prevent/correct vault prolapse in women with procidentia and/or vault prolapse. The procedure is usually performed only on the patient's right but is performed on both sides by some surgeons. The pudendal vessels curve round the ischial spine close to the tip to enter the pudendal canal and care must be taken not to injure these vessels.

Indications The procedure is used in women with large enterocele or procidentia to prevent recurrence of prolapse. It is also used to repair posthysterectomy vault prolapse.

Instruments Since the sacrospinous ligament is located high up, it cannot be easily reached with the usual needle holders and forceps. Special ligature carriers and Miya hook are used to pass the suture through the ligament and pull the thread (Fig. 34.17).

Procedure

Steps are the same as for posterior colporrhaphy until the dissection of posterior vaginal wall from rectum.

- Right ischial spine is palpated and by finger dissection, the pararectal space can be entered and rectal pillars broken.

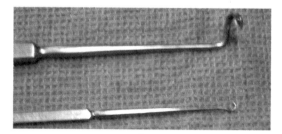

a.

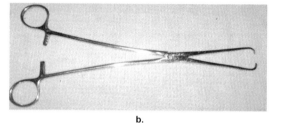

b.

Figure 34.17 Instruments used for sacrospinous colpopexy. **a.** The needle carrier and Miya hook are used for placement of sutures. **b.** The tenaculum forceps are used to hold the sacrospinous ligament.

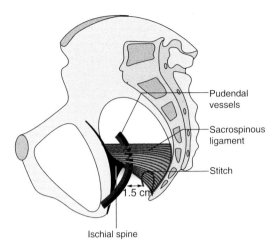

Figure 34.18 Placement of stitch in sacrospinous colpopexy. The pudendal vessels curve round the tip of the ischial spine. The stitch should be 1.5–2 cm medial to the tip of the spine to avoid puncturing the vessels.

- The rectum is retracted towards the left ischial spine and sacrospinous ligament is visualized. The ligament is held with a long Allis clamp or tenaculum forceps.
- A delayed absorbable suture (silk) or nonabsorbable suture is used for fixation. A stitch is taken through the ligament using a long-handled needle holder, 1.5–2 cm medial to the tip of the spine, in order to avoid puncturing of the vessels (Fig. 34.18).
- The ends of the suture are brought out through the vaginal vault.
- One more suture may be placed the same way. These, when tied at the end of the surgery, fix the apex of the vault towards the sacrospinous ligament.

Complications These are listed in Box 34.11.

Manchester–Fothergill operation

This is the conservative surgical procedure performed for correction of POP. The essential components of this surgery are as follows:

- Amputation of the cervix
- Approximation of the cardinal ligaments in front of the amputated cervix in order to shorten the ligaments
- Anterior colporrhaphy; posterior repair, if required

Box 34.11 Complications of sacrospinous colpopexy

- Haemorrhage
  - Injury to pudendal vessels
- Haematoma in the ischiorectal fossa
- Infection
- Dyspareunia
  - Change in angle of vagina

Indications

The only indication is POP in women of reproductive age. Most common cause of POP in this age group is pregnancy and childbirth. Because of traction on the cardinal and uterosacral ligaments during childbirth, supravaginal portion of the cervix elongates and contributes to the descent. The cardinal/uterosacral ligaments that keep the cervix in place are also stretched. Hence, amputating the cervix to reduce the length, shortening the cardinal ligaments by approximating them anterior to the cervix and correcting the associated anterior vaginal wall prolapse would be the appropriate surgery. This procedure was popular two decades ago but has now been replaced by other conservative surgical procedures such as abdominal and vaginal slings and use of mesh. The disadvantages of Fothergill repair, the most important being high rate of recurrence, are listed in Box 34.12.

Procedure

Anaesthesia, antibiotic prophylaxis and patient position are as for vaginal hysterectomy. Bladder should be catheterized.

- D&C is usually performed.

Box 34.12 Disadvantages of Fothergill surgery

- High rate of recurrence
- Cervical incompetence
  - Recurrent miscarriage
  - Preterm labour
- Cervical stenosis
  - Dysmenorrhoea
  - Haematometra
  - Infertility
- Changes in the cervical mucus
  - Infertility

- Length of cervix is measured and the level of amputation decided, to leave behind 2.5 cm of cervix.
- Four Allis clamps are placed on the Fothergill points. These are as follows:
  - Just below the external urethral meatus
  - At the posterior fornix, in the midline
  - Two lateral points that, when approximated, would result in a vagina of appropriate depth [the vaginal wall beyond this point would be excised (Fig. 34.19)]

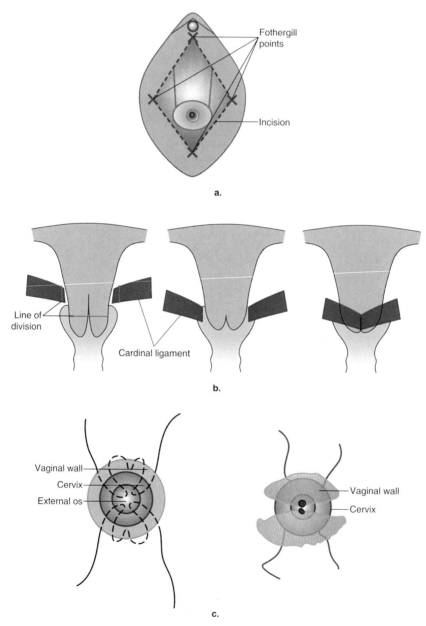

a.

b.

c.

Figure 34.19 Diagrammatic representation of Fothergill operation. a. Fothergill points are marked and joined to make a rhomboidal incision. b. The cardinal ligaments are cut at the attachment to the cervix. Amputation of the cervix to the desired length (2.5 cm) is done. Cardinal ligaments are sutured to the anterior aspect of the cervix. c. The cervix is covered by Sturmdorf sutures.

- A rhomboid-shaped incision is made connecting the four points. The vaginal wall distal to the incision is dissected from the bladder and posterior cervix and removed.
- Vesicocervical ligaments are cut and the bladder is pushed up.
- Cardinal ligaments are clamped with straight clamps, cut and ligated.
- Cervix is amputated at the desired level.
- Cardinal ligaments are brought forward and approximated in front of the cervix with sutures. They are then sutured to the anterior part of the cervix.
- Anterior colporrhaphy is performed.
- The anterior part of the vaginal incision is closed vertically.
- The amputated end of the cervix is covered by vaginal mucosa using Sturmdorf sutures. Two sutures are taken through the vaginal wall at 12 and 6 o'clock points and the ends are left long. The two ends of the anterior sutures are taken over the anterior cervical lip, through the canal, to emerge at the two Fothergill points laterally. Pulling the two ends of the stitch brings the anterior vaginal wall over the anterior lip of the cervix and covers it. The same procedure is repeated posteriorly and the sutures are made to emerge posterolaterally.
- If posterior defects are present, appropriate repairs are done.
- Vagina is packed.

Complications

Late complications are already listed under disadvantages (Box 34.12). Immediate complications include haemorrhage, urinary tract infection and occasional bladder injury.

Abdominal surgical procedures

All abdominal surgical procedures are performed under general or regional anaesthesia. Patients have to be hospitalized, counselled and prepared for surgery. Antibiotic prophylaxis is essential when peritoneal cavity is entered through the vagina or vice versa (*see* Chapter 33, *Preoperative preparation and postoperative management*).

Position

Patients are usually placed in supine position. Bladder is catheterized.

Abdominal hysterectomy

Removal of the uterus through the abdominal route is one of the most common surgical procedures in gynaecology. With the availability of several modalities of medical treatment for abnormal uterine bleeding, myomas and endometriosis and with the increasing use of vaginal hysterectomy in recent years, the need for abdominal hysterectomy has declined, but it still remains the most common major gynaecological surgery. Abdominal hysterectomy is easier than vaginal hysterectomy since the organs can be well visualized and tissue planes are easy to obtain. As abdominal surgery is associated with more morbidity, vaginal hysterectomy is recommended whenever feasible.

Types

Hysterectomy is classified into types I–V. Types I–III are commonly used (Fig. 29.14). Types IV and V refer to pelvic exenteration procedures and are not within the scope of this book.

- *Type I:* It refers to **simple hysterectomy**, which is usually extrafascial.
- *Type II:* It is also known as **modified radical hysterectomy** and includes removal of uterus with parametrium medial to widely displaced ureters. It is used in cervical cancer stage IA2.
- *Type III:* This is **radical hysterectomy** where parametrium up to the pelvic wall is removed. This is indicated in cervical cancer stages IB and IIA.

Subtotal versus total hysterectomy

In subtotal hysterectomy, the cervix is retained and the uterus above the level of internal os is removed. Current evidence does not support the view that removal of cervix can interfere with sexual orgasm and bladder function. When cervix is retained, follow-up with Pap smear is mandatory in women with intact uterus. Some gynaecologists core out the inner layers of the endocervical canal and part of the ectocervix to remove the transformation zone and endocervical glandular epithelium in order to obviate the need for repeated Pap smears, but this is controversial. Therefore, subtotal hysterectomy is now reserved for situations where the cervix cannot be removed without injury to adjacent organs, as in extensive endometriosis.

Oophorectomy at hysterectomy

When to remove normal ovaries at hysterectomy has been a point of debate. Removing the ovaries before menopause leads to surgical menopause characterized by acute symptoms such as hot flushes and sleep disturbances and long-term effects such as osteoporosis. This necessitates oestrogen replacement therapy. Retained ovaries in the perimenopausal or postmenopausal woman can become malignant, although the chances of malignancy are the same as in the general population. The patient should be informed about the positive and negative impacts of removing/retaining the ovaries. Guidelines do not recommend removal of normal-looking ovaries before menopause. In general, ovaries are retained in premenopausal women but after discussion with the patient.

Indications

Gynaecological indications for abdominal hysterectomy are listed in Box 34.13. Obstetric indications and caesarean hysterectomy are beyond the purview of this book.

Instruments

The same instruments are used as for vaginal hysterectomy—Spencer Wells, Heaney, Kocher, Allis and Kelley clamps. Some or all of these instruments are used in all abdominal surgical procedures as well.

Box 34.13 Indications for abdominal hysterectomy

- Benign diseases
  - Large or multiple uterine myomas
  - Adenomyosis
  - Endometriosis
  - Pelvic inflammatory disease
  - Abnormal uterine bleeding
  - Endometrial hyperplasia
- Malignant diseases
  - Microinvasive cervical cancer
  - Endometrial cancer
  - Ovarian cancer
  - Gestational trophoblastic neoplasia

Procedure

See Fig. 34.20.

- A transverse incision (Pfannenstiel incision) is usually preferred unless the uterus is very large, extensive adhesions are anticipated or the surgery is being undertaken for a gynaecological malignancy.
- The uterus, tubes, ovaries, pouch of Douglas and pelvic and abdominal viscera are inspected first. Bowel loops are packed away from the operating field.
- Two straight Kocher or Spencer Wells clamps are applied on each side on the round ligaments, fallopian tubes and ovarian ligaments, close to the uterine cornu. These clamps are used to hold the uterus up.
- Round ligaments are clamped with Spencer Wells clamps, cut and ligated on both sides.
- If oopherectomy is to be performed, infundibulopelvic ligaments are clamped with two Kelley clamps and cut between the clamps. If ovaries are to be retained, ovarian ligaments and tubes are clamped, cut and ligated.
- Uterovesical peritoneum is opened from one round ligament to the other and the bladder is pushed down.
- Uterine vessels are clamped with two Heaney clamps placed horizontally, cut between the clamps and ligated on both sides. Care should be taken to stay clear of the ureter.
- Cardinal ligaments and uterosacral ligaments are clamped individually or together with Spencer Wells clamps, cut and ligated on both sides.
- Vaginal angles are clamped with Kelley or Heaney clamps, placed horizontally, cut and ligated. This opens the vaginal vault. Vagina is then cut around the cervix and uterus is removed.
- Vaginal cuff is held with long Allis clamps and closed with interrupted or continuous sutures.
- Abdomen is closed.

Complications

Complications of abdominal hysterectomy vary with the indication for which it is performed. The complications are listed in Box 34.14.

Oophorectomy

Oophorectomy is the removal of the ovary. It may be removal of a normal ovary or ovary with benign or malignant lesions.

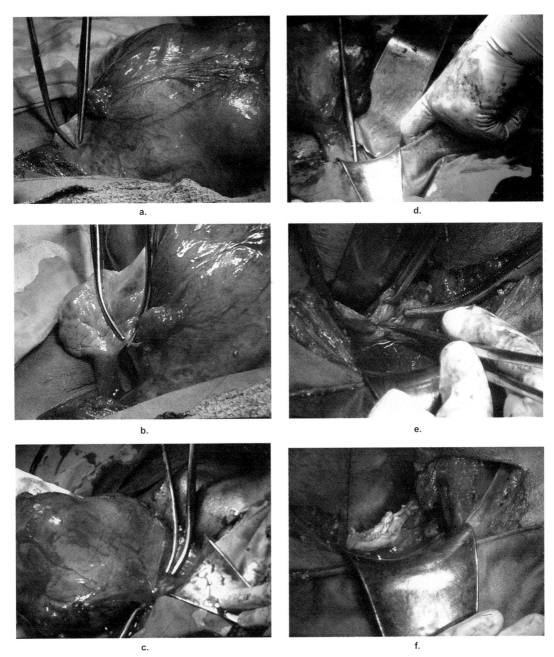

Figure 34.20 Abdominal hysterectomy. The uterus is enlarged with multiple myomas. **a.** Round ligament has been clamped with straight and Kelley clamps and is being cut. **b.** The ovarian ligament and the tube are clamped with Kelley clamps. **c.** The uterine vessels have been clamped with Heaney clamps. The clamps are placed at right angles to the uterus. **d.** The cardinal ligament is clamped parallel to and as close to the cervix as possible. **e.** Vaginal angles are clamped at right angles to the vagina. **f.** Vaginal vault is being sutured.

Indications

Indications for oophorectomy are given in Box 34.15.

Procedure

Abdomen is opened by Pfannenstiel, Maylard or vertical incision depending on the size of

Box 34.14 Complications of abdominal hysterectomy

- Haemorrhage
  - Primary
  - Secondary
- Infection
  - Peritonitis
  - Urinary tract infection
- Paralytic ileus
- Injuries
  - Injury to ureter
    - While clamping infundibulopelvic ligament
    - While clamping uterine vessels
    - At the vaginal vault injury to bladder
- Thrombosis and pulmonary embolism

Box 34.15 Indications for oophorectomy

- Normal ovary
  - At hysterectomy in postmenopausal women
  - Prophylactic oophorectomy in familial ovarian cancer
- Benign diseases
  - Dermoid cyst
  - Endometrioma
  - Epithelial tumours
  - Tubo-ovarian mass/abscess
  - Sex cord-stromal tumours
- Malignant tumours
  - Epithelial
  - Germ cell
  - Sex cord-stromal

the ovarian tumour/cyst (Fig. 34.21). If possibility of malignancy is high, vertical incision is recommended.

- Once the abdomen is opened, the tumour is assessed for features of malignancy such as solid tumours, solid areas in a cystic tumour, fixity, bilaterality, papillary excrescences, multiloculation, ascites and peritoneal deposits.
- If none are present, the ovary with the cyst is pulled upwards to expose the ovarian ligament, mesovarium and infundibulopelvic ligaments.
- Series of Kelley clamps are applied; ligaments and mesovarium are cut and ligated.
- Ovary is removed.

Complications Haemorrhage from the ovarian vessels can occur if the infundibulopelvic ligament is not ligated with care.

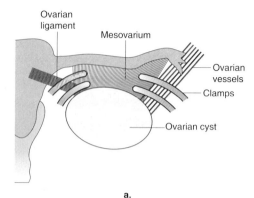

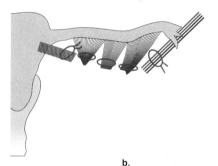

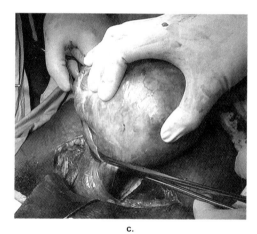

Figure 34.21 Diagrammatic representation of oophorectomy. a. The infundibulopelvic ligament, mesovarium and ovarian ligament are clamped. b. Stumps of ligaments and mesovarium after ligation. c. Oophorectomy for a solid ovarian tumour. Kelley clamps have been placed on the ligaments and mesovarium.

Ovarian cystectomy

Removal of ovarian cyst and retaining the normal ovarian tissue is referred to as ovarian cystectomy. This is the procedure of choice in young

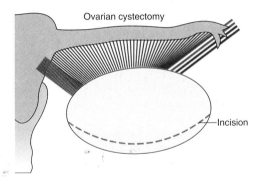

Figure 34.22 The incision for ovarian cystectomy. Incision must be made on the dome of the cyst.

women in whom fertility and hormonal function are desired, even when the lesion is unilateral. When the cysts are bilateral, every effort should be made to conserve as much ovarian tissue as possible. The normal ovarian tissue can be identified by inspecting the ovary carefully and by palpation.

Indications

Indications for ovarian cystectomy include benign epithelial cysts, cystic teratoma and endometriosis.

Procedure

- The incision should be made on the ovarian capsule on the dome of the cyst cautiously with diathermy or knife (Fig. 34.22).
- Incision is deepened till the cyst wall is reached, taking care not to enter the cyst.
- The cyst is separated from the normal ovarian tissue by blunt and sharp dissection and removed.
- Excess ovarian capsule is excised.
- Haemostasis should be achieved by cauterizing the bleeding points.
- The capsule and the ovarian bed are sutured.

Complications

Haemorrhage from the cut edge of the capsule of the cyst or the ovary can occur. Meticulous haemostasis should be achieved by cauterization and ligation of bleeding points during surgery.

Abdominal sling operations for prolapse

These are procedures by which the cervix is pulled up and attached to various structures using fascia or synthetic tapes. Sling procedures are performed in young women where preservation of fertility is desired or in women with vaginal vault prolapse after hysterectomy. There are three commonly used procedures (Fig. 34.23), viz.:

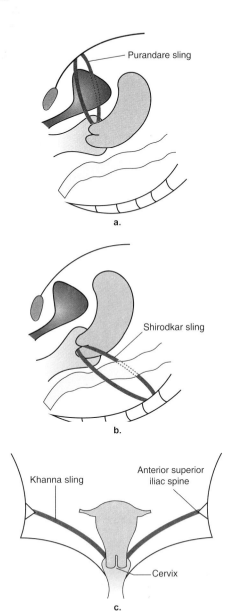

Figure 34.23 Diagrammatic representation of sling operations for prolapse. a. Purandare sling. The cervix is attached to the anterior abdominal wall. b. Shirodkar sling. This attaches the cervix to the first or second sacral vertebra. c. The cervix is fixed to the anterior superior iliac spine.

- *Purandare sling procedure*: The anterior aspect of the isthmus or vaginal vault is fixed to anterior abdominal wall using strips of rectus sheath. The rectus strips are attached to the lateral part of the abdominal incision. Medial end is taken between the layers of the broad ligament and stitched to the anterior part of the cervix at the isthmus.
- *Shirodkar sling procedure*: Mersilene tape is used to fix the posterior part of the isthmus to the sacrum. Special precautions must be taken on the left side to avoid the ureter.
- *Khanna sling procedure*: Mersilene tape is used to fix the anterior part of isthmus to anterior superior iliac spine.

Currently, sacrocolpopexy and sacrohysteropexy using Prolene mesh are used as alternatives to sling operations.

Abdominal sacrocolpopexy/sacrohysteropexy

This procedure is used to correct posthysterectomy vault prolapse or prolapse in young women. A synthetic, macroporous mesh is used. This is fixed to the anterior longitudinal ligament at S1 or S2 and to the vault of the vagina or cervix.

Indications Indications for this procedure include posthysterectomy vault prolapse and prolapse in young women in whom fertility preservation is desired.

Position Low lithotomy position is preferred—Supine position with the patient brought to the edge of the table, the thighs in the same plane as abdomen but abducted a little, and knees semi-flexed and supported by stirrups. The assistant pushes the vaginal vault up with a sponge holding forceps.

Procedure

- Abdomen is opened by Pfannenstiel incision.
- Posterior peritoneum over the S1 and S2 is incised and posterior longitudinal ligament is identified. Two or three sutures of nonabsorbable material are taken through the ligament, one below the other, and the ends are left long.
- Vaginal vault is held with Allis clamps and peritoneum at the vault opened. About 4–5 cm of anterior and posterior vaginal walls is dissected and exposed.

- A Prolene mesh of about 6 inches in length is chosen; lower 2 inches is cut in the middle, forming a 'Y' (Fig. 34.24).
- The anterior arm of 'Y' is sutured to the anterior wall of vagina with four or six stitches of Prolene. The posterior arm is sutured to the posterior vaginal wall.

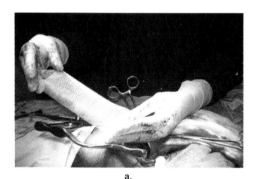

a.

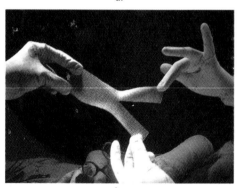

b.

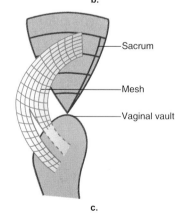

c.

Figure 34.24 Sacrocolpopexy. **a.** Prolene mesh used for sacrocolpopexy. **b.** Mesh is cut to form a 'Y'; the two limbs of the 'Y' to be attached to the anterior and posterior vaginal walls. **c.** The mesh attaching the vaginal vault to sacrum.

- The mesh is then passed posterior to the peritoneum and directed towards S1/S2 on the right side of the rectum. The ends of the sutures placed earlier are used to fix the mesh to the anterior longitudinal ligament.
- In case of sacrospinous hysteropexy, the anterior and posterior aspects of the supravaginal cervix are fixed to the sacrum.

Complications Injury to sacral vessels and mesh erosion are the complications to be kept in mind.

Radical hysterectomy and pelvic lymphadenectomy

This is also known as Wertheim hysterectomy. The uterus, cervix, tubes, vaginal cuff and parametrium up to pelvic side wall are removed in radical hysterectomy. Uterine artery is cut at its origin from internal iliac. Ovaries are usually removed except when the woman is young.

Pelvic lymphadenectomy includes removal of internal, external and common iliac nodes, obturator nodes and the lymphatics along the vessels.

Indications Indication for this surgery is cervical cancer stages IB and IIA.

Preoperative evaluation and preparation

Clinical staging is mandatory. Imaging may be required in some women. Magnetic resonance imaging (MRI) is useful for excluding minimal parametrial infiltration. Decision regarding surgery should be taken based on age, stage of disease and associated comorbidities. Appropriate investigations including chest X-ray are essential.

Preoperative anticoagulation is mandatory as discussed in Chapter 33, *Preoperative preparation and postoperative management.* Pneumatic cuffs should be used during surgery to prevent venous thrombosis. Two units of blood should be available for transfusion. The surgery is usually performed under general anaesthesia. Supine or low lithotomy position may be used. Prophylactic antibiotics must be administered.

Procedure

- Abdomen is opened with vertical midline or transverse muscle cutting (Maylard) incision.
- The pelvis and the abdomen must be inspected and palpated for gross metastatic disease.
- Round ligaments are clamped, cut and ligated as for type I hysterectomy.

- Retroperitoneum is opened taking care to stay lateral to the ureter.
- Paravesical and pararectal spaces are created by finger dissection so that the parametria can be palpated between the fingers.
- Infundibulopelvic ligaments are clamped, cut and ligated. If ovaries are to be retained, ovarian ligaments are clamped, cut and ligated.
- Lymphadenectomy may be performed first. The external, internal and common iliac nodes and lymphatics along the vessels are dissected and removed (Fig. 34.25).
- The uterine artery is ligated at its origin from internal iliac artery.
- Dissection is continued into the obturator fossa and the tissues and nodes above the obturator nerve are removed.
- Bladder is pushed down by sharp dissection. Ureter is pulled up and the ureteric tunnel is opened. Ureter is mobilized from the tunnel.
- Cardinal ligament and parametrium are clamped laterally, cut and ligated.
- Dissection is completed on the other side.
- Uterosacral ligaments are clamped posteriorly, cut and ligated.
- Rectovaginal peritoneum is opened. Vagina is clamped to include 3- to 4-cm cuff.
- All the tissues dissected out, including the cuff of vagina, are removed.
- Vault is closed; abdomen is closed in layers.

Complications

Complications are listed in Box 34.16. Intraoperative haemorrhage is the most common complication.

Modified radical hysterectomy (type II)

The differences between radical and modified radical hysterectomy are given in Table 34.1.

Myomectomy

Surgical removal of myomas is called myomectomy. It is usually performed abdominally but can be performed vaginally or through the laparoscopic/hysteroscopic approach.

Indications

Asymptomatic myomas do not require surgical intervention unless they are large. In older women, symptomatic myomas can be dealt with

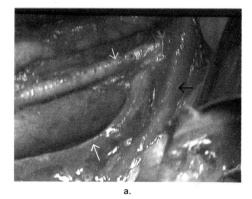

a.

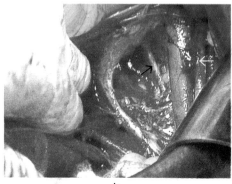

b.

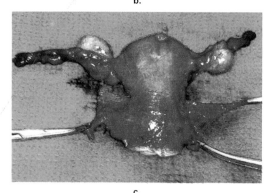

c.

Figure 34.25 Radical hysterectomy and pelvic lymphadenectomy. **a.** Pelvic node dissection. Bifurcation of the common iliac artery (blue double arrow) into external iliac artery (yellow arrow) and internal iliac artery (white arrow). Ureter can be seen crossing the bifurcation (black arrow). The external iliac vein is also seen in the figure (blue arrow). **b.** Obturator fossa has been cleared of nodes. The obturator nerve (black arrow) and external iliac vessels (yellow arrow) are visible. **c.** Radical hysterectomy specimen with parametria divided at the pelvic wall.

by hysterectomy. Indications for myomectomy are listed in Box 34.17.

Box 34.16 Complications of radical hysterectomy and pelvic lymphadenectomy

- Intraoperative
  - Haemorrhage
  - Injury to
    - Vessels
    - Ureter
    - Bladder
- Postoperative
  - Urinary infection
  - Peritonitis
  - Urinary fistulae
  - Lymph cyst formation
  - Bladder dysfunction
  - Paralytic ileus
- Thrombosis and pulmonary embolism

Table 34.1 Differences between radical and modified radical hysterectomy

Radical hysterectomy	Modified radical hysterectomy
Uterine artery ligated at internal iliac	Uterine artery ligated where it crosses the ureter
Cardinal ligament divided at pelvic wall	Cardinal ligament only medial to ureter removed
3–4 cm of vaginal cuff removed	Only 2–3 cm of vaginal cuff removed
Uterosacral divided close to sacrum	Uterosacral divided more anteriorly

Box 34.17 Indications for myomectomy

Young women with myomas and
- Abnormal uterine bleeding
- Large uterus (>14–16 weeks)
- Infertility
  - Submucous myoma
  - Intramural distorting cavity
  - Cornual occluding tube
  - All other causes excluded
- Pressure symptoms

Choice of route for myomectomy depends on the number, size and location of myomas. Multiple myomas, ≥5 in number and larger than 10 cm, and cervical myomas are removed by abdominal approach. If they are smaller than 10 cm, three to four in number and subserous or intramural in location, laparoscopic route may be chosen. Submucous myomas <5 cm in size are removed hysteroscopically. If they are large, preoperative gonadotropin-releasing hormone (GnRH) can be used to reduce the size. Vaginal myomectomy is rarely performed except during vaginal hysterectomy or when the myoma protrudes into the vagina.

Abdominal myomectomy

Preoperative preparation

Clinical evaluation, ultrasonography and counselling are essential (Box 34.18). GnRH analogues may be administered to reduce the size of myoma and minimize bleeding. However, GnRH analogues may obliterate the tissue plane under the pseudocapsule and make the dissection difficult. Moreover, small myomas may become tiny and be left behind and increase the risk of recurrence.

Box 34.18 Preoperative preparation for abdominal myomectomy

- Clinical evaluation
  - Symptoms
  - Size of uterus
  - Mobility
- Ultrasonography
  - Number of myomas
  - Size of myomas
  - Location of myomas
- In couples with infertility
  - Hysterosalpingography
  - Semen analysis
- Blood cross-matched and kept ready
- Counselling
  - Possibility of complications
  - Possibility of conversion to hysterectomy
  - Possibility of postoperative adhesions

Anaesthesia and position

Myomectomy is performed under general or regional anaesthesia. Position should be supine. Bladder should be catheterized.

Instruments

Apart from the usual instruments, myoma screw is used (Fig. 34.26a). Rubber tubes or Foley catheter are used as tourniquet.

General guidelines

These are given in Box 34.19. Myomas are vascular tumours and myomectomy is associated with bleeding. To minimize blood loss, tourniquet or local vasoconstrictors are used. Incisions on the uterus should be preferably on the anterior wall. Posterior wall incisions cause more adhesions involving tubes and ovaries. Midline incisions are better since they minimize blood loss and avert extension of incision to uterine vessels. After the myoma is enucleated, the brisk haemorrhage from the myoma bed must be meticulously controlled.

Procedure

- Abdomen is opened by Pfannenstiel, Maylard or vertical incision depending on the size of the uterus and myomas. Large uterus >24 weeks may require vertical incision.
- The size of uterus, number and size of myomas and their location should be assessed.
- A rubber tube is used as tourniquet to occlude uterine vessels. A hole is made in both broad ligaments just above the level of the isthmus. The tourniquet is passed around the lower uterus, including the uterine vessels, and tied. This is released every 20 minutes to restore blood supply to uterus. Alternatively, 20 mL of vasopressin (0.05 U/mL) may be infiltrated along the line of incision. Both techniques used together can further reduce bleeding. Ovarian vessels should also be occluded by atraumatic clamp or tourniquet.
- Procedure of myomectomy after this step is the same as in abdominal, vaginal and laparoscopic approaches.
- Incision is made on the myoma and deepened till the pseudocapsule is incised and myomas

---

Box 34.19 General guidelines in myomectomy

- Blood loss should be minimized with tourniquet/ vasopressin
- Incision should be on anterior wall
- Avoid posterior wall incisions
- There should be midline vertical incision to avoid vessels
- There should be tunnelling incisions for smaller myomas
- Ensure good haemostasis

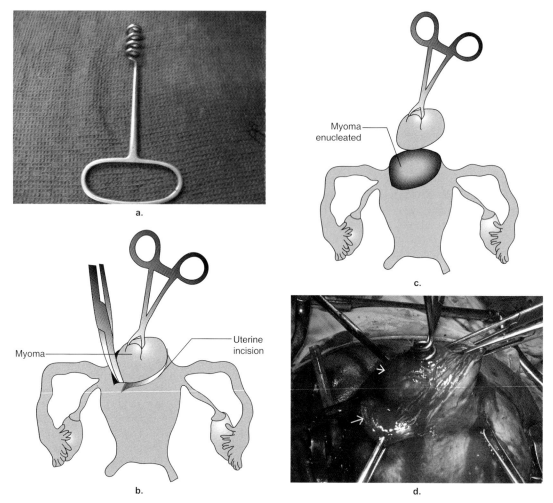

Figure 34.26 Abdominal myomectomy. a. Myoma screw—Used for fixing and holding the myoma. b. Diagrammatic representation of myomectomy. Incision has been made on the pseudocapsule, down to the myoma. c. Myoma being enucleated from the capsule. d. Myomectomy. Arrows indicate myoma screw inserted into the myoma (blue arrow), myoma (white arrow) and pseudocapsule (yellow arrow).

are visible. There is a plane of dissection between the myoma and the pseudocapsule.

- The pseudocapsule is held with Allis clamps and myoma is held with myoma screw for traction. The myoma is enucleated by blunt dissection using a knife handle or finger (Fig. 34.26b–d).
- Tunnelling incisions are made through the myometrium to approach the smaller myomas, which are enucleated through the same incision.
- Submucous myomas >5 cm are removed by opening the cavity. If <5 cm, they can be removed hysteroscopically before the abdominal procedure.

- Posterior intramural myomas can be removed by transcavitary approach, incising the anterior uterine wall and then the posterior uterine wall.
- Subserous posterior myomas are removed by direct posterior incision on the myoma.
- After enucleation, the myoma bed is sutured with series of mattress sutures with delayed absorbable suture material.
- The tourniquet is released to find additional bleeding points that need attention.
- Abdomen is closed.

Complications These are listed in Box 34.20. The most common complication is haemorrhage.

- Immediate
  - Haemorrhage
  - Infection
- Late
  - Pelvic adhesions
  - Infertility
  - Scar rupture in labour
  - Recurrence of myoma

Endoscopic surgery

Endoscopic procedures are currently popular for diagnostic and therapeutic purposes. They have several advantages over open procedures. Endoscopic surgery may be performed by laparoscopy or hysteroscopy.

Laparoscopy

This is also called keyhole surgery. Telescope with fibre-optic cable introduced through a port is used to visualize the abdominal and pelvic contents. Operating instruments are introduced through separate ports.

Advantages of laparoscopy over laparotomy

These are listed in Box 34.21.

Indications

Laparoscopy can be diagnostic or operative. Indications are listed in Box 34.22. With increasing expertise, laparoscopic surgical procedures are becoming popular.

Anaesthesia and position

General anaesthesia is preferred. Position should be low lithotomy. Bladder is catheterized.

Instruments

The instruments used are Veress needle, trocars and sleeves, laparoscope, cables, light source, insufflation system and operative laparoscopic instruments (Fig. 34.27).

Veress needle has a longer blunt inner stylet attached to a spring device and a sharp outer sheath. The blunt spring-loaded stylet bounces back once the abdomen is entered, preventing laceration of viscera and blood vessels.

Trocars are of varying sizes, usually 5, 7.5, 10 and 12 mm in diameter. They are used for telescopes of similar sizes.

Box 34.21 Advantages of laparoscopy over laparotomy

- Avoids large incisions
- Less blood loss
- Less postoperative pain
- Shorter hospital stay
- Early return to normal activity
- Minimal risk of incisional hernia

Box 34.22 Indications for laparoscopy

- Diagnostic
  - Infertility
  - Endometriosis
  - Acute/chronic pelvic pain
  - Ectopic pregnancy
  - Evaluation of adnexal mass
- Operative
  - Sterilization
  - Ectopic pregnancy
  - Endometriosis
  - Ovarian/paraovarian cysts
  - Adhesiolysis
  - Tubal anastomosis
  - Myomectomy
  - Hysterectomy
    - Simple
    - Radical
  - Retroperitoneal lymphadenectomy
  - Sacrocolpopexy
  - Burch colposuspension

Procedure

- Umbilical site is most commonly used for gynaecological procedures. A small incision is made at the lower border of the umbilicus. Size of incision depends on the size of scope to be used.
- A Rubin cannula is inserted into the uterus for uterine manipulation and chromoperfusion. If hysterectomy is planned, uterine manipulator should be inserted.
- The Veress needle is inserted through the incision.
- Alternatively, an open entry method may be used. In this method, rectus sheath is pulled up with Allis clamps through the skin incision and incised. The trocar is inserted directly.
- Carbon dioxide insufflation is started with a flow rate of 1 L/minute. Once percussion confirms intra-abdominal gas, flow rate can be increased in order to maintain an intra-abdominal pressure of 10–12 mmHg.

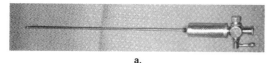

a.

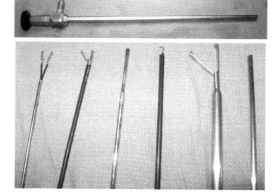

b.

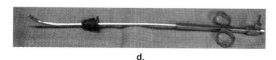

c.

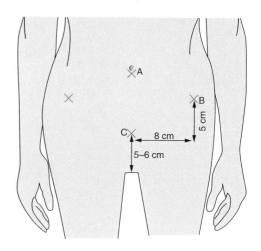

Laparoscopic ports

Figure 34.28 Trocar insertion points. Point A: Umbilical port. Point B: Lateral ports 5 cm superior to and 8 cm lateral to pubic symphysis. Point C: Suprapubic port—Two fingerbreadths (5–6 cm) superior to pubic symphysis.

d.

Figure 34.27 Instruments for laparoscopy. a. Veress needle used for creating pneumoperitoneum. It has a slightly short, sharp outer sheath and a spring-loaded, blunt inner stylet. b. Trocars used for laparoscopy. The scope and other instruments are inserted through the trocars. c. Telescope and operative laparoscopy instruments. d. Rubin cannula. This is used for steadying and anteverting the uterus and injecting dye for checking tubal patency. It has a guard that can be adjusted to uterocervical length.

- Once pneumoperitoneum is sufficient (3–5 L), head-down tilt allows good visualization of pelvis.
- The secondary trocars for introduction of operating instruments are introduced (Fig. 34.28). The usual points are as follows: (a) lateral ports—5 cm above the pubic symphysis and 8 cm lateral to midline (care must be taken to avoid inferior epigastric vessels); (b) suprapubic port—5–6 cm (2–3) fingerbreadths above pubic symphysis.
- The pelvic viscera are visualized and operative procedures are performed (Fig. 34.29).
- Gas should be allowed to escape after the completion of the procedure. Rectus sheath is sutured.

Complications

Complications are fewer with laparoscopy, but they do occur. These are listed in Box 34.23.

Hysteroscopy

Visualization of the endocervical canal and uterine cavity through an endoscope is known as hysteroscopy. Hysteroscopy can be used for diagnostic purposes and therapeutic procedures.

Indications

Indications are listed in Box 34.24. As with laparoscopy, indications are changing and increasing with increasing expertise and new innovations in hysteroscopy.

Instruments

The instruments for hysteroscopy are instruments used for D&C, diagnostic sheath, operative

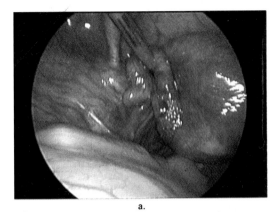

a.

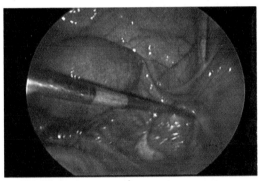

b.

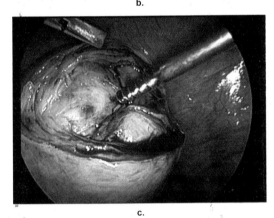

c.

Figure 34.29 Laparoscopy. a. Spill of dye. b. Normal uterus, ovary and tubes. c. Laparoscopic myomectomy.

sheath, hysteroscope, rectoscope, loop, rollerball and needle electrodes, uterine insufflation unit and distension medium (saline or glycine) and light source (Fig. 34.30).

Hysteroscopes vary in diameter from 3 to 4 mm. The angle of view may be 0 or 30 degrees. The diagnostic sheath is 5 mm in diameter and allows insufflation medium to enter the uterus. The operating sheath is 8–10 mm in diameter.

Box 34.23 Complications of laparoscopy

- At needle and trocar entry
  - Injury to vessels
    - Inferior epigastric
    - Aorta/vena cava
  - Injury to bowel
  - Injury to other organs
- Pneumoperitoneum
  - Subcutaneous emphysema
- Laparoscopic surgery
  - Injury to vessels
  - Injury to viscera
  - Injury to bowel
  - Injury to ureter/bladder

Box 34.24 Indications for hysteroscopy

- Diagnostic
  - Endometrial polyp
  - Submucous myoma
  - Abnormal uterine bleeding
  - Postmenopausal bleeding
  - Uterine anomalies
  - Missing IUCD
  - Endometrial cancer
  - Intrauterine adhesions
- Operative
  - Polypectomy
  - Lysis of intrauterine adhesions
  - Removal of IUCD
  - Resection of uterine septum
- Removal of submucous myoma
  - Endometrial resection/ablation
  - Tubal cannulation
  - Hysteroscopic sterilization

IUCD, intrauterine contraceptive device.

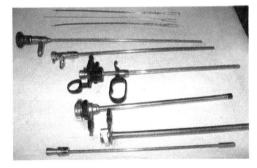

Figure 34.30 Hysteroscopy instruments. From above downwards—Wire loop and rollerball cautery, telescopes, operating sheath, diagnostic sheaths (inner and outer) and obturator.

Distension media

Saline is used as hysteroflation medium for diagnostic hysteroscopy, but since it is a good conductor of electrons, it cannot be used with diathermy. High-viscosity media such as Hyskon or low-viscosity media such as glycine or sorbitol are used for operative procedures. Carbon dioxide can be used as gaseous distension medium.

Anaesthesia and position

Diagnostic hysteroscopy can be performed as an office procedure since diagnostic sheath is only 5 mm in diameter and does not require cervical dilatation (Fig. 34.31a). Operative hysteroscopy requires admission and general anaesthesia. The patient is placed in dorsal lithotomy position.

Procedure

- Vaginal wall is retracted with speculum; cervix is held with vulsellum and uterocervical length is measured with uterine sound.
- Diagnostic sheath and telescope are assembled, and saline and optic cables are connected. The scope with sheath is introduced into the uterus.
- With uterine distension, the cavity, fundus and tubal ostia can be visualized. Cervical canal is visualized while introducing and withdrawing the scope.
- If operative hysteroscopy is planned, cervix is dilated to 8–10 Hegar. Glycine is connected to the operating sheath. Scope and operating attachments are assembled and introduced into the cavity.
- Uterine cavity is visualized and operative procedures are performed (Fig. 34.31b–d).

Complications

Complications are listed in Box 34.25. They are minimal in experienced hands.

Other operative procedures in gynaecological oncology, pelvic reconstructive surgery and endoscopic surgery are beyond the scope of this book.

Box 34.25 Complications of hysteroscopy

- Haemorrhage
  - Intraoperative
  - Postoperative
- Uterine perforation
- Electrolyte disturbances due to distension media
- Infection

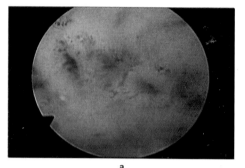

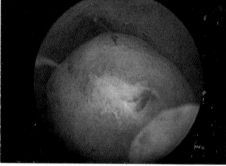

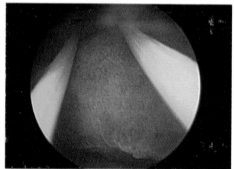

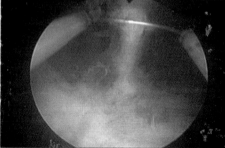

Figure 34.31 Hysteroscopy—Diagnostic and operative. a. Normal tubal ostium. b. Endometrial polyp. c. Resection of endometrial polyp. d. Resection of uterine septum.

Key points

- Gynaecological surgical procedures can be performed through the abdominal, vaginal or laparoscopic approach. Vaginal route is unique to pelvic surgery.

- Preoperative discussion with the patient regarding the procedure, informed consent and documentation are mandatory.

- Several diagnostic and therapeutic vaginal procedures can be performed as office procedures under intravenous or oral analgesia or paracervical block.

- The most common office procedures include cervical biopsy, cervical polypectomy, loop electroexcision procedure (LEEP), endometrial biopsy, dilatation and curettage and endometrial thermal ablation.

- All vaginal surgical procedures are performed with the patient in dorsal lithotomy or low lithotomy positions. Catheterization of bladder and pelvic examination to assess the size, shape and version of uterus are essential preliminary steps.

- Cold knife conization, vaginal hysterectomy and pelvic reconstructive surgery are performed under general or regional anaesthesia after admitting the patient.

- Conization may be performed with knife or LEEP. The cone may be deep or shallow depending on the location and extent of cervical lesion.

- Vaginal hysterectomy has several advantages over abdominal hysterectomy. This should be the approach for hysterectomy whenever feasible.

- Vaginal hysterectomy is contraindicated in women with gynaecological malignancies, when adhesions are anticipated or when the uterus is large.

- Pelvic reconstructive procedures are performed with or without vaginal hysterectomy as and when indicated. Anterior vaginal wall prolapse is repaired by anterior colporrhaphy or site-specific repair, enterocele by McCall culdoplasty, rectocele by posterior colporrhaphy and deficient perineum by perineorrhaphy.

- Manchester–Fothergill operation has now been largely replaced by sacrohysteropexy. It used to be the procedure of choice in young women with pelvic organ prolapse (POP). The essential components are amputation of cervix, shortening of cardinal ligaments and anterior colporrhaphy. The recurrence rate of POP after this surgery is high and amputation of cervix is associated with obstetric complications.

- Abdominal surgical procedures include type I, II or III hysterectomy, oophorectomy, ovarian cystectomy abdominal procedures for POP and myomectomy.

- Abdominal hysterectomy may be total or supracervical. Oophorectomy at hysterectomy has to be carefully considered.

- Type III hysterectomy or radical hysterectomy with lymphadenectomy is performed in women with stage IB and IIA cervical cancer. Structures removed are uterus, cervix, cuff of vagina, tubes, ovaries, internal iliac, external iliac, common iliac, obturator and sacral lymph nodes.

- Oophorectomy is indicated in benign diseases of the ovary and malignant tumours. Ovarian cystectomy is performed in younger women with benign lesions.

- Abdominal myomectomy is indicated in young women with large and multiple symptomatic myomas. Blood loss at myomectomy should be minimized by tourniquet and/or injection of vasopressin. General guidelines for myomectomy should be followed.

- Abdominal sling procedures and sacrocolpopexy or sacrohysteropexy procedures are indicated in young women with POP when fertility preservation is desired.

- Laparoscopic surgery is otherwise known as keyhole surgery. It has several advantages such as no large incisions, short hospital stay, early return to work, less postoperative pain and minimal risk of incisional hernia.

- Laparoscopic procedures may be diagnostic or therapeutic. Indications include evaluation of infertility, endometriosis, ectopic pregnancy, chronic pelvic pain, tubal sterilization, ovarian cystectomy, oopherectomy and hysterectomy.

- Hysteroscopy can also be used for diagnostic and therapeutic procedures. Visualization of endometrial cavity and surgical procedures within the endometrial cavity are performed using hysteroscopy.

Self-assessment

Case-based questions

Case 1

Mrs VA, 35, presented with a history of mass descending per vaginum. She had a 5-year-old girl and was keen on having another child. She wanted a surgical procedure that will enable her to retain the uterus but correct the prolapse.

1. What are the conservative surgeries for prolapse?

2. Which surgery is associated with late reproductive complications and what are the complications?

3. If this was a 40-year-old lady with three children, what surgery would you advise and why?

Case 2

A 31-year-old nullipara presented with a history of heavy menstrual bleeding and inability to conceive after 4 years of marriage. Examination revealed a large myoma at the fundus.

1. What surgery would you advise and why?
2. What is the preoperative preparation?
3. What are the complications of this procedure?

Answers

Case1

1. Manchester–Fothergill operation, abdominal sling procedures, abdominal sacrohysteropexy.
2. Manchester–Fothergill operation. Recurrent miscarriage, preterm labour, infertility.
3. Vaginal hysterectomy and pelvic reconstruction. Conservative surgeries are associated with a high rate of recurrence. If the lady is 40 years old, it is better to perform a definitive procedure with low recurrence rate.

Case 2

1. Abdominal myomectomy or laparoscopic myomectomy.
2. Preoperative ultrasonography to know the number and location of myomas, hysterosalpingography to confirm tubal patency, husband's semen analysis, haemoglobin. She should also be counselled regarding possibility of complications and conversion to hysterectomy.

3. Immediate complications are haemorrhage and infection. Late complications include pelvic adhesions, infertility, rupture of scar during labour and recurrence of myoma.

Long-answer question

1. Mention the various indications for abdominal hysterectomy and discuss in detail the complications.

Short-answer questions

1. Dilatation and curettage
2. Complications of vaginal hysterectomy
3. Indications for hysterectomy
4. Intraoperative complications of hysterectomy
5. Technique of vaginal hysterectomy
6. Preoperative preparations for hysterectomy
7. Structures removed in Wertheim hysterectomy
8. Principles of myomectomy
9. Prerequisites for myomectomy
10. Diagnostic laparoscopy—Indications, procedure and complications
11. Hysteroscopy

Index

SYMBOLS

5-fluorouracil 409, 412, 512
5α-reductase 280, 281, 282, 285, 288, 340, 342
5α-reductase deficiency 28, 255, 259
5α-reductase inhibitors 288, 341, 342
11-hydroxylase defects 259–260
21-hydroxylase 259, 272, 281, 283, 284
β-hCG 177, 502–510, 512, 513

A

Abdominal procedures 366, 380, 394, 523,
Abdominal sacrocolpopexy/
    sacrohysteropexy 366, 367, 550–551
Abdominal uterosacral suspension 366, 367
Ablative procedures 120, 427, 430
Abnormal uterine bleeding (AUB) 92–93, 110–125
Abscess 9, 58, 70, 73, 94, 106, 138, 140, 185–186,
    200–206, 383, 524, 526
Acanthosis nigricans 259
Acetowhite epithelium 427, 428
Acquired abnormalities 307, 308
Actinomycin D 504, 511– 513
Activin 39, 48
Abdominal pain
    acute 100, 494, 495
Acute pelvic/lower abdominal pain 81, 100–101
Add-back therapy 132, 164, 331
Adenocarcinoma 115, 140, 404, 405, 409, 410,
    419, 422, 424, 425, 430, 436–438, 452, 459, 460,
    478, 535
Adenofibroma/cystadenofibroma 174
Adenomas 266, 281, 345
Adenomatous without atypia, complex 125
Adenomyosis 68, 69, 79, 82, 87, 103, 113, 117–119,
    123, 125, 147, 149–153, 217, 235–238
    localized 150, 151
Adjuvant therapy 439, 466, 467, 487, 490, 495
Adnexa 10, 68, 69, 78, 85, 160, 207
Adnexal mass 69, 70, 86, 96, 99, 169, 175, 177,
    200, 237, 482

Adolescents 114, 116, 123, 141, 218, 244–252
    lower abdominal mass in 96, 99
Adrenal adenoma 289
Adrenal hyperandrogenism 283, 284
Adrenarche 247, 250, 251
Adrenalectomy 289
Alcock's canal 17, 18
Alternative therapies 131, 132, 246, 302
Ambiguous genitalia 28–29, 141, 272, 331
Amenorrhoea 32, 41, 59, 60, 94, 100, 114, 115,
    119, 130, 131, 176, 212, 228, 264, 266, 267, 271,
    272, 274, 278, 291, 296, 307, 308, 346, 456, 508,
    primary 28, 30, 62, 131, 250, 254–263, 307, 308
    secondary 41, 62, 174, 211, 212, 256–259,
    264–276, 281, 306, 307, 332, 338
American Institute of Ultrasound Medicine
    (AIUM) 77
American Society of Anesthesiologists 520
Ampullary 9
Anagen phase 280
Anal canal 5–6, 13, 25, 26, 395
Analgesia 523, 524, 531
Anal sphincter injury 106, 383, 395–398, 527
Anastrozole or testolactone 252
Anatomy of the bladder and urethra 26
Androgen-insensitivity syndrome 28, 61, 256,
    260, 493
Androgens 25–28, 40, 44, 45, 48, 61, 152–153,
    256–257, 259, 260, 280–283, 285, 287– 289, 293,
    294, 322, 337, 340– 342, 497
    anti 288, 339, 341–342
    receptor antagonists 342
    physiology 280
Androstenedione 44–46, 115, 248, 280, 282, 284,
    340, 458
Anorexia nervosa 255, 266, 307
Anovulation 114, 117, 118, 265, 266, 269,
    306–307, 318, 320
Anovulatory DUB 114
Anterior colporrhaphy + Kelly stitch 379
Anterior vaginal wall prolapse 358, 359, 362, 365,
    539

Antifibrinolytics   115, 118
Antigonadotropin   120, 163, 165, 228, 341
Antimicrobial prophylaxis   520–521
Anti-Müllerian hormone   24, 27, 256, 293, 306
Antioestrogens   133, 335–336
Antiprogestins   339, 340
Antisperm antibodies   308, 309, 317
Aphthous ulcers   140
Apical/vault prolapse   355
Arachidonic acid   111, 118
Arcuate artery   17
Arcus tendineus   13, 14, 358, 362, 375, 539
    fascia rectovaginalis   14
Aromatase inhibitors   153, 252, 320, 321, 336–337, 457
Aromatization   44, 45, 252, 336, 340
Artificial insemination   325–326
Ascites   63–65, 80, 85, 98, 174, 176, 177, 212, 235, 322, 461, 482–486, 488, 489, 548
Asherman syndrome   211, 272, 274, 275, 308
Aspermia   324
Assisted fertilization techniques   326
Assisted reproductive techniques   229, 305, 326–327
Asthenospermia   324
Atypical vessels   428
Augmentation cystoplasty   382, 384
Auscultation   63, 65, 502
Autologous transfusion   522
Autonomic innervation   18, 19
Ayre spatula   71, 72, 420
Azoospermia   309, 319, 324, 325

B

Bacterial vaginosis   71, 94, 188–189, 191, 199
Bartholin
    adenitis and abscess   185
    gland cysts   139
    glands   3, 4, 66, 138, 185, 188
Basal body temperature (BBT) chart   313
    basal layer   48, 78, 149, 150, 272
Behçet disease   141
Bethesda system   71, 416, 424
Bimanual examination   67–69, 92, 96, 101, 105, 444, 509
Biofeedback   381
Bisphosphonates   302
Bivalent vaccines   419
Bladder drill   381
    bladder sulcus   7, 8, 99, 361, 362, 363, 537
Bleeding, arrest of   111
Bleeding during childhood   123, 246
Blood-stained discharge   92, 246
Blood transfusion   120, 522–523
Boari flaps   390

Body mass index   61, 116, 118, 218, 268, 295, 312, 320, 360, 377, 455, 519
Botryoides sarcoma   247, 410
Bowel preparation   396, 519, 522
Bowel symptoms   106, 359, 363, 482
Brachytherapy   450, 466, 467
BRCA gene mutations   474
Breast
    examination   62, 63, 273, 286, 297, 312, 463, 483
    tanner staging   62, 248, 249
Breast–ovarian cancer syndromes   61, 476
Bulbospongiosus   3–7, 66
Burch colposuspension   380, 555

C

CA 125   98, 177, 178, 224
Cabergoline   275, 321, 332
Calcitonin   302
Candida   67, 71, 94
Candida vaginitis   71, 94
Capillary fragility inhibitors   118, 119
Carcinomas   284
    adenocarcinoma   404, 410
    clear cell   222, 459, 462, 467
    mixed   438
Cardiovascular adverse effects   299, 300
Cascade   50, 111, 219
Catagen phase   280
Catamenial seizures   133
CDC Guidelines for Diagnosis of Acute PID   203
Cellulitis   185, 186, 199, 525
Central defect   358, 360, 365, 539, 541
Cervical cancer   67, 71, 86
    cytology   71, 419–421
    factors   436
    intraepithelial neoplasia   419
    polypectomy   532
    punch biopsy   452
    test   422
Cervicitis   71, 94, 144
Cervix
    benign diseases   144–145
    developmental anomalies   32–35
    hypertrophic elongation   99
    supravaginal   8
    Stenosis 433
Chancroid   183, 187
Chemoprevention   476
Chemoradiation   408, 447, 448
Chemotherapy   412, 448
    high-risk GTN   511, 513, 514
    low-risk GTN   511, 512
Chief complaint   57
Chlamydial infection   67, 71, 83, 236, 308

Chlamydia trachomatis   94, 192
   infection   192
Choriocarcinoma   493, 500, 505
Chronic illnesses   265, 266
Chronic inversion   363
Cisplatin   451
Clinical staging   461
Clitoris   3
Clitoromegaly   29, 279
Cloacal membrane   25
Clomiphene citrate   318, 320
Clonidine   302
Clue cells   71, 95
CO_2 laser   403, 404
Coagulation disorders   61, 123
Coccygeus   13
Coelomic metaplasia theory   218
Cognitive dysfunction   294
Cold-knife conization   430, 432
Colour Doppler   81, 82
Colporrhaphy
   anterior   366, 379
   posterior   541
Colposcopy   135, 364
Colpotomy or laparotomy   73
   posterior   205
Combination oral contraceptives (COCs)   343
Combined oral contraceptive pills   228, 505
Common gynaecological symptoms   91
Complete androgen-insensitivity syndrome   256
Complete mole   501–503
Complete/total vaginal agenesis   29
Computed tomography   83–85
Condyloma acuminata   139
Congenital
   abnormalities   307, 30
   adrenal hyperplasia/late-onset 21-hydroxylase
     deficiency   283–284
Congestive   127
Conization   430, 432
Consent   522–523
Conservative surgery   120–122
Contraception   130
Conventional cytology   420
Corona radiata   42
Corpus albicans   43
Corpus Luteum   43
   cysts   80, 170
Cortex   41, 199
Cosmetic therapies   287
Counselling   205, 227, 274
Cryomyolysis   166
Cryoprobes   430, 431
Cryotherapy   430, 431
Cryptomenorrhoea   30, 257
Culdocentesis/colpocentesis   72–73

Cumulus oophorus   42
Curette   72, 533
Cusco speculum   66, 67, 532
Cushing disease   266, 272, 284
Cyclical progestogens   130
Cyproterone acetate   288, 342
Cytoreductive surgery
   primary   487, 488
   secondary   491
Cyst aspiration   180
Cystic teratoma, benign   174
Cystocele   353, 354
Cystometrography   378
Cystometry   378
Cytobrush   420, 423
Cytotrophoblasts   501

D

Danazol   120
Danazol-loaded intrauterine devices   153
Decidualization   50
Decreased ovarian reserve   306
Decubitus ulcer   359, 360
Deep infiltrating endometriosis   220
Deep perineal muscles   14
Deep transverse perinei   5
Definitive surgery   153, 164
Definitive treatment   118
Degenerative changes   158
Dehydroepiandrosterone (DHEA)   248, 280
Dementia   295, 296
Demonstration of stress incontinence   376
Depot medroxyprogesterone acetate   346, 347
Dermatitis   104
Dermatoses   138
Dermoid cysts   173
Detrusor   371
Detrusor myectomy   382
Detrusor overactivity   381, 382
Devascularization   387
Diffuse adenomyosis   150
Dihydrotestosterone   280
Dilatation and curettage   205
Diploid   468
Direct extension   405, 438
Disorders of
   adolescence   57
   childhood   57
   neonatal period   244
   growth   250
Distension media   558
Documentation   530
Dopamine   38, 267
Doppler flow studies   483
Doppler technology   82

Dorsal lithotomy position   65
Dorsal position   65, 66
Drug-induced hirsutism   285
Dual-energy X-ray absorptiometry (DEXA)   295, 298
Dysgenetic gonad   493
Dysgerminoma   96
Dysmenorrhoea   98, 101
    primary   103
    secondary   103
Dysontogenetic cysts   143
Dyspareunia   143
    deep   105, 106
    superficial   105

E

Early onset PCOS   256, 258
Early stage disease   408
Eflornithine hydrochloride cream   287
Elevated FSH   271
Elevated LH and LH/FSH ratio   269
Embryo cryopreservation   326
Emergency contraception   340, 348–349
Endocervical curettage   425
Endocrinological abnormalities   269
Endometrial
    ablation   120–122
    abnormalities   79
    biopsy   202
    biopsy curette (Novak curette)   533
    cancer   461
    cycle   41
    sampling   72
    thermal ablation   535
Endometrioid
    adenocarcinoma   459
    cystadenoma   172
Endometriosis   153
    staging of   88
Endopelvic fascia   354
Endophytic   436
Endosalpingitis and interstitial salpingitis   211
Endoscopic bladder suspension   380
Enterocele   538
Epidermal growth factor   48
Epithelial ovarian cancer   224
    advanced-stage   487–490
    early-stage   487
    spread of   460–461
Epoophoron   10, 25
Epsilon-aminocaproic acid   118
Equine   120, 262
Erectile dysfunction   310, 324
Ethamsylate   119, 120

Ethinyl oestradiol   120, 130, 288
Examination of the abdomen   63–65
Exophytic   436
Exosalpingitis   211
Extended-field radiation   442, 451
External genitalia   2–3
    development   25–26
External os   67, 144
External pelvic radiation   466–467
External radiation   412, 450
Extrapelvic endometriosis   221
Extraurethral incontinence   383

F

Fallopian tubes   472–497
    benign diseases   175
Falloposcopy   316
Fecundability   305
Female factors   306–309
Female gonads   10
Female pseudohermaphroditism   28
Ferning   50, 318
Fern-like pattern   50
Ferriman–Gallwey scoring   62, 286
Fertile period   312, 319
Fertility-sparing   487
Fibroblast growth factor   111
Fibroma   140
Fimbrioplasty   323
Finasteride   342
First-generation ablation techniques   121
'First-pass' effect   333, 343
Fitz-Hugh–Curtis syndrome   200
Flap-splitting surgery   394
Fluid and electrolyte management   523
Flutamide   288, 342
Folinic acid   512, 513
Follicle
    antral   42, 306, 307
    primary   42
    secondary   42
    tertiary   42
    graafian   11, 42
Follicular cysts   114
Follicular phase   84, 314
Follicular-stimulating hormone   292, 306
Folliculitis   137
Follistatin   38, 48
Fornices   69, 363
Fothergill or Manchester procedure   365
Fourchette, posterior   3, 405
Fractional curettage   465, 534
Frankenhauser plexus   11, 12, 19
Frequency volume chart   378

Frozen pelvis   200, 207, 212
FSH and LH (hCG)   321
Fulvestrant   335, 336
Functional cysts   170, 178
Functional incontinence   382, 383
Functional layer   48, 49

G

Gamete intrafallopian transfer   326
Gartner cyst   363
   duct cysts   143
Gastrointestinal complications   488, 527
General examination   312
Genetic factors and molecular defects   218–219
Genetic testing   319, 476
Genital
   atrophy   141, 294
   folds   26
   herpes   140
   hiatus   357
   swelling   26
   tubercle   26
   tuberculosis   61
   ulcer   184, 186–187
   warts   184
Genital tract, diseases of   203
Genitofemoral nerves   19, 237
Gestational trophoblastic
   disease   500–514
   neoplasia   503
Gestrinone   228
Glycine   121, 558
GnRH agonists   132, 164, 228
   with add-back therapy   228
GnRH analogues   153
GnRH antagonists   229, 326, 331
Gold standard   224, 238
Gonad, development of   29
Gonadal   28, 247
   dysgenesis   258
Gonadarche   247
Gonadotropins   39–40
Gonadotropin-releasing hormone   39
Gonadotrophs   38, 40
Gonococcal   71, 94, 191
Graafian follicle   11, 42
Granuloma inguinale   187
Granulomatous lesions   211, 266
Granulosa cells   247, 292
Groove   69, 70
Gynaecological
   causes   81, 106
   history   56–73
   surgery   59

Gynandroblastoma(s)   283

H

Haemangioma   137, 138
Haematocolpos   257, 260
Haematogenous spread   405, 438
Haematometra   145, 257
Haematosalpinx   31, 257
Haemorrhage   266, 334, 449
Haemostasis   111, 432, 520
Hair growth cycle   280, 287
Haploid   43
hCG alone   332
hCG-H   505
Heaney clamps   537, 539, 546
Heavy menstrual bleeding (HMB)   110, 112
Hegar dilators   534
Hereditary non-polyposis colorectal cancer   61, 459, 474
Hereditary ovarian cancers   474
Hidradenomas   140
High levels of progesterone   43
High-risk HPVs   416
Hirsutism   497
Histological grades   479
Histological grading   438
History of presenting complaints/illness   57–58
Hormonal treatment   118, 119
Hormone receptors   460
Hormone therapy   468
Hot flushes   294
HPV
   DNA testing   422
   infection   422, 436
   vaccines   419
Human chorionic gonadotropin   321
Human papillomavirus   416–418
Human parathormone   302
Hyaline degeneration   158
Hydatidiform mole   171, 500
Hydrocolpos   244
Hydrosalpinx   307
Hydroureteronephrosis   160, 440
Hymen   3
Hyperandrogenism   268, 278
Hypergonadotropic hypogonadism   307
Hyperinsulinaemia   268, 269
Hyperplasia
   atypical   118, 269
   congenital adrenal   272
   endometrial   174
   late-onset congenital adrenal   259
   microglandular   144, 145
   squamous cell   403

Hyperprolactinaemia   41, 160
Hypertrichosis   280
Hypogonadotrophic hypogonadism   307
Hypospermia   324
Hypothalamic causes   265–266
Hypothalamic–pituitary function   319
Hypothalamic/pituitary lesions   259
Hypothalamus   37–38, 47
Hypothyroidism   267, 272
Hypovolaemic shock   525
Hysterectomy   526, 536–539
    abdominal   539
    management of POP   365
    modified radical   552
    modified radical (type II)   446, 448, 551,
    radical   552
    radical (type III)   545, 552
    simple   446
    simple (type I)   448
    total   488, 545–546
    type II   446
    vaginal   521
Hysterosalpingogram   33
Hysterosalpingography   35, 76
Hysteroscopic
    cannulation   323
    polypectomy   324
    resection   162
Hysteroscopy   275

I

Idiopathic
    hirsutism   285
    Iliococcygeus colpopexy   366
Ilioinguinal   19
Imaging-guided procedures   87
Imiquimod   403
Imidazoles   341
Immunological
    factors   309
    theory   218
Imperforate hymen   257, 260
Implantation   306
Implantation theory   218
Incessant ovulation   473–474
Inclusion cysts   140
Induction theory   218
Inferior hypogastric plexus   19, 20
Inferior rectal   16, 17
Infertility
    primary   305
    secondary   305
Infestations   104, 184–185
Inflammatory bowel disease   201, 237

Inflammatory diseases   235
Informed consent   518, 522–523
Infracolic omentectomy   466, 487, 488
Infundibulum   9
Inguinofemoral lymphadenectomy   408
Inhibin   496
Injectable progestins   346–348
Injectable progestogens   119
Inner circular   7, 9
Insomnia   131
Inspection   179
Insulin-like growth factors   48
Insulin resistance   268, 269
Intermediate effects   294
Intermediate trophoblasts   501
Intermenstrual bleeding   112, 113
Intermittent self-catheterization   382, 383
Internal genital organs   2, 7
    development   24–25
Internal iliac (hypogastric) vessels   16–17
Internal os   17, 72
Internal pudendal artery   16, 17
International Society for the Study of Vulvar
    Disease (ISSVD)   402
Interstitial   121, 211
Interstitial cystitis   236
Intertrigo   104
Interval cytoreductive surgery   490–491
Intracavitary radiation   450
Intracervical   325
Intracytoplasmic sperm injection   326
Intraoperative inspection   388
IP chemotherapy   489
Intrauterine insemination   230, 323, 325
Intrauterine system   228
Intravenous chemotherapy   489
Intravesical therapy   382
Intrinsic sphincter   370
    deficiency   376
Invasive mole   500, 502
In vitro fertilization   230
Irritable bowel syndrome   236
Ischiocavernosus   4, 5
Isolated GnRH deficiency   255, 258
Isthmus   322
IUCD-related bleeding   59

K

Kallman syndrome   258
Kegel exercises   378
Kelley clamps   537
Keratinizing type   404
Ketoconazole   341
Khanna sling procedure   366, 550

L

Labial adhesions   141, 245, 246
Labia
   majora   256
   minora   246
Lanolin   394
Lantern on St. Paul's cathedral appearance   161
Laparoscopic and vaginal surgery   551
Laparoscopic
   colposuspension   380
   surgery   229
Laparoscopy   226
   diagnostic   178, 179
Laparotomy   179
Large cell keratinized   438
Large loop excision of the transformation
   zone   431, 532
Laser ablation   409
Laser conization   432–433
Last menstrual period (LMP)   58
Lateral fusion
   anomalies   29
Lateral vaginal sulcus   360
Latzko procedure   394
Left lateral (Sims') position   66
Leiomyoma and pregnancy   160
Letrozole   252, 320
Levator ani   354
Levonorgestrel   348, 457
   intrauterine system   457
Lichen
   planus   104, 105, 137
   sclerosis   246
   simplex or neurodermatitis   137
Lifestyle modification   118
Ligaments
   broad   128, 155
   cardinal or Mackenrodt   11
   infundibulopelvic   11
   ovarian   12
   pseudo or false broad   157–158
   pubocervical   12
   round   12
   triradiate   12
   uterosacral   12
Lipoid cell tumours   283, 289
Liquid-based cytology   71, 421
Lithotomy position   531, 537
Longitudinal vaginal septum   30
Long-term effects   294–296
Loop electroexcision procedure   409
Lower abdominal mass   99, 485
   reproductive years   99
   peri- and postmenopausal years   99

Low-risk HPVs   416, 417
Lumbosacral trunk   19
Luteal phase defect   49, 223
Luteinization   170, 311
Luteinized unruptured follicle syndrome   223,
   310
Luteinizing hormone   307
Luteolysis   339
Luteoma of pregnancy   282
Lymphatic   218
Lymphatic drainage   18, 19
Lymphogranuloma venereum (LGV)   183, 184,
   187
Lymphovascular space invasion   439
Lynch II syndrome   459

M

Magnetic resonance–guided focused ultrasound
   surgery   166
Magnetic resonance imaging   152, 177
Male Factor   306–309
Male Pseudohermaphroditism   28
Malignancy   11
Malignant masses   11
Mammography   297
Mammotrophs   38
Manchester–Fothergill operation   543–545
Marshall–Marchetti–Krantz procedure   380
Marsupialization   140
Mass descending per vaginum   359
Mayer–Rokitansky-Kuster-Hauser (MRKH)
   syndrome   29
Maylard   547, 551, 553
McCall culdoplasty   365–367, 538, 539–540
McCune–Albright syndrome   251, 252
McIndoe operation   31
Medical and surgical history   60–61
Medical management   118–120
Medical treatment   152, 163
Medications   132, 141, 215
Medulla   10, 11
Mefenamic acid   118–119, 163
Meigs syndrome   174
Menarche   218
Menopausal
   history   57, 60
   transition   292, 293
Menopause   291–302
   premature   271, 291
Menorrhagia   112
Menstrual cycle, normal   118
Menstrual parameters   112, 116
Menstruation   112
   diary   116

history   58, 116
  migraine   132–133
  symptoms   159
Metabolic syndrome   269, 285, 287
Metastatic disease   484, 488, 508, 509
Metformin   275, 321
Methotrexate   504, 511–513
Metropathia haemorrhagica   114
Metrorrhagia   112
Microinvasive adenocarcinoma   452
Microinvasive carcinoma   446, 492
Microsurgical procedures   323
Midcycle pain   58, 127, 311, 312
Midluteal serum progesterone   312–314
Midposition   68
Mifepristone   163, 165, 229, 339, 340, 347–349
Mild dysplasia   415, 424
Minipills   346, 347
Mirena   338, 348
Mixed incontinence   375, 378, 382
Moderate dysplasia   415
Molar pregnancy with coexisting foetus   505
Molluscum contagiosum   139, 184
Mons pubis   2, 3, 12, 19, 66, 136, 248, 249
Mood disturbances   131, 164, 293, 294
Mood swings   60, 131, 291, 293, 296, 299, 329
Morning after pill   348
Mosaic   28, 258, 259, 261, 307, 426, 427, 428, 493
Moskowitz procedure   365
Mucinous carcinoma   438, 459
Mucinous cystadenoma   69, 81, 97, 172, 173
Mucocolpos   30
Mucopus   95, 101, 191, 194
Mucosal lesions   67
Mucous cysts   139, 140, 143
Müllerian ducts   24, 25, 30
  anomalies   30, 256, 257
  tubercle   25
Multimodal Screening   474–476
Multiple drug therapy   214
Mural granulosa cells   42
Myomas   58, 65, 69, 76, 79, 82, 83, 96, 99, 113, 117,
  125, 145, 149, 152, 154–155, 156–167, 308, 316,
  317, 324, 335, 336, 340, 380, 382, 383, 387, 440,
  462, 475, 486, 536, 537, 545–547, 551–555, 557
  adenomyoma   87, 97, 98, 149–153, 165, 469
  asymptomatic   162, 163, 551
  broad-ligament   155–160, 165, 387
  cervical   145, 155–157, 159–161, 164, 165, 382,
  383, 552
  intramural   112, 118, 119, 129, 145
  screw   553, 554
  submucous   83, 103, 113, 117, 324, 552–554,
  557
  subserosal   156, 157, 159, 165
  surgical management   164–167

Myomectomy   118, 154, 164–166, 324, 392,
  551–555, 557
  abdominal   553–555
  hysteroscopic   165–166
  laparoscopic   165, 324, 557
Myometrial
  invasion   79, 82, 87, 460–462, 465–468
  reduction   153
Myometrium   9, 77–79, 111, 128, 147, 149–152,
  154, 156, 162, 198, 211, 217, 239, 459, 461–463,
  506–508, 510, 554

N

Nabothian cysts   67, 144, 145, 428
Neisseria gonorrhoeae   144, 185, 191, 192, 199,
  200, 203, 309
Neoadjuvant chemotherapy   451, 484, 488–489
Neoplastic lesions, benign
  complications   180–181
Neosalpingostomy   323
Neovagina   31
Nerve entrapment   234, 237
Nerve supply   19–20
Neuropathic pain   234, 237
Newer interventional techniques   153
Newer methods of treatment   166
New medical approaches   228
New squamocolumnar junction   417
Non-contraceptive benefits   343, 344
Non-hormonal treatment   118–199
Non-keratinized   188, 438
Non-metastatic disease   508, 509
Non-specific vulvovaginitis   94, 245–246
Non-steroidal anti-inflammatory agents   118, 130,
  227
Non-surgical treatment   31, 378, 379
Norethindrone enanthate   346
Normal ultrasonographic findings   78
Normogonadotropic hypogonadism   307
Norplant   338, 347–348

O

Obesity   58, 60, 114–118, 125, 138, 140, 142, 159,
  190, 250, 265, 266, 268, 269, 271–273, 281–287,
  295, 318, 355, 356, 376, 377, 387, 447, 455, 456,
  458, 459, 463, 464, 474, 522
Obliterative procedures   364, 366
Obstetric history   57, 59, 116, 273, 311, 360, 377,
  501
Obstetric injury   392, 395
Occult stress incontinence   363, 364, 366, 376
Occupational and social history   61
Oestradiol, oestrone and oestriol   46, 333

Oestrogen   9, 24, 39, 40, 42–50, 60, 67, 70, 92, 94, 95, 96, 105, 111, 114, 116, 118, 119–121, 123, 130, 132, 133, 142, 143, 148, 149, 152, 154, 158, 163, 165, 170, 173, 174, 188, 219, 222, 227–230, 236, 244–248, 251, 252, 256, 258, 262, 266–269, 271, 273, 274, 282, 283, 285, 291–296, 299–302, 308, 318, 320–321, 330–340, 342–348, 356, 358, 360, 364, 372, 374, 376, 379, 381–383, 416, 455, 456, 458–461, 463–464, 468, 496, 497, 521, 522–523, 546
  conjugated equine oestrogen   120, 262, 274, 301, 333
  receptors   47, 120, 133, 149, 154, 163, 229, 294, 295, 301, 320, 333, 334–335, 340, 468
Oestrogen/implant/patch/gel   334
Oestrogen–progestin combinations   118, 130, 299, 343–346
Oestrogen–progestogen combination   119
Oestrogen vaginal creams   379
Office procedures   531–535, 558
Oligomenorrhoea   212, 285
Oligozoospermia   324
Once-a-month injections   343, 346
Oocyte   23–25, 41–44, 48, 50, 262, 271, 292, 306, 307, 326, 496
Oophorectomy   15, 179–181, 205, 215, 227, 229–231, 236, 238, 241, 289, 292, 295, 297, 386, 392, 446, 466, 476, 487, 492, 495–497, 523, 546–548
Oophorectomy/salpingo-oophorectomy   179, 180
Optimal cytoreduction   486, 488, 489, 490
Oral progestins   119, 163, 343, 346
Organic causes   110
Ormeloxifene   118, 120, 163, 165, 335
Osteoporosis   47, 60, 250, 265, 271, 272, 275, 295–298
Outflow obstruction   32, 96, 97, 255, 256, 257, 260, 262
Ovarian cancer   59, 61, 64, 85, 86, 87, 177, 212, 213, 222, 224, 300, 336, 340, 344, 345, 465, 472, 473–476, 481, 484, 486, 487, 489, 491, 548
  FIGO staging   481
Ovarian
  causes   267–271, 275
  cycle   41, 42–43, 48
  cystectomy   180, 487, 548–549
  drilling   316, 322
  endometriosis   219, 220, 225, 257
  hyperandrogenism   281–283, 288
  hyperstimulation syndrome   171, 321, 322
  lesions   80, 176–179, 484
  neoplasms, benign   96, 171–175, 180
  remnant syndrome   236
  vessels   10, 12, 14–18, 41, 387, 461, 548, 553
Ovarian failure, premature   271
Ovaries
  benign diseases   169–174

entrapped ovary syndrome   236
morphology   41–42, 270, 483
neoplastic lesions   81, 179, 180–181
residual   81, 234, 235–236, 240
resistant (savage syndrome)   271, 306
steroid hormones   10, 44–46
Overactive bladder syndrome   381
Overflow incontinence or retention with overflow   382
Ovulation   9, 10, 40, 43–47, 49, 50, 78, 80, 94, 114, 115, 128, 130, 132, 159, 170, 171, 188, 222, 223, 227, 230, 258, 262, 271, 275, 306–309, 312–314
  induction   80, 171, 230, 262, 275, 307, 314, 319–323, 325, 326, 330, 331, 335–337
  test   46
Ovulatory
  DUB   114, 115
  dysfunction   92, 112, 114–116, 119, 123–125, 223, 285, 306–307, 314, 319–322
Oxybutynin   381

P
Packed cells   117, 118, 485, 503, 522, 525
Pain control   523–524
Painful bladder syndrome   106, 371, 384
Palliative
  chemotherapy   448
  radiotherapy   448
Palpation   63, 64, 66, 482, 495, 549
Papillary serous carcinomas   462
Pap smear   56, 66, 67, 71, 92, 95, 96, 189, 190, 194, 297, 363, 364, 407–410, 414, 419–421, 424, 430, 444, 452, 459, 463, 545
  efficacy of   421
Parametrial infiltration   70, 85, 87, 440, 442–446, 551
Parametrium   11, 12, 86, 438, 441, 448–450, 462, 506, 545, 551
Paraovarian cysts   69, 97, 169, 175, 178, 555
Parasitic myoma   156
Parasympathetic   19, 20, 371, 372
Paravaginal defects   358, 360, 362, 365, 539
Paroophoron   10, 25
Partial androgen insensitivity   28, 259, 310, 334
Partial mole   501, 503–506, 514
Partial response   490
Partial vaginal agenesis   30
Partial vulvectomy   408
Pathogenesis   14, 92, 115, 128–129, 131, 133, 149–150, 154, 199–200, 210–211, 218–219, 227, 228, 234–236, 268, 281, 375, 416–418, 436, 458, 473, 476–477
Pathology   2, 70, 83, 84, 103, 105, 117, 122, 127, 128, 129, 131, 148, 150–151, 152, 153, 154, 169, 200, 211–212, 219–222, 237, 256, 274, 287, 312,

362, 363, 374, 378, 382, 384, 403, 404–405, 409,
416, 427, 436–438, 440, 442, 455, 459–460,
477–479, 493–494, 501, 506
Patient-controlled analgesia 520, 524
Patterns of spread 405, 410, 438–439, 460–461,
479, 480, 506, 507
Pediculosis 104, 184, 185
Pedunculated 148, 155–158, 160, 165, 185
Pelvic
abscess 58, 70, 73, 94, 106, 200–202, 204–206,
383, 526
adhesions 205, 207, 212, 234, 235, 238, 239,
311, 555
congestion syndrome 81, 103, 128, 129, 234,
236, 238, 239
diaphragm 13–14
examination 30, 66, 67, 70, 77, 95, 98, 99, 103,
105, 116, 123, 129, 158, 160, 161, 169, 176, 194,
201, 206, 212, 213, 220, 224, 237, 238, 250, 260,
273, 286, 297, 360, 361, 377, 444, 463, 474, 476,
482, 483, 502, 504, 509, 519, 533, 535, 537
floor 13–14, 77, 351, 354–356, 364, 366, 378,
379, 381
lymphadenectomy 446, 448, 449, 466, 524,
551, 552
mass 30, 31, 58, 64, 193, 207, 213, 223, 244,
251, 283, 483–485, 495, 497
pain and menstrual abnormality 212
plexuses 19, 20
ureters 14–16, 160, 387
Pelvic inflammatory disease 59, 69, 81, 94, 103,
115, 177, 189, 198, 211, 240, 308, 309, 475, 523,
524
acute 184, 201–205
chronic 129, 205–207, 235, 236, 238
Pelvic organ prolapse 14, 58, 59, 61, 65, 66, 99,
294, 352–367, 376, 536–539
myomas 58
Pelvic pain 159, 170, 212
acute 81–82, 91, 100–101
chronic 61, 81–82, 91, 101–102, 206, 212, 217,
222, 223, 228, 233–241, 555
Percussion 63, 64, 555
Perimenopause 292
Perineal arteries 16–18
Perineal body 2, 6–7, 14, 66, 69, 357–359,
395–397, 541, 542
Perineal membrane 4, 5, 14
Perineorrhaphy 537, 541–542
Perineum 4–6, 19, 189
deficient 69, 355, 357, 360, 361, 365, 540–541
gynaecological 395
muscles 4, 5, 13, 14, 19, 105, 542
true 4
Peritoneal carcinoma, primary 480

Peritoneal factors 223, 308–309, 314–316,
323–324
Periurethral injection of bulking agents 381
Pessaries and urethral devices 379
Pessary test 363
Pfannenstiel 546, 547, 550, 553
PG synthetase 111
inhibitors 115, 118–120, 130
Physical status classification 520
Physiology of androgens 280–281
Phytoestrogens 302
Pictorial blood loss assessment chart 58, 116
Pigmentary changes 142
Pioglitazone 320, 321
Pipelle 72, 92, 117, 464
Pituitary
adenomas 266
causes 266–267, 275
gland 38–41, 164, 247, 309, 330, 332
necrosis 266, 275
Placental site trophoblastic tumour 500, 507
Platelet plug 50, 111
Point A 2, 450, 451, 556
Point B 450, 451, 556
Polar body 43
Polycystic ovarian syndrome 41, 114, 125, 174,
179, 256–259, 261, 265, 266, 268–271, 274,
281–282, 306, 307, 332, 338, 458
Polymenorrhagia 112
Polyps 67, 83, 113, 144–145, 148–149, 308, 464,
532
adenomyomatous 150
endocervical and cervical 144, 532
endometrial 68, 80, 113, 117, 118, 123, 144,
148–149, 308, 315, 324, 363, 464, 465, 558
endocervical/endometrial 363
POP-Q system 357–358
Portiovaginalis 8, 67, 363
Positron emission tomography 85, 86, 442, 484,
510
Postcoital bleeding 57, 144, 444
Posterior vaginal wall prolapse—McCall
culdoplasty 365, 539–540
Postmenopausal 14, 60, 70, 95–99, 139, 296, 299,
360, 373, 382, 497
bleeding 77, 79, 92, 148, 455, 461–465, 496
Postmolar follow-up 504–505
Postoperative
adjuvant therapy 466, 467
ileus 522, 527
management 394–395, 523–524
monitoring 523
Post-testicular causes 310
Post-treatment surveillance 452
Postvoid residual urine 378, 382

Pouch of Douglas   9, 70, 72–73, 193, 221, 223, 240, 482, 484, 538, 546
Preantral follicle   42
Preclinical carcinoma   446
Precocious pubarche   250
Pregnancy
    after GTD   514
    related conditions   202
    related problems   57
Pregranulosa cells   24
Preimplantation genetic diagnosis   327
Preinvasive disease   402–404, 408–409, 414, 436
Premenstrual syndrome and premenstrual dysphoric disorder   131–132
Preoperative evaluation   230, 396, 485, 518–520, 551
Prepubertal   94, 188
Preservation of prolapsed uterus   365–366
Pressure symptoms   98, 159–160
Pretesticular causes   309, 310
Pretreatment evaluation   440, 445–446, 465–466
Previous menstrual period (PMP)   58
Primordial germ cells   24, 41, 492
Prostaglandin   43, 44, 111, 130, 150, 339, 503
    PGE_2 50, 111
    $PGF2_\alpha$ 49, 50, 103, 111, 114, 115, 128, 130
    PGI_2 50, 111
Progestasert   338, 348
Progestational contraceptives   343, 346–348
Progesterone   43, 44, 46–47, 49, 114, 119, 133, 348, 457, 459, 460, 468
Progesterone challenge test   273, 274, 338
Progesterone intrauterine system   119
Progestins   119, 130, 163, 227–228, 301, 337–339, 346–347
    vaginal ring   348
Progestogens   119, 294, 334, 337
Prognostic factors   394, 407–408, 451, 468
Prolactin   41, 267, 273, 275, 332
Prolactinoma   256, 257, 267
Proliferative phase   41, 48–49, 78
Prophylactic chemotherapy   504
Proteomic patterns   474, 476
Pruritus   94, 103–105, 141, 188
Pseudocapsule   154, 156, 158, 554
Pseudomyxoma peritonei   172, 181, 492
Psoriasis   137, 139, 142
Psychosomatic disorders   101, 237
Puberty   8, 29, 30, 272, 496
    central precocious   250–252, 330
    delayed   250
    disorders   37, 250–252
    peripheral precocious   251, 252
    physiology   247–248
    precocious   246, 247, 250–252, 330, 496

Pubic hair tanner staging   248
Pubourethralis   370, 375
Pubovaginalis   13, 359, 361, 541
Pudendal nerve   19, 20, 371, 372
Pulmonary embolism   521, 526
Pulsatility index   82
Punch biopsy   410, 445, 452, 531
Punctation   427
Purandare sling procedure   550
Pyelonephritis   372, 373, 374, 391
Pyogenic granulomas   139
Pyosalpinx   200, 202, 213

Q

Q-tip test   377–378
Quadrivalent vaccines   419
Quantification   356–358
Quinagolide   332

R

Radial arteries   17
Radiation therapy   448, 491
Radical hysterectomy and pelvic lymphadenectomy   551, 552
Radical local excision   408
Radical trachelectomy   446, 449–450
Radiologically guided cannulation   323
Radiotherapy   271, 381, 408
    with concurrent chemotherapy   412
Raloxifene   163, 165, 229, 301, 334, 335
Recommendations for screening   476
Reconstructive procedures   364, 365, 539, 542
Rectal
    examination   31, 70
    symptoms   159, 160, 359
Rectocele   66, 359–362, 365, 540–541
    repair of   541
Rectovaginal
    examination   69–70, 361, 398, 483
    fistula   106, 395, 396, 397–398
Recurrent urinary tract infections   236
Red or carneous degeneration   158
Resistance index   82, 177, 474, 483
Retropubic tape procedures   379
Retroversion   68
Rhabdosphincter   370
Ring pessary   364
Risk scoring   508, 511
Risk stratification   521
Rokitansky–Mayer–Küster–Hauser (RMKH) syndrome   256
Routine pelvic examination   30, 474
Rubin cannula   555

S

Sacral vessels   17–18, 551
Sacrocolpopexy
   abdominal   366, 367, 550–551
   laparoscopic   366
Sacrohysteropexy
   abdominal   366
Sacrospinous colpopexy   366, 367, 542–543
Saline infusion sonography   82–83, 315, 316, 317
Satisfactory colposcopy   427
Scabies   104, 184
Screening/diagnostic procedures   71–73
Screening guidelines   424
Screening modalities   419
Sebaceous cysts   139, 140, 143
Second-generation ablation techniques   121
Second-line chemotherapy   489, 490, 491
Second-look surgery   490
Secretory phase   48–50, 78
Selective oestrogen receptor modulators   120,
   133, 229, 301, 334–335, 468
Selective progesterone receptor modulator   163,
   165, 229, 339–340
Selective salpingography   83, 323
Selective serotonin reuptake inhibitors   132, 379
Semen analysis   318, 319, 324
   abnormal   324
Sentinel node biopsy   407–408, 442, 466
Serosa   9, 155, 156, 198, 461, 506, 539
Serotonin   132, 267, 294, 379
   reuptake inhibitors   132, 302
Serous
   adenocarcinoma   479
   carcinoma   460, 467, 473, 478
   cystadenoma   81, 96, 97, 172
Sessile   148, 156
Severe dysplasia   415, 424
Sex hormone–binding globulin   46, 268, 280, 342
Sexual dysfunction   237, 293, 294, 448
Sexual hair   280
Sheehan syndrome   266, 268, 307
Shirodkar sling procedure   366, 367, 550
Sims speculum   66–68, 360, 362, 533, 535, 537
Sinovaginal bulbs   25, 26, 29, 30, 143, 409
Site-specific repair   365, 367, 539, 541
Skene
   duct cysts   143
   glands   3
Sling operations   549–550
Small bowel obstruction
Snow storm appearance   524, 527
Somatic Innervation   19
Somatic nerve   19, 371, 372
Sonohysterography   82, 117, 149
Sonohysterosalpingography   82, 315

Sonosalpingography   82, 129, 205, 463, 464
Space of Retzius   16
Spasmodic dysmenorrhoea   58, 103, 159, 311
Specific vulvovaginitis   94, 246
Speculum examination   66–68, 71, 95, 96, 116,
   161, 194, 408–409, 423
Spencer-Wells clamps   537, 539, 546
Sphincter urethra   370, 371
Spinnbarkeit   50, 51, 318
Spironolactone   132, 288, 337, 342
Squamocolumnar junction   67, 416, 427
   original   417
Squamous cell carcinoma   404, 405, 409, 410, 436,
   437
Staging   11, 84, 85, 87
   laparotomy   479
   endometrial cancer   461, 462, 535
   vulvar cancer   405, 406
Steroid biosynthesis   44, 281
Strassman metroplasty   35
Streak gonads   28, 259
Stress   123, 258
   incontinence   59, 294, 356, 359, 362, 366–367,
   375–383
Stromal hyperthecosis   281, 283, 289
Stromal luteomas   282
Structural abnormalities   67, 92, 112, 113
Subcutaneous injections   343, 347
Subdermal implants   343, 347–348
Subfertility   159, 160
Submeatal sulcus   7, 362
Suboptimal cytoreduction   488, 490
Substance abuse   60, 237, 310, 311, 312
Superficial endometriosis   219, 224, 228, 229
Superficial perineal muscles   4, 5
Superficial transverse perinei   4, 5, 6
Superior hypogastric plexus   19, 20
Surgical
   management   31, 35, 118, 120–122, 153,
   164–167, 228–230, 240
   staging   405, 442, 443, 466, 486–487, 492
Suspension procedure   365, 366
Sympathetic supply   371, 372
Sympathetic system   19, 20, 371
Syncytiotrophoblasts   501, 505–507
Syndromic approach   95, 194, 195
Synthetic and biologic mesh   367
Synthetic pregestational agents   337
Syphilis   95, 186, 187, 201
Systemic diseases   141, 265

T

Tamoxifen   79, 149, 252, 334–336, 456, 459, 521
Tandem   450
Tanner staging   62, 248, 249, 260

Tears and lacerations   67
Telogen phase   280
Tenderness   201, 203, 237, 373
Tenesmus   58, 106, 201
Tension-free vaginal tape   379
Teratoma, immature   173, 493, 494, 495
Teratozoospermia   324
Terminal hair   268, 278, 280
Tertiary or antral follicle   42
Testicular causes   309, 310
Testosterone   24, 28, 256, 282, 284, 309, 340–342
Theca externa   42
Theca lutein cysts   80, 170, 171, 178, 502, 508
Thecomas   174, 497
Thelarche   247, 250, 251
    precocious   250
Theories of development of endometriosis   218
Thermal balloon ablation   121, 122, 535
Thermoablation   430
Thermomyolysis   166
Thromboprophylaxis   521, 522
Thromboxane A$_2$ 111
Thyrotropin releasing hormone   41, 267
Tibolone   302, 331
Tolterodine   381
Torsion   81, 82, 158, 180, 181
Traditional sling procedures   380
Tranexamic acid   118, 119
Transabdominal   77, 79, 117
Transdermal patch and transvaginal ring   346
Transformation zone   67, 71, 416, 427, 432, 545
Transition   292, 299
Transmitted mobility   69
Trans-obturator tape   379, 380
Transperineal   77, 396
Transrectal   77, 319
Transureteroureterostomy   388–390
Transvaginal   73, 77
    layered method   396
    sonography   73, 312–314, 459, 483
    ultrasonography   34, 84, 117, 129, 149, 202, 314, 440
Transverse vaginal septum   30, 86, 244, 257
Transverse vaginal sulcus   7, 362
Treatment   31, 117
    modalities   110, 130, 378, 430–433, 491
    advanced disease   408, 489
    early stage disease   446–448
Trichomonas   94, 189, 191, 245
    vaginitis   94
Trigger points   237
Trilaminar endometrium   78, 314
Triploid   503, 504
Trocars   555, 556
True hermaphroditism   28
Tubal factors   306, 307, 315, 322–323

Tubal and peritoneal factors, tests for   314–316
Tubal sterilization   10, 59
Tuberculosis (TB) of the genital tract   210–215
Tuberculous peritonitis   212
Tubocornual anastomosis   323
Tubo-ovarian
    abscess   81, 100, 200, 205
    mass   69, 81, 175, 200, 202, 207, 213, 235, 238, 239
Tumours   44, 80, 497
    adrenal   44, 284, 289
    androgen-producing   271, 282–283
    benign epithelial   97, 172–173
    borderline   180, 491–492
    Brenner (transitional cell)   173, 477
    endodermal sinus   493, 494, 495
    endometrioid   459, 460, 468, 477
    epithelioid trophoblastic   500, 507
    germ cell   173–174, 492–495
    granulosa cell   96, 247, 496
    Krukenberg   479
    Leydig cell   282, 496, 497
    markers   99, 177, 443, 493
    mesonephroid (clear cell)   172, 173
    mucinous   477, 478, 492
    neuroendocrine   438
    placental site trophoblastic   507
    rare   173, 283, 507
    secondary   98, 479
    Sertoli–Leydig   282, 497
    sex cord stromal   174, 496, 497
    small-cell   438
    steroid-cell   282, 283
    stromal   174, 496–497
    transitional   cell   173, 477
Tumours, hamartomas and cysts   145
Turner mosaic   258, 307
Turner syndrome   28, 63, 256, 258–259, 307
Two-cell two-gonadotropin theory   45

U

Ulcerative   187, 436, 437, 444
    lesions   140
Ultrasonography   31, 32, 34, 77–81, 83, 92, 117, 129, 161
Ultrasound-guided aspiration   178, 205
Upper genital tract
    infections   183, 198, 199
Ureteric
    injuries   387–390, 391
    tunnel   11, 12, 387
Ureteroileal interposition   338
Ureteroneocystostomy   388, 390
Ureteroureterostomy   388–390
Ureterovaginal fistula   393

Urethra   5, 13, 14
   dilatation   160, 383
   diverticulum   143
   fistula   393, 394
   groove   26
   hypermobility   359, 375, 376, 378
   orifice   3, 66, 357
   pressure profilometry   378
   sphincter   4, 5, 13, 376
   syndrome   101, 236, 374
   Urethrocele   14, 66, 357
Urethrovaginal fistulae   14, 354, 357
Urge incontinence   381–382
Urinary
   diversion   382, 394
   incontinence   375–383
   LH   312–314, 319, 320
   retention   257, 382, 383, 526–527
   symptoms   58, 106
   tract infections   236, 372–374
Urodynamic effects   294
Urodynamic study   378, 382
Uroflowmetry   378
Urogenital canal   25, 26
Urogenital diaphragm   5, 19, 408
Urogenital sinus   25, 26, 30, 143
Urologic problems, common   370, 371
Urorectal septum   25, 26
Uterine
   arteries   167
   artery embolization   87–88
   corpus   438
   factors   306–308
   leiomyomas   154
   perforation   315, 533, 534
   sarcomas   469
   sound   533, 534, 558
   versus adnexal mass   69
Uterosacral ligament suspension   366
Uterovaginal agenesis   256
Uterus   163, 256
   abnormalities   79
   benign diseases   147–167
   bicornuate   33, 34, 79
   developmental anomalies   32–35
   prolapsed, preservation   365–366
   retroverted   70, 105, 106
   septate   34, 308, 318
   supports   14
Uterine bleeding
   abnormal   59, 88, 92–93
   dysfunctional   112

V

Vabra aspirator   117

Vagina   94
   benign diseases   143–144
   development   25
   developmental abnormalities   29, 30
   infections   59, 95, 188–191
   supports   14, 354–355
Vaginal adenosis   410
Vaginal agenesis   29–30
Vaginal bleeding
   abnormal   57, 201
Vaginal brachytherapy   466, 467
Vaginal carcinoma   409, 410, 411
Vaginal discharge   188, 202, 359
   children   94
Vaginal dryness   60, 294, 301
Vaginal infections   59, 95, 188–191
Vaginal intraepithelial neoplasia   409
Vaginal length, total   357, 358
Vaginal orifice   3
Vaginal ovoids   450
Vaginal pessary   364
Vaginal procedures   379, 391, 394, 531
Vaginal reconstruction   31, 35
Vaginal septum, transverse   29, 30, 86, 257
Vaginal sulcus, transverse   7, 362
Vaginal surgical procedures   531–535
Vaginal vault   366, 433, 525, 539, 540, 542, 543, 547
Vaginismus   59, 60, 105
Valsalva leak point pressure   378
Varicocele   310, 324
Vasoconstriction   50, 111, 532
Vasodilator   50, 111, 133
Vasomotor symptoms   293, 294
Vellus hair   280
Venous and lymphatic dissemination   218
Venous thromboembolism   300, 335, 338, 521
Veress needle   555, 556
Vertical fusion
   anomalies   29, 30
Verrucous carcinoma   410
Vesico-psoas hitch   390
Vesicouterine fistula   395
Vesicovaginal   393, 395
Vesicovaginal and urethrovaginal fistulae   393
Vestibular bulbs   3
Vestibule   3, 7
Viral infections   184
Virilization   287
Visual inspection
   after acetic acid   422–423
   after Lugol's iodine   423
Vitamin D   275, 296, 297
Voiding diary   378, 381
Vulsellum   533, 534, 535
Vulva   2–3, 17
   benign diseases   135–143

carcinoma   405, 407
endometriosis   139
infections   187–188
Paget disease   404
pruritus   188, 404
secondary infection   184, 187–188
Vulvar intraepithelial neoplasia   402, 403
Vulvovaginitis   94, 104, 187–188

W

Wedge biopsy   407
Wertheim hysterectomy   446, 551
Whole abdominal radiation   466, 467
Whorled appearance   154, 155, 162
Withdrawal bleeding with progesterone
   positive   271

Wolffian ducts   24

X

X–ray, chest   213, 440, 465, 510
XX/XY gonadal dysgenesis   258

Y

Yuzpe method   349

Z

Zinc oxide cream   394
Zona pellucida   42, 43, 326
Zygote intrafallopian transfer   326, 327